Ovarian Carcinoma

THIRD EDITION

Hugh R.K. Barber

Ovarian Carcinoma

Etiology, Diagnosis, and Treatment

THIRD EDITION

Foreword by Felix Rutledge

With 84 Illustrations

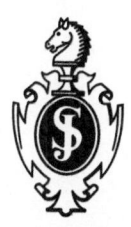

Springer-Verlag
New York Berlin Heidelberg London Paris
Tokyo Hong Kong Barcelona Budapest

Hugh R.K. Barber, M.D.
Director
Department of Obstetrics and Gynecology
Lenox Hill Hospital
100 East 77th Street
New York, NY 10021-1883 USA

Library of Congress Cataloging-in-Publication Data
Barber, Hugh R.K., 1918–
    Ovarian carcinoma / Hugh R.K. Barber.—3rd. ed.
    p. cn.
    Includes bibliographical references and index.

    1. Ovaries—Cancer. I. Title.
    [DNLM: 1. Ovarian Neoplasms. WP 322 B234o]
    RC280.08B34 1992
    616.99'465—dc20
    DNLM/DLC
    for Library of Congress   92-2187

Printed on acid-free paper.

Production managed by Ellen Seham; manufacturing supervised by Rhea Talbert.
Typeset by Asco Trade Typesetting Ltd., Hong Kong.

9 8 7 6 5 4 3 2 1

ISBN-13:978-1-4613-9234-7   e-ISBN-13: 978-1-4613-9232-3
DOI: 10.1007/978-1-4613-9232-3

Foreword

This highly successful book has again been revised and updated by the author. This third edition retains much from the other two; however, in this edition a new chapter on biologic response modifiers discusses a group of promising new therapies for ovarian cancers. These are the exciting new discoveries for curing cancer according to the lay literature. Biologic response modifiers are already in clinical trials and are rapidly proving an important new treatment or a method to potentiate cancericidal drugs. Although some of the products are still investigational, not yet released for general clinical use, physicians should become knowledgeable about these new therapies. This chapter presents a readable overview of this topic.

The FIGO staging has been updated according to modifications announced in their most recent publication. There has been much activity in tumor marker research and clinical application. The chapter on tumor markers in ovarian cancer has been updated by adding markers that have been identified since the second edition. Dr. Barber provides a perspective on the usefulness and contributions these researches have yielded.

The excellent section on embryology has been made more valuable and unique by identifying the time and development of the ovary from which ovarian tumors probably arise. This excellent tracing of the developmental anatomy of the genital organs and the stage of maturity when stem cells are sequestered for later carcinogenesis fits well with the classification of tumors of the ovary. The complex genesis of the many various ovarian tumors that have so long been confusing to students is explained in a manageable order.

The section on chemotherapy of ovarian carcinoma in the second edition, which discusses the platinum-containing regimens, is retained here with some additions. Cis-platinum and its analogues are still the mainstay of chemotherapy of ovarian cancer; and although a variety of dosage schedules and routes of administration have been tested, the basic information has changed little. The new drugs noted by Dr. Barber are still being tested clinically for their usefulness and tolerance.

The attraction of this book, in addition to the ease of reading and comprehension that has not been lost in this revised version, is Dr. Barber's experienced assessment of the literature. He is able to distinguish for the reader information that has been confirmed. As the book's author he can be discriminating about expressing unproved opinions. Because of his extensive experience as a gynecologic oncologist and researcher in the field, he qualifies as an author, which today is special as most books of this type are produced by editors.

Dr. Barber's easy, relaxed, and conversational writing style and his manner of reemphasizing major points from chapter to chapter are excellent communication tools. There are some favored expressions he seems to enjoy. As he speaks of early detection of cancer of the ovary, such statements as "early diagnosis is a matter of chance rather than scientific discovery" add a note of sincerity. These statements are sometimes referred to by his colleagues as "Barberisms" and fortunately have not been lost in this revised edition.

Barber's first edition provided a long awaited volume on this subject and his second was well received. Those two volumes have been invaluable for students and for informing all physicians who treat women patients. This third edition will also be an important textbook and reference for all gynecologists' libraries.

Felix Rutledge, M.D.
Emeritus Head, Department of Gynecology
M.D. Anderson Hospital and Tumor Institute
Houston, Texas

Preface

It has been 13 years since the first edition of this book was published and 10 years since the second edition. During that time many advances have been made in the epidemiology and treatment of ovarian cancer, but there has been no significant contribution to early diagnosis. Progress in the field of ovarian cancer has been slow but steady. Work being carried out with immune complexes, serologic studies using an immunologic approach for early diagnosis, new drugs and technology and an aggressive plan of management, and the potential presented by hybridoma research promises to change the gloom and doom of the last four decades for managing patients with ovarian cancer to one of optimism for the 1990s.

Ovarian cancer is the most frustrating problem in gynecology today. It is not possible to diagnose it (60–70% are in stages III and IV when treatment is undertaken), and it is not possible to predictably treat it for cure, as evidenced by the approximately 30% survival rate.

The cause of death with ovarian cancer has always been contributed to the repeated bouts of intestinal obstruction accompanied by the inanition and actual starvation of these patients. With the introduction of hyperalimentation, however, a challenge has been raised to this concept. It appears that many of these patients are compromised immunologically and succumb to infections.

It is evident that ovarian cancer is really a disease of the gastrointestinal tract. Despite the fact that these patients have a carcinomatosis ileus with vomiting, they are often ravenously hungry and thirsty, although any attempt to give them food or water aggravates the vomiting. The other disturbing feature is that these patients often remain alert up to the moment of death, and it is difficult to deal with them clinically. It is a time when the art of medicine must take over from the science of medicine. The one lesson we have learned is that we should never give up on these patients—many have had their disease palliated for long periods.

Gynecologic oncology has developed as a subspecialty of obstetrics and gynecology. On April 5, 1974, the Division of Gynecologic Oncology of the American Board of Obstetrics and Gynecology examined candidates for the first time for special competence in gynecologic oncology; for those passing written and oral examinations, a diploma was awarded. The diploma is less than the certificate that is associated with the rank of Diplomate of the Specialty Board, but it does indicate recognition of the increasing importance of special knowledge, techniques, and skills within the discipline of obstetrics and gynecology.

With the exception of ovarian cancer patients, most women having a gynecologic malignancy today can be cured with well structured and planned treatment. Although the profession has not been able to make an early diagnosis, it has achieved the goal of making diagnoses earlier than formerly. The use of hyperalimentation, Swan-Ganz catheter, and aggressive management with combination anticancer chemotherapy and surgery plus new and potent antibodies has added significantly to the longevity of these patients. Ovarian cancer vaccines are being studied, and hopefully genetic engineering will help advance the potential for their use in therapy. On the basis of one survey it was reported that about 1 of every 70 newborn girls (1.4%) develop cancer of the ovary at some time during their lives. It accounts for 4% of all cancers among women.

The definition of cancer of the ovary is difficult because of the diversity of the histogenetic types of cancer originating in the ovary. Ovarian cancer has been and is still considered a family of malignancies. The ovary is complex in terms of its embryology, histology, steroidogenesis, and potential for malignancy. It is made up of mesothelial cells, germ cells, and gonadal stromal cells. Each has its own potential to form a tumor. The ovary is unique in that it not only gives rise to a great variety of malignancies but is a favorite site for metastases from many other organs.

Ovarian cancer is now the leading cause of death from gynecologic cancer in the United States. It was anticipated that there would be more than 21,000 new cases and more than 13,000 deaths due to ovarian cancer in 1992. The results of therapy in 1991 were no better than they were during the previous two decades. However, patients with ovarian cancer are living longer and more comfortably at present.

The management of patients with ovarian cancer presents a constant challenge to the physicians. This challenge is reflected not so much in the incidence of disease (25% of gynecologic cancers) but, rather, in its high mortality rate (approximately half of all deaths from cancer of the genital tract). Thus whereas 10 of every 1000 women in the United States over age 40 develop ovarian cancer, only one or two can be cured. The remainder suffer repeated bouts of intestinal obstruction as the tumor spreads over the surface of the bowel; they develop inanition, malnutrition, and literally vomit themselves to death. This pathology, described as carcinomatosis ileus, is one of the few indications for the intermittent use of a nasogastric tube as definitive therapy to decompress the bowel. Those therapeutic nihilists who plead that patients should be left to die with dignity must face a dilemma when forced to apply their philosophy to the care of women with advanced ovarian cancer.

Because cancer of the ovary is such a frustrating problem for the clinician, I have attempted to assimilate, in a concise form, the prevailing opinions as an overview to ovarian cancer. I hope that I have achieved this goal without being superficial.

Each chapter has a conclusion that not only covers pertinent material presented but includes ideas not covered in the chapter. The glossary and an index follow the last chapter. The glossary was included to define terms discussed in the text and to provide a ready reference for those pursuing the subject in more detail in other articles and textbooks.

The references at the end of each chapter are not meant to cover the entire field; they have been selected for their historical value or because they represent an original or significant contribution. In general, the references consist principally of recent articles, reviews, monographs, and books. The book has been developed from these sources.

Acknowledgments

I want to express my appreciation to Dr. Sheldon C. Sommers for the help he has given me in this undertaking. He has been particularly helpful in selecting material to illustrate histologic and nuclear grading as well as stromal reactions.

Dr. Margaret Long has kindly supplied illustrations and material from her large collection of photographs of ovarian tumors. Dr. Harry Ioachim and Research Associate, Brent Dorsett, have been most helpful in collecting material for this study. I would like to thank Margaret Ryon-Uibel for having supplied illustrations that were presented in the first two editions and for those carried over to this edition. Patricia Kuharic has worked with me to provide additional illustrations for the third edition, and I am most grateful for her help.

Rosemarie Spitaleri and her assistant, George Tanis, have provided the photographic illustrations; and for their superb help I express my sincere appreciation.

For taking time from a busy schedule that includes practice, research, teaching, lecturing, and administrative duties, I am most grateful to Dr. Felix Rutledge for reading the text and writing a foreword.

As always, I am most grateful to Marcia Miller and Ruzena Danek for their help in writing this book. I have relied on them for their skilled typing, for locating and photocopying articles, for making suggestions, and, most important, for assisting me with their editorial expertise. Marcia Miller has been particularly helpful in proofreading the manuscript. These contributions lightened my burden and allowed me to concentrate on writing the book.

Elizabeth Armour has skillfully and expeditiously retyped the entire book, carefully deleting outdated material and inserting up-to-date additions as requested by the author. I thank her for her help.

A special thank you to my wife, Mary Louise, for her patience during the revision of this book.

I want to thank Bridie McGuire and Ann McGuire for their wonderful aid in helping me to maintain my private practice during the time I spent working on this book.

I am most appreciative of the help and support of the entire Lenox Hill family—doctors, nurses, paramedics, administrators, and trustees. The house staff on obstetrics and gynecology at Lenox Hill Hospital has been most helpful with their suggestions and the stimulation they supplied through their interest. I would particularly like to thank Shirley Dansker, Chief Librarian, and Julia Chai, who have been extremely helpful in collecting material from the literature for inclusion in this book.

I express my gratitude to Doctor Irving Buterman for covering my private practice while I was working on this book.

To my colleagues, I want to express my appreciation for encouraging and stimulating me to revise the book and write a third edition.

Contents

1

Introduction

The purpose of this book is to collect in a single volume pertinent material about ovarian malignancy that is either new or in which there has been a change in traditional concepts in terms of contemporary findings and knowledge. To accomplish this goal, it was necessary first to identify the problems associated with ovarian cancer and then to suggest solutions in light of the present phase of medical development. This chapter identifies problems related to ovarian cancer but does not discuss them in detail. The detailed discussions are included in the appropriate chapters.

It is my hope that the information collected and presented here will satisfy the goals of this book as well as suggest new avenues for meeting the constant challenge presented by ovarian cancer. More than 13,000 women die from ovarian cancer each year in the United States, and the results for the early 1990s are no better than those of the previous two decades. These figures mean that more than 130,000 women at the height of their social and economic productivity die from ovarian cancer within a decade. It is hoped that patients with ovarian cancer are living longer now and more comfortably than previously, but at this point the 5-year survival remains dismally low.

Incidence

Cancers of the ovary account for roughly 4% of all cancers among women and about 27% of the cancers of the female reproductive system. Estimates of cancer incidence show that cancer of the ovary is the fifth leading cancer in women. In age groups from 40–44 years to 80–84 years, it is the fourth, and fifth, leading cause of cancer death. At lower ages the incidence is somewhat lower. Only cancers of the skin, breast, colon and rectum, uterus, and lung account for more new cases of female cancer than cancer of the ovary. In 1973 the National Cancer Institute (NCI) began a new and larger program than the National Cancer Survey, gathering data from 11 population-based registries. It is called SEER (for surveillance, epidemiology, and end results). On the basis of the SEER data, about 1 of every 70 newborn girls (1.4%: for whites 1.5%, or 1 in 67; for blacks 1.0%, or 1 in 100) develop cancer of the ovary at some time during their lives. It was estimated that in 1992 there would be 21,000 new cases of cancer of the ovary. Carcinoma of the ovary is now the leading cause of death from gynecologic cancer.

The age-specific incidence rate for ovarian cancer rises steadily up to age 77, then drops off slightly in the older age group. It is obvious that the ovary becomes too old to function but never too old to form a cancer. By applying these rates to the estimated population for 1992, it was possible to determine the distribution of cases by age. The greatest number of cases are found in the age groups 50–59 years. The mean age is 59.5 and the median age 60.0.

The trends by age through the years have shown that the age-adjusted rate for all ages has remained about the same throughout the period from 1940 to 1991. All age groups have generally shown the same trend as the rates for all ages.

The age-specific incidence rates for ovarian cancer rise steadily to age 77 and then drop off slightly in older ages. The greatest number of cases were in the age group 60–64 years. The mean age was 61.5 and the median age 61.8 years.

The trends for ovarian cancer by age from 1935 to 1983 show that the age-adjusted rate for all ages remained about the same throughout the period. All individual age groups have shown the same trend, in general, as the rates for all ages.

The incidence trends by age group for white females in the NCI surveys show that all age rates have been stable during the years with only slight fluctuations. The rates for ages 30–39 have shown some fluctuations, and the rates for ages 40–49 and 50–59 have decreased slightly in recent years. The age groups above 60 years have been increased slightly since the earliest period.

In black females the rate for all ages combined decreased between 1969 and 1977 but has increased in recent years. The rates by age fluctuate considerably but show no noticeable pattern.

The death rate by age for cancer of the ovary shows a steady increase as the population at risk gets older. The nonwhite rates are lower than the white rates in each group for those over 30 years of age. The trends in age-standardized death rates for major sites show the rate for ovarian cancer increased until recent years and then dropped off.

Cancer of the ovary accounted for approximately 5% of all cancers among women. In this study ovarian cancer accounted for 27% of the genital cancers among white women and for 12% among black women.

Analysis of ovarian cancer by histologic type indicates notable racial variations. Although papillary serous cystadenocarcinomas made up about one-fourth of all ovarian cancers in both races, a high percentage of these tumors were classified as localized in more black women than white women (34% versus 26%). Papillary carcinomas occurred more frequently among white than black women and were more

often diagnosed in the localized stage among white women (27% versus 19%). There was a much higher percentage of papillary cystadenocarcinomas of the ovary among black women (15%) than among white women (2%); 31% of these lesions were localized among white women and only 16% among black women.

Detection of ovarian cancer when it was confined to the ovaries occurred in only one-fourth of the patients. One-half to two-thirds of the patients had distant metastases when first diagnosed. The only noticeable change over time was an increase in distant disease with the corresponding decrease in regional spread, probably an artifact reflecting only a shift in the classification definition for the extent of disease.

Mortality

Deaths due to cancer of the ovary have increased from 10,002 in 1973 to 13,000 in 1992 (Fig. 1.1). The mean age at death was 65.0 years and the median age 65.2 years.

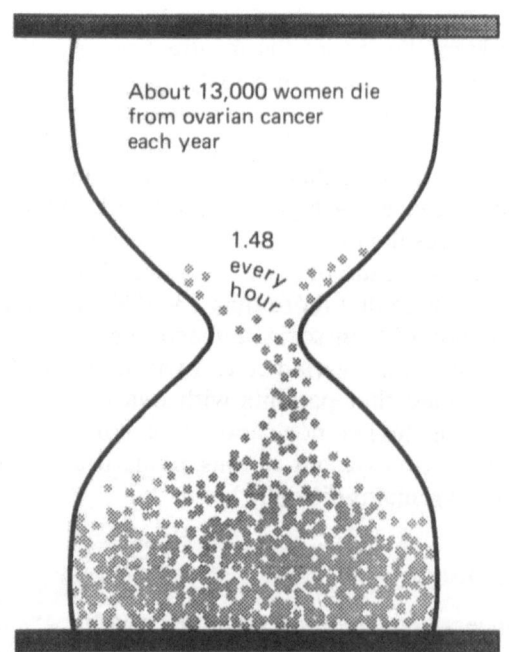

About 13,000 women die from ovarian cancer each year

1.48 every hour

FIGURE 1.1. Ovarian cancer is the leading cause of death due to gynecologic cancer.

Common epithelial ovarian cancers are more frequent in older women. Consequently, the relatively favorable median survival at diagnosis for women under age 45 years reflects the survival experience of only 17% of all patients. For all older women, it is important to compare the observed and relative survival rates. The poor results are not nearly as dreary when the observed survival rate is compared to the relative survival rate. For women diagnosed with localized disease, the age gradient is relatively weak.

Cancer of the ovary is the fifth leading cause of *cancer* death in women. In age groups from 40–44 to 80–84, it is the fourth, and fifth, leading cause of cancer death. At older ages it is lower.

The death rates by age for cancer of the ovary show a steady increase as the population at risk gets older. The rates for nonwhites are lower than those for whites in each age group over age 30 years.

The observed median survival time by age for white patients for all ages is 1.6 years; under age 45 it is more than 5 years; at age 45–54 it is 1.9 years; at age 55–64 it is 1.5 years; at age 65–74 it is 0.9 years; and at age 75 and over it is 0.6 years.

The observed median survival time by age among blacks for all ages is 0.9 years; under age 45 it is over 5 years; at age 45–54 it is 2.0 years; at age 55–64 it is 0.7 years; at age 65–74 it is 0.5 years; at age 75 and over it is 0.4 years.

Stage at Diagnosis

In most reported series, ovarian cancer when first diagnosed is in stages III and IV in about 60 to 70% of the cases. The End Results Section of the National Cancer Institute has reported that the proportion of cases diagnosed with distant metastases has continued to increase since the early 1950s, after a decrease from the 1940s cases to the 1950s cases. After increasing from the 1940s cases to the 1950s cases, the proportion of cases with regional involvement has continued to decrease since the 1950s. The number of cases diagnosed as localized remained approximately the same until recently, when there was a slight decrease. The distribution by stage is now almost the same for blacks and whites.

Treatment

The extent of disease or stage for each ovarian cancer patient seems to be the main determinant for choice of therapy. A surgical attack is considered the backbone of therapy, to either completely eradicate the disease or debulk the cancer. The fourth End Results in Cancer report revealed that surgery alone was the most frequently used treatment for patients with localized disease diagnosed during 1955 to 1964, but the favorable survival rates for such patients given chemotherapy in addition to surgery seem to have guided clinicians to choose this combination therapy almost as often as surgery alone during 1965 to 1969. For patients with regional disease, surgery plus irradiation was used most often during the earlier period, but for 1965 to 1969 the addition of chemotherapy to surgery plus irradiation was used as frequently as the earlier treatment. Although survival rates are poor for patients with distant metastases, the use of chemotherapy in combination with surgery seems to yield more favorable results. Currently, irradiation is being chosen only for a highly selected indication, discussed later.

Survival

The survival rate in 1991 was only slightly better than it was during the previous two decades. This improvement may reflect better management of the complications, earlier cases, and the judicious use of chemotherapy. The overall 5-year survival rate in most series of patients with invasive common epithelial ovarian cancer runs between 15% and 35%.

Pertinent Considerations

Embryology

Ovarian cancer has been considered a family of malignancies within the ovary rather than as a single entity. The ovary is complex in terms of its embryology, histology, steroidogenesis, and potential for malignancy. It is composed of germ cells, gonadal stromal cells, and cells of the mesenchymal tissue, each with its own potential to form a tumor. Although sex is determined genetically at fertilization, the ovary passes through its early phases as an indifferent organ with parallel development that could allow it to become an ovary or a testis. Alterations or imbalances during these steps of development may provide the setting for later cellular malfunctioning that produces endocrine imbalances as well as malignancy. The ovary is unique in that it not only gives rise to a great variety of malignancies but is itself a favorite site for metastases from many other organs. The embryology of the ovary is discussed in greater detail in Chapter 2.

Phylogenic Development

A review of the phylogenic development and comparative anatomy of the ovary seems indicated in a study devoted to ovarian cancer. It is hoped that a clue might be found that could serve as the Rosetta stone for unraveling the mystery of new growths in the ovary. There are many interesting reports of work done in this field. A brief summary of these condensed reports is incorporated in this discussion.

The protozoan genera plasmodia reproduce, but it is not until the metazoan genera are reached that an identifiable ovary makes its appearance. The amphioxus has gonadal tissue distributed in various tissues of its body, but the lowest form in which the ovary is concentrated in one ovary is the lamprey. The female vertebrate species have ovaries, and the process of fertilization becomes more complex.

The ovaries in the bird are interesting in that the left ovary develops into an adult ovary, and the right atrophies (Fig. 1.2). Among fowl the most common spontaneous tumors are lymphosarcoma, leukemia, carcinoma of the ovary, and adenocarcinoma of the intestine. Generally, ovarian tumors affect most species of mammals and birds. Ovarian tumors that develop spontaneously in these animals are epithelial tumors and resemble those found in the human. However, artificially produced

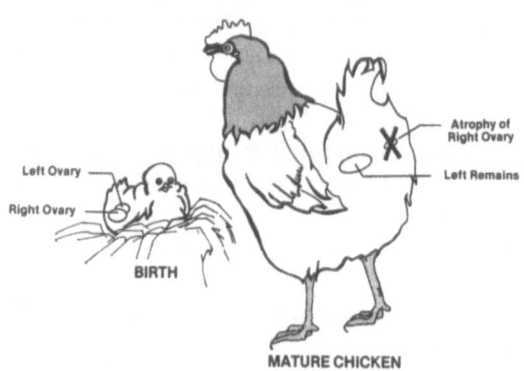

COMPARATIVE ANATOMY: CHICKEN

FIGURE 1.2. In birds and chickens the left ovary and oviduct develop to maturity, and the organs on the right side atrophy. Adenocarcinomas and cystadenocarcinomas reported in birds are histologically similar to those found in humans.

ovarian cancers are always of the granulosa cell tumor type.

It is interesting that one of the most common solid tumors in the bird is carcinoma of the ovary. The peculiar postnatal course of the ovary in the bird makes the problem doubly interesting. Whether there is an abnormal steroidogenesis or a faulty feedback mechanism is difficult to ascertain from the literature. Transferring animal data to interpret a process in the human is fraught with danger, but there are areas that supply a common ground for consideration. Because ovarian cancer is difficult to diagnose and deadly in its prognosis, every avenue of approach must be thoroughly investigated.

Conservation or Prophylaxis

Although cancer of the endometrium is the most common malignancy in the female pelvis, ovarian cancer is now the leading cause of death from gynecologic malignancy. In the United States six or seven of each 100 women require surgery for an ovarian cyst or tumor during their lifetime. One woman in 100 over age 40 develops a malignancy of the ovary; or, to put it another way, 9 or 10 women in each 1000 develop a malignancy and only one or two can be cured. Randall and colleagues have reported that about 30 women in 100,000 develop ovarian cancer before age 45, and that the rate increases to 281 per 100,000 between ages 45 and 60 years. Eight of every nine malignancies of the ovary develop after the patient's 50th birthday. The ovary may be too old to function, but it is never too old to form a cancer. The reports by Randall cover a period when ovarian cancer was not the serious problem it is today. Current reports show that the incidence of malignancy in an adnexal mass ranges between 50 and 80% in the postmenopausal patient.

A report by Gibbs is more current and documents the problem in a precise manner. From 1949 to 1969, a total of 236 cases of ovarian cancer were seen at the Butterworth Hospital in Grand Rapids, Michigan. Of these cases, 85.6% had their onset in women over age 41. At the time of diagnosis 69% of the ovarian cancers were in stages III and IV. The overall 5-year survival for all stages was 15.7%. Previous operations had been performed in 126 patients. Twenty-eight patients had had hysterectomies. The expected incidence of ovarian carcinoma following hysterectomy was observed. Ovarian cancer may develop in patients who had had prior irradiation to the ovaries and breast or gastrointestinal malignancy. Gibbs suggested that a radical approach to pelvic operation (hysterectomy and bilateral salpingo-oophorectomy) beyond age 35 could prevent 20% of all ovarian carcinomas seen.

Barber and Graber have reported an early sign of ovarian cancer that has been most valuable in diagnosis: the postmenopausal palpable ovary (PMPO) syndrome. Simply stated, palpation of *what is interpreted as a normal-sized ovary in the premenopausal woman represents an ovarian tumor in the postmenopausal woman.* This does not imply that anything palpated in the adnexal areas is abnormal, because small atrophic ovaries may be felt in certain thin, relaxed women. However, patients with the PMPO syndrome should not be simply followed and reevaluated; the presence or absence of an ovarian tumor must be determined promptly. To save more women and diminish the mortality due to ovarian cancer, more liberal indications for operation must be accepted. Waiting until one feels a solid tumor mass of up to 5 cm in size and then expecting a cure is an exercise in fancy and futility. As with other cancers, early diagnosis is the most effective way to increase survival rates among women with ovarian cancer. These figures have a sobering effect and emphasize the responsibility shouldered by physicians who are charged with the care of women. Constant vigilance and reevaluation must be pursued.

Early Diagnosis, Treatment, and Terminal Care

The problem of ovarian cancer is best divided into three primary categories: early diagnosis, treatment, and terminal care of patients with advanced or recurrent cancer. Because it is almost impossible to diagnose ovarian cancer in its early stages, it is impossible to treat it with any predictable degree of certainty for cure. With the present state of knowledge, early diagnosis is the key to successful treatment. The logical question, then, is how can we ensure early diagnosis? A high degree of suspicion reinforced by knowledge of the natural history of ovarian cancer is important. Early ovarian cancer is a disease found more often in community hospitals than in large medical centers. In cases in which cancer is diagnosed in its early stage, it is considered a surgical disease. The standard treatment is total hysterectomy, bilateral salpingo-oophorectomy, omentectomy, appendectomy, para-aortic and pelvic node sampling, and washings from the upper abdomen and pelvis for cytologic examination. There has been no significant study clearly demonstrating that removal of the omentum is desirable or necessary. The arguments advanced for its removal are that it may contain microscopic cancer and that the cancer is then in a more advanced stage. In addition, after removal any instilled radioactive substance is better able to come in contact with the peritoneum and therefore to provide better control of ascites. Treatment is covered in detail in other chapters of this book.

Ovarian Tumors in Children

Ovarian tumors comprise about 1% of all new growths in the field of pediatric gynecology. The problem of diagnosis is surpassed only by the problem and confusion about treatment. In this age group it is difficult to accept the diagnosis of ovarian cancer and even more difficult for the physician to carry out surgery that will deprive a child of her reproductive potential. Fortunately, more than one-third of ovarian tumors in children are benign cystic teratomas. This problem can be handled by simple excision of the cyst with preservation of that ovary in most instances. Dysgerminomas and solid teratomas have been found more frequently in children than later in life.

In general, the types of ovarian tumor seen in children are not dissimilar from those in adults. Therapy must be tailored to the patient and the extent of disease. A malignancy that has spread beyond the ovary should undergo radical extirpative therapy. If there is any doubt about the type of tumor or if it is malignant, it is better to perform a salpingo-oophorectomy on the side of the tumor if the tumor has an intact capsule and is freely movable. If the tumor proves to be highly malignant, the abdomen may be reopened and the remaining reproductive organs excised if this treatment appears to be the best course. With certain low-grade malignancies the previously performed treatment may be considered sufficient to ensure cure.

Effect of Spill

Often the question is raised of how the prognosis is affected by rupture of the cyst or tumor, resulting in spill. The smooth, freely movable cyst that is ruptured accidentally as a result of poor technique or a thin wall probably has little unfavorable effect on prognosis. The exception may be the mucinous cyst. The nature of the fluid content varies from a stringy, sticky, mucoid secretion to one with the consistency of wet glue. The gelatinous material is tenacious and sticks to everything it touches. It is this adhesive property that creates the pseudomyxoma peritonei sometimes described

after rupture or spillage from the cyst. However, a poor prognosis can be anticipated with rupture in the presence of a soft vascular ovarian tumor that is densely adherent and directly infiltrating. It is obvious that this poor prognosis is not due solely to the rupture of the cyst but, rather, to the advanced stage of the disease. The new staging of ovarian cancer upstages the cancer in stages I and II if the capsule is ruptured. In the new FIGO clinical staging, stages IC and IIC include rupture of the capsule of the ovary. This will supply the statistical data necessary to answer the question about spill at the time of surgery.

Role of Node Dissection

Should a node dissection be part of planned definitive therapy? The consensus is that it should not. A survey of its usual spread when the nodes are involved indicates why there has been little enthusiasm for a node dissection in ovarian cancer. The iliac nodes are involved about one-fourth as often as with cancer of the cervix, or in about 7% of cases. The usual nodal spread is to the upper abdomen. Because the ovary embryologically arises at about T10, it is not surprising that the retroperitoneal nodes in the upper abdomen located around the duodenum, kidney, and celiac axis are involved. From here the spread advances to the mediastinal and then the supraclavicular areas. Retrograde extension to the inguinal nodes is infrequent. The natural history of the disease, because it spreads widely throughout the abdomen, contraindicates a node dissection in most instances. However, lymph node sampling of the pelvis and paraaortic areas is now part of the staging process. Unless nodes are sampled from the paraaortic and pelvic areas, the lesion has not been adequately staged.

Radioactive Substances

After all gross disease tissue is removed, a decision must be made about the instillation of radioactive phosphorus (^{32}P). Impressive as the results have been at Memorial Hospital (New York) for the early stages of cancer, most series have not been able to confirm their results. In the presence of positive cells in the pelvis, however, or perhaps after rupture of a cyst, it may have therapeutic value. Because ^{32}P emits only beta rays, it causes little bowel reaction, whereas the gamma rays of radioactive gold have been associated with late bowel necrosis. The greatest benefit of radioactive substances is that they control ascites. Their main contribution is their use as palliatives. When nodules are 2 cm or larger, palliation cannot be anticipated. Radioactive substances exert their greatest benefit in the presence of free-floating cells.

Prophylactic Therapy

Guidelines for the use of prophylactic irradiation when all gross tumor has been removed are sought constantly. The value of prophylactic irradiation cannot be established from a survey of the literature. It has been recommended, however, that radiation therapy be given for highly anaplastic cancers or if there is ascites with positive cells, rupture of a cyst, any question about the complete removal of the tumor, excrescence on the surface of the ovary, or difficulty establishing planes of dissection. It is reported that a recurrence is biologically more potent, and maximum therapy should be attempted to prevent persistence of disease or recurrence. With dysgerminoma that is histologically and serologically proved by a negative pregnancy test, local paraaortic irradiation is advisable. Increasing knowledge of the natural history of common epithelial ovarian cancer and the limitation of radiation therapy in controlling ovarian cancer have stimulated an interest in chemotherapy. The plan is to use prophylactic chemotherapy for stages I and II when the disease has been removed and therapeutically for stages III and IV when the disease persists.

A prospective randomized trial is under way at the Princess Margaret Hospital in Toronto. The physicians have structured a program for the moving-strip technique that is slightly different from that normally employed. The central figures for abdominal pelvic irradiation at the hospital have been published and are discussed later in the book.

External therapy has a place in the treatment of germ cell and gonadal stromal tumors. These tumors are more responsive to external radiation therapy than are the common epithelial ovarian tumors; and they have a natural history and pattern of metastases that make them suitable for such treatment.

Whether chemotherapy can improve the 5-year survival rate for ovarian cancer is difficult to estimate, but it has certainly made life more comfortable for a great number of patients with cancer of the ovary and has increased their survival time. Each center has its own criteria; but, in general, patients with metastases and ascites have been given chemotherapy. The indications are becoming more liberal. Chemotherapy, given in a well-controlled manner, does not produce as much morbidity as occurred with radiotherapy when it was applied to the upper abdomen. The most commonly used first-line drugs are the platinum drugs. When there is a recurrence or if the tumor plateaus or fails to regress, the decision regarding the type of management becomes more difficult. There are a variety of combinations that are being used, and none has proved to be superior including the intraperitoneal use of cis-platinum.

Widespread Disease

When the abdomen is opened and widespread disease has been found, should as much cancer as possible be removed? Hoskins (1989) reports that the amount of cytoreductive surgery influences the tumor-free interval. Residual tumors greater than 2 cm in diameter decrease the chances for prolonged survival. Removing large masses helps improve metabolic and symptomatic status; it also places remaining tumors into a more rapid growth phase, producing better effect with chemotherapy. The tumor blood supply improves, bringing the chemotherapy drugs to the remaining tumor in greater concentrations. The consensus, however, is that as much cancer as possible should be removed without violating good surgical and clinical judgment. Because ovarian cancer is known to spread to the upper abdomen and rarely remains confined to the pelvis, it lends

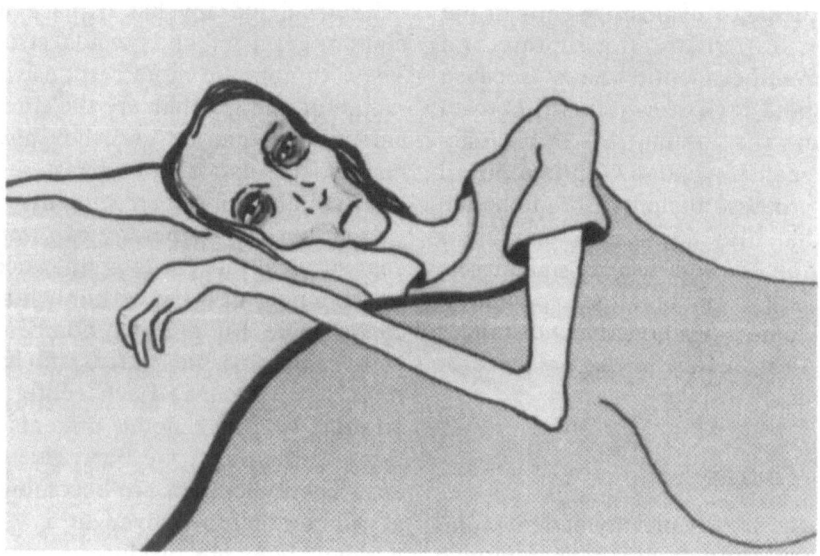

FIGURE 1.3. The patient with advanced or recurrent ovarian cancer often has a distended abdomen, atrophic extremities, and loss of facial fat. These patients are frequently ravenously hungry, but one bite of food induces marked vomiting.

itself to pelvic exenteration only if it violates its natural history.

Terminal Ovarian Cancer

The patient with recurrent and far-advanced cancer presents a real challenge. A balance must be struck between doing too much and doing too little. Therapy should be aimed at relieving symptoms. Because the patient undoubtedly has undergone several modalities of therapy, including surgery, additional surgery should be reserved for the relief of an intestinal obstruction, drainage of an abscess, or relief from a fistula. Indeed, most of the symptoms arise from the intestine, and the problem is best managed by a physician trained in gastrointestinal surgery.

The patient with advanced or recurrent ovarian cancer presents a characteristic clinical picture of inanition and malnutrition. The abdomen is greatly distended, and the extremities are thin, giving the impression that the bones are covered with skin with no intervening muscle tissue. The muscle and fat are missing from the hands, resulting in a skeleton-like appearance. The fat has been lost from around the face, and the patient seems to have a sardonic smile. The tissue around the eyes has atrophied, and the eyeballs appear sunken. The clinical picture is not unlike that associated with the advanced starvation of Nazi concentration camp victims (Fig. 1.3). Often spot radiation therapy can relieve pain in the terminal patient. In addition, wisely administered chemotherapy may also achieve palliation. Because the goal is palliation toxicity must be avoided.

Steroidogenesis in Ovarian Tumors

There has long been a belief that the finding of abnormal steroidogenesis might supply a key to early diagnosis and management of ovarian cancer, but to date there has been no concrete evidence to support this hypothesis. Cholesterol is considered the keystone on which steroids are built up from acetate; and for steroid synthesis, endogenous cholesterol is considered the important factor. Preformed cholesterol is reported to play a minor role, but this contention has been challenged. The process of steroidogenesis in the adrenal, testis, and ovary is the same up to the point of progesterone formation. At this point the three glands complete the synthesis of their steroids along individual patterns. Androstenedione and testosterone are synthesized as final steps before estrone and estradiol are produced as the main steroids of the ovary. Anything that disturbs the delicate balance of the pituitary-ovarian axis could alter the final step in the formation of estrogens and thus cause an accumulation of intermediate products in the ovary. The Japanese have a low rate of ovarian cancer, whereas in Denmark the rate is high. The increase of ovarian cancer among Japanese immigrants to the United States may provide a lead to unravel the complex interplay that occurs in steroidogenesis. Since World War II the Japanese have westernized their diet, which now includes more cholesterol and fatty acids, and they have reduced the number of children they have. Whether it is cause or effect, there is an increased incidence in carcinoma of the ovary, endometrium, and breast among the Japanese compared to the pre-World War II days.

Clinical leads often come from animal laboratory experimentation. Biskind and Biskind, working with rats, and Furth and Sobel, working with mice, transplanted the gonads into the spleen and produced granulosa cell tumors. Although the menopausal human female has a similar pattern of increased excretion of pituitary gonadotropins, the malignancies formed in the human ovary are not usually the granulosa cell type. The results from animal experimentation are difficult to correlate with clinical findings in the human. When ovarian cancer is produced in animals, the result is usually a functioning tumor, most commonly a granulosa cell tumor, and is associated with continuous unopposed stimulation of the pituitary. In the human, granulosa cell tumor occurs in the young age group and may be accompanied by a high estrogen titer with a feedback to control the pituitary. Only about 25% of the granulosa thecoma tumors function and produce estrogen. Most ovarian cancers in the human are epithelial tumors and are different from those artificially produced in animals.

Survival Factors

Further evaluation of factors affecting the survival of patients with ovarian cancer may help in the quest for early diagnosis. Often retrospective studies indicate a point in time when the ovary started its malfunction, much like a cam running off center. A study reported by Wynder, Dodo, and Barber included data that seemed to bear out this statement. The incidence of spontaneous abortion, dysmenorrhea, heavy flow, postmenopausal bleeding, and swelling of the breasts was higher than in control series. Sometimes benign cysts show progressive changes toward precancer and finally cancer. There are reports in the literature of small areas of localized malignancy in benign multilocular cysts. One theory of cystoma etiology reports that there is an invagination of small fragments of the surface germinal epithelium much as in the formation of inclusion cysts. It results in a cyst lined with low cuboidal epithelium, as seen in serous cysts, or with a tall columnar epithelium of the mucinous type. These cysts develop pseudostratification with papillary processes and finally a complex cystadenoma.

Histologic Classification and Clinical Staging

There was no common language for the histologic classification or clinical staging until the International Federation of Gynecology and Obstetrics (FIGO) established them. There had been as many histologic classifications and clinical stagings as there were hospitals in the United States until FIGO in 1971 announced their classifications, which are now well accepted.

The histologic type and grading provide the microscopic character of the tumor. The tumor is named from its most differentiated portion and graded from the least differentiated parts. The clinical staging, which is determined clinically, estimates the extent of disease and the size of the tumor. Staging and detailed histologic studies serve as a guide for understanding the natural history of disease. The heterogeneous nature of cancer makes it difficult to establish criteria for histologic grading. Establishing a common language for histologic classification and clinical staging was an important step in understanding ovarian carcinoma. The difference in reported 5-year survival rates usually reflects the different criteria used when reporting the material. More attention has been directed to establishing rigid histologic clinical staging for ovarian cancer. Progress will be slow until we establish more accurate histologic criteria that not only help identify the various tumors but make it possible for different institutions to compare their material meaningfully.

Borderline Malignancy (Carcinoma of Low Malignant Potential)

It is important to make an accurate diagnosis of the malignant potential of the ovarian tumor. No matter how potent the epithelial cells appear and no matter how they are stratified, the epithelial elements must invade the stroma of the tumor before it can be considered invasive. Because the low malignant potential tumor is often parvilocular and multilocular, it is essential that careful scrutiny does not reveal the tumor cells penetrating the basement membrane of the tumor. An absolute requirement for the diagnosis of an ovarian epithelial carcinoma of low malignant potential is the lack of destructive invasion of the underlying stroma. The height of the cells is no longer considered when evaluating the low malignant potential (LMP) tumor. These LMP common epithelial ovarian cancers are defined as having some, but not all, of the morphologic features of malignancy. Those features include, in varying combinations, stratification of the epithelial cells, apparent detachment of cellular clusters from their sites of origin, mitotic activity, and nuclear abnormalities intermediate between those of clearly benign and unquestioned malignant tumors of a similar cell type; on the other hand, obvious invasion of the adjacent stroma is lacking. Tumors with epithelial cell proliferation or atypicality of a minor degree should be placed in the benign category. It is imperative that a pointed reference be made to the fact that benign, borderline, and malignant forms of any of the neoplastic types may coex-

ist in any one tumor. Therefore it is important to have multiple representative sections before making the diagnosis of a so-called borderline or low malignant potential tumor. At least one tissue section for every 1 cm of maximal tumor diameter should be obtained for microscopic examination.

Role of Immunology

Although immunology has grown to maturity in the field of bacteriology, it is in its embryonic phase in the field of tissue transplant and oncology. Of any of the avenues now being pursued, this approach, though exotic, has the greatest potential for effecting a cure or prophylaxis against the development of a malignancy.

The long haul to produce a vaccine that could be used as therapy as well as prophylaxis has now been realized. Active programs are under way for lung cancer vaccine, melanoma vaccine, colonic tumor vaccine, and others. Genetically engineered vaccines are being studied, but there are no progress reports available at this time.

A variety of tumor markers are available. CEA, beta human chorionic gonadotropin, alpha-fetoprotein, CA 125, CA 15-3, polypeptide antigen (TPA), CA 19-9, NB/70K (DM/70K), and LASA-P. Currently, CA 125 is being used to monitor therapy in patients with common epithelial ovarian cancer. However, it is neither highly sensitive nor specific; moreover, it may be elevated in the presence of endometriosis, infection, a menstrual period, inflammation, pregnancy, and a variety of other tumors.

The problem of multiple drug resistance and cancer is being explored. Currently, an ancient pump protein that flushes toxins out of cells may be to blame when cancer chemotherapy fails. Its identification offers hope that multiple drug-resistant cancers might be made vulnerable again. A P-glycoprotein has been found in the membrane of the cell that is apparently responsible for the failure of cancer chemotherapy to control the growth of the cancer. A great deal of work is under way, and scientists have turned to tools of molecular biology that hopefully will give them a close look at the structure and ultimately the function of the molecule itself.

A great deal of work is being done with monoclonal antibodies directly as therapy and as carriers for chemotherapeutic drugs and radioactive substances in the attack on ovarian cancer. Genetic engineering has provided a large number of substances that are included under the heading of biologic response modifiers. Early work seems promising, and there are a variety of biologic response modifiers that will play an increasingly important role in the management of cancer in the future.

Cancer immunology may now be at the threshold of an era for the prevention and treatment of cancer not unlike that in which the conquest of some major infectious disease was achieved. Current studies in the immunology of cancer have the following objectives.

1. To determine the antigenic properties of cancer cells
2. To understand the details of the mechanisms of immune reactions, particularly those evoked by cancer cells
3. To contribute to the knowledge of the etiology of cancer
4. To create new and better diagnostic methods to increase the effectiveness of all forms of therapy
5. To develop new therapeutic methods based on an immunologic approach
6. To establish guidelines for selecting patients to undergo immunoprophylaxis, rather than immunotherapy
7. To develop methods to monitor the volume of disease in a patient while under treatment

Bibliography

Barber HRK: CA 36(3):149, 1986.

Barber HRK: Foreword—ovarian tumors. Clin Obstet Gynecol 12:292, 1969.

Barber HRK, Graber EA: The PMPO syndrome (postmenopausal palpable ovary syndrome). Obstet Gynecol 38:921, 1971.

Barnhill DR, O'Connor DM: Management of ovarian neoplasms of low malignant potential. Oncology 5(4):21, 1991.

Bennington JL, Ferguson BR, Harber SL: Incidence and relative frequency of benign and malignant ovarian neoplasms. Obstet Gynecol 32:627, 1968.

Biskind MS, Biskind GR: Development of tumors in rat ovary after transplantation into the spleen. Proc Soc Exp Biol Med 55:176, 1944.

Cancer Facts and Figures 1991. American Cancer Society, Atlanta.

Furth J, Sobel H: Neoplastic transformation of granulosa cells in grafts of normal ovaries into spleens of gonadectomized mice. J Nat Cancer Inst 8:7, 1948.

Gibbs EK: Suggested prophylaxis for ovarian cancer: a 20-year report from cases at Butterworth Hospital. Am J Obstet Gynecol 111:756, 1971.

Heintz APM, Hacker NF, Berek JS, et al: Cytoreductive surgery in ovarian carcinoma: feasibility and morbidity. Obstet Gynecol 67:783, 1986.

Hollinshead AC: Analysis of soluble melanoma cell membrane antigens in metastatic cells of various organs and further studies of antigens present in primary melanoma. Cancer 36:1288, 1975.

Hoskins WJ: The influence of cytoreductive surgery on progression-free interval and survival in epithelial ovarian cancer. Baillieres Clin Obstet Gynecol 3:59, 1989.

James PD: Epidemiology of ovarian cancer. Lancet 1:412, 1974.

Jones TC, Gilmore CE: The ovaries in animals. In The Ovary. Grady HG, Smith DE (eds): Williams & Wilkins, Baltimore, 1963, p. 255.

Lingeman CH: Etiology of cancer of the human ovary. J Natl Cancer Inst 53:1603, 1974.

Myers NA, Gloeckler Ries LA: Cancer patient survival rates: SEER program results for 10 years of follow up. CA 39(1):21, 1989.

Oran TJ: Is the appendectomy essential in the treatment of ovarian cancer? Surg Forum 39:469, 1988.

Randall CL, Hall DW, Armenia CS: Pathology in the preserved ovary after unilateral oophorectomy. Am J Obstet Gynecol 84:1233, 1962.

Silverberg E, Lubera JA: Cancer statistics 1989. CA 39(1):3, 1989.

Stone ML, Weingold A, Sanford S, Sonnenblick B: Factors affecting patients with ovarian carcinoma. Surg Gynecol Obstet 116:351, 1963.

Terz JJ, Barber HRK, Brunschwig A: Incidence of carcinoma in the retained ovary. Am J Surg 113:511, 1967.

West RO: Epidemiologic studies of malignancies of the ovaries. Cancer 19:1001, 1966.

Wynder EL, Dodo H, Barber HRK: Epidemiology of cancer of the ovary. Cancer 23:352, 1969.

2

Anatomy, Embryology, and Comparative Anatomy

The ovaries are solid, slightly nodular, pink-gray bodies with the approximate proportions of unshelled almonds. They are situated on either side of the uterus, behind and below the uterine tubes. The human ovary undergoes marked changes in size, shape, and position during its lifetime in addition to the histologic changes brought about by various endocrine stimuli. It is important to appreciate the changes in size, shape, and consistency of the ovary that occur at different ages as well as during any given menstrual cycle. The ovaries are usually not symmetric, with the right ovary often larger than the left.

The size of the ovaries increases slowly but progressively between birth and the seventh or eighth year of life. During this period the ovaries lie with their superior poles at the brim of the pelvis and their inferior poles near the uterus. They descend to their final position, which is considerably lower, near the time of menarche. In general, there is no remarkable change in their gross appearance until 3 or 4 years before the menarche, when the pituitary gonadotropins induce increased ovarian function.

The ovary of the newborn is an elongated structure approximately 1.5 cm long and 0.5 cm wide, and it varies from 1.5 to 3.5 mm in thickness. The ovarian surface is pinkish-white, smooth, and glistening. It weighs about 0.3 to 0.4 g. The ovary gradually grows larger and changes shape and position between birth and puberty. It is developed between the tenth and twelfth segments on the posterior wall near the kidney, then slowly moves into the true pelvis and enlarges to about $3.0 \times 1.8 \times 1.2$ cm. The weight of both ovaries at puberty is between 4 and 7 g.

The premenopausal ovary measures $3.5 \times 2.0 \times 1.5$ cm. The menopausal ovary tends to atrophy and shrink when the graafian follicles and ova disappear. The ovary eventually becomes an inert residue that consists of connective tissue, and it clings to the posterior leaf of the broad ligament. Its pink color becomes pure white. It shrinks to $2.0 \times 1.5 \times 0.5$ cm, and in some it may be as small as $1.50 \times 0.75 \times 0.50$ cm. Its wrinkled surface resembles the gyri and sulci of the cerebrum. At this point it is almost impossible to palpate it on examination.

In the nullipara the ovary lies in a shallow peritoneal fossa on the lateral pelvic wall known as the fossa ovarica of Waldeyer. Its long axis lies in the vertical plane, so it has an upper and a lower pole, an anterior and a posterior border, and a medial and a lateral surface. The fossa of the ovary lies immediately below the bifurcation of the common iliac artery; and one of the most important relations of the ovary is the ureter, which lies immediately behind it.

During pregnancy the ovaries are lifted out of the true pelvis as the uterus enlarges. During the early part of the first trimester the corpus luteum may be large and protrude above the ovarian surface. At the time of cesarean section the ovaries are in a resting state and are covered with a shaggy pink material, which is a decidual reaction.

Each ovary has two extremities, two surfaces, and two borders. The ovary is attached to the posterior layer of the broad ligament by the mesovarium, to the lateral pelvic wall by the infundibulopelvic fold, and to the uterus by the ovarian ligament. The posterior border is free. The uterine extremity, or lower pole, is directed inferiorly and is connected through the ovarian ligament to the lateral margin of the uterus. The tubal extremity, or upper pole, is attached to the peritoneum of the lateral pelvic wall by the infundibulopelvic ligament. The medial surface faces inward and to a great extent is covered by the fimbriated extremity of the fallopian tube. Usually the lateral surface is in direct contact with the parietal peritoneum overlying the shallow ovarian fossa in the angle between the diverging external iliac and hypogastric vessels. The position of the ovary is therefore likely to be influenced by the move-

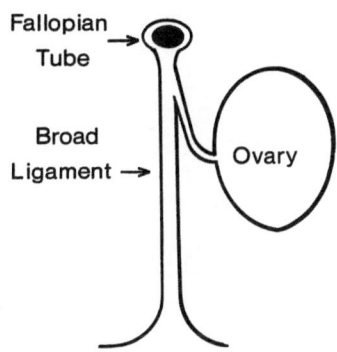

FIGURE 2.2. Attachment of the ovary to the broad ligament.

ments of the broad ligament and the uterus under normal circumstances (Fig. 2.1).

The relations of the ovary may be described as follows.

1. The anterior border is attached to the posterior layer of the broad ligament by a double layer of peritoneum, which forms a mesentery for the ovary. It is known as the mesovarium, and between its two layers the ovarian vessels and nerves enter the hilum of the gland (Fig. 2.2).
2. The posterior border is directed backward and is free. The ovary is separated from the ureter and the hypogastric artery by peritoneum.
3. The superior border, or tubal pole, is in direct contact with the ampulla of the uterine tube, and the infundibulopelvic fold is attached to it.
4. The inferior border, or uterine pole, is directed toward the uterus and is attached to it by the uteroovarian ligament.
5. The medial surface is in contact with the abdominal ostium and fimbriae of the tube.
6. The lateral surface is in contact with the abdominal ostium and fimbriae of the tube.

Blood Supply

The blood supply of the ovary is from the ovarian artery, a branch of the abdominal aorta, which arises immediately below the renal artery. From here it crosses the inferior vena cava and ureter on the right, and on the left it

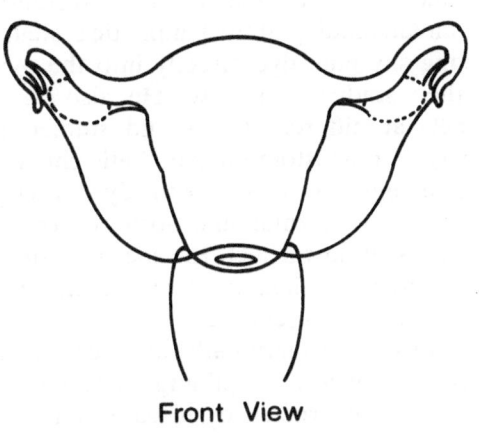

Front View

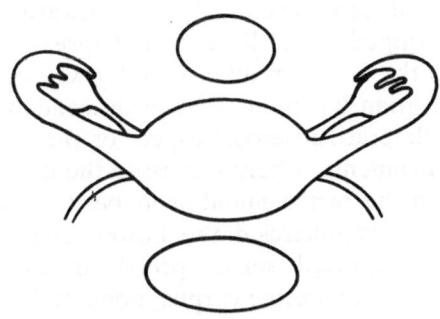

Front View — from the top

FIGURE 2.1. Relation of the ovaries to the tube and uterus.

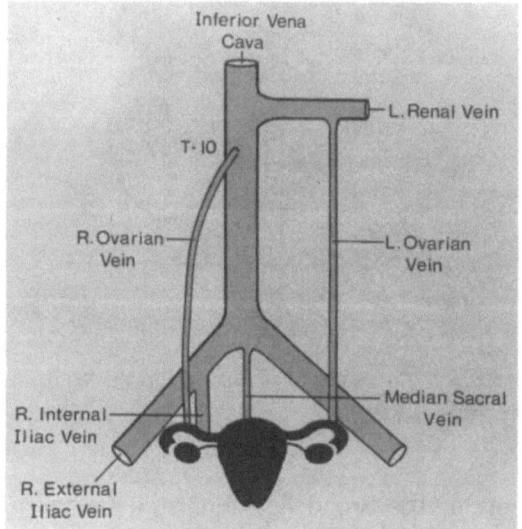

FIGURE 2.3. Inferior vena cava and its tributaries constitute the ovary's venous drainage system.

crosses the ureter and the left psoas muscle. Having reached the pelvic brim it crosses the common or external iliac artery and runs between the two layers of the infundibulopelvic fold and enters the broad ligament. It reaches the hilum of the ovary by passing between two layers of mesovarium.

The venous drainage is into a pampiniform venous plexus from which the ovarian vein emerges. On the right side the ovarian vein enters the inferior vena cava at an oblique angle below the renal vein, and on the left side it enters the left renal vein at a right angle (Fig. 2.3). A hypernephroma arising in the left kidney may metastasize in a retrograde manner along the left ovarian vein and present in the pelvis or the vagina.

The nerve supply comes from the level of the tenth thoracic segment. It is derived from the lateral column of gray matter in the spinal cord at this level. The ovarian artery and vein, nerves, and lymphatic vessels enter the infundibulopelvic fold (ligament), broad ligament, and mesovarium to reach the hilum of the ovary.

Vestigial remnants of the mesonephric duct and tubules persist within the peritoneal layers of the broad ligament as the epoophoron, the

paroophoron, and the duct of Gartner. The epoophoron consists of a longitudinal duct and 8 to 20 small tubes at right angles to it, situated in the lateral aspect of the mesosalpinx. The paroophoron refers to a few scattered tubules medial to the epoophoron and nearer the uterus. The lower end of the mesonephric duct may persist along the lateral margin of the uterus or vagina as Gartner's duct.

Lymphatic System

Lymphatic drainage is into the lateral aortic lymph nodes near the kidney, which represents the level of the embryologic origin of the ovary. On the left side, primary nodes may be situated between the left ovarian and left renal veins. On the right side they may be found between the right renal vein and the inferior vena cava. Shorter lymphatic pathways may also lead to the hypogastric nodes (Fig. 2.4).

Eichner has made a significant contribution to an understanding of the lymphatic system by injecting sky blue dye directly into the ovary and then studying its flow. He also ligated channels at different levels and studied the drainage into anastomotic lymphatic channels. On injecting the ovary with dye, Eichner observed that normal unobstructive ovarian lymphatics drain through the mesovarian and infundibulopelvic ligaments and then follow the ovarian vessels cephalad.

The various primary pathways were serially ligated to show how lymph might drain if these routes were obstructed by disease. When the infundibulopelvic ligament was ligated, a new pattern of flow developed. The forward progress stopped at the ligature and spread mesially to the fallopian tube, then by way of the uteroovarian ligament. It then descended the posterolateral subserosal aspect of the uterosacral ligaments, where it crossed the midline, involved the rectosigmoid at its peritoneal reflection, and encircled the bowel. Although Eichner reported some spread toward the midline on the uterine corpus, none of the dye crossed the midline.

After both the infundibulopelvic and uteroovarian ligaments were obstructed surgically, the dye spread through the broad ligament to

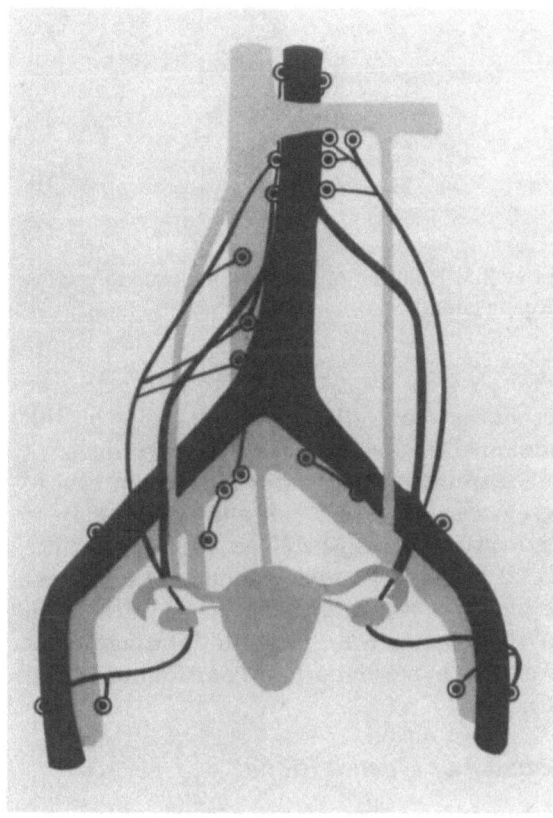

FIGURE 2.4. Lymphatic drainage of the ovaries. The dark vessels indicate the arterial system and the light vessels the venous system.

Plentl and Friedman summarized the accumulated data on the intrinsic as well as the extrinsic lymphatic supply of the ovary. They reported that the parenchymal lymphatics of the ovary comprise a rich network, and that their origin is irregular and mutable, paralleling the cyclic histologic changes of this organ. The tunica albuginea is essentially devoid of lymphatics. The cortex, particularly in the vicinity of the developing follicle, demonstrates a lymphatic network and appears to be dependent on theca externa cellular activity. The lymphatic network in the vascularis and the medulla formed small collecting tubes that converge on the hilus without apparent relation to the blood vessels.

Plentl and Friedman also reported that the lymph from the ovary is drained peripherally by six to eight large collecting chains that leave the ovary by way of the hilus to form the subovarian plexus. Efferent vessels from this plexus drain in a cephalad direction, passing through the infundibulopelvic fold along with the ovarian vessels to the lateral periaortic lymph nodes. On the left side, primary nodes may be situated between the left ovarian and left renal veins. On the right side, they may be found between the right renal vein and the inferior vena cava. Shorter lymphatics may also lead to the hypogastric nodes.

Eichner stated that he was not able to force dye from an ovarian injection into the endometrium. Serosal and superficial myometrial stain could be made at will by forcing the dye, but he failed to produce deeper penetration. He also stated that similar attempts to force extension of endocervical injection into the endometrium, or of endometrial injections to the cervix, were unsuccessful.

The spread to retroperitoneal lymph nodes takes place by three routes of lymphatic drainage. The tunica albuginea of the ovary is probably devoid of lymphatics, but the parenchyme is enriched with a dense lymphatic network. Lymphatic capillaries and vessels of the parenchyme converge on the hilus of the ovary to form the subovarian lymphatic plexus. From here the main route continues by a group of six to eight large collecting trunks that ascend bilaterally along the ovarian blood vessels and

the round ligament or into the depths of the vessels. The ureteral adventitia was occasionally stained by the latter route. This observation is interesting. In a study of palliative therapy of advanced ovarian cancer in 67 women at Memorial Hospital, Lewis found that the clinical problem requiring admission for therapy among five patients was related to the genitourinary tract. Three of the patients were admitted for symptomatic obstruction of one ureter, and in two others the indication for admission was hemorrhagic cystitis with urinary retention due to clots.

Among patients in whom both the uteroovarian and infundibulopelvic ligaments were ligated, the obturator and hypogastric nodes as well as the peritoneal reflection of the rectosigmoid and the roots of the uterosacral ligaments were always stained.

terminate in the paraaortic group of lymph
nodes between the bifurcation of the aorta and
the renal arteries. In fewer than half of women
there is a second route, the accessory efferent
lymphatic trunks, which cross within the broad
ligament toward the lateral and posterior pelvic wall and terminate in the upper most external iliac and hypogastric nodes. From here the
lymph drains along the external, internal, and
common iliac vessels into the paraaortic region. The third group of efferent lymphatic
drainage from the ovaries that has been
demonstrated experimentally in humans runs
along the round ligament and drains into the
external iliac and inguinal group of lymph
nodes. Drainage by this route seems to occur
infrequently and accounts for the rare but significant incidence of ovarian carcinoma that
metastasizes into the inguinal nodes.

Embryology

Functionally, the urogenital system can be divided into two entirely different components:
(1) the urinary system, which excretes waste
products and excess water by means of an intri-
cate tubular system in the kidneys; and (2) the
genital system, which ensured continuation of
the human race by producing germ cells.

Because the urinary and genital systems are
so closely related anatomically, and more particularly embryologically, it is difficult to study
one and not the other. Both develop from a
common ridge formed by proliferation of

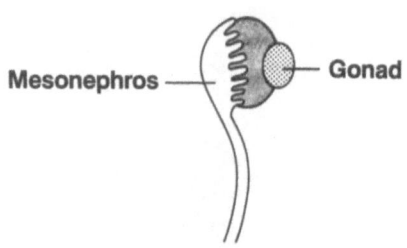

FIGURE 2.5. Relation of the mesonephros to the developing gonad.

mesoderm along the posterior wall of the
abdominal cavity, and the excretory ducts of
both systems initially enter a common cavity,
the cloaca. However, only the embryology of
the ovary and testis will be considered here
(Fig. 2.5). During the development of both excretory and reproductive organs, mesoderm
plays the major role, but entoderm and ectoderm also make important contributions (Fig.
2.6).

Gonadal or Genital Ridge

Initially, the gonads appear as a pair of longitudinal ridges (gonadal or genital ridges), located
on each side of the midline along the posterior
wall of the embryo between the mesonephros
and distal mesentery. They are formed by a
proliferation of the coelomic epithelium and
condensation of the underlying mesenchyme.
There are no germ cells in the gonadal ridge
until the sixth week of development (Fig. 2.7).

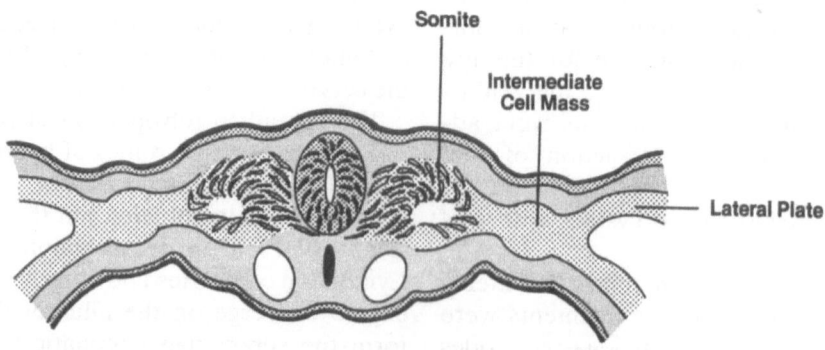

FIGURE 2.6. Cross section of the embryo (adapted from chick embryo) showing
the position of the intermediate cell mass (nephrotome) between the somite
and the lateral plate.

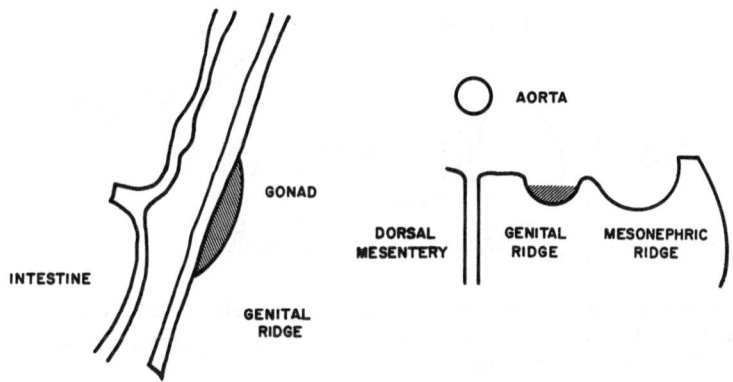

FIGURE 2.7. Genital or gonadal ridges. (From Barber HRK: Embryology of the gonad with reference to special tumors of the ovary and testis. *J Pediatr Surg* 23:967, 1988, with permission.)

Primordial Germ Cells

In mammalian and human embryos, the primitive germ cells appear at an early stage of development (human embryo, 21 days) among the endodermal cells in the wall of the yolk sac close to the allantois. Primitive germ cells migrate by ameboid movement along the dorsal mesentery of the hindgut. The route of the migrating germ cells is called the *keimbahn*. By the sixth week of development, the primitive germ cells enter the gonadal ridges. They are located jointly in the coelomic epithelium and partly in the underlying mesenchyme. It is accepted that the primitive germ cells have an inductive influence on the development of the gonad, as their failure to reach the gonadal ridge results in a lack of development of the gonad. Germ cells never persist outside the genital ridge (Fig. 2.8).

Indifferent Gonad

During and just before the arrival of primitive germ cells in the gonadal ridges, changes occur that make it impossible to distinguish whether the gonad will be male or female in its morphology. The coelomic epithelium undergoes marked proliferation and some of the cells penetrate the underlying stroma. Continued growth of these cells produces a series of irregularly shaped cords. They are the primitive sex cords. At this stage of development, the

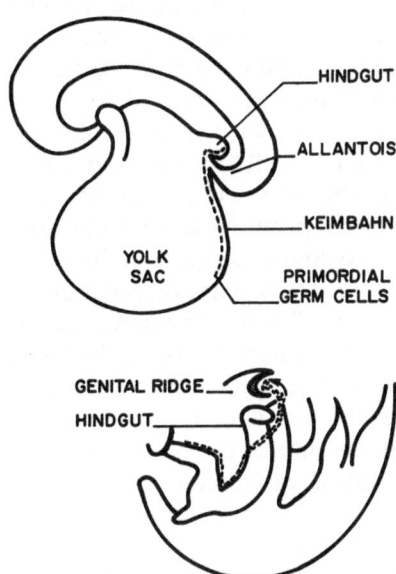

FIGURE 2.8. Primordial germ cells' migration to the genital ridge. (From Barber HRK: Embryology of the gonad with reference to special tumors of the ovary and testis. *J Pediatr Surg* 23:967, 1988, with permission.)

primitive sex cords join the coelomic surface epithelium. The connection of the primitive sex cords in the surface epithelium produces a gonad that cannot be identified as male or female; at this stage it is referred to as the "indifferent gonad." Dysgerminomas and seminomas probably arise in cells at this level of development (Fig. 2.9).

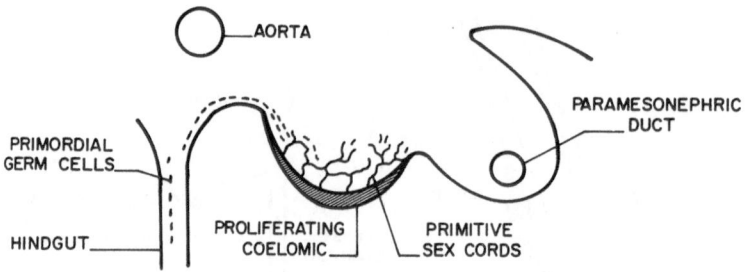

FIGURE 2.9. Indifferent gonad. (From Barber HRK: Embryology of the gonad with reference to special tumors of the ovary and testis. *J Pediatr Surg* 23:967, 1988, with permission.)

Testis

The Y chromosome influences the continued and increased development of the primitive sex cords. The cords penetrate toward the hilus of the gonad lying in the medulla. At this stage of development they are referred to as testis, or medullary cords. The cords break up into a network of tiny cell strands, and the strands give rise to the tubules of the rete testis.

In the testis, primitive testis cords are cut off from the coelomic epithelium by a layer of mesenchyme. The separation is completed by a dense layer of fibrous connective tissue called the tunica albuginea, a distinguishing feature of the testis. The epithelium on the surface of the testis flattens and disappears, which explains the absence of the development of common epithelial carcinoma in the testis. The tunica albuginea forms the capsule of the testis. There is no similar structure in the ovary.

During the fourth month of development, the testis cords are composed of primitive germ cells and sustentacular cells of Sertoli, which are derived from the surface of the gonad. These cells have an origin similar to that of follicular cells of the ovary. Sertoli cells in the fetal testis produce a nonsteroidal substance, known as müllerian inhibiting substance, which produces regression of the paramesonephric ducts.

The interstitial, or Leydig, cells develop from mesenchyme located between the testis cords and are particularly abundant from the fourth to the sixth month of development. The gonad is now identified as a testis with the capability of influencing the sexual differentiation of the fetus (Fig. 2.10).

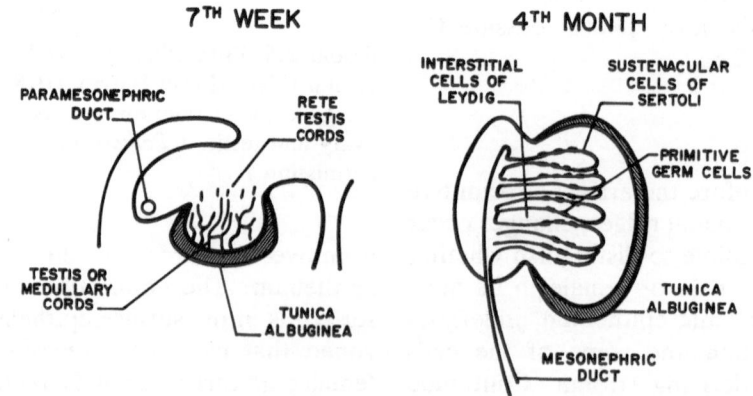

FIGURE 2.10. Testis at the seventh week and the fourth month. (From Barber HRK: Embryology of the gonad with reference to special tumors of the ovary and testis. *J Pediatr Surg* 23:967, 1988, with permission.)

7TH WEEK   4TH MONTH

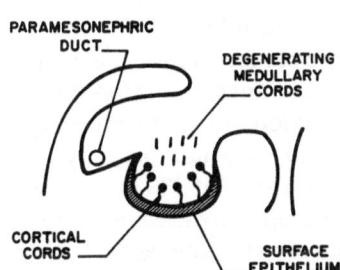
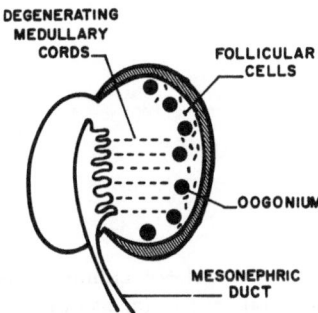

FIGURE 2.11. Ovary at the seventh week and the fourth month. (From Barber HRK: Embryology of the gonad with reference to special tumors of the ovary and testis. *J Pediatr Surg* 23:967, 1988, with permission.)

Ovary

The primitive sex cords are broken up in the female embryo, and the difference between female and male gonads begins to emerge. The sex cords in the female ovary break up into cell clusters. These clusters are located mainly in the medulla and contain groups of primitive germ cells. They disappear, and the highly vascular stroma remains. This structure is the ovarian medulla.

A significant difference begins to appear during the seventh week. The coelomic epithelium of the female continues to proliferate, but this stage does not occur in the male. The proliferation of surface epithelium in the female gives rise to a second set of cords. Because these cords are mainly in the cortex of the gonad they are referred to as cortical cords. The epithelium of the cortical cords penetrates the underlying mesenchyme but remains close to the surface. The cortical cords break up into isolated cell clusters, each surrounding one or more germ cells. This step occurs during the fourth month of differentiation. The germ cells then develop into oogonia. The surrounding epithelium arises from the surface epithelium and has an origin similar to that of sustentacular cells of Sertoli. This epithelium gives rise to the follicular cells.

The oogonia undergo mitoses with great frequency and are most numerous during the fifth month, when their estimated number is eight million plus. The oogonium becomes an oocyte when it enters into the first of two meiotic divisions. The first oocytes can be recognized at about 8 weeks and are most numerous at about the fifth month. At the time of birth no oogonia remain, and oocytes have been reduced to 2 million. By the seventh postnatal year, only about 300,000 oocytes remain (Fig. 2.11).

Embryology of the Ovary and Testis: Summary

The sex of the embryo is determined at the time of fertilization and depends on whether the spermatocyte carries an X or Y chromosome. In embryos with an XX chromosome configuration, medullary cords of the gonads regress, and the second generation of cortical cords develop. In embryos with XY chromosome complex, medullary cords develop into testis cords, and secondary cortical cords fail to develop. The tunica albuginea, a tough layer of fibrous tissue that separates the testis cords from the surface epithelium, is characteristic of the testis. Later the surface epithelium (mesothelium) completely disappears in the testis.

Descent of the Fetal Ovary to Its Adult Position

The fetal ovary is suspended to the posterior abdominal wall by a mesentery, a double layer of peritoneum containing vessels and nerves. This mesentery is attached to the upper pole of

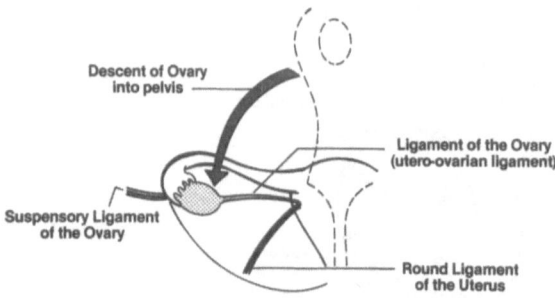

FIGURE 2.12. In females the gubernaculum forms and the gonad descends (but not as far as does the testis in males). The gubernaculum is caught up in the condensed mesenchyme that forms the wall of the uterus, and thus it is divided into two parts: the ligament of the ovary passing from the ovary to the uterus, and the round ligament of the uterus that ends in the outer genital swelling or labium majus. The ligament of the ovary shortens as the ovary takes up its adult position in the pelvis.

the gland and later becomes the infundibulopelvic fold and the mesovarium. Attached to the lower pole of the kidney is a fibromuscular cord called the gubernaculum, which is also attached to that part of the ventral body wall that eventually becomes the large labia. In the female, after the gubernaculum forms the ovary descends, but not as far as does the testis in the male. The gubernaculum is caught up in the condensed mesenchyme that forms the wall of the uterus and becomes divided into two parts: The ligament of the ovary passes from the ovary to the uterus (uteroovarian ligament), and the round ligament of the uterus ends in the outer genital swelling or labium majus. The ligament of the ovary shortens as the ovary assumes its adult position in the pelvis (Fig. 2.12).

The ovary is developed between the tenth and twelfth thoracic segments, on the posterior abdominal wall near the kidney, which accounts for its long attenuated blood supply, its venous drainage, its nerve supply from a plexus adjacent to its origin, and its lymphatic drainage into nodes lying adjacent to the renal veins.

A supernumerary ovary is one that is independent of and the same size as the normal ovary. Its occurrence is rare.

An accessory ovary is usually attached to the normal gland by peritoneal bands in the mesovarium or adjacent part of the broad ligament, near the hilum of the ovary. These structures have clinical significance if they undergo pathologic changes or when bilateral oophorectomy is carried out; their presence may result in continued ovarian activity. Accessory ovaries occur in about 3% of women.

Ectopic ovaries may be congenital or acquired, but the acquired type is much more common. Congenital displacement may be caused by nondescent of the ovary, which remains above the pelvic brim. It may also result when the ovary is pulled into the inguinal canal or labium majus by the gubernaculum. The acquired type of displacement is common and liable to occur after pregnancy, when the ovary may prolapse into the cul-de-sac.

Special Tumors of the Ovary and Testis

Teilum has presented material on the comparative pathology of special tumors of the ovary and testis as well as related extragonadal neoplasms. This study led to the concept of classifying identical tumors in the male and female.

Common epithelial tumors develop from embryonic surface epithelium, called mesothelial tissue. The types of tumor formed are serous, mucinous, endometrioid, clear cell, and Brenner cell tumors, mixed epithelial tumors, undifferentiated carcinomas, squamous cell carcinomas, and unclassified epithelial tumors.

Embryonic gonadal tissue, which is often called sex cord epithelium, gives rise to the granulosa cell tumor and the Sertoli-Leydig cell tumor. These lesions are now accurately called gonadal-stromal tumors rather than sex cord tumors. Primitive germ cells, which are present in the adult, represent the oogonia and oocytes and give rise to embryonic tumors. The most common malignant embryonic tumor is the dysgerminoma, which arises at the indifferent stage of the development of the ovary (Fig. 2.13). Extraembryonic cells, which are associated with the yolk sac, give rise to endodermal sinus tumors; and syncytial and cytotrophoblast, which make up the trophoblastic tissue, give rise to choriocarcinoma. This chorio-

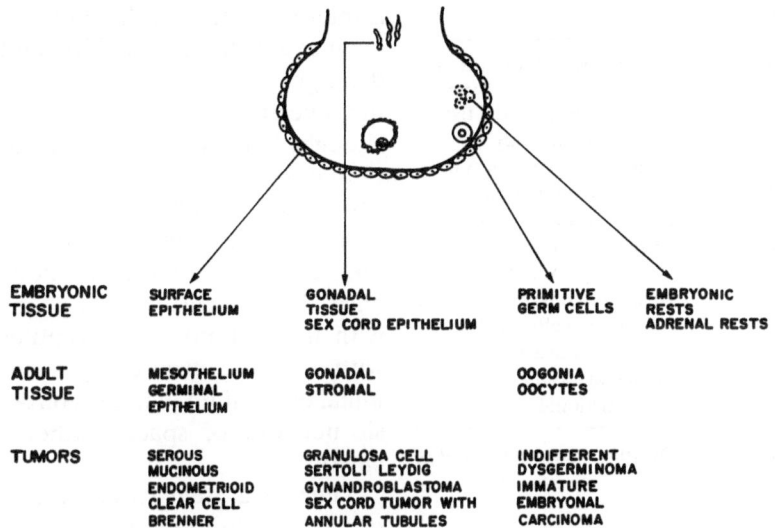

EMBRYONIC TISSUE	SURFACE EPITHELIUM	GONADAL TISSUE SEX CORD EPITHELIUM	PRIMITIVE GERM CELLS	EMBRYONIC RESTS ADRENAL RESTS
ADULT TISSUE	MESOTHELIUM GERMINAL EPITHELIUM	GONADAL STROMAL	OOGONIA OOCYTES	
TUMORS	SEROUS MUCINOUS ENDOMETRIOID CLEAR CELL BRENNER	GRANULOSA CELL SERTOLI LEYDIG GYNANDROBLASTOMA SEX CORD TUMOR WITH ANNULAR TUBULES	INDIFFERENT DYSGERMINOMA IMMATURE EMBRYONAL CARCINOMA	

FIGURE 2.13. Histogenesis of primary ovarian neoplasms. (Modified from Barber HRK: Embryology of the gonad with reference to special tumors of the ovary and testis. *J Pediatr Surg* 23:967, 1988, with permission.)

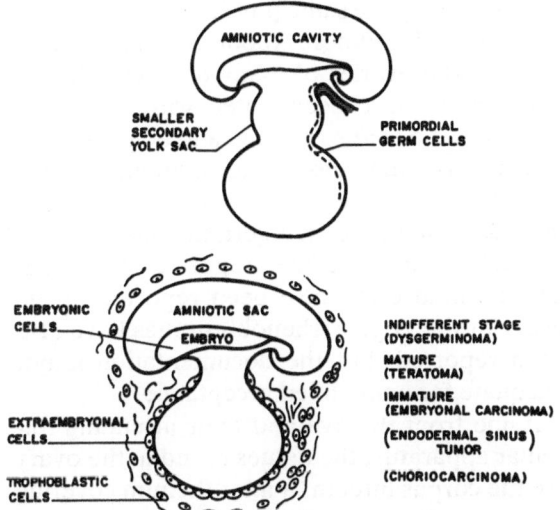

FIGURE 2.14. Extraembryonic ovarian tumor. (Modified from Barber HRK: Embryology of the gonad with reference to special tumors of the ovary and testis. *J Pediatr Surg* 23:967, 1988, with permission.)

carcinoma is a teratoma and is folic acid-independent, which differentiates it from the gestational trophoblastic choriocarcinoma (Fig. 2.14).

The ovary forms common epithelial ovarian tumors, gonadal-stromal tumors, and germ cell tumors. The testis does not form common epithelial tumors because the surface mesothelial cells disappear when the tunica albuginea forms. The testis does produce gonadal-stromal and germ cell tumors that are similar to those found in the ovary.

Phylogenic Development of the Ovary

Jones and Gilmore briefly reviewed the phylogenic development and comparative anatomy of the ovary. The phylogenic development is covered first here (Table 2.1).

One functional role of the ovary, the production of gametes, is accomplished by some of the protozoa even though they have no organ comparable to the vertebrate ovary. The protozoa can reproduce sexually, alternating with multiplication by fission. In contrast, the simplest metazoa reproduce asexually by budding as well as sexually by the union of morphologically distinct gametes (sperm and ovum). In the more complex metazoan organisms the reproductive organs become more elaborate, and the sexes as well as their gametes become more

TABLE 2.1. Ovaries in Animals

Phylogenic development	Comparative development
Protozoa genera: sexual forms and fission	Amphioxus: gonadal tissue scattered in body
Metazoan organisms: ovary becomes an identifiable organ	Lamprey: lowest form with ovary in one organ
All vertebrates: have ovaries	Higher vertebrates: not segmented; generally intraabdominal
	Birds and monotremes; left ovary develops to maturity; right ovary atrophies
	Some bats: right ovary only is functional

Reprinted with permission of the *International Journal of Fertility*.

distinct. It is in these classes of animals that the ovary becomes an identifiable organ.

All vertebrate species have ovaries and therefore have complex reproductive phenomena. Among the nonmüllerian vertebrates, most species are oviparous; and their large number of eggs, surrounded by an abundant yolk, are in many instances fertilized outside the body of the female, whose external genitalia are poorly developed. Such groups include the birds, fish, and amphibians. Others, such as reptiles, are ovoviviparous; their eggs are covered with a protective shell, have abundant yolk, but the larva still hatch inside the body of the female. Most mammals, on the other hand, are viviparous; they produce fewer ova with scant yolk, fertilization and fetal development occur inside the body of the female, and the external genitalia are well developed. These general characteristics of reproduction through the phylogenic schema of animal life are associated with and perhaps dependent on specialized anatomic features of the ovary.

Comparative Anatomy

Jones and Gilmore have reported that the amphioxus has gonadal tissue distributed in various tissues of its body, and the lowest form in which the ovary is concentrated in one organ is the lamprey. In higher vertebrates the gonads are not segmented and are intraabdominal. It is interesting that in the bird the left ovary and oviduct develop to maturity, and the organs on the right side atrophy, whereas in some bats the reverse is true. Among birds that live long enough, adenocarcinoma of the ovary similar to that found in man is not uncommon. Lower vertebrates generally produce many ova surrounded by an abundant yolk sac, and hence their ovaries are large and nodular in appearance. The ovaries of most mammals have ova with little or no yolk. Reptiles have ovaries with a large central cavity surrounded by germinal epithelium, whereas birds have an intrinsic network of spaces rather than a central cavity.

There is a great variation in size among the ovaries of different animals. The ovary of a whale may reach 40 cm in length and weigh more than 1500 g, whereas a shrew may have an ovary that is less than a millimeter in maximum dimension. Despite this great difference, the ovary in each has similar histologic features and essentially the same physiology.

Jones and Gilmore reported that tumors occur in the ovaries of many animals. Granulosa tumors have been noted with some frequency in the ovaries of cows and dogs. Adenocarcinomas and cystadenocarcinomas have been found in birds—and not infrequently if they live a long life. Dysgerminomas and Sertoli cell tumors have been reported in the dog, and dermoid cysts have been reported in the ovary of the dog. Arrhenoblastomas have also been reported, but the documentation is not adequate for unqualified acceptance.

Aside from the ova and their attending follicular apparatus, the tissues found in the ovary are the corpus luteum, a mesothelium covering the external surface of the ovary, and a stroma comprised of connective tissue, blood vessels, and nerves. In the human ovary the stromal matrix consists of whorls of spindle-shaped cells enmeshed in reticular fibers. The presence of a cortex and a medulla has been established in the ovaries of humans and other mammals. In the cortex a tunica albuginea is represented by a condensation of the stroma just underneath the germinal epithelium. In the medulla only loose connective tissue, elastic fibers, and smooth muscle are found.

Tumors of the Ovary in Animals

A variety of tumors are found in the ovaries of animals. Granulosa cell tumors have been found in the ovaries of a thousand dogs. In birds, adenocarcinoma and cystadenocarcinoma similar to that seen in humans has been frequently reported. Dysgerminomas have been reported in the ovaries of dogs. Dogs also have Sertoli cell tumors of the ovary that are similar to the tumor that arises in the dog's testicle. Dermoid cysts have also been reported in the canine ovary.

Histology

The histology of the ovary is described in detail in standard textbooks on gynecology. However, a resumé of significant points is appropriate here for background purposes. The histology of the ovary must be described with reference to its hormonal function. The ovary produces ova as well as important hormones, i.e., estrogen and progesterone. Because the histologic patterns of the ovary vary with sexual activity and the time of the menstrual cycle, it is not possible to give a simple description of the ovary in all its phases.

The ovary is generally divided into a cortical zone and a medulla. The cortical zone contains stroma, ova, and (depending on age) those bodies (e.g., corpora lutea, corpora albicantia) that form after the discharge or degeneration of the ovum. During reproductive life the cortex is broad and makes up one-half to two-thirds of the depth of the ovary. The stroma is composed of spindle-celled connective tissue, placed compactly. Underneath the germinal epithelium there develops with advancing age a connective tissue layer of increasing density called the tunica albuginea, containing collagenous (van Gieson-red) fibers. These fibers are almost absent from the rest of the cortical stroma, which is peculiar in that, in addition to blood vessels, lymphatics, and nerves, it shows an abundance of short and long spindle-shaped nuclei. The cell bodies to which these nuclei belong are difficult to discern in ordinary sections, and silver methods reveal reticular fibers between them. This richly nucleated stroma is characteristic of the human ovary, is established long before puberty, and remains fairly constant in its nuclear density up to old age.

The ovarian medulla contains many blood vessels, in particular spirally running arteries, lymphatics, and nerves embedded in fibrous tissue; and all of these structures are continuous at the hilum with those present in the mesovarium. Because the medulla may contain such structures as the rete ovarii and hilus cells, many look on it as primarily potentially androgenic instead of estrogenic, simlar to the cortex. In the hilus there are often remnants of certain embryonic structures, especially the rete ovarii and the parovarian tubules. The latter are of wolffian origin and appear as clusters of small lumens lined by cuboidal epithelium and surrounded by a thick muscular zone. The rete tubules are zigzagged in arrangement, lined by flat epithelium, and have no surrounding muscle tissue.

The ovary is covered by a low cuboidal epithelium called the germinal epithelium, which is modified peritoneum. It is derived from the coelomic epithelium and joins the flat serosal cells of the peritoneum at the mesovarium. The epithelium is easily detached on handling the organ and may be found in the postmenopausal ovary, although only in patches. It may be invaginated, and occasionally it penetrates the underlying stroma by tubular formations. Sometimes its cells are cubical or even flat, especially when overlying large, growing structures such as a maturing follicle or a corpus luteum.

The sympathicotropic or hilus cells are often seen in the hilus of the ovary. They are usually polyhedral or ovoid and arranged in a type of mosaic pattern. Because Reinke crystals have been found in these cells and are identical to those found in Leydig cells, a relation between these two cells has been proposed. Tumors arising from these cells have produced a virilizing effect similar to that found with the Sertoli-Leydig (arrhenoblastoma) cell tumors.

The development of the follicles, the formation of a corpus luteum, the atretic follicles, and ovarian changes of pregnancy are discussed in detail in standard textbooks of gynecology.

Summary

Knowledge of the embryology and anatomy is important for understanding the clinical findings and pathologic picture accompanying an ovarian malignancy. The ovary originates at the level of the 10th to the 12th thoracic segments (T10 to T12) and migrates to the pelvis. In prepubertal girls the ovary is an abdominal structure, becoming a pelvic structure only at puberty. The origin of the ovary may offer an explanation for the gastrointestinal symptoms of ovarian cancer and may also explain its propensity to spread to the upper abdomen.

It is interesting that in the bird the left ovary and oviduct develop to maturity, and the right ovary and tube atrophy. In birds that live long enough, an adenocarcinoma similar to that seen in man is not an uncommon finding.

Bibliography

Barber HRK: Embryology of the gonad with reference to special tumors of the ovary and testis. *J Pediatr Surg* 23:967, 1988.

Barber HRK: The ovary—then and now. *Int J Fertil* 34(3):173, 1989.

Dodds GS: *The Essentials of Human Embryology.* 3rd Ed. Wiley, New York, 1947.

Eichner E: In vivo studies on the pelvis lymphatics in women. Meigs, JV and Sturgis, S (eds): *Progress in Gynecology.* Vol. 3. Grune & Stratton, Orlando, FL, 1957.

Fuks A: Patterns of spread of ovarian carcinoma: relation to therapeutic strategies. In Newman CE, Ford CHJ, Jordan JA (eds): *Ovarian Cancer.* Pergamon Press, New York, 1980, p. 39.

Griffith CT: The ovary. In Kistner RW (ed): *Gynecology. Principles and Practice.* 2nd Ed. Year Book, Chicago, 1975, p. 323.

Haines RW, Mohinddin A: *Handbook of Human Embryology.* 3rd Ed. Williams & Wilkins, Baltimore, 1965.

Jacoby F: *Gynecological and Obstetrical Anatomy.* Edward Arnold, London, 1948.

Jost A, Vigier B, Prepin J, Perchellet JP: Studies in sex differentiation in mammals. *Rec Prog Horm Res* 29:1, 1973.

Jones TC, Gilmore CE: The ovaries in animals. In Grady HG, Smith DE (eds): *The Ovary.* International Academy of Pathology Monograph. Williams & Wilkins, Baltimore, 1963.

Langman J: *Medical Embryology.* Williams & Wilkins, Baltimore, 1963.

Lewis JL Jr: Palliative therapy of advanced ovarian cancer. *Clin Obstet Gynecol* 12:1038, 1969.

Netter FH: *The Ciba Collection of Medical Illustrations.* Vol. 2. Ciba Pharmaceutical Products, Summit, NJ, 1954.

Novak E, Jones GS, Jones HW, Jr: *Gynecology. Condensed from Novak's Textbook of Gynecology.* 9th Ed. Williams & Wilkins, Baltimore, 1975.

Novak E, Woodruff JD: *Novak's Gynecologic and Obstetric Pathology with Clinical and Endocrine Relations.* Seventh edition. Philadelphia, WB Saunders, 1974.

Plentl A, Friedman E: *Lymphatic System of the Female Genitalia: The Morphologic Basis of Oncologic Diagnosis and Therapy.* Saunders, Philadelphia, 1971.

Reiffenstuhl G: *The Lymphatics of the Female Genitalia.* Lippincott, Philadelphia, 1964.

Teilum G: *Special Tumors of Ovary and Testis and Related Extragonadal Lesions.* Copenhagen, Munksgaard, 1971, pp. 135, 327.

3

Epidemiology of Cancer of the Ovary

Etiology and epidemiology are often intertwined. Therefore an introductory discussion is devoted to these subjects.

Cancer Etiology

The goal of cancer etiology is cancer prevention. Three types of agent have now been shown to cause cancers: chemicals, radiation, and viruses. Of these agents, two—chemicals and radiation—clearly cause cancer in humans. The third, viruses, are highly suspect on the basis of present knowledge.

Cancer Epidemiology

Cancer epidemiology seeks to correlate differences in the incidence of various types of cancer with differences in the external or internal environments of persons developing these cancers. The correlation between cigarette smoking and lung cancer is an established example.

Investigations have raised some intriguing questions that call for further study. They include the sevenfold higher incidence of breast cancer and ovarian cancer among Americans compared to Japanese women; the much greater incidence of colon cancer in the United States than in certain areas of Africa; and the spotty geographic distribution of esophageal cancer throughout Africa.

So far the results of epidemiologic research strongly suggest that variations in social practices and in exposure to environmental agents are largely responsible for variations in the incidence of cancers among various groups of people. Therefore if such environmental exposures and social practices could be identified and eliminated, most cancers in man might be prevented. Because of the complexity of the relation between man and his environment and the long latent period of cancer development, the identification of particular cancer-inducing factors is difficult. There is no other area of cancer research, however, that holds more promise for cancer prevention.

The ovary is the sixth leading site of cancer in females in the United States. It accounts for about 5% of all female cancer deaths. Age-adjusted death rates for malignant neoplasms of the ovary show that the Danes have the highest rate and the Japanese the lowest. The white American female is about in the middle of the group. The urban incidence is slightly higher than that in rural areas. Studies among American Indians show that their rates are lower than those of whites and other non-Indians, but this result may be related to the lack of longevity in this group.

A number of epidemiologic factors are suspected of being linked with ovarian cancer. Among them are nulliparity, infertility, marked premenstrual tension, abnormal breast swelling, marked dysmenorrhea, increased abortion rate, early menopause, group A blood, irradiation of pelvic organs, environmental factors, industrial products such as asbestos and talc, high socioeconomic status, celibacy, breast cancer, and resistance to mumps parotitis.

There are 15 major demographic leads.

1. Ovarian cancer, particularly in postmenopausal women, is less common in Japan
   than in the Western world. Compared with
   caucasian women, Oriental women, who
   have a low incidence of breast and ovarian
   cancer, have a high estriol titer between
   ages 15 and 19. It has been accepted that
   estriol acts as an antagonist of carcinogenic
   activity of estradiol-estrone. As each
   group moves toward age 40, the difference
   decreases until it is negligible. Because
   there is little difference at the time that
   cancer in these organs begins to develop, it
   must be concluded that estriol was protecting the immature cell.
2. Ovarian cancer occurs more commonly
   among first-generation Japanese women in
   the United States than in women in Japan.
3. The incidence of ovarian cancer has increased not only in the Western world;
   there has also been some increase in
   Japan.
4. Cancer of the ovary tends to be somewhat
   more common in upper than in lower in-
   come groups in the West.
5. Ovarian cancer in New York City is more
   common among Jews than other religious
   groups, particularly among postmenopausal women.
6. There is a positive correlation between the
   incidence pattern of ovarian, mammary,
   and endometrial cancers.
7. In several studies ovarian cancer is more
   commonly reported among single and nulliparous women.
8. There is a greater incidence of ovarian cancer in the highly industrialized nations.
9. Much of this variation cannot be
   accounted for by racial or genetic differences: Migrants from one country to
   another rapidly acquire rates of ovarian
   cancer prevalent in the country of adop-
   tion; that is, second-generation Chinese
   living in the United States have ovarian
   cancer mortality rates similar to those of
   whites in the United States, whereas first-
   generation Chinese have considerably
   lower rates.

10. It is suggested that some environmental or
    behavioral factor accounted for the inter-
    national variation in ovarian cancer inci-
    dence; that is, life style.
11. The difference in the average size family
    from one country to another may offer a
    reasonable explanation for the difference
    in the incidence of ovarian cancer.
12. Ovarian cancer is most common in profes-
    sionals and executives and least common
    among the lower socioeconomic groups.
13. Comparing Catholic women, Protestant
    women, and Jewish women, it was found
    that the Catholics had the lowest rate and
    the Jewish women the highest, which may
    reflect the fact that the Jewish women, on
    average, had small families and Catholic
    women large families.
14. Ovarian cancer appears to be more com-
    mon in women who had previously had a
    variety of conditions, including breast can-
    cer, endometrial cancer, obesity, gallblad-
    der disease, cervical fibroids, and Peutz-
    Jeghers syndrome.
15. The generation of women of childbearing
    age during the Depression had fewer chil-
    dren but more ovarian cancer than the
    generation of women before and that after
    the Depression.

Trends

Silverberg has shown that the death rates by
age for cancer of the ovary show a steady increase as the population at risk ages. The nonwhites have a lower rate than do the whites in
each group for ages over 30 years. Trends by
age and race since 1930 show that the rates for
all ages in white females rose slowly until the
late 1940s and have remained at the same level
until recent years, when the rates have decreased slightly. The rates for age groups over
55 in general show an increasing trend. In the
age group 30–44 there has been a decrease
since the 1950s. The rates for the nonwhite
females for all ages show the same general
trend as for whites.

Beral and colleagues reported that what is
interesting is that the downward trend in mortality at age 30–34 preceded that at age 30–39,

which in turn preceded that at age 40–44. They raised the question of whether this phenomenon may not be due to the use of the contraceptive pill by these groups. This pattern is consistent with a so-called cohort effect, that is, with different generations of women having a different risk of ovarian cancer throughout their lives. In addition, Beral et al. reported that from the United States and many other countries there is a suggestion that women born during the decade 1900 to 1910 have an especially high risk of developing ovarian cancer—higher than that of women born before or after them. There is a suggestion that this pattern can be explained by the varying average number of children born to women of each generation. Women born during 1900 to 1910 were of childbearing age during the 1930s (Depression Era) and had, on average, smaller numbers of children than their predecessors or successors. This factor might well explain their lifetime high risk of ovarian cancer. It would tend to identify the importance of the repeated stimulation of the ovary by incessant ovulation and the etiology of ovarian malignancy, that is, factors such as pregnancy that suppress ovulation may protect against ovarian cancer. Additional support for this contention is found in the reports that the increasing incidence of ovarian cancer in many Western countries has probably resulted from the decreasing average number of children born to the successive generations of women.

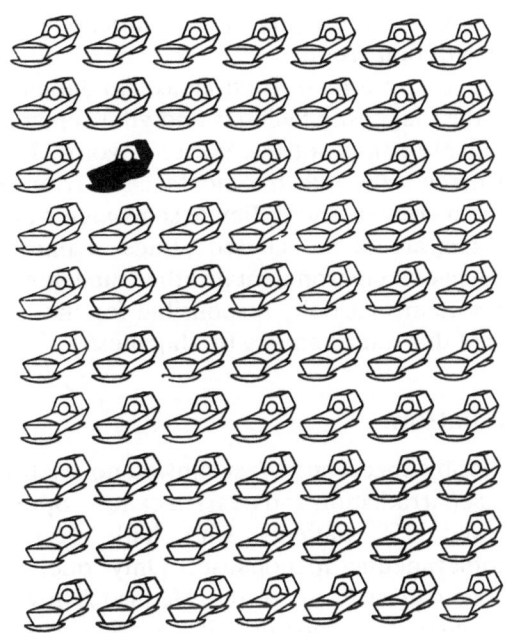

FIGURE 3.1. Third national Cancer Survey found that 1 of every 70 newborn girls (1.4%) will develop ovarian cancer.

Evidence of Incidence

Estimates of the incidence of cancer show that cancer of the ovary is the sixth leading cancer in women. About 1 of every 70 newborn girls (1.4%) develop cancer of the ovary during their lives. The incidence rates are reported in greater detail in Chapter 1 (Fig. 1.1).

It is still questionable whether the observations on the incidence pattern of various cancers are valid. Cancer of the ovary is an inaccessible cancer that is difficult to diagnose. Confirmation of the presence of the disease almost always requires surgery and expert pathologic interpretation. Part of the increase of ovarian cancer in the United States may be attributable to improved diagnostic facilities and increased awareness of the disease. However, when the increases in population and in the age of the population are taken into account, there is still an increase in incidence that has not been explained.

Ovarian cancer appears to be diagnosed more often in individuals for whom better medical care is available, and data on this factor from specific hospitals must therefore be cautiously evaluated in respect to socioeconomic status as well as educational level. For socioeconomic and educational distributions, the vital statistics of a city or a national population are more meaningful than those of any individual hospital.

The incidence among single women is difficult to evaluate, but the effects of other demographic factors have been ascertained. Studies of the death rate in New York City suggest that ovarian cancer is somewhat more common among Jewish women. The data suggest that the disproportionate number of Jewish women with cancer of the ovary may be the result of increased susceptibility in postmenopausal women of that group.

The low rate of ovarian cancer in Japan is real, the diagnostic facilities and vital statistics are equal to those of the Western world. It is also noteworthy that the incidence of ovarian cancer increases among Japanese women when they migrate to the United States, a finding that suggests environmental rather than genetic factors are partially responsible for the low rates of this cancer among the Japanese.

Irradiation

Studies by Speert and West showed no relation between irradiation and ovarian cancer. Speert followed 958 patients who had received radiotherapeutic menopause: Only one developed cancer of the ovary. He also followed 343 consecutive patients with ovarian cancer and 247 consecutive patients with cystadenomas of the ovary. Of these 590 women, 17 had a record of previous pelvic irradiation for benign conditions. One of the variables examined by West was the milliroentgens delivered to ovaries by diagnostic and therapeutic x-irradiation. The results of his study did not warrant the conclusion that exposure to x-rays, particularly diagnostic x-rays, influences the production of ovarian malignancies. West noted that calculations were based only on whether the patient and the control had received x-irradiation over the abdomen; the question of who may have had a higher dose was not considered. On this scale there was no significant difference between the patients and the group with benign ovarian tumors.

Endocrinologic Considerations

The apparently normal endocrinologic status of the ovarian cancer patient stands out more than any marked variation from the general female population. Wynder and associates challenged this observation. However, the few marked differences that were shown by their study, particularly in menstrual history, even if real, provide less of a lead than the different rates among ethnic groups and especially the changing rates among non-Americans who have immigrated to the United States.

The ovary is complex in its embryology, histology, steroidogenesis, and potential for malignancy. It is made up of germ cells, cells of sex cord, and cells of the mesenchymal tissue. Although sex is genetically determined at fertilization, the ovary passes through its early phases as an indifferent organ with parallel development that could allow it to become a testis or an ovary. Alternations or imbalances during these steps of development may provide the setting for later mesenchymal functioning, and cell nests may give rise to a clinically dramatic picture.

Clinical leads often come from animal experimentation. Biskind and Biskind (working with rats) and Furth and Sobel (with mice) transplanted the gonads into the spleen and produced granulosa cell tumors. Although menopausal women have a similar pattern of increased excretion of pituitary gonadotropins, the malignancies formed in the human ovary are not usually the granulosa cell type.

In addition to our findings on the rarity of ovarian cancer among women in Japan and its increase among Japanese immigrants to the United States, another important epidemiologic clue comes from the facts that prostatic cancer is also increasing among Japanese immigrants and that mammary cancer appears to be increasing much more slowly. Japanese immigrants provide much data to suggest that environmental factors may affect the development of the steroid-related cancers.

Cholesterol is considered the keystone on which steroids are built. It is apparently built up from acetate, and endogenous cholesterol is the important factor for steroid synthesis. Prefabricated cholesterol is reported to play a minor role.

Bulbrook's findings in this area merit attention. Among female Japanese immigrants living in Vancouver, the more Canadian food they eat, the more similar their $5\alpha/5\beta$ testosterone ratios become to those of Canadian women. (The 5-derivatives are not androgenic; however, the 5α-derivative is potent. Indeed, dihydrotestosterone (DHT), the 5α-derivative, is probably the principal androgenic hormone formed in target tissue from testosterone. Thus testosterone has been reduced to a prehormone, the circulating precursor for DHT.

Short has suggested that a higher nutritional plane increases multiple ovulation, which in turn enhances the amount of estrogen and progesterone produced, an effect mediated through the pituitary.

The process of steroidogenesis in the adrenal, testis, and ovary is the same up to the point of formation of progesterone. At this point the three glands complete the synthesis of their steroids along individual patterns. Androstenedione and testosterone are synthesized as final steps before estrone and estradiol are produced as the main steroids of the ovary. Anything that disturbs the delicate balance of the pituitary-ovarian axis could alter the final step in the formation of estrogens and thus cause an accumulation of intermediate products in the ovary. A number of publications document that these intermediate products are not innocuous, but their exact role in the problem under discussion remains to be seen.

Dysmenorrhea, heavy menstrual flow, and relatively early onset of menopause were the only gynecologic findings in which there were any differences between study and control patients. Dysmenorrhea is a complex disorder that can be divided into two classifications. Primary dysmenorrhea is characterized by an absence of recognizable pathology and characteristically is rarely seen in the absence of ovulation. It may appear spontaneously or persist without change. Secondary dysmenorrhea is related to discernible pathology and frequently gets progressively worse, as in endometriosis.

The many theories advanced to explain the mechanism of dysmenorrhea substantiate the subtle nature of this problem. All investigators agree that a strong psychogenic factor makes it difficult to compare the severity of dysmenorrhea.

This study suggests some relation of dysmenorrhea to ovarian cancer, although the findings may be related to an artifact. Ovarian cancer patients tended to experience dysmenorrhea both before and during menstrual flow, whereas the controls were affected more often during flow. However, a considerable number of women with ovarian cancer gave no history of dysmenorrhea. We must also consider if our findings may have been influenced by

a greater awareness of gynecologic complaints among women with ovarian cancer than among those without gynecologic disease.

Certain observations by Bell and Loraine are relevant to a discussion of dysmenorrhea. Among patients with intractable dysmenorrhea, these investigators found lower estrogen excretion levels than in women without intractable dysmenorrhea. The total gonadotropin levels, however, were within the normal range for women during reproductive life. It is interesting to speculate on the significance of low estrogen excretion in the presence of dysmenorrhea.

Although there was a higher incidence of heavy vaginal bleeding among the ovarian cancer patients, the subjective interpretation associated with this finding makes it difficult to evaluate. The bleeding was of average duration.

The age of spontaneous menopause among the ovarian cancer patients is slightly earlier than in the controls and in other controls reported in the literature. Could this finding reflect an earlier reduction of estrogen production? It is important to establish the age of menopause so there is a point of reference. Speroff, Glass, and Kase report that the median age of the menopause in the United States is 51.4 years. Data published by the National Center for Health Statistics (NCHS) report the last mentioned period at 50 years, plus or minus. A further breakdown of data from the NCHS indicates that natural menopause occurred in 25% of women by age 47, in 50% by age 50, in 75% by age 52, and in 95% by age 55. The exact 50% point for age at natural menopause is 49.7 years. This study also revealed that 25 to 30% of women in the United States undergo surgical menopause.

A major point of interest is the relative incidence of ovarian cancer in Japanese and American women. Among postmenopausal Japanese women in particular, there is little ovarian cancer. Further study of this finding should include a review of the known endocrinology during the postmenopausal period. The observation in postmenopausal women, for whom there is more repeatedly confirmed evidence, is that there is estrogen hypoexcretion and excess gonadotropin excretion. Although estrogen excretion may persist in reduced amounts for a considerable time after menopause, daily vaginal smears indicate that the cyclic patterns disappear within 6 months after the last menstrual period.

Randall and coworkers have found that women experiencing normal menopause appear to have a better estrogenic status than those who have undergone oophorectomy. Oophorectomy in postmenopausal women did not alter estrogen levels, but adrenalectomy in previously oophorectomized women resulted in a rather prompt, pronounced decrease in estrogen. The reduction in urinary estrogen excretion following oophorectomy in the premenopausal woman and the further decrease after adrenalectomy establish the ovary and adrenal as the main sources of estrogen secretion.

Knobil and Reid found that gonadotropin secretion tended to be stimulated by low doses of estrogenic substances and to be suppressed by larger doses. Between ages 60 and 70 (late menopause) there is marked reduction in gonadotropin excretion, related to the length of time after menopause, and this reduction is undoubtedly a pituitary reflection of progressive generalized tissue senility. Gonadotropins in the menopausal patient are quantitatively more potent with regard to follicle-stimulating hormone than luteinizing hormone activity. There is also a diminished output of 17-ketosteroids and 17-hydroxycorticosteroids in this age group. Thyroid function decreases a little but is not reflected in the protein-bound iodine values or basal metabolism rates. However, ^{131}I uptake decreases after menopause.

Melorum and Colleagues have shown that the postmenopausal ovary appears to secrete predominantly androgens rather than estrogens. The postmenopausal ovary does not always produce estrogen per se, but it is more frequently indirectly involved in estrogen production in the adrenals by adding significant amounts of estrogen precursors, androgens, to the plasma pool.

Because ovarian cancer is bilateral in at least 50% of cases and appears to be more in the nature of simultaneous primaries than metastases, a common endocrine denominator influencing the etiology must be sought. West reported that the second variable in his study was the unusual interest in the therapeutic increase of hormone levels. Particular interest was directed during the interview toward eliciting any history of natural or synthetic hormones including estrogen, progesterone, testosterone, thyroid, adrenocorticotropic hormone (ACTH), and cortisone or its derivatives. He concluded that there is no significant difference in the use of cortisone or thyroid; and when all endocrines are considered together, significant differences are not apparent.

Oral Contraceptive Use

There is growing evidence that oral contraceptive use decreases the risk of ovarian cancer. Moreover, the longer the use of the pill, the lower the risk of ovarian cancer.

Mumps

West suggested that mumps might offer some protection against ovarian cancer. He interpreted his data in two ways: (1) Having mumps during childhood may help to protect against getting an ovarian cancer in later years. (2) Some unknown factor that gives a patient resistance against a clinically recognizable case of mumps at the same time decreases one's resistance to ovarian malignancy. In a study by Wynder, Dodo, and Barber, no meaningful difference was noted. However, it was concluded that because of the relation of the mumps virus to the gonad, this disease deserves further exploration.

Role of Stress

A considerable amount of literature has linked stress to hormonal secretion as mediated via the hypothalamus in humans and experimental animals. No precise evidence of increased stress could be deduced from marital status and occupation background in a study group by Wynder and coworkers, although these factors were not investigated in detail. The role of stress deserves further controlled study.

Double Primaries

Observations of women with multiple primary neoplasms contribute to the evidence that cancers of the ovary and breast share common etiologic determinants. Women with breast cancer have twice the risk of subsequently developing a separate primary cancer of the ovary. Death rates among patients with cancer of the ovary and breast have a positive correlation. The greater tendency for mammary cancer to be antecedent probably reflects the better chance of survival with this disease than with ovarian cancer. It has been reported that most double primary ovarian cancers involved antecedent mammary cancer. Although this point cannot be evaluated in terms of relative risks for the general population, the breast–ovary cases appear more numerous when compared with the frequency of double lesions involving ovarian and other types of cancer. During analysis it is important to consider the age distribution and the relatively poor survival of ovarian cancer patients as well as the admission practices of a hospital.

Causative Carcinogens

The search for causative carcinogens should logically be focused on the immediate environment, such as food, personal customs, or other influences that have been introduced to an affluent, pleasure-oriented American society.

Several chemical carcinogens have been shown to induce ovarian cancer in rodents, but there is no firm evidence that these substances cause cancer in women. Cancer of the ovary is not among those neoplasms reported in the few women exposed industrially to dyes, tars, soots, and other products containing anthracenes and related compounds that have resulted in cancer. Of the main industrial products known or suspected to have human carcinogenic activity, only asbestos and talc have been seriously considered as possible causes of ovarian cancer. Could these substances be introduced by means of contraceptive diaphragms that have been dusted with talc that may contain asbestos? The millions of women who have been exposed in this manner would logically produce more cancers if it were a cause-and-effect relation. Studies of women with occupational exposure indicate that the observed rate is slightly higher than the expected rate of cancer of the ovary as well as of the lung and mesotheliomas of pleura and peritoneum. Evidence linking ovarian cancer to asbestos exposure is disputed because of the few women studied and the difficulty distinguishing primary carcinoma of the ovary and peritoneal implants from mesotheliomas originating in the peritoneum.

Family History

Several reports describe families in which girls and women of the same or succeeding generation develop similar neoplasms of the ovary. Most of these neoplasms were serous carcinomas, but other types were also observed. Cancers of breast, colon, and other sites were also found in female and male members of two of these families.

Women with ovarian cancer are more likely than are controls to have relatives with ovarian cancer. Furthermore, where families with ovarian cancer have been described, the link between affected individuals has always been through the maternal line, suggesting vertical transmission. Fraumeni et al. reported on six families prone to ovarian cancer, which were mainly serous cystadenocarcinomas. Three families had concomitant aggregation of breast cancer, suggesting genetic determinants common to both tumors. The exceptional cancer risk in these families prompted prophylactic oophorectomy in 14 asymptomatic women from four families. Review of the original microscopic sections from eight women revealed that three, representing two families, had abnormalities of ovarian surface epithelium and mesothelial tissue, which may be of etiologic significance and portend neoplastic changes. To enable early detection and prevention of ovarian cancer, new diagnostic techniques and etiologic studies should be applied whenever possible to high-risk families.

The Familial Ovarian Cancer Registry has been established at the Roswell Park Memorial

Institute, New York State Department of Health in Buffalo, and is supervised by Steven Piver and Trudy R. Baker. Their *Newsletter* of April 1989 gave a registry update. The Familial Ovarian Cancer Registry established in 1981 continues to accession families that contain two or more relatives with ovarian cancer. The number of families registered is 176 and the cases 413. These physicians stated that they are made aware almost weekly of cases that require consultative counseling for proposed prophylactic oophorectomy in the family with two or more first degree relatives who have had ovarian cancer.

Their newsletter contained interesting information on genetic counseling for prophylactic oophorectomy. They stated that genetic counseling for prophylactic oophorectomy should be done at the time when the woman has completed her family but not later than age 35. This age is crucial to all women with a family history of ovarian cancer because the disease occurs most commonly in sister/sister and mother/daughter pedigrees. Sisters and daughters in families with a history of ovarian cancer have a 50% chance for developing the disease, which compares with 1.4% in women without this family history, or 1 of every 70 newborn females in the United States.

They further stated that because of this 50% risk that first-degree relatives could develop ovarian cancer genetic counseling should begin during the early twenties, and actual physical surveillance should begin during the early thirties. Physical surveillance consists in pelvic and abdominal examinations and a CA 125 assay every 6 months and pelvic ultrasonography every year.

Fucosidosis is an autosomal recessive lysosomal storage disease due to a deficiency of α-L-fucosidase activity in tissue and body fluids. The quantity of α-L-fucosidase activity in serum of humans apparently is determined by heredity. An individual may inherit low, intermediate, or high activity of α-L-fucosidase in serum. About 8% of the general population have low enzyme activity in serum. The low enzyme activity is less than 100 units of α-L-fucosidase/ml serum. Intermediate activity is 100 to 274 units/ml serum, and high activity is 275 units/ml serum.

It has been shown that females with low α-L-fucosidase activity in serum were threefold more prevalent among ovarian cancer patients than healthy females. This finding suggests that low α-L-fucosidase activity in serum of females may be a hereditary condition associated with increased risk for developing ovarian cancer. It may be concluded that investigation of the properties of α-L-fucosidase in sera of healthy females and ovarian cancer patients may contribute to an understanding of the disease process.

They also pointed out that there have been reports of women with a family history of ovarian cancer developing intraabdominal carcinomatosis, also known as extraovarian papillary carcinoma of the peritoneum, after a prophylactic oophorectomy, but this occurrence appears to be rare. Many sections of all ovaries removed prophylactically should be prepared to rule out the presence of a small, early ovarian cancer.

Blood Group

Osborne and DiGeorge have reported on the ABO blood groups and neoplastic disease of the ovary. They selected diseases of the ovary for their study of the ABO blood group because (1) the ovaries are subject to a great variety of benign and malignant neoplasms; (2) mucinous cysts of the ovary contain the ABO (H) group-specific substances in women who also secrete these substances in their saliva; and (3) carcinoma of the ovary has been reported to associate with the ABO blood group system.

In a volunteer donor control they found that the frequency of blood group O is 42.82% and that that of blood group A is 38.58%. In patients with ovarian disease the proportion of group O is 39.97% and that of group A is 44.04%. The 1.22% frequency of ovarian disease in group A relative to the 1% frequency in group O is statistically significant ($p = 0.025$). When analyzing the 19 classifications of ovarian disease, Osborne and DiGeorge observed that only six classifications (four benign and two malignant) contribute to the increased frequency of ovarian disease in women of blood group A. They are mucinous cysts, endometriosis cysts, dermoids, simple cysts, papillary adenocarcinoma, and secondary carcinoma.

The conclusions drawn from this study are that ovarian neoplasms that associate with blood group A have a glandular type of epithelium. In contrast, the ovarian diseases that do not appear to associate with blood group A are solid rather than cystic and, if of an epithelial origin, they are entirely of an ovarian type. There is one finding that, if verified, is significant: There is a four- to sixfold excess of secondary carcinomas of the ovary in women of blood group A compared to women of blood group O.

It is interesting to review the correlation between carcinoembryonic antigen (CEA) and blood group A. Scientists have been taking apart bits of the CEA molecule to find out why its activity appears to be similar to that of blood group A substance. When the CEA molecule is split enzymatically, the fractions with high CEA activity seem also to have a high level of group A activity. By breaking down the molecule chemically, a Montreal group under the direction of Gold has found a repeating unit of *n*-acetylglucosamine—a substance familiar to blood group chemists—which seems to be partly responsible for the antigenicity of CEA.

Nutrition and Cancer

The relations of nutrition, diet, and cancer can be viewed from three perspectives: (1) diet as a factor in cancer causation; (2) the effect of cancer and its treatment on nutritional status; and (3) nutritional management of the cancer patient. Various types of study (epidemiologic, animal, case control) have described a number of highly suggestive associations between diet and cancer in humans, but there is as yet no absolute proof of a direct cause-and-effect relation. The role that ingestion of food-borne carcinogens or carcinogen precursors has in causing major human cancer remains to be determined. It is likely that diet has an indirect role, modifying carcinogenesis. Several mechanisms are advanced to explain this effect. For example, it is theorized that excess dietary fat may promote carcinogenesis via its influence on altering bile acid production or gut microflora development in colon cancer and secretion of endocrine glands in breast cancer and possibly ovarian cancer. Although there is probably no specific preventive diet for cancer, it may be advisable to eat a variety of foods, adjust energy intake to energy expenditure, and avoid moldy food, deficiency of certain nutrients (i.e., vitamin A), and known dietary carcinogens (e.g., alcohol and cigarettes).

It is becoming apparent that there are dietary associations with particular cancers. Logically, much of a country's cancer risk must be attributable to diet. It is accepted that no major cancer is common everywhere in the world. More importantly, we know that high rates are rarely genetic, because migrants from one culture to another characteristically evidence a shift in cancer patterns once they have settled in the new country. An increased incidence of skin cancer has been reported among Europeans migrating to Australia due to new working habits and new sexual mores. It has been reported that migrants to the United States develop more bowel cancer, and eventually more breast, endometrial, ovarian, and prostate cancer when they come from less affluent regions where these cancers are uncommon. These cancers alone comprise more than 40% of all nonskin cancers in the United States, so priority is being given to the investigation into what environmental factors produce this high level of risk.

Ovarian cancer, breast cancer, and endometrial cancer follow bowel cancer as the most common problems in the affluent westernized populations. Environmental factors are involved because migrants from low-risk countries eventually acquire high risks in highly industrialized countries. Naturally, there is a correlation between risk for these cancers and the average consumption of dietary protein and fat.

Because cancers in each of these target organs can be produced in animals by specific carcinogens, the possibility of a dietary carcinogen or precursor certainly must be considered. On the other hand, no chemical produces ovarian, endometrial, and breast cancers in animals. An alternative possibility, for which there is no direct animal parallel, is that the same factors that produce growth and early menarche in Americans also overstimulate the endocrine target epithelium to make the ovary particularly vulnerable to cancerous change. Much work remains to be done on the correlation between nutrition and ovarian cancer.

The endometrium, ovary, and breast constitute the upper genital tract. These organs have a great deal in common and are all related to the endocrine system. Because a great deal of work has been done on mammary cancer, it is thought that it may be applicable to ovarian cancer. It has been shown that high-fat intake stimulated mammary tumor in dimethyl-benzanthracene-treated (DMBA) rats. More importantly, direct evidence obtained by radioimmune assay techniques indicated that serum prolactin titers are increased at the proestrous-estrous stages of the estrous cycle by high-fat diets. Hence the tumor-enhancing effects of high-fat intake may be mediated in part via the endocrine system by transitory elevations in serum prolactin. It has been established that estradiol at levels higher than 1 μg/ml is inhibitory to cell growth. However, the inhibitory effect of estradiol can be counteracted by high doses of prolactin. These experimental findings suggest that simulation and inhibition of growth of rat mammary tumor cells may depend on the prolactin/estrogen (P/E) ratio rather than on the absolute concentration of the individual hormones. Put in its simplest form, it is proposed that if the serum P/E ratio lies below a certain threshold, tumor growth is inhibited; if it lies above it, growth is stimulated. It has been reported that the P/E ratio may influence the adenyl cyclase system, which is known to respond to a variety of regulatory polypeptide hormones by increasing or decreasing the intracellular levels of cyclic adenosine monophosphate (AMP), a potent molecule regulating proliferation and differentiation.

It may be significant that an altered P/E ratio may induce changes in the binding capacity or the synthesis and degradation of intracellular estrogen receptors. It could also influence the rate of cell proliferation. DMBA-induced breast cancer in rats suggests that perhaps in man there may be a system where a nonhormonal agent initiates breast cancer, which is then promoted by hormonal factors. It is in-teresting to speculate on whether cholesterol in an alkylating form or as an oxide could be such an agent. One attractive aspect of this hypothesis is that it provides a physiologically meaningful explanation for the abrupt upward hook seen in cancer incidence curves when populations of pre- and postmenopausal women from Japan and United States are compared. The question must be asked whether one can hypothesize that, particularly in post-menopausal women with low estrogen titers, the prolactin-elevating effect of high-fat intake may push the P/E ratio beyond a critical threshold point, with the result that growth of a preneoplastic lesion may be enhanced. The hypothesis does suggest a plausible explanation for the finding that postmenopausal women receiving estrogen therapy have been reported to have delayed onset of breast cancer and decreased mortality when compared with un-treated controls.

Cancer of the ovary appears to be on the increase in the highly industrialized nations. However, Japan is one of the most highly in-dustrialized nations, and the incidence of ovar-ian cancer was low until just after the end of World War II, despite the fact that it had been a highly industrialized nation prior to World War II. In searching for an explanation for the increased incidence of ovarian cancer as well as that of breast and endometrial carcinoma in the Japanese, it is suggested (but not conclu-sive) that the change in the diet following World War II may offer an explanation. Prior to World War II the Japanese had a diet that was low in cholesterol. However, after the war, particularly as they became more affluent, the Japanese took on a more westernized diet and shifted from a low cholesterol diet to one that was high in fat. Obviously there were other changes in their life style, but this factor and the decrease in the size of their families stand out as areas that need further investigation.

Epidemiologic Limitations

The major epidemiologic difficulties of an ovarian cancer study relate to certain subjec-tive questions, mostly in the gynecologic area, as well as to the appropriate choice of controls.

Questions relating to menstruation—for example, a history of dysmenorrhea and the amount of menstrual bleeding—are subjective. Though this condition applies to both study subjects and controls, it could be that the patient with an ovarian cancer has a bias different from that of other comparison groups. Reliability of recall must also be considered. Where the comparison groups are concerned, benign ovarian diseases might have been chosen. Some factors may apply to all ovarian diseases, however, so they may not be appropriate controls. Patients with other hormone-related and gynecologic cancers obviously do not comprise adequate control groups. These restrictions reduce the number of available controls in a cancer hospital. When choosing controls from other hospitals, certain diseases, such as rheumatoid arthritis, particularly in the young, have an unusual epidemiologic background and therefore cannot be included. Also, when subjects are drawn from a cancer detection center they may represent a biased population because of their socioeconomic and religious background and their medical and surgical histories, particularly of gynecologic disorders. To reduce bias, data from one control group were compared with those from another before they were combined. Ideally, women from the general population should be interviewed, but it is difficult to find an appropriate group willing to answer the questions required in this study.

As Lingeman pointed out, epidemiologic evidence strongly suggests that environmental variables are major etiologic factors in ovarian cancer. The finding that the highest rates for ovarian cancer are recorded in highly industrialized countries suggests that physical or chemical products of industry are major causes of these neoplasms. A major exception is highly industrialized Japan, which has one of the lowest rates in the world. Thus the causative factors must be postulated to be more highly concentrated in the U.S. environment than in that of Japan. This higher concentration is evident from the increased rates of cancer of the ovary in Japanese migrants to the United States and their offspring.

A problem in most epidemiologic studies is the number of cases available for analysis. Although most studies are large enough to permit analysis of single variables, the modules in a study of a relatively uncommon disease are usually too small to permit an adequate crossing of variables. A large-scale relation may appear, but it is less likely that a small association can be statistically verified.

Future Studies

Future investigations into the epidemiology of ovarian cancer should interrelate the epidemiologic findings with chemical data on steroid excretion. Because the progress of the disease may alter the steroid pattern, it is worthwhile to obtain more steroid data prospectively, as Bulbrook and Hayward are now trying to do. Pathologists might also more carefully examine the adrenal and pituitary glands of patients who have died from ovarian malignancies.

Additional laboratory investigations should include routine blood cholesterol levels and glucose tolerance tests. It would be particularly interesting to conduct prospective studies to follow the incidence of ovarian cancer among women on long-term oral contraception.

Steroid excretion patterns should be explored in greater detail in women of different weights. The relation of diet to steroid formation based on the major leads provided by studies on Japanese immigrants in the United States should be studied also because an increase in the overall fat consumption in this group is paralleled by increased blood cholesterol levels, an increase of hormone-related cancers, and an increase of other diseases suspected to be related to dietary fats.

Another area that merits more detailed exploration is that of target-organ response. Certain women have a different response in each breast after the administration of either endogenous or exogenous hormones. Should no major hormone differences be determined for ethnic groups who have different rates of hormone-related cancers, the target organ response to a given hormone or its intermediary products might be explored with success. Target organ responses may be influenced by a change in diet, especially in lipid components.

Summary

Epidemiology of ovarian cancer depends primarily on accurate diagnosis. For example, a specific tumor, a specific histologic type within a single organ, may point to a particular causal factor. Epidemiologic work is handicapped, when accurate diagnosis is not possible, and Berg and Baylor have disclosed just such a situation in ovarian cancer. Nowhere is accurate diagnosis more important than with ovarian tumors. These tumors are difficult to manage and have a high mortality rate. Moreover, ovarian cancers differ from country to country, and it is from these differences that important etiologic factors may emerge. The Danes have a high incidence of ovarian cancer, whereas Japanese women in their homeland have relatively low rates. The Danes eat a high dairy product diet and therefore a high cholesterol diet, whereas the Japanese diet is low in cholesterol. Studies of nutrition and hormones among these two groups have contributed little toward finding a possible etiologic factor. The descendants of the Japanese who have moved to the United States have an increased rate of ovarian cancer, and in some reports it is higher in their offspring than in American women.

Many personal characteristics are identified with a high risk of ovarian cancer, including reproductive history, marital status, social class, and religion. Many of them are interrelated in terms of the importance of the women's reproductive history in determining her risk for ovarian cancer. It seems that married patients in low socioeconomic groups and practicing Catholics have large families, which may be an explanation for their lower incidence of ovarian cancer. It seems that pregnancy protects against ovarian cancer. The same observation has been made in animals; that is, egg-laying hens, particularly if they are made to ovulate more frequently, have exceptionally high rates of ovarian cancer, whereas broiler hens (which ovulate less frequently) have lower rates. The explanation that an increased number of ovulatory cycles in a lifetime should bring about this change is difficult to prove. However, it is known that the germinal epithelium can be invaginated at this time, becomes pinched off, and is lined within the stroma. It represents normal tissue in an abnormal position and may increase its risk for developing a neoplastic process. Casagrande et al. reported growing evidence that oral contraceptive use decreases the risk of ovarian cancer. Moreover, the longer the use of the pill, the lower is the risk of ovarian cancer.

An acceptable classification is needed for correlation of all parameters associated with ovarian cancer. Despite the lack of agreement in classification, remarkable differences between populations are evident. In one collected series the overall incidence varies from 14.4 to 3.3 per 100,000 per annum, as well as varying in tumor types. Reports suggest that Africans are affected much more commonly than others by Burkitt's lymphoma involving the ovary. They have more dysgerminomas, granulosa cell tumors, and Brenner tumors as well as embryonal rhabdomyosarcomas. The biggest obstacle when studying ovarian cancer is the lack of uniform classification and nomenclature for tumors and a comprehensive, precise definition of terms.

Wynder, Dodo, and Barber reported that ovarian cancer patients often have a long history of heavy periods, more premenstrual tension, more breast swelling, more miscarriages, and early menopause. It seems that the ovary is like a cam running off center—never completely normal.

Cancer of the ovary accounts for about 4% of all female cancers. The urban incidence rate is slightly higher than the rural rate. Studies among American Indians show lower rates than for whites and blacks.

A number of epidemiologic factors are suspected of being linked with ovarian cancer. Among them are nulliparity, infertility, endometriosis, adenocarcinoma of the endometrium, group A blood, and irradiation of pelvic organs. There are reported cases of women developing ovarian cancer whose mothers or sisters also developed this cancer.

Lingeman pointed out that epidemiologic evidence strongly suggests that environmental factors are major etiologic factors in ovarian cancer. The highest rates for ovarian cancer are recorded in highly industrialized countries, which suggests that industrial, physical, or chemical products are major causes of these neoplasms. The major exception is highly industrialized Japan, which has one of the lowest rates in the world. The causative factors must be postulated to be in higher concentrations in the U.S. environment than in that of Japan. The ovarian cancer rate in Japanese immigrants to the United States and their offspring are higher than for native Japanese. Thus search for causative carcinogens could be focused on the immediate influences that change gradually due to Americanization.

Single women have higher rates than married women. Cancer of the ovary is found in children and teenagers at a higher rate than all other gynecologic cancers including breast cancer.

Observations of women with multiple primary neoplasms contribute to the evidence that cancers of the ovary and the breast share common etiologic determinants. Women with breast cancer have twice the risk of subsequently developing a separate primary cancer of the ovary. Death rates for cancer of the ovary and breast show a positive correlation in different countries. Israeli and Parsi women with ovarian cancers share histories of late marriage and first pregnancy at older ages. The relatively high incidence of ovarian and breast carcinoma in these women contrasts with the relatively low incidence of cancer of the cervix. The rates are highest in the high socioeconomic group and lowest in the low socioeconomic group.

Bibliography

Bell ET, Loraine JA: Hormone excretion patterns in patients with dysmenorrhea. *Lancet* 2:519, 1966.

Beral V, Fraser P, Chilvers C: Does pregnancy protect against ovarian cancer? *Lancet* 1:1083, 1978.

Berg JW: Nutrition and cancer. *Semin Oncol* 3:17, 1976.

Berg JW, Baylor SM: The epidemiologic pathology of ovarian cancer. *Hum Pathol* 4:537, 1973.

Biskind MS, Biskind GR: Development of tumor in rat ovary after transplantation into the spleen. *Proc Soc Exp Biol Med* 55:176, 1944.

Buell P: Changing incidence of breast cancer in Japanese-American women. *J Natl Cancer Inst* 51:1479, 1973.

Bulbrook RD, Hayward JL: Abnormal urinary steroid excretion and subsequent breast cancer: a prospective study in the island of Guernsey. *Lancet* 1:519, 1967.

Carroll KK, Khor HT: Dietary fat in relation to tumorigenesis. *Lipids Tumors* 10:308, 1975.

Casagrande JT, Lowe EW, Pike MC, et al: "Incessant ovulation" and ovarian cancer. *Lancet* 2:170, 1979.

Cook PJ, Burkitt DP: Cancer in Africa. *Br Med Bull* 27:14, 1971.

Doll R, Muir C, Waterhouse J (eds): *Cancer Incidence in 5 Continents*. Vol. 2. International Union Against Cancer. Springer Verlag, Berlin, 1972.

Fathalla MF: Factors in the causation and incidence of ovarian cancer. *Obstet Gynecol Surv* 27:751, 1972.

Fine PEM: Analysis of family history data for evidence of non-mendelian inheritance resulting from vertical transmission. *J Med Genet* 14:399, 1977.

Fraumeni JF, Grundy GW, Creagan ET, Everson RB: Six families prone to ovarian cancer. *Cancer* 36:361, 1975.

Gold P, Freedman SO: Demonstration of tumor-specific antigens in human colonic carcinomata by immunologic tolerance and absorption techniques. *J Exp Med* 121:439, 1965.

Graham J, Graham R: Ovarian cancer and asbestos. *Environ Res* 1:115, 1967.

Haenszel W: The United States network of cancer registries. *Recent Results Cancer Res* 50:52, 1975.

Higginson J, Muir CS: Epidemiology. In Holland JF, Frei E. (eds): *Cancer Medicine*. Lea & Febiger, Philadelphia, 1973, pp. 241–306.

Hinderson WJ: Talc and carcinoma of the ovary and cervix. *J Obstet Gynaecol Br Commomu* 78:266, 1971.

Jackson SM: Ovarian dysgerminoma in three generations. *J Med Genet* 4:112, 1967.

James PD: Epidemiology of ovarian cancer. *Lancet* 1:412, 1974.

Joly DJ, Libenfeld AM, Diamond EL, Bross IDJ: An epidemiologic study of the relationship of reproductive experience to cancer of the ovary. *Am J Epidemiol* 99:190, 1974.

Keal EE: Asbestosis and abdominal neoplasms. *Lancet* 2:1211, 1960.

King H, Haenszel W: Cancer mortality among foreign and native born Chinese in the United States. *J Chronic Dis* 26:623, 1973.

Knobil E: The neuroendocrine control of the menstrual cycle. *Recent Prog Horm Res* 36:53, 1980.

Kolstad P, Beecham JC: Epidemiology of ovarian neoplasia. In: *Proceedings of the American-European Conference on the Ovary, Montreux, Switzerland.* International Congress Series No. 364. Excerpta Medica, Amsterdam, 1974, p. 56.

Leung BS, Saski GH, Leung JS: Estrogen-prolactin dependency in 7,12-dimethylbez(a)anthracene-induced tumors. *Cancer Res* 35:621, 1975.

Lewis AC, Davison BC: Familial ovarian cancer. *Lancet* 2:235, 1969.

Li FP: Familial ovarian carcinoma. *JAMA* 214:1559, 1970.

Liber AF: Ovarian cancer in mother and five daughters. *Arch Pathol* 49:280, 1950.

Lingeman CH: Etiology of cancer of the human ovary. *J. Natl Cancer Inst* 53:1603, 1974.

Lynch HT, Krush AT: Carcinoma of the breast and ovary in three families. *Surg Gynecol Obstet* 133:644, 1971.

MacMahon B, Pugh TF: *Epidemiology: Principles and Methods.* Little Brown, Boston, 1970, p. 1.

McCrann DJ, Marchant DJ, Bardawil WA: Ovarian carcinoma in three teenage siblings. *Obstet Gynecol* 43:132, 1974.

Meites J: Relation of prolactin and estrogen to mammary tumorigenesis in the rat. *J Natl Cancer Inst* 48:1217, 1972.

Meites J, Cassell E, Clark J: Estrogen inhibition of mammary tumor growth in rats, counteraction by prolactin. *Proc Soc Exp Biol Med* 13:1225, 1971.

Melorum DR, Davidson BJ, Tataryn IV, Judd HL: Changes in circulating steroids with aging in postmenopausal women. *Obstet Gynecol* 57:624, 1981.

Miller DS, Reid R.L., Cetel Ns, Rebar RW, Yen SG: Pulsatile administration of low-dose gonado-tropin-releasing hormone. *JAMA* 250(21):2937, 1983.

Molloy WB: Identical ovarian malignant disease in two sisters. *Aust NZ J Obstet Gynaecol* 10:265, 1970.

Newhouse ML: A study of the mortality of female asbestos workers. *Br J Ind Med* 29:134, 1972.

Osborne RH, DiGeorge FV: The ABO blood groups in neoplastic disease of the ovary. *Am J Hum Genet* 15:380, 1963.

Randall CL: Ovarian Conservation. In: Meigs JV ed. *Progress in Gynecology.* Vol. 4. New York, Grune and Stratton, 1963, p. 457.

Randall CL, Hall DW, Armenia CS: Pathology in the preserved ovary after unilateral oophorectomy. *Am J Obst Gynecol* 84:1233, 1962.

Silverberg E: *Statistical and Epidemiological Information on Gynecologic Cancer.* American Cancer Society Professional Education Publications, New York, 1980.

Speert H: The role of ionizing radiations in causation of ovarian tumors. *Cancer* 5:478, 1952.

Speroff L, Glass RH, Kase NG (eds): *Clinical Gynecologic Endocrinology and Infertility.* Third Edition. Baltimore/London, Williams & Wilkins, 1982.

Staszewski J: Cancer registry data versus mortality data. *Recent Results Cancer Res* 50:103, 1975.

West RO: Epidemiologic study of malignancies of the ovaries. *Cancer* 19:1001, 1966.

Wynder EL, Chan P, Cohen L, Hill P: Overview—nutrition and breast cancer; breast; diseases of the breast. *Diagn Management Res* 2(2):11, 1976.

Wynder EL, Dodo H, Barber, HRK: Epidemiology of cancer of the ovary. *Cancer* 23:352, 1969.

4

Histologic Classification of Ovarian Tumors

One of the prerequisites for comparative studies is agreement on histologic criteria for the classification of cancer types and a standardized nomenclature. All too often different terms are used for the same pathologic entity, and indeed the same term is sometimes applied to lesions of different types. It is most important to have an internationally accepted classification of tumor. A committee of the International Federation of Gynecology and Obstetrics (FIGO) formulated a classification of the common epithelial tumors of the ovary, and more recently a group of pathologists appointed by the World Health Organization (WHO) suggested a classification. WHO currently lists 19 cell types and 27 subtypes for benign and malignant primary ovarian tumors based on histogenesis. The histogenetic classification has provided a parameter by which to judge prognosis. Unfortunately, it has not been applicable to all ovarian tumors. Approximately 90% of ovarian carcinomas originate from the epithelial (mesothelial cells) surface of the ovary. These classifications are presented in this chapter.

Most histologic classifications are based primarily on morphology and histogenesis. Although it is admittedly imperfect because of the imprecision of current embryologic knowledge and the difficulty of identifying specific cell types, it has the advantages of grouping together closely related ovarian tumors, which may be mixed or difficult to distinguish from one another, and of separating neoplastic types that have a dissimilar prognosis and require different therapy.

Ovarian tumors are often composed of a combination of several types that may vary in their biologic behavior, and it is important that the diagnostic terms chosen include all the varieties encountered and indicate as accurately as possible the proportion and distribution of each.

Grading of malignant tumors (a neoplasm is named from its most differentiated portion and graded from its least differentiated part) has been widely recommended. In general, it has proved to be of prognostic value for evaluating some but not all ovarian tumors.

The ovarian stroma is specialized and may be stimulated by the growth of a variety of tumors, either benign or malignant, primary or secondary. It can assume the morphologic appearance of steroid-hormone-secreting tissue and may produce androgens, estrogens, and rarely progestogens. Therefore it is important to describe the stroma. When the stroma is endocrinologically active, it has been occasionally designated "tumors with functioning stroma." This term is not included in the present classification.

In 1961 a committee of the FIGO formulated a classification of common epithelial tumors of the ovary that was adopted in 1971. The WHO has also prepared an International Histologic Classification of Ovarian Tumors and made an effort to conform to the classification of common epithelial tumors that had been proposed by FIGO and subsequently used in publications from several large centers. Broad categories of tumors have been divided into numerous subtypes throughout the classification. This subtyping was done to stimulate the investigation of smaller and possibly distinctive groups as well as general classes. In addition to the epithelial ovarian tumors, WHO includes germ cell tumors, hormone-producing tumors (gonadal stromal), and metastatic carcinoma.

A brief outline of the WHO classification with my modifications is presented for purposes of orientation.

I. Tumors of surface epithelium of the ovary
   A. Serous
   B. Mucinous
   C. Endometrioid
   D. Clear cell
   E. Transitional cell tumors
   F. Mixed epithelial tumors
   G. Undifferentiated carcinoma
   H. Unclassified
II. Germ cell tumors
   A. Dysgerminoma
   B. Tumors in the teratoma group
      1. Extraembryonal group
      2. Embryonal teratomas, solid and cystic
      3. Adult teratomas, solid and cystic
      4. Struma ovarii
      5. Carcinoid
III. Gonadoblastoma
IV. Gonadal stromal tumors (sex cord—mesenchymal)
   A. Granulosa
   B. Sertoli-Leydig
   C. Sclerosing stromal tumor
   D. Sex cord tumors with annular tubules
V. Tumors not specific for the ovary
   A. Burkitt's
   B. Lymphoma
VI. Metastatic tumors
VII. Sarcomas

The Cancer Committee of FIGO reported that although ovarian carcinoma is a common malignant tumor it cannot be regarded as a single entity. Therapeutic statistics on ovarian cancer have limited value if attention is not paid to the histologic type of growth. Experience has shown that there is no clear correlation between clinical and histologic malignancy in ovarian tumors. This tenet holds valid for various types of neoplasm but especially for epithelial tumors, granulosa cell tumors, and virilizing tumors.

According to the FIGO recommendations on the histologic classification of ovarian tumors, cases of germ cell tumors, hormone-producing neoplasms, and metastatic carcinomas should be excluded from therapeutic statistics on ovarian epithelial tumors. The FIGO classification is presented below.

FIGO Histologic Classification of the Common Primary Epithelial Tumors of the Ovary (To Be Used from January 1, 1971)

I. Serous cystomas
   A. Serous benign cystadenomas
   B. Serous cystadenomas with proliferating activity of the epithelial cells and nuclear abnormalities but with no infiltrative destructive growth (low potential malignancy)
   C. Serous cystadenocarcinomas
II. Mucinous cystomas
   A. Mucinous benign cystadenomas
   B. Mucinous cystadenomas with proliferating activity of the epithelial cells and nuclear abnormalities but with no infiltrative destructive growth (low potential malignancy)
   C. Mucinous cystadenocarcinomas
III. Endometrioid tumors (similar to adenocarcinomas in the endometrium)
   A. Endometrioid benign cysts
   B. Endometrioid tumors with proliferating activity of the epithelial cells and nuclear abnormalities, but with no infiltrative destructive growth (low potential malignancy)
   C. Endometrioid adenocarcinomas
IV. Mesonephric tumors
   A. Benign mesonephric tumors
   B. Mesonephric tumors with proliferating activity of the epithelial cells and

nuclear abnormalities but with no in-filtrative destructive growth (low potential malignancy)

   C. Mesonephric cystadenocarcinomas

  V. Concomitant carcinoma, unclassified carcinoma (tumors that cannot be allotted to groups I to IV)

It has been proposed that cases, according to the above classification, that are tumors of low malignant potential (i.e., IB, IIB, IIIB, and IVB) are usually referred to as borderline tumors. The Cancer Committee of FIGO cannot accept this term, especially because histologically unquestionably benign tumors of papillary nature may give rise to implantation of metastases that spontaneously disappear after removal of the primary growth. Such tumors should not be included among cases of IB, IIB, IIIB, or IVB. The Cancer Committee is aware of the fact that ovarian neoplasms allotted to the group "low potential malignancy" may exhibit different biologic behavior. However, there is presently no method to subdivide these cases.

A proposed ISGYP-WHO classification of tumors of the ovary will be published with definitions, explanatory notes, and illustrations as part of the Spring WHO Classification Series.

WHO includes not only the common epithelial tumors but also the germ cell tumors, hormone-producing tumors (gonadal stromal), and metastatic carcinomas. The histologic classification of ovarian tumors proposed by WHO follows.

WHO Histologic Classification of Ovarian Tumors

  I. Common "epithelial" tumors
    A. Serous tumors
      1. Benign
        a. Cystadenoma and papillary cystadenoma
        b. Surface papilloma
        c. Adenofibroma and cystadenofibroma
      2. Borderline malignancy (carcinomas of low malignant potential)
        a. Cystadenoma and papillary cystadenoma
        b. Surface papilloma
        c. Adenofibroma and cystadenofibroma
      3. Malignant
        a. Adenocarcinoma, papillary adenocarcinoma, and papillary cystadenocarcinoma
        b. Surface papillary carcinoma
        c. Malignant adenofibroma and cystadenofibroma
    B. Mucinous tumors
      1. Benign
        a. Cystadenoma
        b. Adenofibroma and cystadenofibroma
      2. Borderline malignancy (carcinomas of low malignant potential)
        a. Cystadenoma
        b. Adenofibroma and cystadenofibroma
      3. Malignant
        a. Adenocarcinoma and cystadenocarcinoma
        b. Malignant adenofibroma and cystadenofibroma
    C. Endometrioid tumors
      1. Benign
        a. Adenoma and cystadenoma
        b. Adenofibroma and cystadenofibroma
      2. Borderline malignancy (carcinomas of low malignant potential)
        a. Adenoma and cystadenoma
        b. Adenofibroma and cystadenofibroma
      3. Malignant
        a. Carcinoma
          i. Adenocarcinoma
          ii. Adenoacanthoma
          iii. Malignant adenofibroma and cystadenofibroma
        b. Endometrioid stromal sarcomas
        c. Mesodermal (Müllerian) mixed tumors, homologous and heterologous
    D. Clear cell (mesonephroid) tumors
      1. Benign: adenofibroma

      2. Borderline malignancy (carcinomas of low malignant potential)
      3. Malignant carcinoma and adenocarcinomas
  E. Brenner tumors
      1. Benign
      2. Borderline malignancy (proliferating)
      3. Malignant
  F. Mixed epithelial tumors
      1. Benign
      2. Borderline malignancy
      3. Malignant
  G. Undifferentiated carcinoma
  H. Unclassified epithelial tumors
II. Sex cord stromal tumors
  A. Granulosa-stromal cell tumors
      1. Granulosa cell tumor
      2. Tumors in the thecoma-fibroma group
        a. Thecoma
        b. Fibroma
        c. Unclassified
  B. Androblastomas; Sertoli-Leydig cell tumors
      1. Well differentiated
        a. Tubular androblastoma; Sertoli cell tumors (tubular adenoma of Pick)
        b. Tubular androblastoma with lipid storage; Sertoli cell tumor with lipid storage (*folliculome lipidique* of Lecene)
        c. Sertoli-Leydig cell tumor (tubular adenoma with Leydig cells)
        d. Leydig cell tumor; hilus cell tumor
      2. Intermediate differentiation
      3. Poorly differentiated (sarcomatoid)
      4. With heterologous elements
  C. Gynandroblastoma
  D. Unclassified
III. Lipid (lipoid) cell tumors
IV. Germ cell tumors
  A. Dysgerminoma
  B. Endodermal sinus tumor
  C. Embryonal carcinoma

  D. Polyembryoma
  E. Choriocarcinoma
  F. Teratomas
      1. Immature
      2. Mature
        a. Solid
        b. Cystic
          i. Dermoid cyst (mature cystic teratoma)
          ii. Dermoid cyst with malignant transformation
      3. Monodermal and highly specialized
        a. Struma ovarii
        b. Carcinoid
        c. Stuma ovarii and carcinoid
        d. Others
  G. Mixed forms
V. Gonadoblastoma
  A. Pure
  B. Mixed with dysgerminoma or other forms of germ cell tumor
VI. Soft tissue tumors not specific to ovary
VII. Unclassified tumors
VIII. Secondary (metastatic) tumors
IX. Tumor-like conditions
  A. Pregnancy luteoma
  B. Hyperplasia of ovarian stroma and hyperthecosis
  C. Massive edema
  D. Solitary follicle cyst and corpus luteum cyst
  E. Multiple follicle cysts (polycystic ovaries)
  F. Multiple luteinized follicle cysts, corpora lutea, or both
  G. Endometriosis
  H. Surface-epithelial inclusion cysts (germinal inclusion cysts)
  I. Simple cysts
  J. Inflammatory lesions
  K. Parovarian cysts

Norris and Chorlton have divided the functioning ovarian tumors into five basic categories. The largest group is derived from the specialized gonadal stroma: granulosa cell tumors, thecomas, Sertoli-Leydig tumors, and Sertoli tumors. Most lipid cell tumors, regardless of the cytologic features, arise from stromal cells. Some germ cell tumors qualify as functioning ovarian tumors inasmuch as certain ones give rise to gonadotropin production, and some teratomas form tissues that have an associated endocrine effect. Rare primary epithelial tumors of the ovary have an associated endocrine effect caused by steroid production from adjacent supporting stroma. Some metastatic carcinomas do the same thing. The gonadoblastoma contains elements of both the germ cell and the gonadal stromal tumors in almost equal proportions. Included in this classification is a group of neoplasms that are not derived from germ cells or gonadal stroma and that are associated with a wide variety of paraendocrine syndromes. The classification of functioning ovarian tumors by Norris and Chorlton follows.

Norris and Chorlton Classification of Functioning Ovarian Tumors

   I. Tumors of gonadal stroma
      A. Granulosa-theca tumor
      B. Sertoli-Leydig tumor (arrhenoblastoma)
      C. Sertoli tumor (*folliculome lipidique*)
      D. Lipid cell tumors
      E. Unclassified gonadal stromal tumors
  II. Tumors with functioning stroma
      A. Brenner tumor
      B. Adenofibroma
      C. Cystadenoma
      D. Cystadenocarcinoma
      E. Metastatic carcinoma
 III. Functioning germ cell tumors
      A. Choriocarcinoma
      B. Teratomas with endocrine components
  IV. Mixed germ cell and stromal tumors
      A. Gonadoblastoma
   V. Nonendocrine tumors with endocrine effect
  VI. Tumorous hyperplasias simulating neoplasms
      A. Nodular theca-lutein hyperplasia of pregnancy
      B. Hilus cell hyperplasia

Summary

These classifications are based primarily on the microscopic characteristics of the tumors and thus reflect the nature of morphologically identifiable cell types and patterns. The definitions and discussion of the different categories of tumors are reviewed in Chapter 5.

The main problem in ovarian cancer is that of early diagnosis. At present, early diagnosis is a matter of chance rather than a scientific method. However, until such methods are available it is important to study the natural history of disease by all means available. By accumulating material from many investigators treated by a variety of methods, some progress may be achieved in salvaging additional patients.

It is obvious that the interpretation of data concerning ovarian tumors is difficult and limited by the small number from any one series. However, as the material accumulates and is reported according to stage, grade, and histologic criteria that are universally acceptable, a meaningful and profitable study will result. The acceptance and use of the clinical staging and histologic classification established by WHO and FIGO has helped compare therapeutic results among institutions around the world. It has led to a greater insight into the natural history of ovarian cancer and has resulted in a more rational approach to therapy with anticipated improved results.

Bibliography

Barber HRK, Sommers SC, Snyder R, Kwon T: Histologic and nuclear grading and stromal reactions as indices for prognosis in ovarian cancer. *Am J Obstet Gynecol* 121:795, 1975.

Cancer Committee of the General Assembly of International Federation of Obstetrics and Gynecology. *International Histologic Classification of Tumors Int J Gynecol Obstet* 9:172, 1971.

Jimerson GK: Germ cell tumors of the ovary: the role of pathology in diagnosis and management. *Clin Obstet Gynecol* 17:229, 1974.

Norris HJ, Chorlton J: Functioning tumors of the ovary. *Clin Obstet Gynecol* 17:189, 1974.

Santesson L, Kottmeier HL: General classification

of ovarian tumors. In Gentil F, Junqueira AC (eds): *Ovarian Cancer. U.I.C.C. Monograph Series.* Vol. 2. Springer-Verlag, Berlin, 1968.

Santesson L: Cited by Kraus FT: *Gynecologic Pathology.* Mosby, St. Louis, 1967.

Scully RE: Recent progress in ovarian cancer. *Cancer* 1:73, 1970.

Seerov SF, Scully RE, Sobin LH: Histologic typing of ovarian tumors. In: *International Histological Classification of Tumors, No. 9.* WHO, Geneva, 1974.

Teilum G: Classification of endodermal sinus tumor (mesoblastoma vitellinum) and so-called "embryonal carcinoma" of the ovary. *Acta Pathol Microbiol Scand* 64:407, 1965.

Woodruff JD: Pathophysiology of the ovary. *Clin Obstet Gynecol* 17:169, 1974.

5

Histologic Typing of Ovarian Tumors: Definitions and Discussion

Common Epithelial Ovarian Tumors

The word *common* has been used to describe certain epithelial ovarian tumors because approximately 75 to 80% of ovarian tumors belong in this general category. They arise from the basic germinal epithelium or mesothelium on the surface of the ovary and can be designated mesotheliomas with varying amounts and activities of the gonadal mesenchyme. The latter is known as the ovarian stroma and contains two elements: the potentially functioning element, or theca, and the supporting connective tissue. Thus all ovarian tumors are potentially hormone producing.

The common epithelial ovarian tumors have often been referred to as epithelial-stromal tumors. The explanation is that there are invaginations of the germinal epithelium into the ovarian stoma during adult life, which may be produced by heterotropic alteration of one or more diverse epithelia of the paramesonephric system. These invaginations represent the earliest developmental stage of the simple serous tumors of the ovary. They may also play a part in the development of the other common epithelial ovarian tumors. These epithelial tumors are thought to arise consequent to penetration of the surface epithelium into the underlying stroma to form inclusion glands or cysts, and there is currently support for the belief that repeated or incessant ovulation is an important etiologic factor in the propensity of cells in this epithelium to undergo malignant change.

Between the obviously benign and the obviously malignant there is a common epithelial tumor that is termed a tumor of borderline malignancy or a carcinoma of low malignant potential. No matter how abnormal the epithelium appears, unless it invades the stroma the tumor must be classified as low malignant potential (borderline). The assessment of stromal invasion in serous tumors is usually easy, but the diagnosis in mucinous tumors may present some difficulty. The mucinous tumors are multilocular and parvilocular, and it is difficult to determine if these outpouchings represent invasion. The outpouchings may be pinched off and appear to be islands of tumor in the stroma, and as such they compound the difficulty of making an accurate diagnosis. Differential diagnostic criteria have been proposed that appear to be more reliable than determination of the presence or absence of invasion alone; if there is unquestionable invasion, the tumor is classified as carcinoma. Benign, borderline, and malignant forms of any of the neoplastic types listed below may coexist in any one tumor. An absolute requirement for the diagnosis of an ovarian epithelial carcinoma of low malignant potential is the lack of destructive invasion of the underlying stroma.

Tumors of borderline malignancy occasionally implant on the peritoneum; and although such implants may be invasive, distant metastases are rare. The diagnosis must be morphologically objective, and to have prognostic significance it must be based exclusively on an examination of the ovarian tumor with-

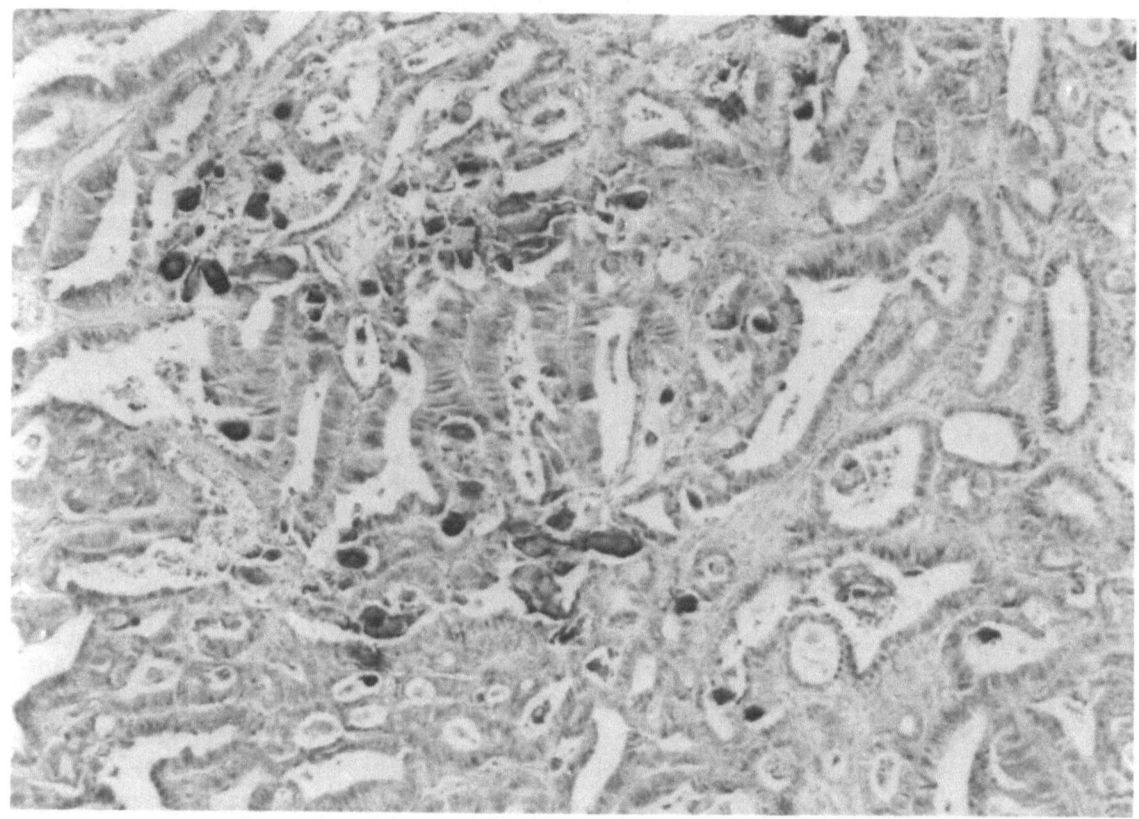

FIGURE 5.1. Serous tumors are composed of epithelium resembling that of the fallopian tube or the surface epithelium of the ovary. Psammoma bodies may be present but do not by themselves indicate malignancy. The tumors cells may produce considerable mucin, which is almost entirely extracellular. They may be unilocular or multilocular.

out consideration of whether spread beyond the ovary has taken place.

The descriptive prefixes *adeno-* and *cystadeno-* and the adjective *papillary* should be added to the more specific designation of a tumor whenever appropriate. The suffix *-fibroma* should be used when a tumor, with the exception of the Brenner tumor, is composed predominantly of stroma derived from the ovarian stroma. If the neoplastic epithelium is growing primarily on the peritoneal surface of the ovary, the word *surface* is an appropriate addition to the diagnostic term. The adjective indicating the epithelial cell type should generally be placed first among the descriptive words.

Serous Tumors

The epithelial cells of the serous tumors resemble to varying degrees those of the fallopian tube. Papillae, ciliated cells, and psammoma bodies are commonly encountered. Ciliated cells are rarely found in the invasive serous carcinomas. The tumors may form mucin, which is extracellular. Psammoma bodies may be present, at times in great perfusion, but they do not by themselves indicate malignancy nor are they always associated with ovarian tumors. Kolstad has reported that the occurrence of so-called psammoma bodies or calcifications in the tumor seem to reflect a specific tumor–host reaction and are seen more frequently in the

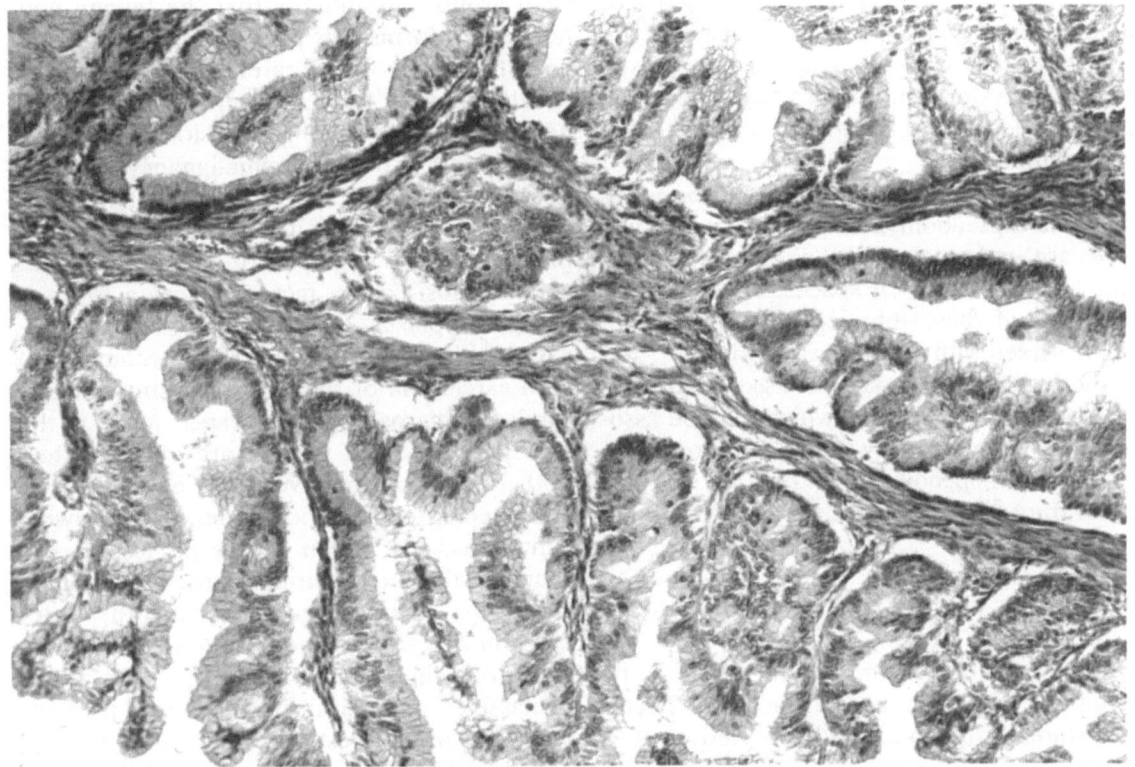

FIGURE 5.2. Mucinous tumors may be unilocular or multilocular. They are lined by tall columnar epithelium resembling that of the cervix or large intestine. Microscopically, the tumor has an outer fibrous capsule from which extend septa supporting the walls of the cyst. The walls are lined by tall columnar epithelium with basal nuclei and contain a gelatinous glycoprotein or mucin. Malignancy in a mucinous cyst is characterized by the formation of areas of solid carcinoma in the wall. The cells are columnar, show mitoses, and tend to form glandular structures.

younger age groups. These authors also reported an increased survival rate in the presence of psammoma bodies.

Julian and Woodruff have indicated there is a borderline low-grade type of papillary malignancy characterized by excessive papillary growth and a tendency to implant on the peritoneal surfaces with the production of ascites, although the lesion would still have to be called histologically benign. They spoke of this lesion as a grade 0 papillary serous cystadenocarcinoma, which is characterized by infrequent mitoses and a remarkably high salvage rate. Salvage decreases as the mitosis count increases (Fig. 5.1).

Mucinous Tumors

The epithelium may resemble endocervical or enteric epithelium and occasionally contains argentaffin cells and Paneth cells. This point raises the question of whether these tumors should be classified with the teratomas. The epithelial elements include prominent components of mucin-filled cells (Fig. 5.2).

Mucinous tumors have been identified as germ cell tumors by some pathologists, as 20% have gastric or intestinal rather than endocervical type of epithelium and 5% are associated with dermoid cysts. Fenoglio et al. concluded, after ultrastructural studies, that the presence of an intestinal type of epithelium in some of the mucinous tumors reflects metaplasia of the surface epithelium as it undergoes neoplastic change. Therefore mucinous tumors continue to be included as part of the common epithelial ovarian tumors.

An unusual variant of the mucinous cystadenoma is pseudomyxoma ovarii. In this type there are extremely thin connective tissue septa between the cystic spaces. There is often disruption of these thin septa with fusion of the cysts filled with mucinous material.

Mucinous tumors may be associated with pseudomyxoma peritonei, which may be associated with a malignancy of the ovary or a mucocele of the appendix. When both are present, the ovarian mass is recorded as the primary tumor.

Endometrioid Tumors

The endometrioid tumor was first described by Sampson. Santesson and Long, and Taylor have studied this tumor and reported on it in detail.

Tumors of the endometrioid group have the microscopic features of one or more of the typical forms of endometrial neoplasm. Some of the endometrioid tumors have been shown to have arisen in endometriosis, but the demonstration of such an origin is not required for the diagnosis.

The histologic criteria used by Long and Taylor to differentiate endometrioid tumors from serous cystadenocarcinomas are as follows: (1) The cellular arrangement is glandular or acinar with varying resemblance to primary endometrial carcinoma, depending on the differentiation of the tumor. (2) Papillae, when present, should be blunt, in contrast to the finer branching papillae of serous tumors. (3) The growing border of the tumor should be even, without the papillary projections of serous tumors. (4) Squamous metaplasia may be present. (5) With differential staining techniques, glycoprotein and nonspecific mucin can be distinguished in the apical regions of the epithelial cell, and abundant extracellular mucin can be seen (Fig. 5.3).

One of the unusual aspects of the endomet-

rioid group of tumors is that the benign and borderline forms are uncommon. Benign endometrioid tumors are rarely encountered and usually take the form of an endometrioid adenofibroma, whereas only occasional endometrioid tumors of borderline malignancy occur. A possible supplement to this apparent rarity of the benign endometrioid neoplasm is the possibility that some examples of apparent ovarian endometriosis do in fact represent a form of benign neoplasia.

One third of these tumors are accompanied by a carcinoma of the endometrium, which is similar in microscopic appearance. Many of the associated uterine tumors are small. When both organs are involved, the evidence suggests separate primaries under the following conditions: (1) When dysplastic lesions are found in the endometrium containing a small carcinoma, the implication is that the latter arose in situ and was not a metastasis from an accompanying ovarian cancer. (2) The lesion is classified as ovarian if the patient presents with clinical manifestations of ovarian cancer, and it is classified as endometrial if the symptoms first relate to the uterus. (3) When the endometrial cancer is less than 2 cm in diameter, well differentiated, and no more than minimally invades the myometrium, it is practically certain that the accompanying ovarian tumor is primary. (4) When the uterine cancer is larger than 2 cm, poorly differentiated, grade III, and more invasive into the myometrium, there is a strong possibility that the ovarian cancer represents a metastasis. (5) Endometrioid cancers of the ovary may have a markedly papillary pattern, which is unusual for carcinomas of the endometrium (Fig. 5.4).

Clear-Cell Tumors (Mesonephroid)

Clear-cell tumors are composed of clear cells containing glycogen and resembling those of renal cell carcinoma (Fig. 5.5). They are large epithelial cells with abundant clear cytoplasm. The cells may be arranged in sheets or cords. The hobnail or peg-shaped cell is considered characteristic of the tumor. The cell is characterized by scant cytoplasm and large nuclei that project into the lumen. The hobnail cell is

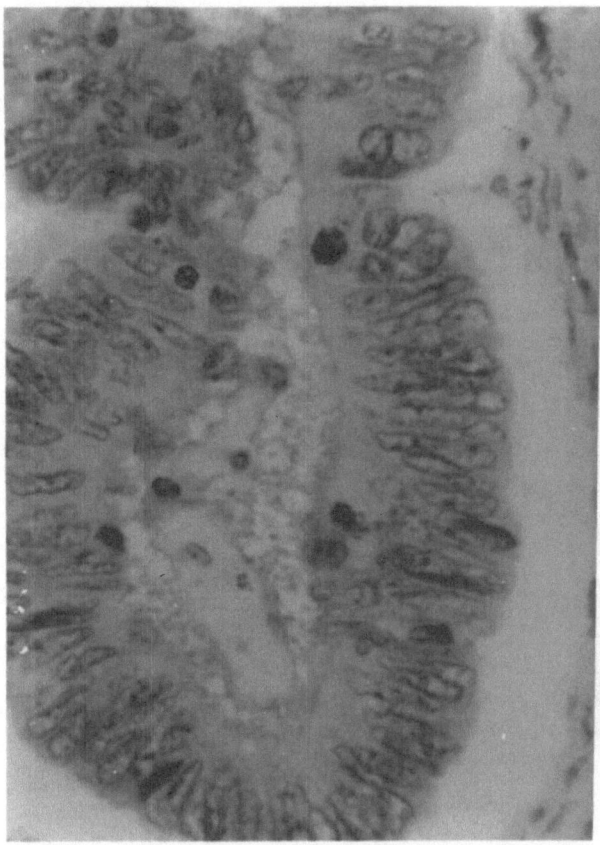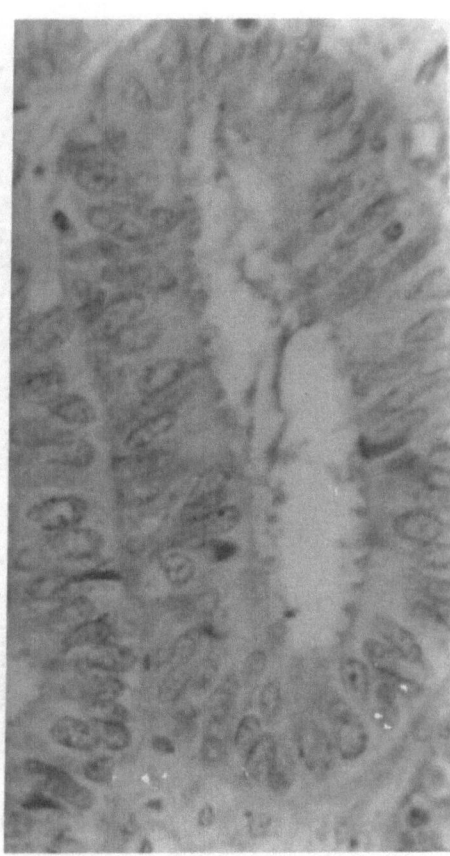

FIGURE 5.3. Endometrioid tumors have the microscopic features of one or more of the typical forms of endometrial neoplasia. They may be adenoacanthomas. These tumors arise in endometriosis, but the demonstration is not required for the diagnosis. Endometrioid carcinomas may have a marked papillary pattern, which is unusual in carcinomas of the endometrium.

a clear cell that may have discharged its contents into a lumen. Mucus may be secreted by neoplastic cells but does not accumulate in their cytoplasm.

Clear-cell tumors of the ovary were at one time considered to be of mesonephric or mesometanephric origin or at least to differentiate in the direction of mesonephric or metanephric derivatives, but now these neoplasms are generally considered to be of müllerian type—and in the genital tract of müllerian origin. The evidence for the modern view of their histogenesis is abundant. Clear-cell-type ovarian carcinomas are often admixed with endometrioid carcinomas and are associated with pelvic and ovarian endometriosis significantly more often than are ovarian carcinomas of any other type, even including the endometrioid carcinoma. A number of examples of clear cell carcinoma have been reported to arise from the epithelium of an endometriotic cyst. The rare clear cell carcinoma of the uterine corpus arises within the endometrium where mesonephric remnants have never been observed and may be intimately admixed with areas of typical endometrial adenocarcinoma. More recently, the development of clear-cell carcinoma has been reported in young females with vaginal adenosis of müllerian type as a consequence of prenatal exposure to diethylstilbestrol. The clear cell cancer is characterized by the presence of tubular and cystic

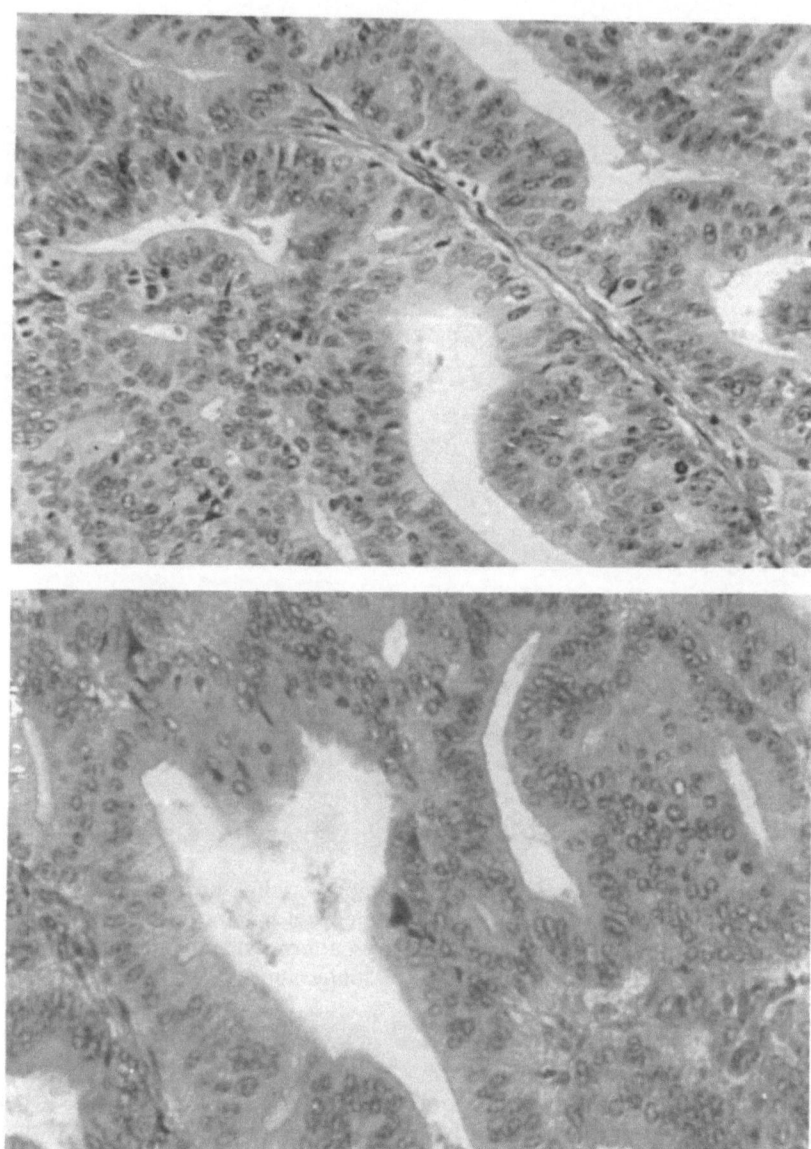

FIGURE 5.4. Endometrioid carcinoma of the ovary and carcinoma of the endometrium are associated in about one-third of cases. In general, they have a similar microscopic appearance. It is difficult to make a judgment about whether a double primary is present or one is primary and the other is metastatic.

structures set in a fibrous stroma, papillary formations that are frequently of a complex pattern, and often relatively large sheets of clear cells. Although these tumors are classically considered to have a mesonephroid origin, there is in fact little to support this view. Electron microscopic studies have tended to suggest that these neoplasms bear a considerable resemblance to a mesothelioma. Moreover, as all of the common epithelial tumors of the ovary are, almost by definition, forms of differentiated mesotheliomas, the so-called mesonephroid tumor can be considered a neoplasm arising from the surface epithelium, that

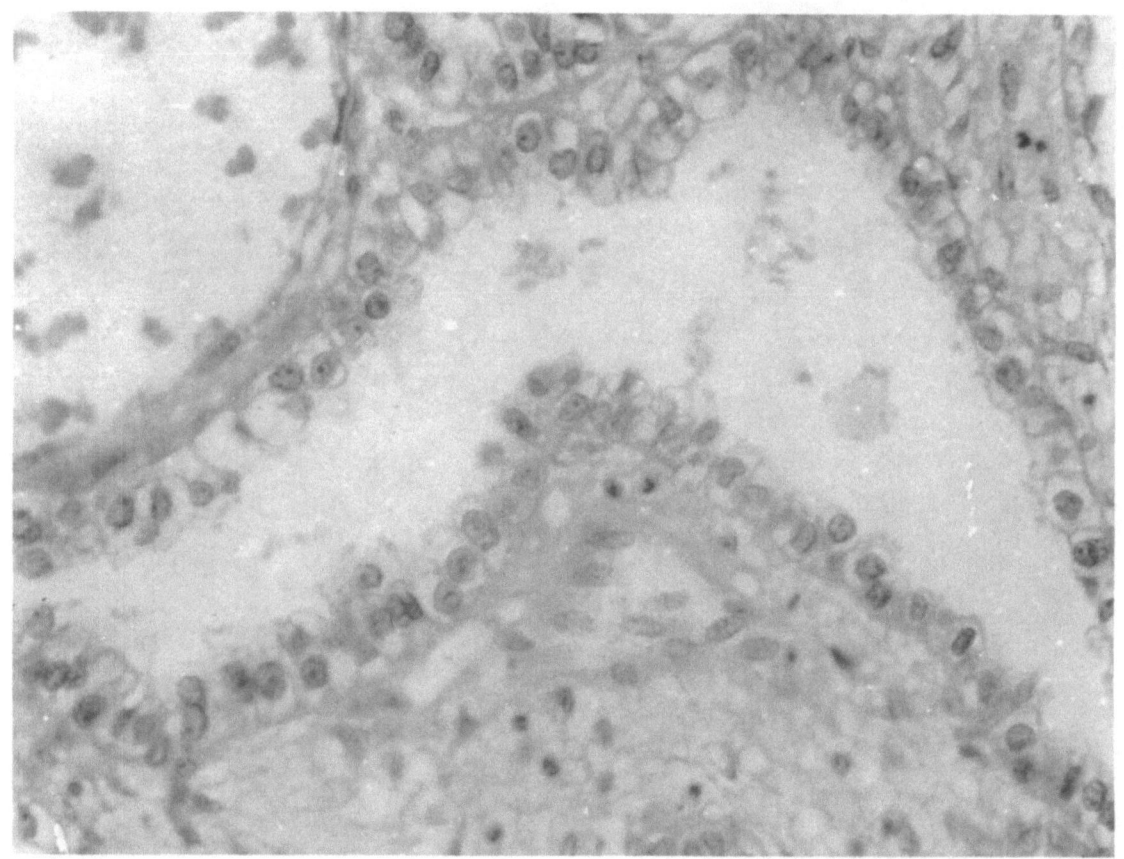

FIGURE 5.5. Clear-cell (mesonephroid) tumors are composed of clear cells containing glycogen and resembling the cells of renal cell carcinoma. They may have hobnail or peg-shaped cells lining small cysts and tubules. Hobnail cells have scant cytoplasm and large nuclei that project into the lumen.

is, a mesothelioma, but one that has failed to show any significant degree of differentiation along either a müllerian or a wolffian pathway.

Occasionally, a renal cell carcinoma metastasizes to the ovary and may be confused with a primary clear cell carcinoma. The tumor must be distinguished from endodermal sinus tumor, the dysgerminoma, and the lipid cell tumor.

Brenner Tumors

Brenner tumor is a fibroepithelial tumor composed of stroma derived from the ovarian stroma and nests of polyhedral or rounded epithelial cells of transitional or uroepithelial type; these cells often contain grooved, coffee-bean nuclei (Fig. 5.6). The nests may form glands or cysts lined by flat, cuboidal, or columnar cells; these cells often contain mucin and are occasionally ciliated. Cells of transitional cell type predominate; squamous cells may also be present.

The Brenner tumor is seen histologically to consist of epithelial islands set in a fibrous stroma: In fact, reconstruction of Brenner tumors has shown that the apparent islands are branches of a treelike structure cut in cross section, and continuity of these branches with the surface epithelium can be traced in many cases. The nature of the epithelium within the Brenner tumor has given rise to much speculation, but there is now widespread agreement, based on electron microscopic studies, that it is virtually identified with

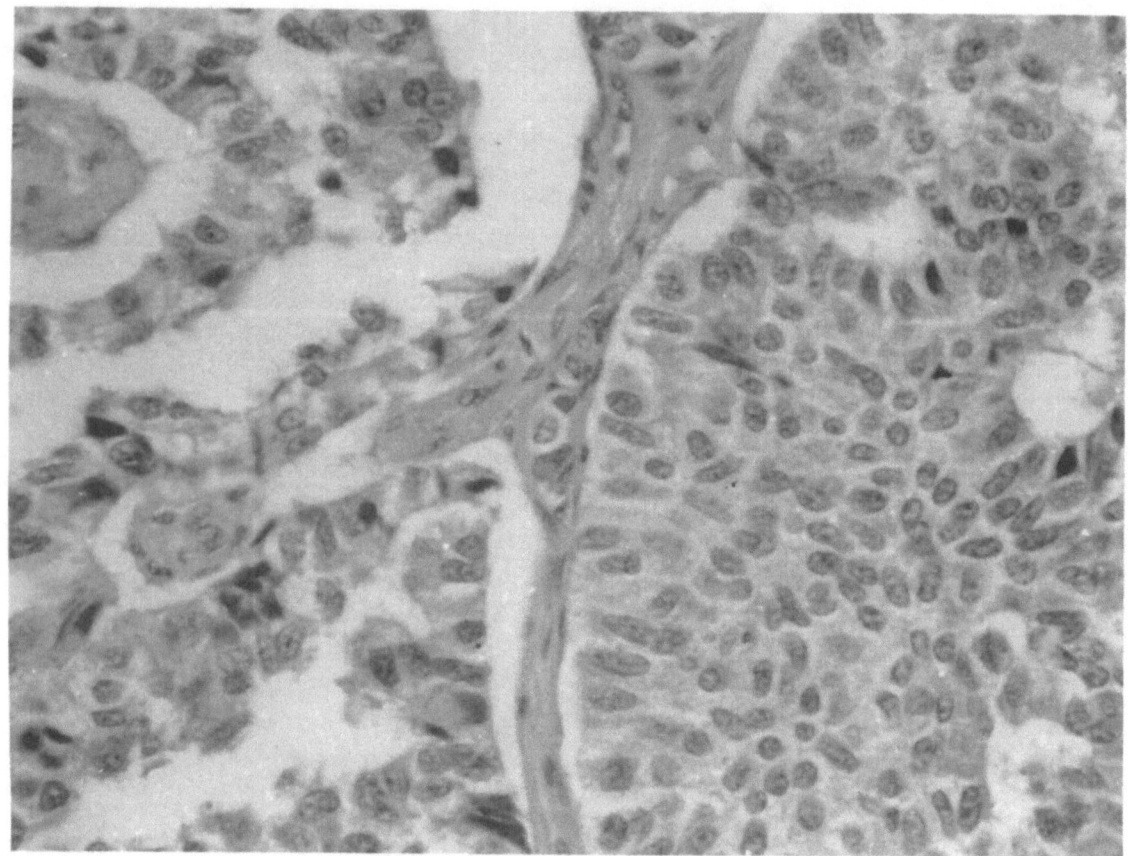

FIGURE 5.6. Brenner tumor is composed of fibrous tissue with small islands of clear epithelial cells of transitional or urethelial type cells. The cells often contain grooved, "coffee bean" nuclei. The term "malignant Brenner tumor" is used when carcinomatous change has taken place in the predominant cell type with the development of either a transitional cell or squamous cell carcinoma.

uroepithelium. It is considered that Brenner tumors usually develop from the surface epithelium by differentiation into uroepithelium. The mucinous change that is seen with some frequency in the Brenner tumors is considered to be the equivalent of the cystitis glandularis that occurs in the urinary bladder.

Scully reported that the Brenner tumor is included in the common epithelial category because (1) the pelvic peritoneum is capable of transitional epithelial metaplasia, (2) the epithelial nests of the tumor have occasionally been demonstrated to be continuous with the ovarian surface; and (3) the tumor contains mucinous epithelium lining glands or cysts in about one-third of cases and ciliated epithelium of serous type on rare occasions. At an ultrastructural level, both the transitional type of epithelial cells that predominate in Brenner tumors and the less common mucinous cells resemble those encountered in the urinary bladder, including urinary bladder tumors, suggesting transitional cell metaplasia of the surface epithelium as the histogenesis of many of these neoplasms; there are also electron microscopic similarities between the epithelial component of the Brenner tumor and Walthard's cell rest, which are thought to arise as a result of transitional metaplasia of the pelvic peritoneum. The term "borderline" seems worth retaining for uniformity of nomenclature within the common epithelial category but only with the understanding that clinical malignancy has not yet been demonstrated.

The designation *malignant Brenner tumor* is used when carcinomatous change has taken place in the predominant cell type, with the development of either transitional cell or squamous cell carcinoma. Idelson has defined fairly rigid criteria for the diagnosis of malignancy in Brenner tumors, and these criteria have rarely been met in reported cases.

Transitional Cell Carcinoma

Transitional cell tumors are usually poorly differentiated ovarian carcinomas and have a histologic appearance similar to that of transitional cell carcinoma of the bladder. They are frequently observed in high-grade, high-stage ovarian carcinomas and should be included in the common epithelial ovarian tumor group.

Most of these high grade, high stage ovarian cancers are found to be aneuploid. Ovarian tumor antigens such as carcinoembryonic antigen (CEA), HMFG2 and CA 125 are clinically useful as serum markers of tumor progression or recurrence. These tumors have a high percentage of complete responses to chemotherapy and improve patient survival with respect to other groups. The DNA content and immunoreactivity to ovarian tumor antigens is similar in transitional cell carcinoma and other types of common ovarian carcinoma.

Mixed Common Epithelial Tumors

Mixed common epithelial tumors should be classified according to the predominant element. In general, the ultrastructural study of various types of ovarian carcinoma has shown heterogeneity within the same tumor with coexistence of more than one cell type and with variations from differentiation to anaplasia. The coexistence of serous and mucinous cells in ovarian carcinoma, also noted by Gondos, can be satisfactorily explained by the histogenetic theory to the multipotential ovarian surface germinal epithelium.

Germ Cell Tumors

Structures of germ cell tumors may be derived from any or all of the three embryonic layers: ectoderm, mesoderm, endoderm. In some tumors extraembryonic structures predominate, whereas in others immature or mature structures may be derived from any or all embryonic layers. There are four main types of germ cell tumor: (1) dysgerminoma; (2) tumors comprised of tissues found in the embryo or adult (teratoma); (3) tumors of dysgenetic gonads (commonly a gonadoblastoma); and (4) tumors of extraembryonic tissues (e.g., choriocarcinoma or endodermal sinus tumors).

Dysgerminoma

The ovarian homologue of seminoma testis is a pure monocellular entity composed of uniform vesicular cells arranged in the form of strands or nests and separated by a variable amount of connective tissue stroma. Stroma and parenchyma commonly show lymphocyte infiltration, one of the most striking histologic characteristics of the tumor. In summary, microscopically it consists of masses of large, clear epithelial cells with large nuclei, resembling primitive germs cells, in the cords or alveoli. Fine connective tissue infiltrated by lymphocytes separates the bundles of epithelial cells. The malignancy varies, but many of these lesions appear to be relatively benign and do not recur. Those in children appear to be more malignant (Fig. 5.7).

The dysgerminoma is considered to arise from the germ cells of the sexually indifferent stage in gonadogenesis. Morphologically and histologically, the dysgerminoma cells are identical with primordial germ cells.

Embryonal Carcinoma

Embryonal carcinoma is generally predominantly solid but may contain many small cysts or be primarily cystic with solid areas in its wall. Microscopically, it is characterized by the presence of embryonal and adult tissues derived from all three germ layers.

The polyembryoma is a form of embryonal

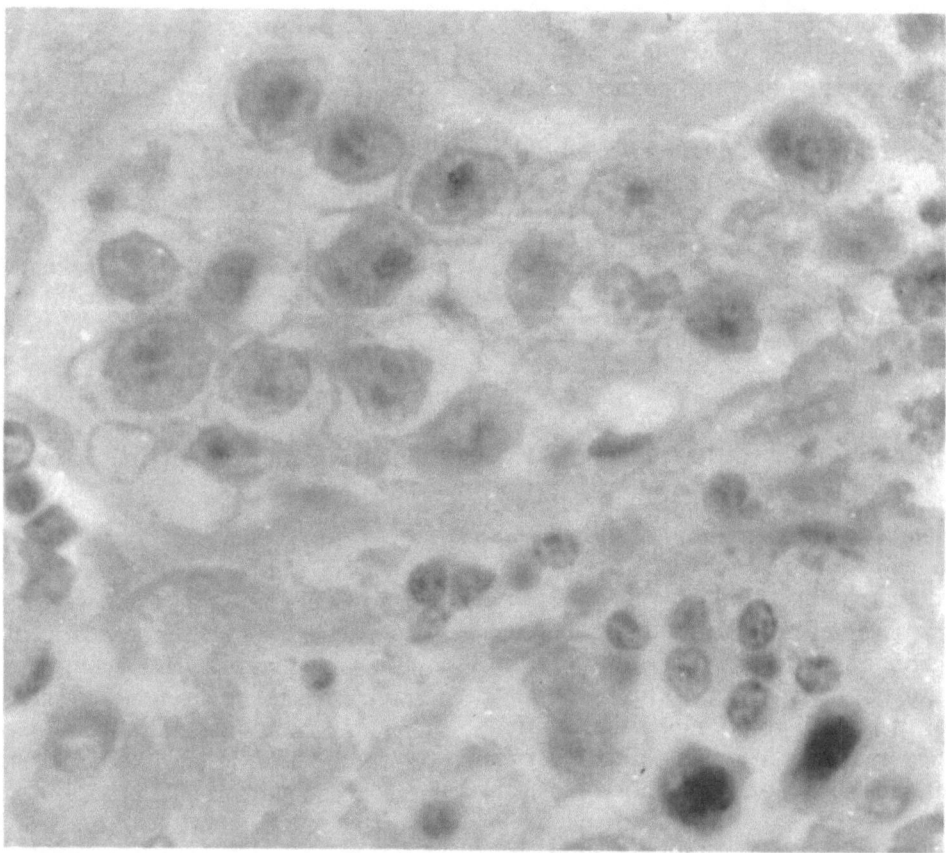

FIGURE 5.7. Dysgerminoma is a tumor of uniform appearance. Microscopically, it consists of masses of large clear epithelial cells with large nuclei, resembling primitive germ cells, in cords or alveoli. Fine connective tissue infiltrated by lymphocytes separates the bundles of epithelial cells; granulomas, which may contain Langhans' giant cells, are often present. The cytoplasm of the tumor cells contains glycogen, the presence of which may be an aid in diagnosis.

carcinoma (polyembryonic embryoma). It is a teratomatous tumor of the gonads containing myriad embryonal bodies comparable to normal presomite embryos (Fig. 5.8).

Extraembryonal Tumors

The germ cell tumor classification includes the extraembryonic mesoderm, an interesting group of tumors. The mesoderm seems to be derived at least in part from the inner surface of the trophoblast, and it differentiates before the endoderm has had time to spread around the anterior of the blastocysts. As a result, the primitive or primary yolk sac has endoderm on its roof only; the remainder of the blastocyst cavity becomes lined with a thin layer of flattened cells (mesothelial in character) representing the inner limiting layer of the extraembryonic mesoderm. It is in continuity with the primitive entoderm around its margins, which then closes the yolk sac. There is controversy over whether this mesoderm is truly mesoderm in origin. It is interesting to note that the primitive yolk sac is eventually converted to a smaller secondary sac. At this point it resembles an hourglass. Part of the mesoderm covering the yolk sac is called the extraembryonal splanchnopleuric (visceral) mesoderm. Yolk sac tumors of the human ovary obvious-

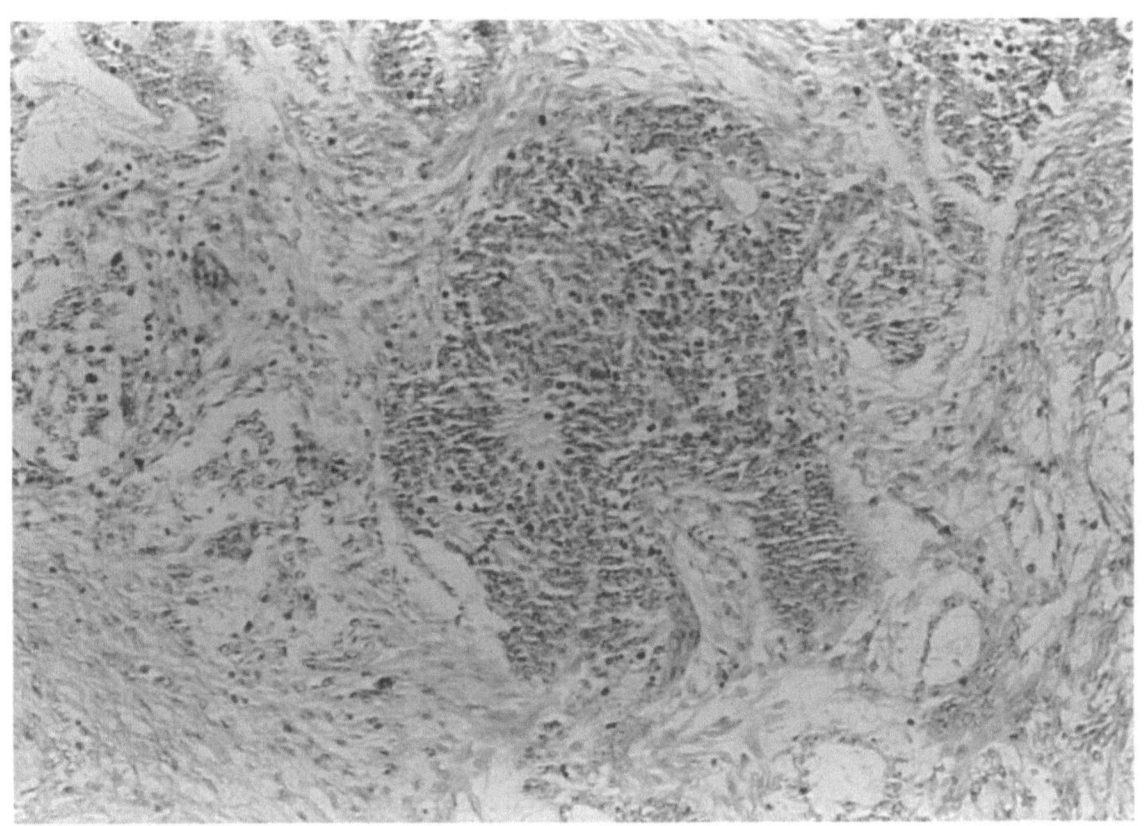

FIGURE 5.8. Embryonal carcinoma is a tumor composed of anaplastic embryonal cells of epithelial appearance growing in a variety of patterns, i.e., acinar, tubular, papillary, and solid. Teilum reported that the term "embryonal carcinoma" is restricted to tumors composed of undifferentiated neoplastic embryonal cells representing the undifferentiated forms of extraembryonic as well as embryonic types.

ly reproduce these transient stages during the embryonic development of the yolk sac. Although the embryonic tumors arise from the embryonic cells, mature cells give rise to teratomas such as cystic or dermoid, whereas immature cells give rise to embryonic carcinomas.

On the other hand, the extraembryonal cells give rise to the endodermal sinus tumors and trophoblastic cells consisting of cytotrophoblasts and syncytial trophoblasts, which in turn give rise to the highly malignant choriocarcinoma. The choriocarcinoma is a fólic acid-independent tumor. The extraembryonal tumors of the ovary are highly malignant and have a counterpart in the testis. Generally, they are not radiosensitive but have shown satisfactory response to triple or combination chemotherapy.

Endodermal Sinus Tumor

The endodermal sinus tumor is a highly malignant germ cell tumor showing a selective overgrowth of yolk sac endoderm intimately associated with the extraembryonic mesoblast. There are distinctive perivascular structures resembling the endodermal sinuses of the rat placenta and both intracellular and extracellular hyaline globules, giving a positive periodic acid Schiff reaction. The hyaline bodies resemble Russell bodies. These tumors are thus extraembryonic derivatives of yolk sac endoderm from embryonal carcinoma (Fig. 5.9).

The yolk sac tumor (endodermal sinus tumor) may contain cysts resembling yolk sac vesicles (polyvesicular vitelline pattern). The polyvesicular vitelline tumor is a distinctive

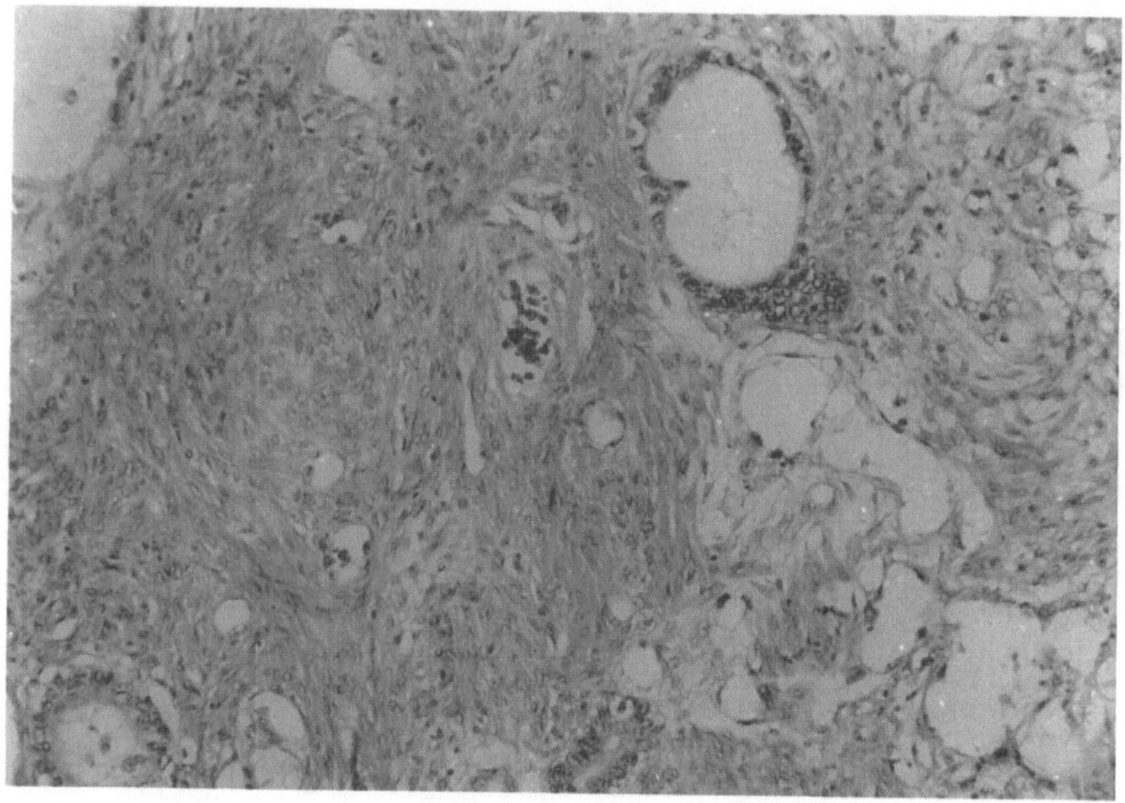

FIGURE 5.9. Endodermal sinus tumor is character-ized by the presence of a loose vacuolated network of embryonal cells and distinctive perivascular struc-tures resembling the endodermal sinuses of the rat placenta. They contain both intracellular and ex-tracellular hyaline globules that give a positive periodic acid Schiff reaction. When it contains cysts resembling yolk sac vesicles, it is said to have a polyvesicular vitelline pattern.

type of highly malignant yolk sac tumor, but histologically it is characterized by myriad blastocyst-like yolk sac (endoblast) vesicles. It is important to distinguish the endodermal sinus tumor from the clear cell (mesonephroid) carcinoma. The clear cell carcinoma has a different pattern and lacks endodermal sinuses and hyaline bodies; it typically occurs in older women and is associated with a much better prognosis.

Choriocarcinoma

Choriocarcinoma; a rare, highly malignant tumor, is composed of both cytotrophoblast and syncytiotrophoblast. It may be associated with sexual precocity. The primarily ovarian choriocarcinoma is a derivative of embryonal carcinoma; and in contrast to the tumor origi-nating in a pregnancy in the uterus, it does not respond well to chemotherapeutic agents (Fig. 5.10). In contrast to the gestational trophoblas-tic diseases, a choriocarcinoma that arises as a teratoma in the ovary is not a folic acid-dependent tumor and therefore is not as easy to treat with chemotherapeutic agents.

Teratomas

Teratomas are generally composed of several types of tissue representing two or three embryonic layers. The structures present may be immature, mature, or both. In occasional cases differentiation is monodermal or may be evidenced by the exclusive or predominant formation of a single highly specialized tissue.

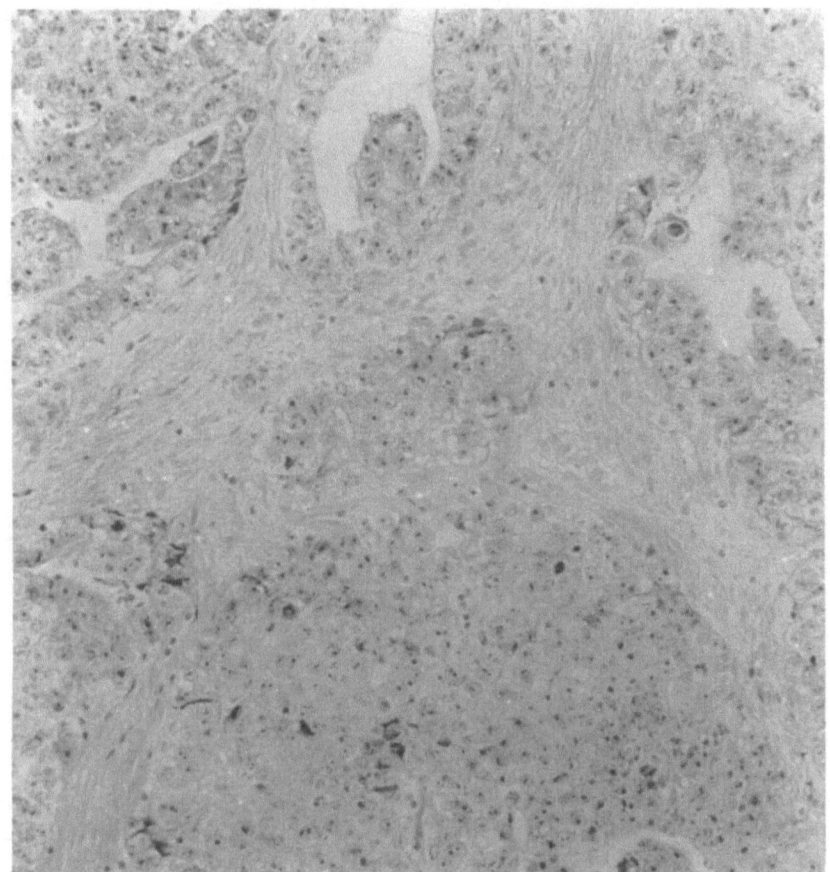

FIGURE 5.10. Choriocarcinoma is a rare tumor of the ovary. Syncytiotrophoblast is always present, but sometimes cytotrophoblast is formed as well. Hormones produced are those normally associated with chorionic tissue, e.g., chorionic gonadotropin and estrogens.

Solid Tumors

It is important to differentiate immature and mature cell teratomas because of their striking difference in prognosis; whereas the former are often clinically malignant, the latter are almost invariably benign. The presence of implants and mature glia as well as mature structures of other types on the peritoneum have not been associated with the malignant clinical course in the reported cases and so do not warrant the diagnosis of malignancy.

The solid adult teratoma is a rare tumor composed entirely of adult tissues derived from all three germ layers. When it is diagnosed according to strict criteria, the results from appropriate therapy are excellent.

Cystic Adult Teratoma

The cystic adult teratoma is composed of all three germinal layers, although ectodermal structures predominate (Fig. 5.11). Studies of nuclear sex chromatin in ovarian teratomas have uniformly shown a female pattern. They are positive for sex chromatin and therefore indicate the presence of XX sex chromosomes, which has been confirmed by chromosome studies. The presence of nuclear sex chromatin also suggests that these cells are haploid. However, a significant portion of teratomas in the male have shown the sex chromatin pattern of females. This discrepancy can be explained if we accept the explanation that teratomas in males are derived from haploid germ cells by a

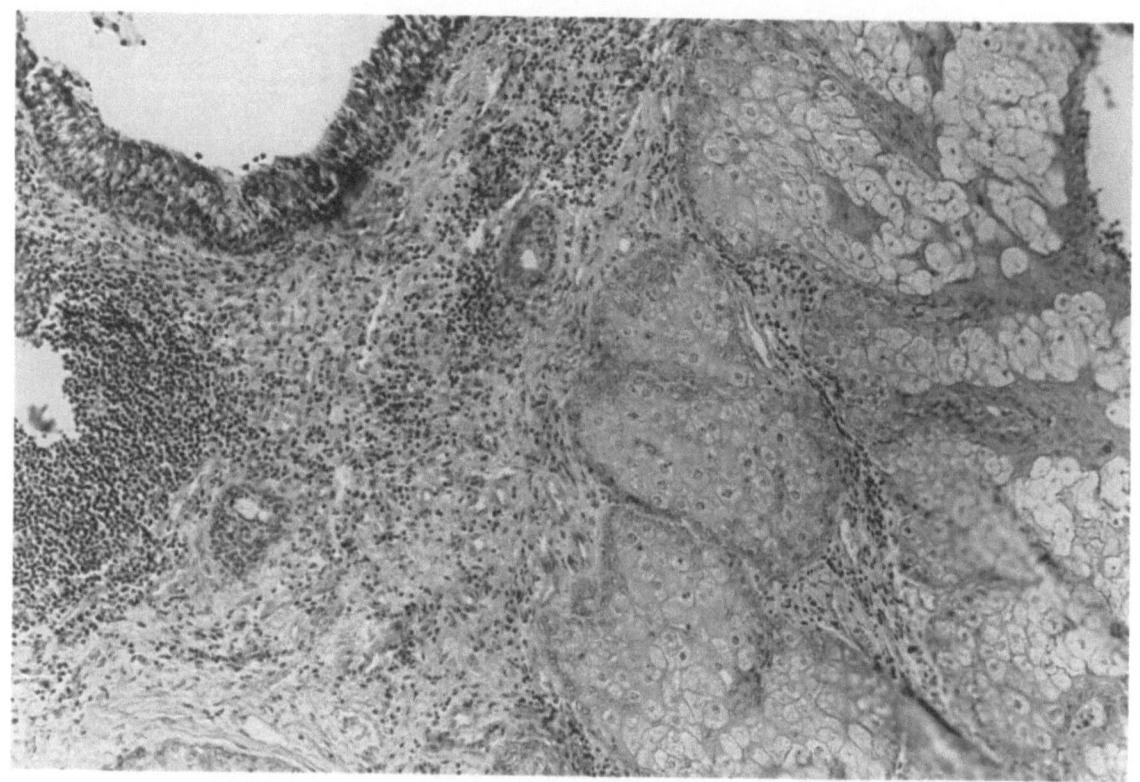

FIGURE 5.11. Cystic adult teratoma (dermoid cyst) is a cyst with a rounded eminence from which hairs grow and on or in which teeth may be found. The eminence may contain sweat glands, teeth, hair, nerve tissues, cartilage, bone, respiratory and intestinal epithelium, and thyroid gland tissue. Thick, yellow sebaceous material fills the cyst. The tumor often contains other ectodermal, especially neuroec-todermal (a derivative), material; elements of endodermal and mesodermal origin are also found with great frequency. Occasionally, respiratory epithelium or glia form a portion of the cyst lining. Squamous cell carcinoma is the usual form of malignant change; adenocarcinoma and sarcoma are much less common, and melanoma is rare.

process of autofertilization or fusion of adjacent haploid cells. The result would be a diploid chromosome number with either XX or XY chromosomes. The same process in the female could result only in XX diploid cells. Some teratomas in the male have shown a mosaic pattern with sex chromatin-positive and sex chromatin-negative cells, suggesting that their origin may be multicentric rather than from a single germ cell. The microscopic examination may reveal all types of mature ectoderm, mesoderm, and entodermal elements. It is not uncommon to find gastrointestinal mucosa, stratified squamous epithelium, hair follicles, sebaceous glands, cartilage, and nerve and respiratory elements. Giant cells and pseudoxanthoma cells are often seen. Occasionally, an overgrowth of thyroid tissue results in a struma ovarii, which may function.

Although 2% of cystic tumors are complicated by malignancy, the malignant change is confined usually to one ovary. Patients with squamous carcinoma within the cyst have a much better survival rate than do patients with the other forms of malignancy, i.e., sarcoma, carcinoids, and adenocarcinoma.

Struma ovarii may complicate a dermoid but is not so designated unless thyroid tissue is the main or sole teratoid component. About 10% of patients with these tumors show evidence of thyrotoxicosis, and only a few of the tumors prove to be malignant.

Carcinoid tumors (argentaffinomas) of the ovary may arise in the wall of a dermoid cyst from either intestinal or bronchial epithelium. The characteristics of the syndrome resulting from this tumor include intermittent flushing, cyanosis, diarrhea, and asthmatic attacks. The clinical manifestations are attributed to the production of excessive quantities of 5-hydroxytryptamine (serotonin) by the argentaffin cells of the tumor. The argentaffin granules may be identified with appropriate silver stains even in neoplasms of apparent bronchial origin. These tumors occasionally metastasize.

Gonadoblastoma

Gonadoblastoma is composed of a mixture of germ cells (dysgerminoma) and gonadal stromal cells (granulosa-Sertoli). Because the tumor had previously been reported only in intersexual individuals, it was called dysgenetic gonadoma. In most cases in which sex chromatin studies have been done, the nuclear pattern has been negative in the patient (46,XY) or may have a sex chromosome mosaicism (XO/XY). Most patients with a gonadoblastoma are intersexual with a phenotype female habitus, are amenorrheic, and may be virilized. Grossly, the tumor ranges from a solid mass of gray to cream-colored, fleshy tissue resembling a dysgerminoma to a firm, fibrous mass. A characteristic feature is calcification, which may be evident on x-ray examination of the pelvis. Microscopically, there are masses of large germ cells that wrap themselves around granulosa-like cells. Between the nests of cells, there are a large number of cells suggestive of Leydig cells. Calcification is often encountered. Bilateral involvement occurs in approximately one-third of cases. The malignant potential of pure gonadoblastoma has not been established, and it may well depend on the mixture of gonadoblastoma with other germ cell tumors present, such as dysgerminoma or endodermal sinus tumor. These patients often reveal eunuchoidal features or signs of Turner syndrome and sterility, and the tumor has the

potential of developing a malignancy (Fig. 5.12).

Gonadal Stromal (Sex Cord-Mesenchyme) Tumors

Female Cell Type

Gonadal stromal (sex cord-mesenchyme) tumors comprise the category of lesions that includes gonadal stromal tumors of the female cell type, e.g., granulosa or granulosa-thecoma type, or of the male cell type, e.g., Sertoli-Leydig cell (arrhenoblastoma) and Sertoli and hilus (Leydig) cell tumors. These lesions are not as common as the germ cell tumors, nor are they as malignant.

Granulosa Cell Tumors

Although approximately 100 granulosa tumors in children have been reported in the literature, only three have proved to be malignant. Barber and Graber have called them the most glamorous of all neoplasms. Granulosa cell tumors in children are infrequent and account for a few cases of precocious puberty. The startling secondary sexual changes they produce in children are dramatic. From 5 to 10% of the tumors occur before the patient reaches the age of puberty. However, they may function and produce a feminine habitus, maturation of the genitalia, and enlargement of the breasts. Pubic hair is scant, and vaginal bleeding may occur. However precocious puberty is usually constitutional, and only about 2% of such cases result from an ovarian tumor. More often the diagnosis is made after an abdominal or pelvic mass is discovered. The tumors are bilateral in about 4% of the cases.

The tumor has a good prognosis. The malignancy rate in adults is about 25% but only 3 to 6% in children. The recurrences are usually local, and distant metastases are rare. Recurrences may occur at any time, but the rate of recurrence is slow, and it often takes many years to develop. The histologic appearance of a tumor of this group is no index of its final behavior (Fig. 5.13).

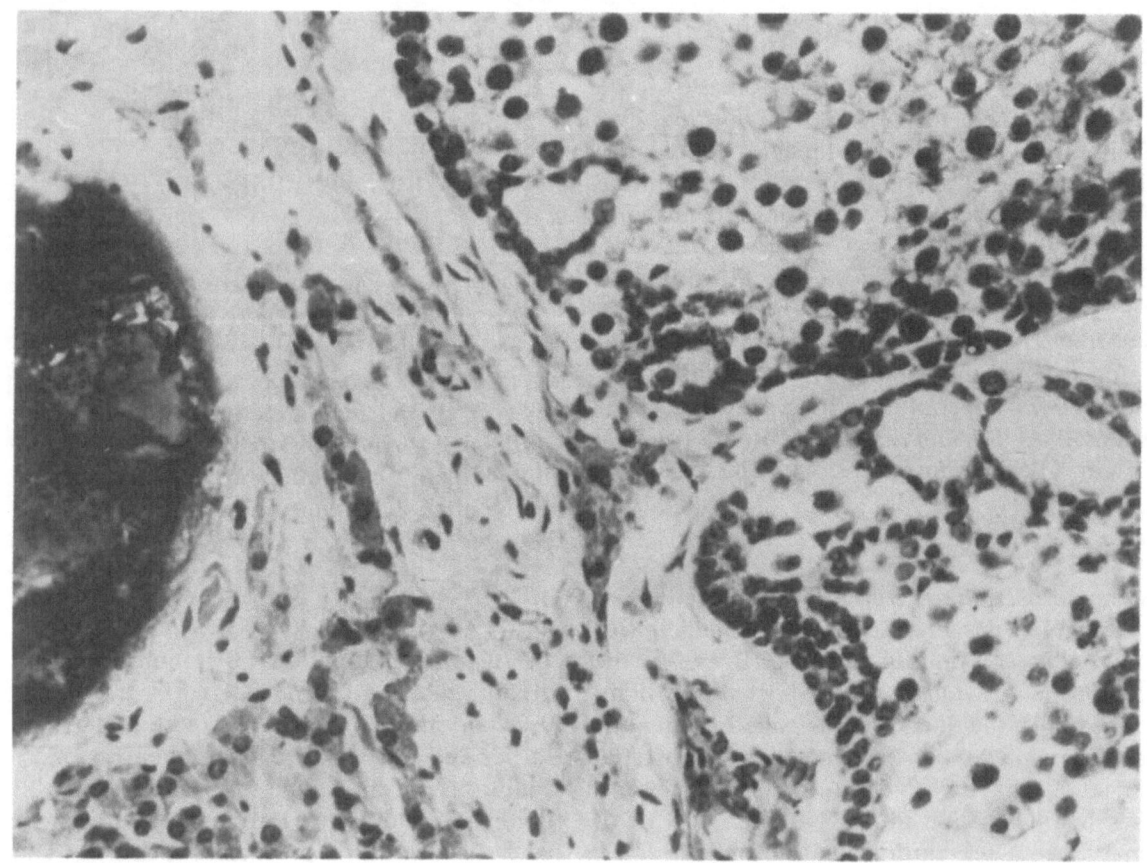

FIGURE 5.12. Gonadoblastoma is a tumor associated with dysgenetic gonads, usually streak gonads. Commonly there is a sex chromosome anomaly such as XO/XY. The patient here is a phenotypic female. The tumor is composed of two types of cell: (1) a large primitive germ cell, and (2) small cells of the granulosa cell type. Call-Exner bodies (small rosettes) may be seen in the latter. These two types of cell form epithelial islands in a stroma that may contain Leydig-like cells. Sometimes the germ cells undergo rapid proliferation and give rise to a dysgerminoma. Some of the dysgerminomas in children arise in this way. (Courtesy of Dr. RE Scully. Reprinted from Scully RE: Ovarian Tumors of Germ Cell Origin. In: *Progress in Gynecology*. Vol. 5. S. Sturgis and M. Taylor, eds. Grune & Stratton, New York, 1970, with permission.)

Juvenile Granulosa Cell Tumor

About 85% of the granulosa cell tumors that occur before the age of puberty have distinctive microscopic features that differ from those of the well-known forms of granulosa cell tumor encountered in older patients. Although these features are observed on rare occasions in specimens from older women, their frequency in tumors in young females has led to the designation juvenile granulosa cell tumors.

On gross examination, the juvenile granulosa cell tumor has as great a variation in appearance as the typical granulosa cell tumor encountered in older patients. Accordingly, it may be uniformly solid or partially solid, sometimes containing blood; or it may be composed predominantly of one or more thin-walled cysts. The neoplastic tissue may be gray, cream-colored, or yellow; occasionally, large areas of necrosis or hemorrhage suggest a high degree of malignancy.

The microscopic examination reveals a number of features that differ from those of a typical granulosa cell tumor seen in older patients. Low-power   examination   characteristically

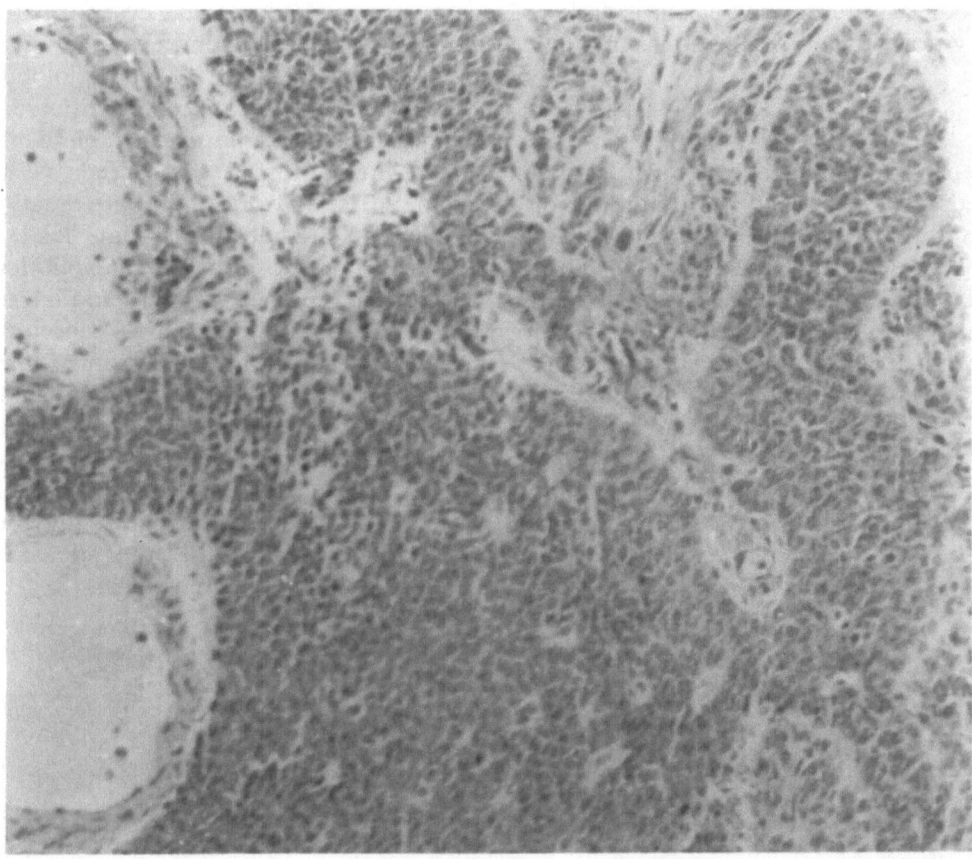

FIGURE 5.13. Granulosa cell tumor is a tumor of female cell type containing more than a small component of granulosa cells. The cells may be arranged in a variety of patterns, including follicular (microfollicular and macrofollicular), trabecular, insular, and diffuse (sarcomatoid). The microfollicular pattern is characterized by the presence of distinctive Call-Exner bodies. The most specific diagnostic feature of the granulosa cell tumor, in addition to its characteristic patterns, is the appearance of its nuclei, which may be either irregular in shape, with their long axes directed haphazardly, or round and uniform. Although mitoses may be numerous, the nuclei typically lack the pleomorphism and hyperchromatism of the nuclei of adenocarcinoma and undifferentiated carcinomas. The presence of nuclear grooving in granulosa cells is often helpful in the differential diagnosis.

shows nodules of neoplastic granulosa cells, which may be solid or contain follicles that are usually round or oval, although they are occasionally irregular in size and shape. Generally, the follicles do not reach the large size of those encountered in the typical macrofollicular form of granulosa cell tumor. Follicles of the juvenile tumor typically contain eosinophilic or basophilic material that may stain with mucicarmine. Thecal cells are often present in varying amounts between the nodules of granulosa cells, which may grow in a diffuse pattern. Occasionally, the granulosa and thecal cells are arranged in a jumbled, disordered fashion. Reticulum stains may help differentiate the two cell types, with fibrils investing the thecal cells individually but surrounding aggregates of granulosa cells. A solid, tubular architecture resembling that of Sertoli cell tumors is encountered focally in occasional cases. In summary, the juvenile granulosa cell tumor occurs before puberty in 50% of cases and is rare after age 30. Immature follicles with mucin secretion are usually present, and Call-

Exner bodies are rare. The nucleus is dark and (rarely) grooved, and luteinization is frequent.

Sclerosing Stroma Tumor

The sclerosing stroma tumor, which has been identified as a distinct entity within the World Health Organization (WHO) category of unclassified tumors and theca-fibroma group, generally occurs at a younger age than the typical thecoma or fibroma. More than 80% of the patients are under 30 years of age. Endocrine manifestation occurs in only about 25% of the patients, and it usually causes abnormal uterine bleeding.

All of the cases of sclerosing stromal tumors have been unilateral. The gross examination reveals typically a well-demarcated, predominantly solid mass that is white with yellow parts; areas of edema and cyst formation are common. The microscopic examination reveals four typical features: (1) pseudolobules of cellular tissue; (2) collagen distributed within the pseudolobules but more abundantly between them often accompanied by marked edema; (3) a network of delicate blood vessels within the nodules that may lead to an erroneous diagnosis of hemangiopericytoma; and (4) the presence within the nodules of two intermingled cell types: spindle cells and round to oval cells with small, dark nuclei in vacuolated cytoplasm containing lipid. The latter cells occasionally resemble signet ring cells and may result in a missed diagnosis of Krükenberg tumor. With the occasionally functioning form of the tumor, the round or oval cells typically have the appearance of luteinizing cells with large nuclei.

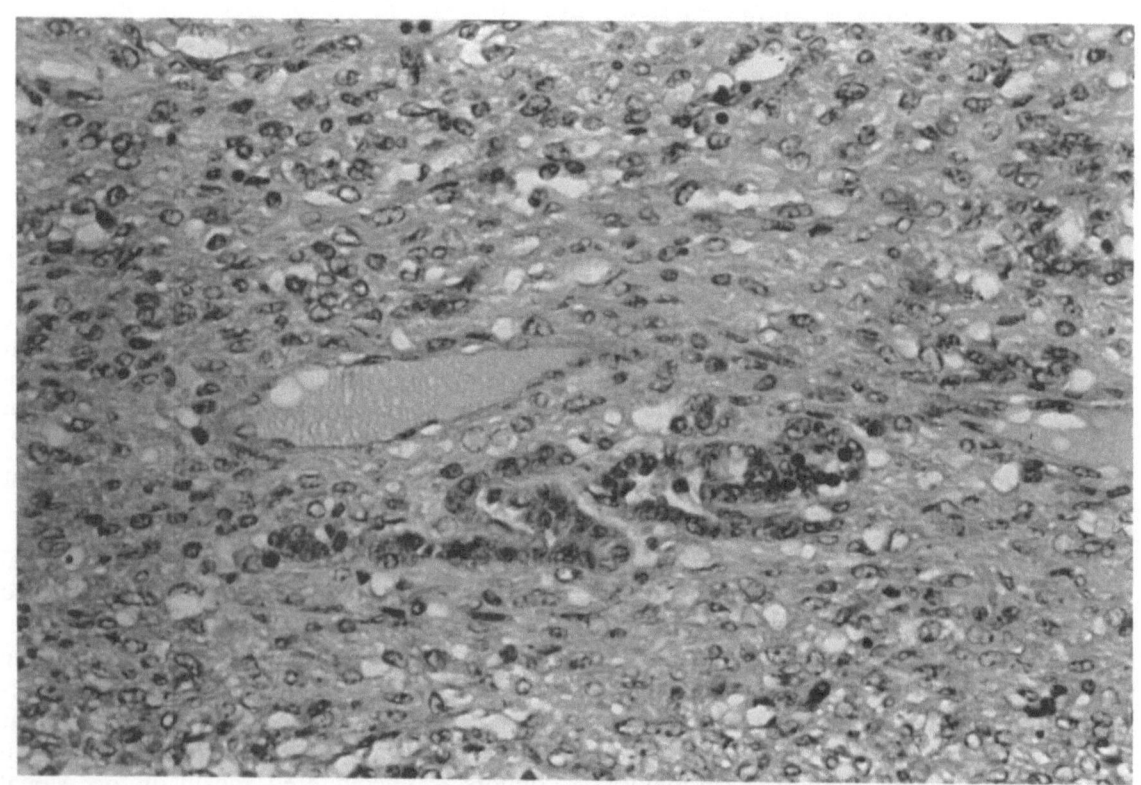

FIGURE 5.14. Sertoli-Leydig cell tumors (arrhenoblastomas) contain Sertoli and Leydig cells of varying degrees of maturity. Histologically, they consist of primitive tubules surrounded by Leydig cells that may be crystalloids of Reinke. The latter are rod-shaped structures in the cytoplasm of Leydig cells and are said to be diagnostic of these cells.

Sertoli-Leydig Cell Tumor

The term "Sertoli-Leydig cell tumor" has been selected instead of the more familiar term "arrhenoblastoma" because many of these tumors are nonfunctioning or have estrogenic effects rather than masculinizing tendencies. In those tumors with a predominance of functioning Sertoli cells, the effect may be that of a feminizing tumor. However, if the Leydig cells are predominant and function, the patient first is defeminized (atrophy of breasts, loss of female contour, amenorrhea) and then masculinized (hirsutism, hypertrophy of clitoris, and voice changes). The tumor usually affects women of childbearing age and is rare during childhood. The tumor is bilateral in only 5% of the cases. From 3 to 20% of these tumors dem-onstrate malignant behavior, which is usually manifested by intraabdominal spread rather than distal metastasis (Fig. 5.14).

Mixed Type Tumor (Gynandroblastoma)

Gynandroblastoma should contain typical aggregates of granulosa cell with Call-Exner bodies and either hollow tubules or Leydig cells containing crystalloids of Reinke. There are no reports of this tumor in children, but there is no reason to believe that its behavior differs from that of granulosa cell or Sertoli-Leydig cell tumors (Fig. 5.15).

Unclassified Sex-Cord Stromal Tumors

In approximately 10% of sex cord stromal tumors it is impossible to be certain whether

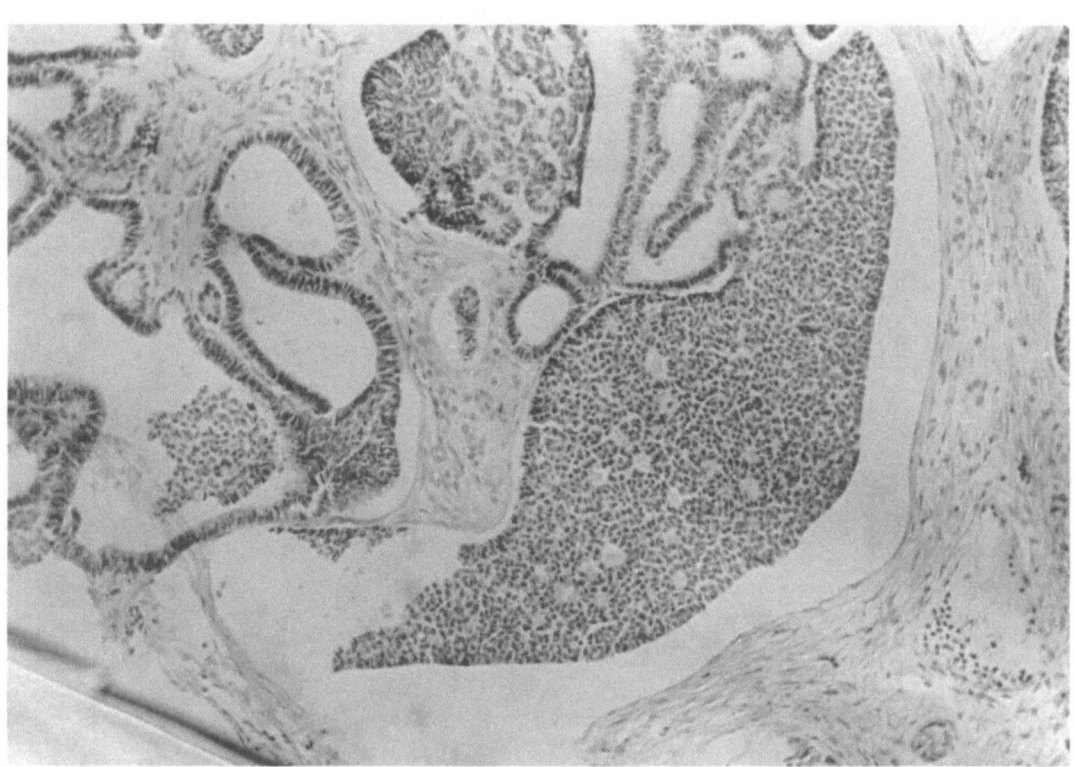

FIGURE 5.15. Gynandroblastoma is a rare tumor in which collections of granulosa cells with typical Call-Exner bodies coexist with hollow tubules lined by Sertoli cells. Although the two cell types need not be present in equal amounts in order to bear the name *gynandroblastoma*, they should be present in at least a 70:30 ratio. This tumor is also know as a sex cord stromal tumor of mixed cell types. (Courtesy of Dr. RE Scully. Reprinted from Scully RE: Androgenic Lesions of the Ovary. In: H. Grady and D.E. Smith, eds. *The Ovary*. International Academy of Pathology Monograph No. 3. Williams & Wilkins, Baltimore, 1962. © International Academy of Pathology, with permission.)

the cells and their patterns of growth are more typical of the female or male gonads; in such cases, the term "sex cord-stromal tumor, unclassified" is used. Such tumors have been placed in the nonclassified category by the WHO.

Sex-Cord Tumor with Annular Tubules

One distinctive subtype within the category of unclassified sex cord-stromal tumors is the sex cord tumor with annular tubules (SCTAT), which is characterized by simple and complex ring-shaped tubules, has a pattern intermediate between that of granulosa cell tumor and Sertoli-Leydig cell, and resembles a gonadal blastoma except for the absence of a germ cell component. The SCTAT may be estrogenic, having been associated with the cystic hyperplasia of the endometrium and isosexual precocity. When it presents pathologically in the form of multiple tumors or tumorlets, the SCTAT is almost always complicated by classification within the tubules and associated with the Peutz-Jegher syndrome, on occasion providing the first evidence of its existence. The tumor is encountered relatively frequently among sex cord-stromal tumors in the canine ovary.

Non-Peutz-Jeghers syndrome-related SCTAT is clinically malignant in at least one-fifth of cases, a much higher degree of malignancy than that associated with Sertoli cell tumors. Unilateral salpingo-oophorectomy is the therapy of choice in a young patient with stage Ia SCTAT who does not have Peutz-Jeghers syndrome because of the rarity of involvement of the contralateral ovary. The possible role of chemotherapy or radiotherapy in clinically malignant cases needs further evaluation.

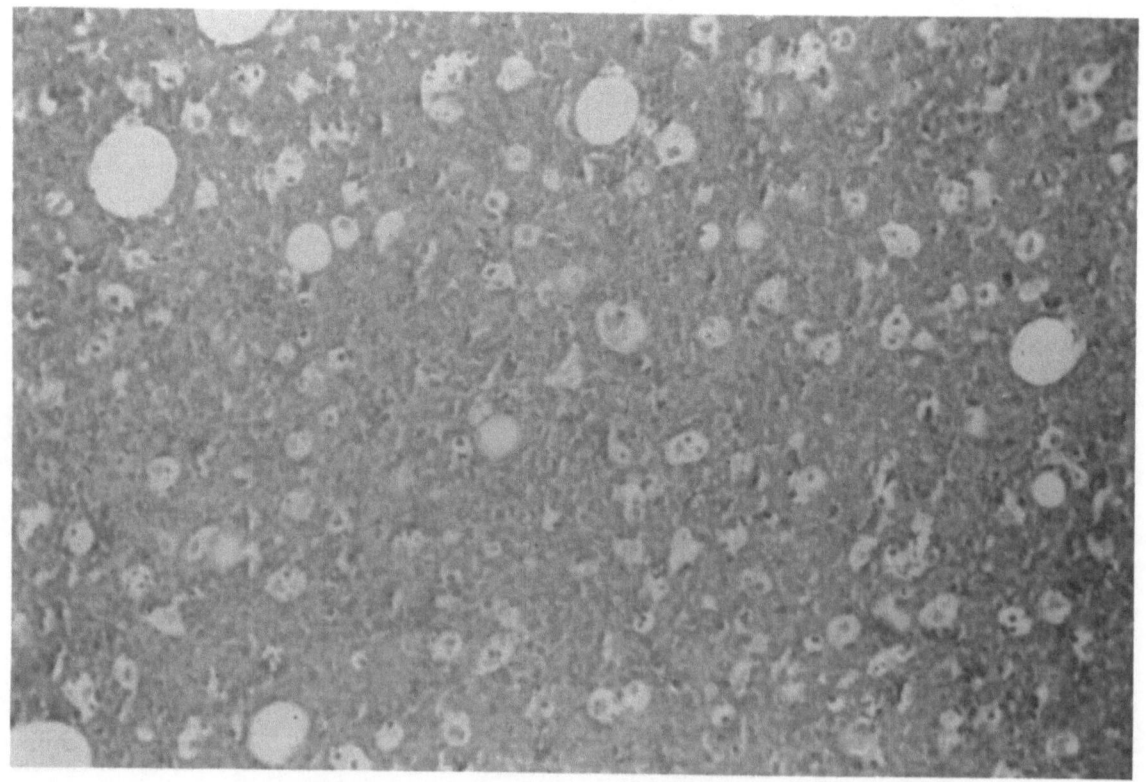

FIGURE 5.16. Burkitt's lymphoma is characterized by proliferation of a primitive lymphoreticular system. It presents a histologic picture of stars in the heavens.

Tumors Not Specific for the Ovary

The ovary may be involved as part of disseminated Hodgkin's disease. These tumors are usually found in adults, but ovarian involvement has been reported among children suffering from Burkitt's tumor. It is interesting that the first virus to be suspected of causing a human cancer was isolated as a result of epidemiologic observations made in populations of tropical Africa, particularly in persons with Burkitt's tumor. The particular distribution of the tumor from the geographic and ecologic standpoint as well as its age distribution were typical of an infectious disease and thus led to the suspicion that Burkitt's tumor may be caused by an infectious agent. A concerted effort resulted in the isolation of a virus (Epstein-Barr virus) from Burkitt's tumor cells (Fig. 5.16). Lymphoma of the ovary is rare (Fig. 5.17).

Miscellaneous Tumors

Fibroma and sarcomas fall into the "miscellaneous" category. Ovarian sarcomas occur more frequently in children than in adults. Grossly, these tumors are solid, lobulated, or soft growths. They grow rapidly and fill the abdomen. The cut surface of the cellular sarcomas are soft and fleshy, whereas the more fibrous ones are firm and somewhat granular when sectioned. Azoury and Woodruff reported on 47 primary sarcomas of the ovary. The most common symptoms were abdominal pain and swelling. Regardless of therapy, survival is poor (Fig. 5.18).

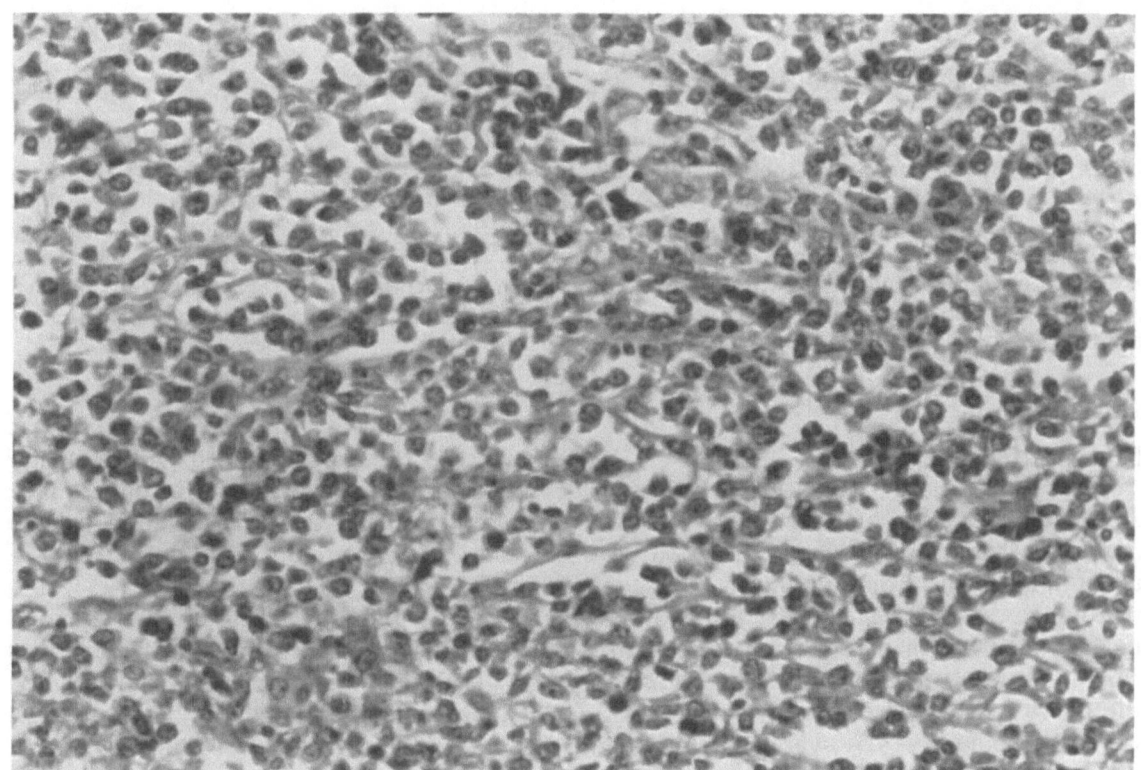

FIGURE 5.17. Lymphoma is a rare tumor of the ovary. It may be mistaken microscopically for a granulosa cell tumor or a dysgerminoma because growth in the dense ovarian stroma may result in a pseudocarcinomatous pattern. It may grow diffusely or in the form of well-defined nests and cords of cells, simulating the pattern of a carcinoma.

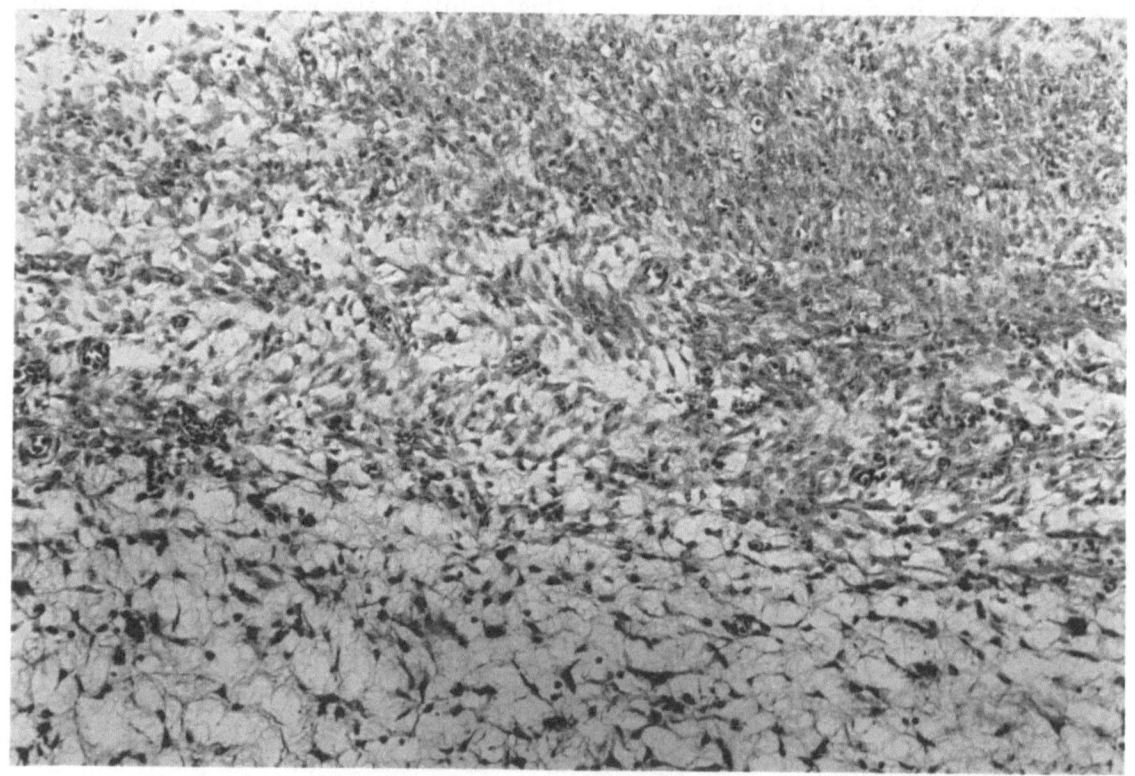

FIGURE 5.18. Sarcoma of the ovary is a rare tumor. Grossly, the tumors are solid, lobulated, or soft growths. The cut surfaces of the cellular sarcomas are soft and fleshy, whereas others are firm and somewhat granular when sectioned. The ovarian sarcomas are divided into three groups: teratoid, mesenchymal, and mixed tumors. The sarcomas have bizarre nuclei; some are larger and more irregular than those seen in normal tissue. The number of mitoses is increased. The entity known as *stromatous endometriosis*, characterized by ectopic endometrial stroma without endometrial glands, is today considered the etiologic factor in ovarian sarcoma, carcinosarcoma, and mixed mesodermal tumors, whether homologous or heterologous.

Metastatic Cancer

Approximately 10% of ovarian cancers are metastatic, and the survival rate is low. Most of those tumors arise from the bowel, breast, or thyroid. Because cancer of the colon is on the increase among women and is the second most common cancer, the incidence of metastasis to the ovary from the colon is also increasing. Careful sectioning of the ovaries has revealed that approximately 25% of patients with colon cancer have metastases to the ovary. Metastatic breast cancer is rarely detected clinically because the patient usually dies from widespread disease before the ovaries have become large enough to produce symptoms. However, the results of prophylactic oophorectomies have disclosed that more than 40% of patients have metastases to the ovary if multiple sections are taken.

Krükenberg tumor is an unusual type of malignancy that usually arises in the gastrointestinal tract and metastasizes to the ovary. It is often bilateral, is typically solid, and retains its shape. There are few cases reported among children. Krükenberg tumors are characterized histologically by large, swollen, signet-ring-like cells that lie in clumps within areas of mucoid degeneration. These cells are scattered throughout an edematous stroma-like matrix.

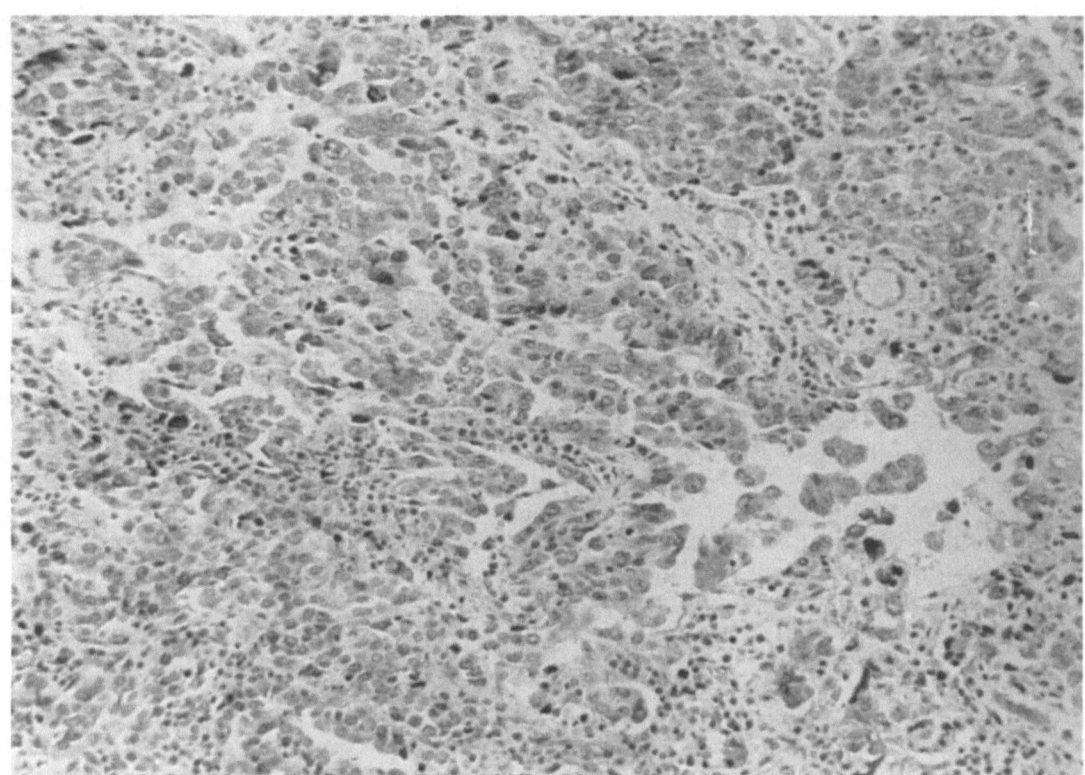

FIGURE 5.19. Krükenberg is a rare secondary carcinoma of the ovary. Histologically, it has a characteristic appearance. There is a highly cellular stroma, resembling a sarcoma, in which large epithelial cells lie singly or in alveoli. These epithelial cells have a clear cytoplasm with a crescentic nucleus pushed to one side, resulting in a typical signet ring appearance. The cytoplasm is full of mucin.

Only tumors meeting these criteria should be so designated (Fig. 5.19).

Summary

Many classifications for ovarian tumors have been proposed over the years. None have been completely satisfactory, and it has been difficult to get the medical profession to adopt a common classification for reporting results. In 1961 a committee of the International Federation of Gynecology and Obstetrics proposed a classification for ovarian tumors, and more recently a committee of the World Health Organization has formulated a more detailed classification. The new classifications have grouped closely related ovarian tumors. Because current embryologic knowledge is imprecise and because it is difficult to identify specific cell types, the present classifications have inherent weaknesses. Despite these shortcomings, the new classifications have been accepted, and material is being reported according to them.

It is important to standardize the parameters used when studying ovarian cancer. Editors of journals should insist on a common method of presenting data. By accumulating material from many investigators using the same parameters for their studies, it would then be possible to identify the best form of treatment, and progress could be achieved in salvaging additional patients.

Bibliography

Agrofojo BA, Gibbs ACC, Langley FA: Histological discrimination of malignancy in mucinous ovarian tumors. *Histopathology* 1:431, 1977.

Arey LB: The origin and form of the Brenner tumor. *Am J Obstet Gynecol* 81:743, 1961.

Azoury RS, Woodruff JD: Primary ovarian sarcoma: report of 47 cases from the Emil Novak ovarian tumor registry. *Obstet Gynecol* 37:920, 1971.

Barber HRK, Graber EA: Gynecological tumors in childhood and adolescence. *Obstet Gynecol Surv* 28:357, 1973.

Barber HRK, Graber EA, Kwon T: *Ovarian Cancer* (monograph). American Cancer Society, Professional Education Publication, 1975, pp 2–21.

Fenoglio CM, Ferenczy A, Richart RM: Mucinous tumors of the ovary: ultrastructural studies of mucinous cystadenomas with histogenetic considerations. *Cancer* 36:1709, 1975.

Fox H, Langley FA: *Tumors of the Ovary*. Heinemann, London, 1976.

Gondos B: Electron microscopic study of papillary serous tumors of the ovary. *Cancer* 27:1455, 1971.

Gondos B: Surface epithelium of the developing ovary: possible correlation with ovarian neoplasia. *Am J Pathol* 81:303, 1973.

Hudson CN: Immunology and immunotherapy of ovarian cancer. *Ovarian Cancer Adv Biosci* 26:211, 1980.

Hudson CN (ed). *Ovarian Cancer*. Oxford, Oxford University Press, 1986.

Idelson MG: Malignancy in Brenner tumors of the ovary with comments on histogenesis and possibly estrogen production. *Obstet Gynecol Surv* 18:246, 1963.

Janovsky NA, Paramanandhan TL: *Ovarian Tumors: Tumors and Tumor-Like Conditions of the Fallopian Tubes and Ligaments of the Uterus*. Saunders, Philadelphia, 1973.

Julian CG, Woodruff JD: Low-grade papillary cystadenocarcinoma of the ovary. *Obstet Gynecol* 40:860, 1972.

Kolstad P: Prognostic indicators and staging. *Ovarian Cancer Adv Biosci* 26:67, 1980.

Long ME, Taylor HC Jr: Endometrioid carcinoma of the ovary. *Am J Obstet Gynecol* 90:936, 1964.

Long ME, Taylor HC Jr: Nucleolar variability in human neoplastic cells. *Ann NY Acad Sci* 63:1095, 1956.

Morris JM, Scully RE: *Endocrine Pathology of the Ovary*. Mosby, St. Louis, 1958.

Robey SG, Silva EG, Gerchenson DM, et al: Transitional cell carcinoma in high-grade, high-stage ovarian carcinoma. *Cancer* 63:839, 1989.

Sampson JA: Endometrial carcinoma of the ovary, arising in edometrial tissue in that organ. *Arch Surg* 10:1, 1923.

Santesson L: Cited By Kraus ET, *Ovarian Cancer*. Gynecologic Pathology. Mosby, St. Louis, 1967.

Santesson L, Kottmeier HL: General classification of ovarian tumors. In: Gentil F Janqueira AC (eds): *Ovarian Cancer*. UICC Monograph Series, Vol. II. Berlin, Springer-Verlag, 1968.

Scully RE: Ovarian tumors: a review. *Am J Pathol* 87:686, 1977.

Scully RE: Recent progress in ovarian cancer. *Hum Pathol* 1:73, 1970.

Serov SF, Scully RE, Sobin LH: Histological typing of ovarian tumors. In: *International Histological Classification of Tumors, No. 9*. WHO, Geneva, 1973.

Silverberg SG: Ultrastructure and histogenesis of clear cell carcinoma of the ovary. *Am J Obstet Gynecol* 115:394, 1973.

Teilum G: *Special Tumors of Ovary and Testis and Related Extragonadal Lesions*. Munksgaard, Copenhagen, 1971.

Teilum G, Albrechtsen R, Nogaro-Pederson B: Immunofluorescent localization of alpha-fetoprotein synthesis in endodermal sinus tumors (yolk sac tumors). *Acta Pathol Microbiol Scand* 82A:586, 1974.

Woodruff JD: The pathogenesis of ovarian neoplasia. *Johns Hopkins Med J* 144:117, 1979.

Young RH, Scully RE: Ovarian sex cord-stroma tumors: recent advances and current status. *Clin Obstet Gynecol* 11(4):93, 1984.

6

Histologic, Nuclear, and Stromal Grading

According to Decker and coworkers, within a given stage of ovarian epithelial carcinoma, regardless of the histologic cell type, the increasingly higher grades have an increasingly poorer prognosis. This finding suggests that more intensive therapy be considered for all patients with ovarian epithelial carcinomas than is currently undertaken. Decker also restated that epithelial ovarian cancer has always been difficult to treat successfully. The concept of a "scale of malignancy" was suggested by Virchow as long ago as 1858, but its application to ovarian carcinoma classification systems has not been implemented. Reports by Decker have demonstrated the value of grading tumors for prognostic significance, and the International Federation of Gynecology and Obstetrics (FIGO) has now recognized that grading has value in the classification of carcinoma of the endometrium. It is anticipated that increased attention will be directed to the grading of ovarian cancers. Barber and associates reported on histologic and nuclear grading and stromal reactions as indices for prognosis in ovarian cancer. That report provides the basis for this chapter.

Ovarian cancer is one of the most frustrating problems in gynecology. Each year about 21,000 new cases are diagnosed in the United States, and almost 13,000 patients die from ovarian cancer. The incidence comprises 24% of all gynecologic cancers, but the dramatic figure is that it causes more than 47% of gynecologic cancer deaths. The challenge presented is that the results in 1981 were no better than they were during the previous two decades. Early diagnosis, of which there is none, and prophylaxis, to which there is resistance, offer the only hope of improving the lot of these unfortunate patients. Until major advances are made in the areas of early diagnosis and treatment with predictable promise for cure, attention must be directed to the study of the natural history of the disease and its histologic patterns, cell type, and stromal reactions. This approach should further validate end results and in the future help improve the survival rate for those with ovarian carcinoma. This chapter explores the relations among the staging, grading, and stromal reactions of the tumors as they relate to survival.

In 1961 a committee of FIGO formulated a classification of common epithelial tumors of the ovary that was adopted in 1971. The World Health Organization (WHO) has also prepared an International Histologic Classification of Ovarian Tumors. WHO tried to conform to the classification of common epithelial tumors that was proposed by FIGO and subsequently used in publications from several large centers. Broad categories of tumors have been divided into numerous subtypes throughout the classification in order to stimulate the investigation of smaller and possibly distinctive groups as well as general classes. In addition to the epithelial ovarian tumors, the WHO classification includes germ cell tumors, hormone-producing tumors (gonadal stromal), and metastatic carcinomas. This classification is discussed in Chapter 4.

The patients treated during the early part of the study were staged in a retrospective manner based on physical examination, laboratory and pathology reports, and operative records. Although it provides an outline for comparison of material among medical centers, it has inherent weaknesses. Cases were included in the invasive group only if there is infiltrative destructive growth into the stroma, regardless of the extent of the proliferative activity of the epithelial cells and nuclear abnormalities. Because mucinous tumors are commonly both multilocular and parvilocular, it is often impossible to determine accurately whether glandular structures lying within the stroma are the result of budding from a larger gland or cyst or they indicate invasion of the stroma. In the study discussed in this chapter an attempt was made to determine if documentation of histologic and nuclear grading and of stromal response would help establish if these tumors are low-grade malignant.

Materials and Methods

The patients reported were those with epithelial ovarian cancers who were treated at Lenox Hill Hospital in New York from 1963 to 1973. During the early part of the study the treatment employed was removal of the cancer or as much as possible, if it could be done, without an inordinate amount of morbidity and death. During those years, postoperative pelvic and abdominal irradiation was added for those patients whose disease was not completely removed or for those considered to be at risk for recurrence because of the size of the tumor. In the last part of the study a protocol had evolved that served as the basis for treatment. Most of the patients were treated by a small

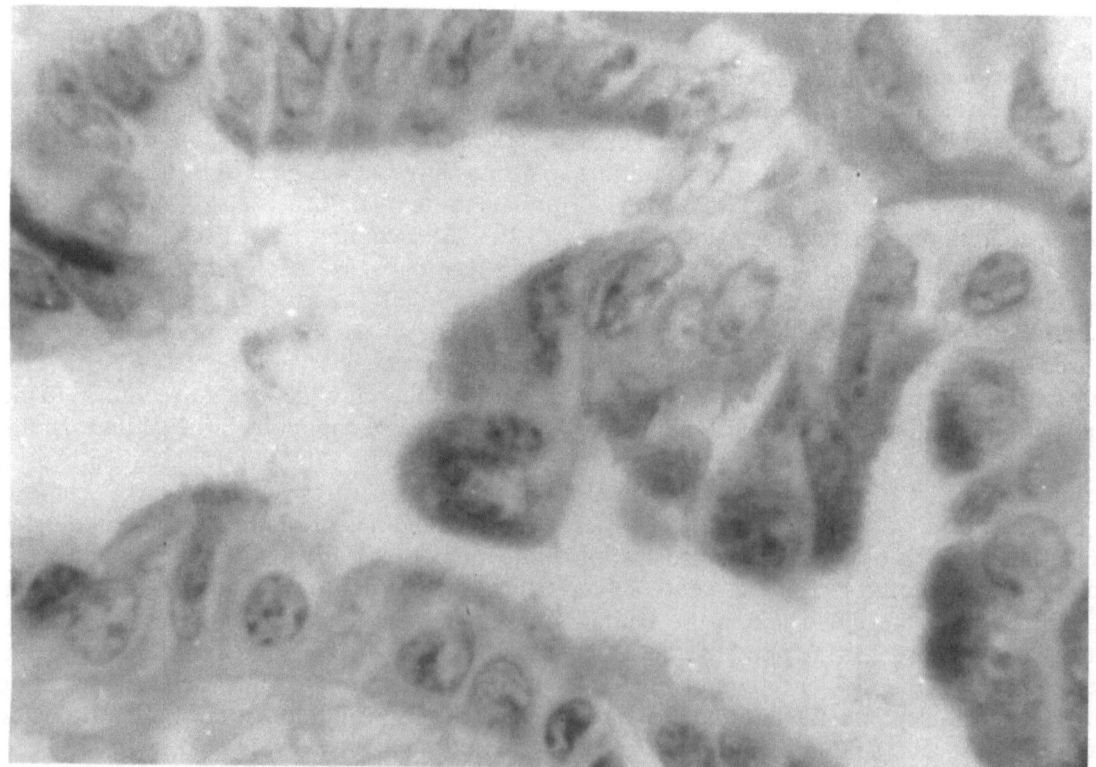

FIGURE 6.1. Grade I is the most highly differentiated cell type. The cells are fairly uniform, the nucleus is regular, and there is little increase in the number of nucleoli.

group of gynecologists and by only two radiation therapists. Currently, external x-ray therapy has been phased out, and chemotherapy is the adjuvant therapy employed.

Histologic Grading

The Broders classification, devised by A. C. Broders of the Mayo Clinic, consists of four numerical grades (I, II, III, IV) for both epidermoid carcinoma and adenocarcinoma of the cervix. It is the most commonly used classification in the United States. The basis for this classification is the well-known observation that the degree of malignancy keeps pace with the degree of cell differentiation; thus grade I is the most highly differentiated and grade IV the most immature.

The original Broders grading method was cumbersome, because as many as 13 cytologic characteristics had to be observed and evaluated. When estimating the grade of an epidermoid carcinoma, the following factors are recorded for each grade: epithelial pearls, individual keratinized cells, intercellular bridges, tumor giant cells, and mitosis per high-power field. It is obvious that pathologists differ in the weight they assign to each of these factors. One axiom in use is that a neoplasm is named from its most differentiated portion and graded from its least differentiated parts. Most pathologists now use a simplified version.

Ewing influenced many pathologists when he presented his material using only three grades. In Ewing's scheme, Broders' grades III and IV are combined and called grade III. It is this his-

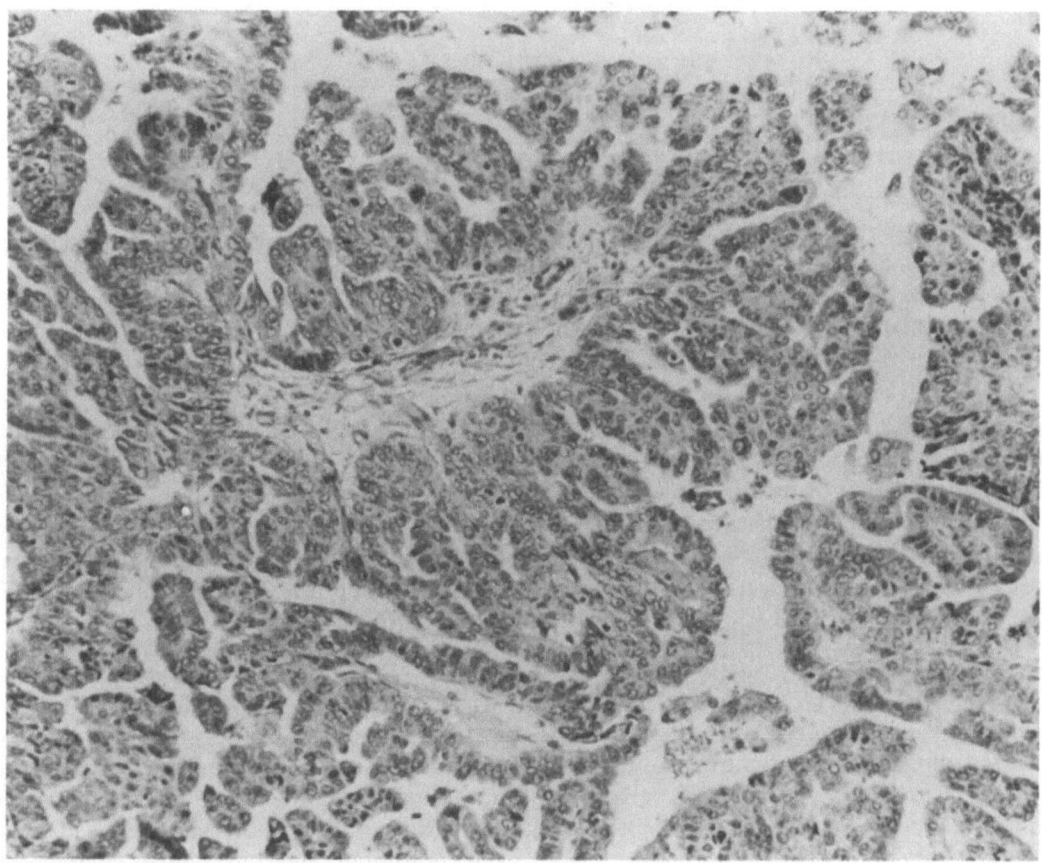

FIGURE 6.2. Grade II is intermediate between grade I, which is near normal, and grade III, in which the cells are immature.

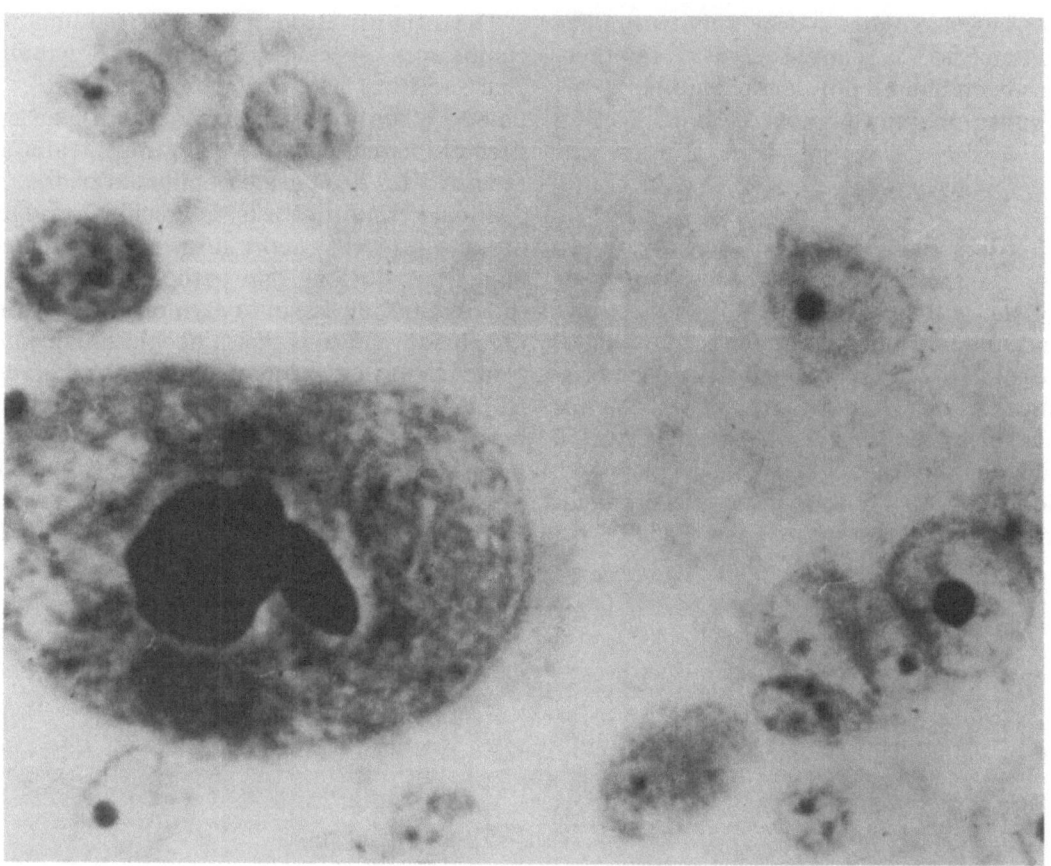

FIGURE 6.3. Grade III combines Broders' grades III and IV into one grade, grade III. In this grade the cells are immature and lack uniformity, the nucleus is irregular and enlarged, and the nucleus/cytoplasm ratio is altered so the nucleus makes up a large part of the cell. The number and size of the nucleoli are increased, as is the number of mitoses per high-power field.

tologic classification that is followed herein. It is based on (1) the uniformity or lack of uniformity of the cells; (2) whether the nucleus is regular; and (3) the nucleus/cytoplasm ratio, the number and size of the nucleoli, and the number of mitoses per high-power field (Fig. 6.1, 6.2, 6.3).

Nuclear Grade

The nuclei of the tumor cells were graded from 1 to 3 according to the classification of Black and Speer: grade 1—markedly enlarged, irregular in outline with chromatin clumping and prominent nucleoli; grade 2—intermediate degree of differentiation; grade 3—similar in size and appearance to each other and to normal ovarian tissue when present. It should be noted that with histologic grading the better differentiated tumors are grade I and the least differentiated grade III, whereas when grading the nuclei grade 1 is the most anaplastic and grade 3 the least anaplastic (Fig. 6.4, 6.5, 6.6).

Stromal Reactions

Chabon, Takeuchi, and Sommers employed a stromal evaluation method in a breast study, and we have adapted this method for grading the ovarian cancers in this study. The stroma of each epithelial ovarian cancer was graded according to the number of lymphocytes, plasma cells, and polymorphonuclear leukocytes

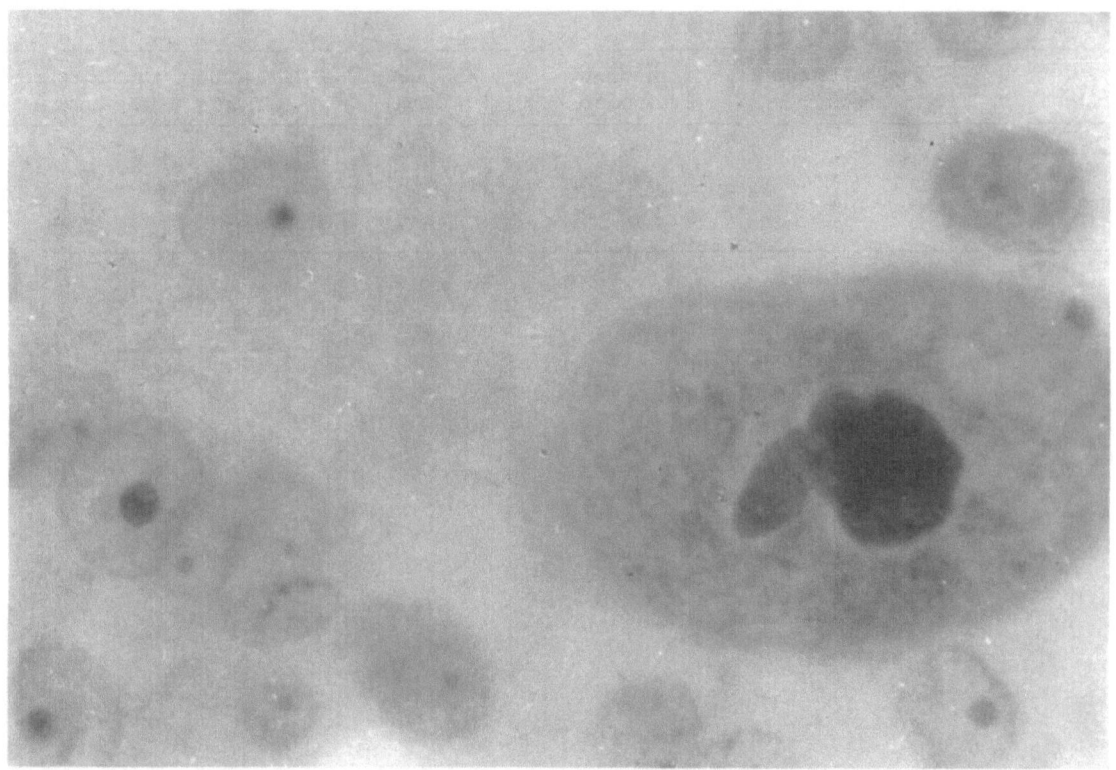

FIGURE 6.4. Nuclear grade 1 is characterized by nuclei that are markedly enlarged and irregular in outline, with chromatin clumping and prominent nucleoli. It is the most anaplastic grade.

present. Lymphocytes, plasma cells, and polymorphonuclear infiltration in the stroma and around small veins were graded 0 to 3: 0—none; 1—minimal; 2—moderate; and 3—marked (Fig. 6.7, 6.8, 6.9).

Results

The ovarian cancers studied were in 182 patients seen from 1963 to 1973. Eight patients were lost to follow-up, so only 174 could be followed for the entire study. However, five of the eight were available for 2 years of the study. Because therapy for and prognosis of ovarian cancer depend largely on the extent of disease and penetration of the capsule, all patients have been staged according to the stage grouping for primary epithelial cancer of the ovary as established by FIGO. The staging is discussed in Chapter 11. Although the major part of this chapter is related to prognosis relative to the findings of staging and grading, a discussion of the overall material is indicated. The type and number of epithelial cancers were as follows: serous 88, mucinous 26, endometrioid 38, clear cell 10, undifferentiated 20. The age distribution of the 182 patients is listed in Table 6.1.

Each slide was reviewed by a panel of pathologists consisting of not fewer than two or more than four members. If there was any disagreement about whether a tumor was invasive, or if discussion indicated that clear-cut criteria for cancer were not evident, the case was not included in the study. Many slides contained more than one cell type and were included in the group having the predominant histologic type.

The study included only patients with epithelial ovarian tumors who received their primary treatment at Lenox Hill Hospital. A few who had exploratory laparotomies and biopsies

TABLE 6.1. Age distribution of ovarian cancer

Parameter	Papillary serous cystadenocarcinoma	Mucinous cystadenocarcinoma	Endometrioid cancer	Clear cell cancer	Undifferentiated cancer
Mean age alive	54.6	51.9	50.5	58.3	64.0
Mean age dead	58.6	61.0	65.0	60.6	62.9
Total	57.4	56.9	59.5	59.9	63.1
Range	20–81	23–78	32–86	35–87	46–82

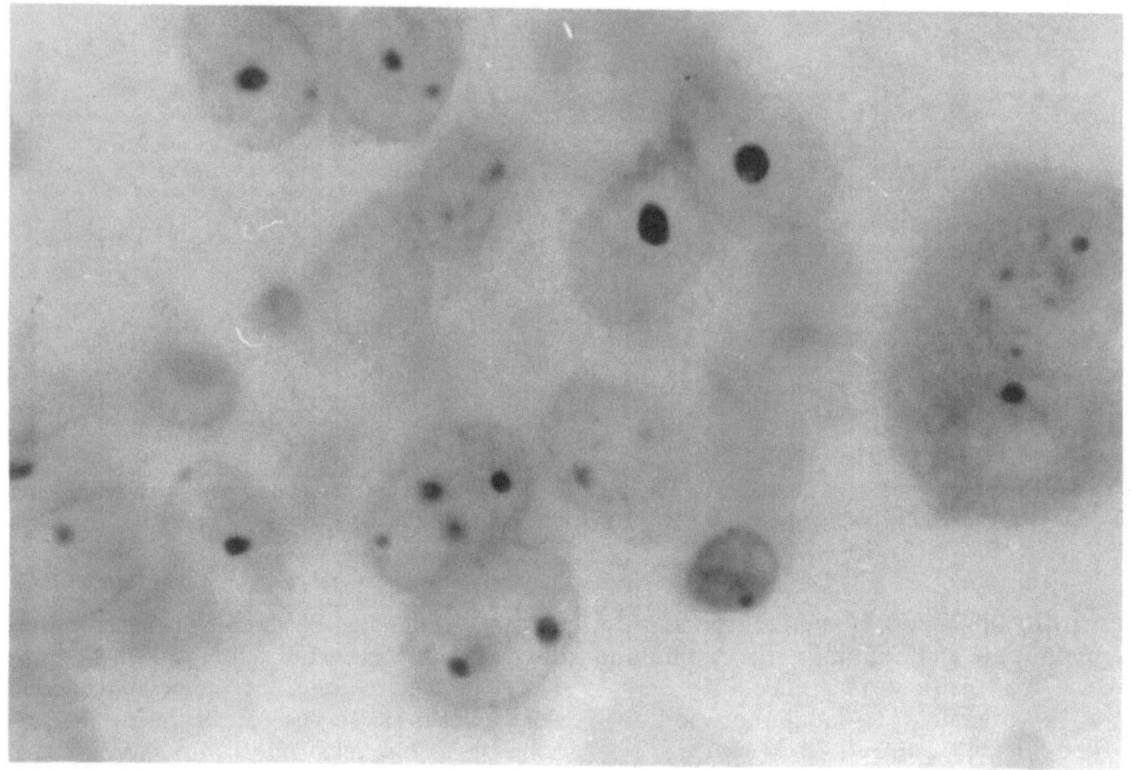

FIGURE 6.5. Nuclear grade 2 is intermediate in differentiation between grades 1 and 3.

elsewhere and were then referred on for definitive therapy are included as fresh cases. The patients with recurrent epithelial tumors that were referred for additional treatment as well as those with nonepithelial ovarian cancers are not included in this study.

Survival Related to Histologic and Nuclear Grading and Stromal Reaction

The histologic grades range from I to III, with III being the least differentiated; and the nu-clear grades range from 3 to 1, with 1 being the most anaplastic. The histologic and nuclear grades for serous cystadenocarcinoma are outlined in Table 6.2. Among those patients with histologic grades I and II, 29 were living at 2 years or more, and 23 died during this interval. In the group of patients with the less favorable histologic grade III, 5 of 30 were living at 2 years or more, and 25 were dead. There were 52 patients with the more favorable histologic grades I and II; among those with nuclear grades 3 and 2, there were 24 were living at 2

TABLE 6.2. Serous cystadenocarcinomas—all patients

Histologic grade	Nuclear grade	Stage I			Stage II		Stage III	Stage IV	Total
		IA	IB	IC	IIA	IIB			
I	3	2	2	1				(1)	5 (1)
	2	2 (1)					1		3 (1)
	1								
II	3						1		1
	2	3	1	(1)	3 (1)	1	6 (9)	1 (3)	15 (14)
	1	3 (1)			(1)		2 (2)	(3)	5 (7)
III	3								
	2				1 (1)		(6)	(3)	1 (10)
	1		2		1 (1)		1 (8)	(6)	4 (15)
Total		16 (3)			6 (4)		11 (25)	1 (16)	34 (48)

Patients in parentheses were dead at 2 years. Six were lost to follow-up and not included.

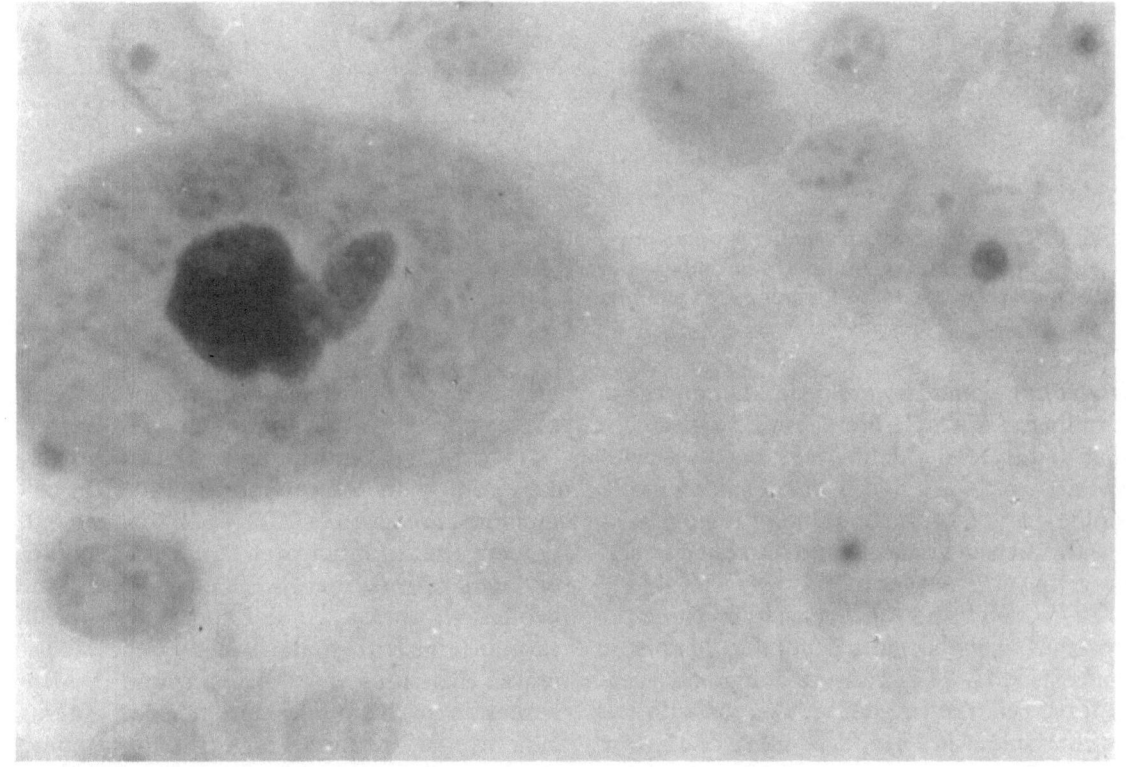

FIGURE 6.6. Nuclear grade 3 is characterized by nuclei that are of similar size and appearance, and similar to nuclei of normal ovarian tissue, when present.

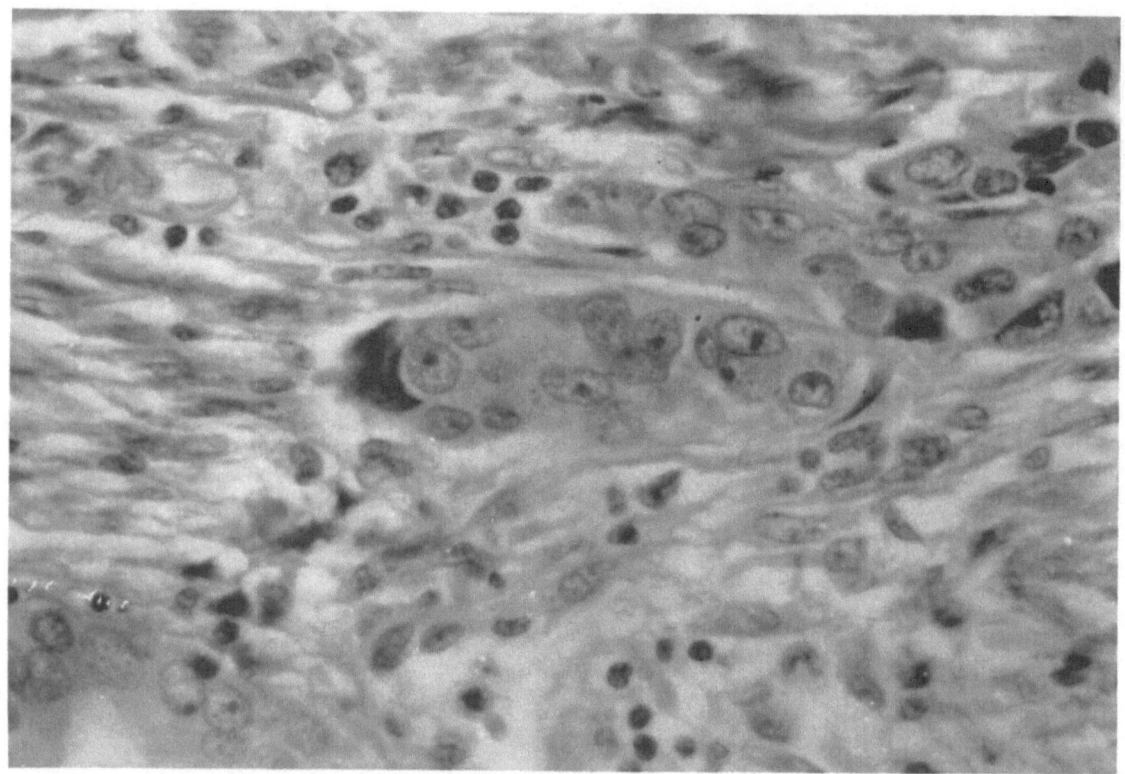

FIGURE 6.7. Lymphocytes, plasma cells, and poly-morphonuclear infiltration in the stroma and around small veins were graded 0 to 3 = none; 1 = minimal (Fig. 6.7); 2 = moderate (Fig. 6.8); and 3 = marked (Fig. 6.9).

years or more, and 16 were dead. Among those with nuclear grade 1, there were 5 who were living and 7 dead. There were no cases with favorable nuclear grade 3 in the unfavorable histologic grade III group. One of ten and 4 of 15 with nuclear grades 2 and 1, respectively, were living at 2 years or more.

The endometrioid cancers listed in Table 6.3 show that with the more favorable histologic grades I and II, 14 of 26 were living at 2 years or more, and 12 were dead; whereas with the less favorable histologic grade III, 2 of 12 were living at 2 years or more, and 10 were dead. With histologic grades I and II, 20 of 26 patients had nuclear grades 2 and 3; 11 were living at 2 years or more, and 10 were dead. With nuclear grade 1, there were 3 of 5 patients living, and 2 were dead. With the less favorable histologic grade III there were no cases with the favorable nuclear grade 3. Of 12 patients

with nuclear grades 2 and 1, there were 2 living at 2 years or more, and 10 were dead.

The results in mucinous cystadenocarcinoma, undifferentiated carcinoma, and clear cell carcinoma are listed in Tables 6.4, 6.5, and 6.6, respectively. As anticipated among the undifferentiated cancers, there were no cases with the favorable histologic grade I and none with the favorable nuclear grade 3 among the 20 patients. This study did not determine if documentation of histologic and nuclear grading and stromal response might help establish whether a given mucinous carcinoma is of low-grade malignancy. However, among the 24 cases, only one had the less favorable histologic grade III and only two had the unfavorable nuclear grade 1, results suggesting that these tumors are less aggressive than the other epithelial ovarian cancers.

The stromal reaction is reported in Table

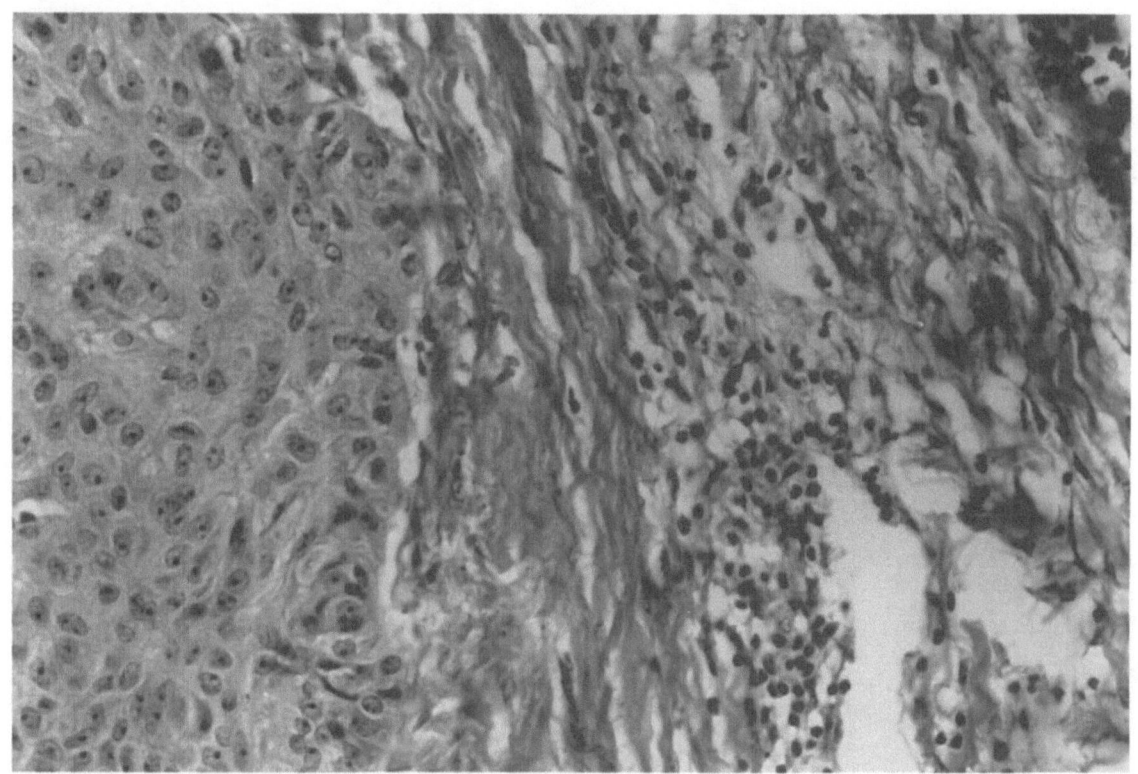

FIGURE 6.8. Moderate infiltration. (See legend to Figure 6.7.)

TABLE 6.3. Endometrioid cancers—all cases

Histologic grade	Nuclear grade	Stage I			Stage II		Stage III	Stage IV	Total
		IA	IB	IC	IIA	IIB			
I	3	1					(1)	(1)	1 (2)
	2	1							1
	1								
II	3								
	2	4	1 (1)				4 (4)	(3)	9 (8)
	1	1					1 (1)	1 (1)	3 (2)
III	3								
	2						(4)	(1)	(5)
	1	2					(3)	(2)	2 (5)
Total			10 (1)		0 (0)		5 (13)	1 (8)	16 (22)

Patients in parentheses were dead at 2 years.

6.7. Among those dead before 2 years, 23 had no lymphocytes and 61 no plasma cells. It should be noted that there is overlap among these groups because some patients had neither lymphocytes nor plasma cells in their stroma. Of those patients living 2 years or more, 15 had no lymphocytes in their stroma and 45 had no plasma cells. An evaluation of Table 6.7

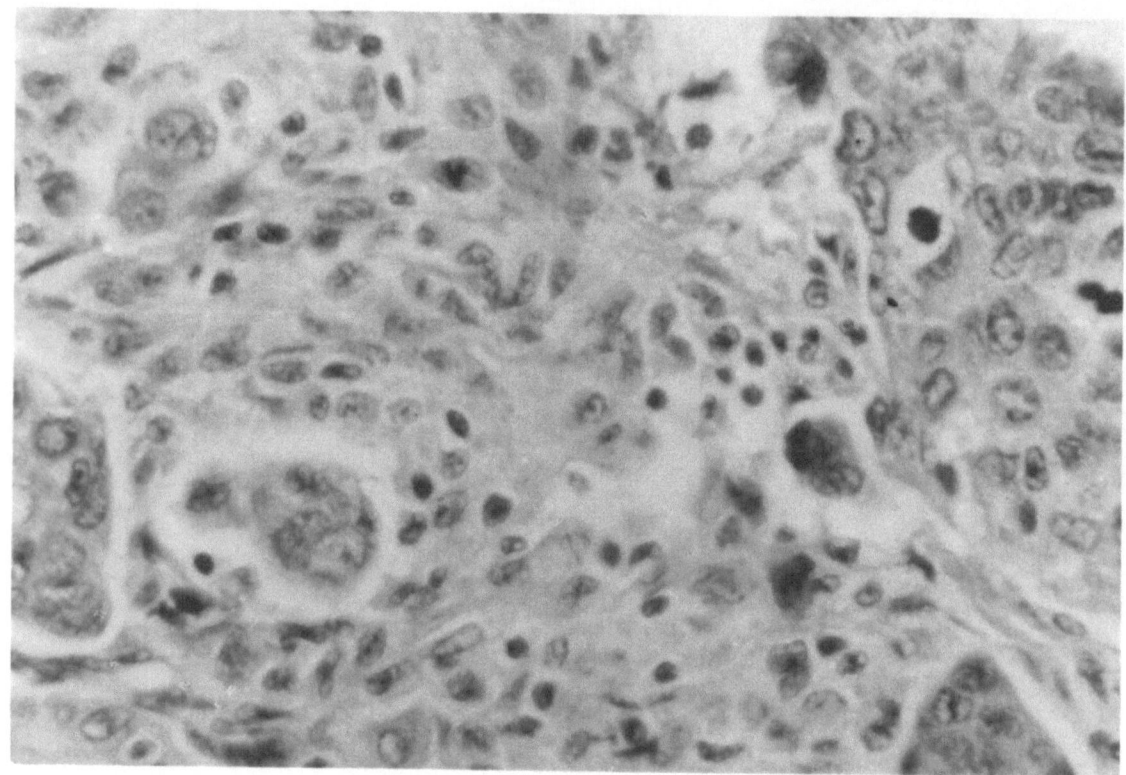

FIGURE 6.9. Marked infiltration. (See legend to Figure 6.7.)

TABLE 6.4. Mucinous cystadenocarcinoma

Histologic grade	Nuclear grade	Stage I			Stage II		Stage III	Stage IV	Total
		IA	IB	IC	IIA	IIB			
I	3	2			1			1	4
	2	3					1		3 (1)
	1	1							1
II	3						1 (1)		1 (1)
	2	3				(1)	2 (3)	(2)	5 (6)
	1	1							1
III	3								
	2							(1)	(1)
	1								
Total		9			1 (1)		4 (5)	1 (3)	15 (9)

Patients in parentheses were dead at 2 years. Two were lost to follow-up and not included.

shows that in the early stages there was less combined lymphocyte and plasma cell reaction than in the more advanced stages. Although stromal reaction with lymphocytes and plasma cells is considered a favorable reaction, the results in this series did not bear out this observation. There may be other factors that are more important, or perhaps the ovary does not

TABLE 6.5. Undifferentiated carcinoma—all cases

Histologic grade	Nuclear grade	Stage I			Stage II		Stage III	Stage IV	Total
		IA	IB	IC	IIA	IIB			
I	3								
	2								
	1								
II	3								
	2								(1)
	1				(1)				
III	3								
	2	(1)					(2)		(3)
	1				(1)	(1)	2 (4)	(8)	2 (14)
Total		(1)			(2)	(1)	2 (6)	0 (8)	2 (18)

Patients in parentheses were dead at 2 years.

TABLE 6.6. Clear-cell carcinoma

Histologic grade	Nuclear grade	Stage I			Stage II		Stage III	Stage IV	Total
		IA	IB	IC	IIA	IIB			
I	3	(1)							(1)
	2	1							1
	1								
II	3								
	2				(1)	1			1 (1)
	1			(1)			1 (1)		1 (2)
III	3								
	2			(1)					(1)
	1						(2)		(2)
Total		1 (1)		(2)	(1)	1	1 (3)	0 (0)	3 (7)

Patients in parentheses were dead at 2 years.

attract lymphocytes and plasma cells to the degree that tumors in other organs do, at least in the early stages. The number of cases may not be sufficient to permit study of the stromal reaction, but in a group this size it is anticipated that the heterogenicity of the immune state should indicate that the body defenses are active. The lack of documentation may be attributable to the failure of the ovary to mobilize its immune defense as rapidly as defenses are mobilized in breast cancer. However, the stromal reaction among the ovarian cancers did increase with the stage of disease. Although the stromal reaction was minimal during the early stages when each histologic type was grouped together (stages I through IV), marked lymphocyte, plasma cell, and stromal reactions were observed.

Certain observations can be made from Tables 6.4 through 6.7. The greatest number of survivals were of patients with the more favorable histologic grades I and II and the more favorable nuclear grades 3 and 2. The least anaplastic histologic and nuclear grades are found in the early stages and the more anaplastic tumors in the more advanced stages. The correlation is particularly evident among the undifferentiated tumors. In this group the fact

TABLE 6.7. Stromal reactions (overall)

Stromal reactions	No. of reactions, by stage							Total
	IA	IB	IC	IIA	IIB	III	IV	
Lymphocytes								
0	7 (2)	1 (1)	(2)	(2)	1	5 (13)	1 (3)	15 (23)
1+	21 (1)	3	(1)	3 (2)	1	10 (26)	1 (17)	39 (47)
2+	2 (1)	2	1	3 (2)	(2)	7 (13)	1 (15)	16 (33)
3+				(1)				(1)
Plasma cells								
0	22 (4)	4 (1)	(3)	3 (4)	2	12 (32)	2 (17)	45 (61)
1+	6	1	1	(1)	(1)	3 (8)	(9)	11 (19)
2+	2	1		3 (2)	(1)	6 (9)	1 (9)	13 (21)
3+						1 (3)		1 (3)
Polymorphonuclear leukocytes								
0	24 (4)	5 (1)	1 (2)	6 (5)	2 (2)	18 (37)	2 (35)	58 (86)
1+	4	1	(1)	(1)		2 (10)		7 (12)
2+	2			(1)		2 (4)	1	7 (5)
3+						(1)		(1)
Total	90 (12)	18 (3)	3 (9)	18 (21)	6 (6)	66 (156)	9 (105)	210 (312)

Patients in parentheses were dead at 2 years.

that there were no cases in the favorable histologic grade I or favorable nuclear grade 3 confirmed the malignant potential of this histologic type. Although the histologic and nuclear grades and stromal reaction added little to determining the degree of malignancy for a given mucinous cancer, the grading and stromal reaction did indicate that as a group the mucinous cancers are less aggressive tumors than the other epithelial ovarian cancers. For the common epithelial ovarian tumors, grading correlated with prognosis during the early stages but was less reliable for the more advanced cancers. There were differences in the malignant potential among cancers in the same stage of disease.

Our results parallel those reported by Decker. He presented his material by graph for each stage, grouping the tumors into grades 1, 2, and 3. He commented that the importance of grading tumors to date has been controversial. Analysis of the data presented by him supports the following conclusions: (1) All epithelial ovarian carcinomas are equally lethal when compared by stage and grade. (2) The low-grade tumors become increasingly lethal as the stage increases. (3) High-grade, low-stage tumors should be treated differently from low-grade, low-stage tumors. (4) When therapy is uniform within a stage, grading is of prognostic value to both patient and physician. In general, mucinous cystadenocarcinomas and endometrioid adenocarcinomas tend to be low grade and low stage, and serous cystadenocarcinomas and solid adenocarcinomas tend to be high grade, high stage. In the past when tumors were evaluated only by histologic features without regard to stage and grade, greater malignant potential was erroneously attributed to a tumor type. Decker's conclusions are summarized in the following paragraphs. We agree with his conclusions.

We have included a fourth category—the "solid" tumor—in our evaluation of epithelial ovarian tumors. This tumor probably represents one of the other three that has been prolific enough to have obliterated any cystic component.

These studies from the literature and results of the present analysis indicate that valid and reliable evaluation of ovarian carcinoma cannot be achieved unless both grade and stage are considered. A specific, carefully performed staging regimen should be adhered to. The extent of peritoneal involvement, nodal involvement, subdiaphragmatic surface status, and peritoneal cytology also should be noted carefully at the initial surgery. Such detailed analysis probably would (1) lead to the finding of more high-stage lesions, (2) explain some of the poor results with low-stage lesions, and (3) lead to more appropriate treatment than has heretofore been offered to these patients.

Histologic grading of tumors should be routine, and such grading would have significant prognostic value regardless of the stage or histologic cell type, especially when the lesion is a low-stage lesion. If the criteria specified by Malloy and colleagues are applied strictly, the borderline lesion category should be eliminated. A useful addition to the FIGO classification is grading by either the Broders scale or a similar grading system with designations by stage, substage, and grade. Once this type of classification has been adopted, the effectiveness of therapeutic modalities can be compared within an institution and among institutions.

The histologic type of the tumor has been included in the FIGO classification in which the common epithelial tumors of the ovary are concerned. The serous, mucinous, and endometrioid lesions are well defined. The unclassified group—the group we designated "solid" lesions—represents one of the other groups of epithelial malignancies that has lost its structural identification, which is consistent with the finding of more higher-grade lesions in this category.

The data presented here show that, in general, low grade is associated with low stage and that more mucinous and endometrioid lesions than serous or solid lesions are low grade and low stage. Furthermore, if serous and mucinous lesions are compared stage for stage and grade for grade, they are of equal lethal potential. There were insufficient data to develop such comparisons for the endometrioid or solid lesions. The data suggest that more intensive treatment than is currently being given for stage I disease is indicated for all histologic cell types when the lesion is other than FIGO stage

1A, Broders' grade 1, intracystic, nonruptured, nonadherent, and without extracystic excrescences.

Our current approach to therapy of all epithelial ovarian carcinomas is dictated by the stage and, in some instances, by the grade of the lesion. For lesions of stage IA/grade 1, that are intracystic, nonadherent, and nonruptured, a unilateral oophorectomy with biopsy of the contralateral ovary may be offered if childbearing is important. Otherwise, total abdominal hysterectomy and bilateral salpingo-oophorectomy (TAH-BSO) with omentectomy, without further therapy, are done. For all other stage I lesions, TAH-BSO with omentectomy are performed, followed by intraperitoneal radioisotopes or chemotherapy for 6 months, depending on the specific situation.

For stage II disease, TAH-BSO with omentectomy are performed, followed by 12 months of therapy with an alkylating agent. Reexploration is performed at 12 months; and if the patient is clinically free of disease and absence of disease is confirmed, chemotherapy is stopped. If disease is demonstrated, chemotherapy is continued.

For stages III and IV disease, treatment involves TAH-BSO with omentectomy and removal of as much tumor as possible. These procedures were originally followed by chemotherapy with an alkylating agent and after 1979 with combination intravenous anticancer chemotherapy. If the patient is clinically free of disease, and if it is confirmed at reexploration at 6 to 9 months, one more treatment is given in the hospital and then therapy is stopped. Demonstrated disease by clinical or laboratory methods warrants further chemotherapy. Patients who do not respond to first-line drugs are then shifted to a second line of combination chemotherapy.

Thus concludes the report by Decker.

Cases Grouped Together: Stages I–IV

An overall view is possible by grouping together the cases from stages I through IV in order to study the percentage of histologic and nuclear grades and stromal reaction within each type of epithelial ovarian cancer (Table

TABLE 6.8. All stages

Cancer	Histologic grade						Nuclear grade						Stromal reaction			
	I		II		III		1		2		3		Lymphocytes + plasma cells (L+P+)		Polymorpho-nuclear leukocytes (P+)	
	No.	%	No.	%	No.	%	No.	%	No.	%	No.	%	No.	%	No.	%
Clear cell carcinoma	2	20	5	50	3	30	5	50	4	40	1	10	4	40	1	10
Undifferentiated carcinoma			1	5	19	95	16	80	4	20			17	85	3	15
Serous cyst-adenocarcinoma	10	12	42	51	30	37	32	39	43	52	7	9	65	79	13	16
Endometrioid carcinoma	4	11	22	58	12	32	12	32	23	61	3	8	30	79	3	8
Mucinous cystadeno-carcinoma	9	38	14	58	1	4	2	8	16	67	6	25	18	75	5	21

6.7). Thus there are enough cases to study serous cystadenocarcinoma and endometrioid carcinoma. The percentage distribution by histologic grade, nuclear grade, and stromal reaction are similar. In each instance, histologic grade II and nuclear grade 2 account for 51 to 61% of the cancers. From the data in Table 6.8, it is not possible to determine if the nuclear and histologic grades are closely correlated for a given case.

Relatively speaking, mucinous cystadenocarcinoma was characterized by the greatest percentage of highly differentiated tumors (38% histologic grade I and 25% nuclear grade 3).

The relation of stage, histologic grade, nuclear grade, and stromal reaction in short-term survivors compared with longer-term survivors was reviewed in the two groups with the more adequate sample sizes: serous cystadenocarcinoma ($n = 88$) and endometrioid carcinoma ($n = 38$). There were only three survivors with endometrioid carcinoma at 5 years, and thus detailed study of multiple prognostic factors was impossible.

When the 88 patients were divided into subgroups by stage of disease, neither histologic grade, nuclear grade, nor stromal reaction, when analyzed independently, is significantly predictive of long-term survival (5 years or more). When the cases are grouped together, however, grading did correlate with prognosis.

Life-Table Method for Analyzing Survival

Table 6.9 summarizes the material from this study. The direct method for calculating a survival rate does not utilize all information available. The actuarial, or life-table, method utilizes all survival information accumulated up to the closing date of the study and describes the manner in which the patient group was depleted during the total period of observation. This method provides a better insight into the nature of the disease and the effect of therapy than does one specified endpoint. For example, the overall 5-year survival by the direct method does not tell whether all patients died at 1 year or 4 years or by a fixed percentage rate for each year during the 5-year period. However, with the life-table method it is obvious that of the patients who died after treatment, most were dead at 2 years. The number alive between 5 and 10 years is not appreciably different from the percentage surviving 5 years.

Figure 6.10 shows the survival rates for stages I through IV, including the entire group

TABLE 6.9. Computation of the 5-year survival rate and standard error

Years after treatment	Alive at beginning of treatment	Died during interval	Lost to follow-up	Withdrawn alive during interval	Effective no. exposed to risk of dying	Proportions dying	Proportion surviving	Cumulative proportion surviving[a]
0–1	182	68	3	2	179.5	0.379	0.621	0.621
1–2	109	32	2	2	107.0	0.2990	0.701	0.435
2–3	73	3	3	10	66.5	0.045	0.955	0.416
3–4	57	6	0	10	52.0	0.115	0.855	0.355
4–5	41	1	0	6	38.0	0.026	0.974	0.346
5–6	34	3	0	6	31.0	0.097	0.903	0.313
6–7	25	2	0	4	23.0	0.087	0.913	0.285
7–8	19	1	0	2	18.0	0.056	0.944	0.269
8–9	16	0	0	9	11.5	0.000	1.00	0.269
9–10	7	0	0	2	6.0	0.000	1.00	0.269

[a] Cumulative proportion surviving from beginning of treatment through end of interval.

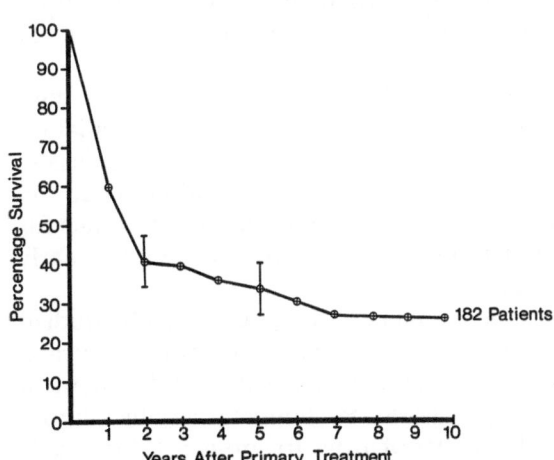

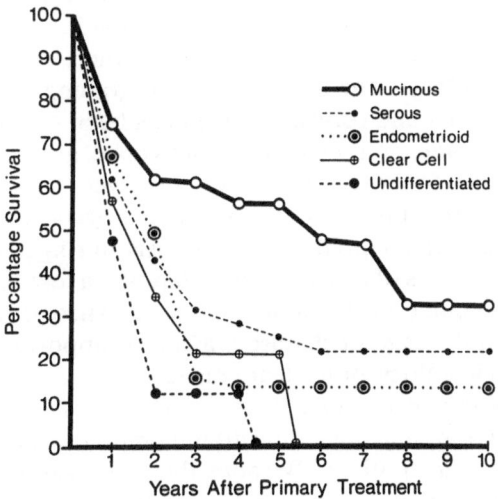

FIGURE 6.10. Survival for all stages, with 95% confidence limits expressed at 2 and 5 years.

FIGURE 6.11. Survival for all stages according to life-table analysis of survival.

of 182 patients. The survival rate at 2 years is 43.5% and the standard error ±3.7%. The survival rate at 5 years is 34.6% and the standard error ±3.7%. When the standard error is multiplied by 2, and when this number in each instance is added and subtracted from the survival rates at 2 years (±7.3%) and 5 years (±7.2%), respectively, the 95% confidence limit is established. Enough cases were studied at 2 and 5 years to allow us to make a valid statement about the findings. Figure 6.11 summarizes the survival time for each group of epithelial tumors according to the life table method of analyzing survival rates.

Comment

The main problem in ovarian cancer is early diagnosis. At present, early diagnosis is a matter of chance rather than a scientific method. However, until such methods are available it is important to study the natural history of the disease by all means available. By accumulating material from many investigators treated by a variety of methods, some progress may be achieved in salvaging additional patients.

It is obvious that interpretation of data is difficult and limited by the small numbers from any one series. However, as the material accumulates and is reported according to stage, grade, and histologic criteria that are universally acceptable, a meaningful and profitable study will result. The acceptance and use of the clinical staging and histologic classification established by WHO and FIGO have helped compare therapeutic results among institutions around the world. It has led to greater insight into the natural history of ovarian cancer, resulting in a more rational approach to therapy with anticipated improved results. In addition, careful grading of the tumor for both epithelial elements and stroma should validate the results.

The material reviewed indicates that staging and grading are both important and should be used to establish therapy. It is obvious that they are not competitive but, rather, complementary. The importance of grading endometrial and cervical cancers has been established and accepted, but a universal grading system for ovarian cancer has yet to be adopted. This study shows that the grade was important for predicting prognosis during the early stages of ovarian cancer but was a less reliable guide for the more advanced cancers. In general, stage of disease was more important than histologic or nuclear grades.

Within each stage there is a great deal of variation, making it difficult to compare results among institutions. Because there are varying degrees of malignancy in groups of a particular stage, it is important to examine tumor tissues microscopically to determine their grade or degree of malignancy according to the histologic and nuclear grade as well as the stromal reaction. Staging is determined clinically and estimates the extent of the disease and the size of the tumor, whereas histologic type and grading provide its microscopic character. The present study has indicated that in any stage there is considerable variation, and it is suggested that certain tumors are more potent than others within a given stage. Accepting this finding as valid, treatment should be tailored to the cancer rather than to the stage of disease.

Host resistance is considered an important factor in cancer control. It can be studied by examining the lymphocytes and plasma cells that infiltrate the area where the tumor is growing. A marked lymphocyte and plasma cell response is interpreted as the body's mounting a defense against the tumor. For certain tumors, especially breast cancer, this situation has been repeatedly confirmed. In the present series the lymphocytes and plasma cells were not as numerous as anticipated with stage I lesions, especially as this stage had the best survival rate. However, the number of lymphocytes and plasma cells increased as the disease became more advanced, which may indicate that the tumor has to grow to a certain volume or a certain potency before it can stimulate a local immune response. If a correlation is observed between lymphocytic and plasma cell response and long-term survival when large series are accumulated, perhaps immunotherapy can be employed to stimulate an immune response of this type.

The histologic grade remained fairly constant in a given tumor, and cell differentiation suggested the degree of malignancy, especially in the early stages. Classification based on tumor grade provided a satisfactory means for the determination of prognosis in the early stages.

Large numbers of subgroups must be studied for many years before there is enough information to make a statistically valid statement about prognosis. By lumping variables into a small number of arbitrary groups, a statistically significant number of patients can be amassed for study in each group. However, the information on a single or individual factor is lost. To study a great number of variables in a small group of patients as presented here would be statistically invalid. It is difficult for any one institution to accumulate a large number of untreated ovarian cancers. Generally, when cases from various institutions are pooled there are so many variables that findings become useless in terms of adapting therapy for a given stage and grade of ovarian cancer. Not infrequently, within each institution treatment is subject to change during any given 5-year period. However, as the microscopic criteria become more widely accepted and groups of institutions agree to work from a common protocol, some of the confusion will be resolved. In this way meaningful statistics with multiple variables will be available to guide clinicians in their management of ovarian cancer. Documentation of the histologic and nuclear grades and the stromal reaction adds another parameter for establishing treatment.

Summary

Among the prerequisites for comparative studies of cancer, particularly ovarian cancer, are international agreement on histologic criteria for the classification of cancer types and a standardized nomenclature. An internationally agreed upon classification of ovarian tumors acceptable to gynecologists, pathologists, radiologists, and statisticians would enable workers in ovarian cancer in all parts of the world to compare their findings, thereby promoting collaboration.

It was mutually agreed by a committee appointed by the WHO to have three separate classifications: (1) anatomic site; (2) histologic type; and (3) degree of malignancy. In 1963 the WHO International Reference Center for Histological Classification of Ovarian Tumors was established.

It is obvious that the classification will require study and modification as experience accumulates. Although there is disagreement on certain points, it provides an overall classification and a starting point for an internationally agreed upon classification of tumors. The classification is based primarily on the microscopic characteristics of the tumors and thus reflects the nature of morphologically identifiable cell types and patterns. Previously used and widely accepted terms have usually been retained, unless they were considered to be seriously misleading. Occasionally, it was necessary to adopt controversial histogenetic designations when they were the most convenient terms available. WHO has made an effort to conform to the classification of common epithelial ovarian tumors proposed by FIGO and used by many of the large centers. The classification has subdivisions to include the obviously benign and the obviously malignant tumors, as well as a large group of potentially malignant (borderline) tumors. WHO has expanded the classification to include germ cell tumors, gonadal stromal tumors, gonadoblastomas, tumors not specific for the ovary, unclassified tumors, and secondary metastatic tumors.

The material in this chapter directs itself to the histologic and nuclear grading and stromal reactions as indices for prognosis in ovarian cancer. The neoplasm was named from its most differentiated portion and graded from its least differentiated parts.

It was observed that certain tumors are more potent than others within a given stage and that undifferentiated cancers were generally in the unfavorable histologic grades. Studies at Lenox Hill Hospital determined that it was in the best interest of the patient to tailor the treatment to the cancer rather than to have a standard treatment for a given stage of ovarian cancer. Although the histologic grade and nuclear grade are important for determining prognosis, stage of disease was the most important parameter.

The use of life-table analysis, particularly the slope of the curve as opposed to the relative 5-year survival result, is a significant advance. This slope-survival comparison is most important when studying the results of various therapeutic modalities in the management of ovarian cancer.

A plan for standardizing the parameters used for studying ovarian cancer should be proposed and adopted. The editors of the journals could insist on a common method of representing data. By accumulating material from many investigators using the same parameters for their studies, some progress may be achieved in salvaging additional patients.

A new ISGYP-WHO classification of tumors derived from the ovaries will be published with definitions, explanatory notes, and illustrations as part of the Springer *WHO Classification Series*.

Bibliography

Barber HRK, Sommers SC, Snyder R, Kwon T: Histologic and nuclear grading and stromal reactions as indices for prognosis in ovarian cancer. *Am J Obstet Gynecol* 121:795, 1975.

Broders AC: Carcinoma: grading and practical application. *Arch Pathol* 2:376, 1926.

Chabon AB, Takeuchi SJ, Sommers SC: Histologic

differences in breast carcinoma of Japanese and American women. Cancer 33:1577, 1974.

Decker DG, Malkasian GD, Jr, Taylor WF: Prognostic importance of histologic grading in ovarian cancer: symposium on ovarian carcinoma. *J Natl Cancer Inst Monogr* 42:1, 1975.

Dyson JL, Beilby JO, Steele SJ: Factors influencing survival in carcinoma of the ovary. *Br J Cancer* 25:237, 1971.

Long ME, Sommers SC: Staging, grading and histochemistry of ovarian epithelial tumors. *Clin Obstet Gynecol* 12:937, 1969.

Long ME, Taylor HC Jr: Nucleolar variability in human neoplastic cells. *Ann NY Acad Sci* 63:1095, 1956.

Malkasian GD Jr, Decker DG, Webb MJ: Histology of epithelial tumors of the ovary: clinical useful-ness and prognostic significance of the histologic classification and grading. *Semin Oncol* 2:191, 1975.

Malloy JJ, Dooherty MB, Welch JS, Hunt HB: Papillary ovarian tumors: I Benign tumors and serous and mucinous cystadenocarcinomas. *Am J Obstet Gynecol* 93:867, 1965.

Report presented by the Cancer Committee to the General Assembly of FIGO: New York, April 1970. *Int J Gynecol Obstet* 9:172, 1971.

Silverberg E: *Gynecologic Cancer: Statistical and Epidemiological Information.* Professional Education Publication. American Cancer Society, Atlanta, 1975.

Sommers SC, Long ME: Ovarian carcinoma: pathology, staging, grading and prognosis. *Bull NY Acad Med* 49:858, 1973.

7

Symptoms, Signs, and Diagnosis

It is commonly stated that ovarian malignancies are frequently asymptomatic; subjective complaints occur only after complications arise or, in the case of carcinoma, after dissemination is widespread. Therefore it is accepted that of all aspects of ovarian cancer the symptomatology is the least satisfactory. If there are no early symptoms of malignant ovarian tumors, this fact is partly responsible for the poor results achieved, because one of the important factors in prognosis in ovarian cancer is the extent of disease at the time of treatment. Specific symptoms depend on the size, location, and type of tumor, as well as on such complicating factors as torsion, hemorrhage, infection, or rupture. Among the germ cell or gonadal stromal tumors, symptoms may relate to the hormone secreted by the tumor.

The usual presenting symptoms of patients with ovarian cancer are pain or discomfort, abdominal swelling, abnormal uterine bleeding, and gastrointestinal and urinary complaints. Unfortunately, these symptoms and signs appear late.

The insidious onset of ovarian cancer needs no elaboration. It is time, however, to change the generally accepted notion that there are no early symptoms of ovarian cancer. Symptomatology includes vague abdominal discomfort, dyspepsia, increasing flatulence, a sense of bloating, particularly after ingesting food, mild digestive disturbances, and pelvic unrest that may be present for several months before diagnosis. Unfortunately for the patient, a workup at the time, including a gastrointestinal series or a barium enema, often reveals no definitive information. Continued symptoms without a definite diagnosis frustrates both patient and doctor. All too often the patient is considered a middle-aged crock who goes to too many cocktail parties and eats too many hors d'oeuvres. Thus many ovarian cancers are nurtured in a sea of bicarbonate of soda and antacids. It is imperative therefore to rule out ovarian cancer in women over age 40 who present with persistent gastrointestinal symptoms that cannot be definitely diagnosed. In terms of function it must be emphasized that a variety of paraendocrine effects, such as hypercalcemia, hypoglycemia, and Cushing syndrome, as well as disorders such as hemolytic anemia, may be related, though rarely, to the presence of an ovarian tumor.

The peak incidence of the common epithelial ovarian cancer in women is at about age 77 years. The ovary may become too old to function, but it is never too old to form tumors. Women at high risk usually have a long history of ovarian imbalance or dysfunction, including increased premenstrual tension, heavy menstruation with marked breast tenderness, a tendency for spontaneous abortion, infertility, and nulliparity, as well as an early menopause. The ovary is like a cam running off center.

I have established a triad that serves as a guide for making an early diagnosis of ovarian cancer.

1. Patients over age 40 are in the high risk group to develop ovarian cancer.

2. There is a history of ovarian dysfunction characterized by increased premenstrual tension, heavy menstruation with marked breast tenderness, a tendency to spontaneous abortion, infertility, and nulliparity, and an early menopause.
3. The patient has vague abdominal discomfort and mild digestive symptoms that persist, including dyspepsia, flatulence, and distension, especially after ingesting food. These symptoms are helped only to a slight degree by antacids and bicarbonate of soda.

When this triad is present it is important to think of the diagnosis of ovarian cancer and systematically to carry out all diagnostic measures that are outlined elsewhere in the book (see Chapter 8).

There is no definite and specific explanation for the early gastrointestinal symptoms that so often accompany early ovarian cancer. Cancer of the ovary spreads over surfaces, and in the advanced stages it coats the bowel and interferes with peristalsis. However, in the early stage this problem is not present. McGowan has reported that, compared with the peritoneal fluids from women with benign ovarian tumors, those from women with ovarian cancer had significantly higher indexes for calcium, inorganic phosphorus, urea nitrogen, uric acid, cholesterol, total protein (not albumin), total bilirubin, lactic dehydrogenase (LDH), and glutamic oxaloacetic acid transaminase (G-OT), and a pH of 7.43. The altered peritoneal fluids may irritate the bowel. Another point that may be relevant concerns the embryologic origin of the ovary. It arises at about the level of the 10th thoracic vertebra (T10) and migrates to the pelvis. Pain originating in the ovary may be referred to the abdomen and secondarily give rise to gastrointestinal symptoms. This explanation is theoretical and lacks documentation at this time. It is interesting to speculate whether the origin of the primitive germ cells in the fetal yolk contributes to the early gastrointestinal symptoms in ovarian cancer. As stated in Chapter 2, primitive germ cells migrate by ameboid movement along the dorsal mesentery of the hindgut. The route of the migrating germ cells, called the *keimbahn*, supports the often quoted association of ovarian malignancy with gastrointestinal malignancy and vice versa. Unless the primitive germ cells are able to migrate to the ovary, there is lack of ovarian development.

Diagnosis

The early diagnosis of ovarian cancer is a matter of chance and not a triumph of the scientific approach. The means of early detection are limited. In most cases finding a pelvic mass is the only available method of diagnosis, with the exception of functional tumors, which may manifest endocrine activity even with minimal ovarian enlargement. In some cases the pelvic findings are uncertain even late in the disease. The tumor may be deep in the pelvis, and the patient may be obese, heavily muscled, and uncooperative. The elderly patient may have an inelastic and conical vagina complicated by marked atrophy. Occasionally, there are widespread metastases in the presence of minimal pelvic findings. The usual signs and symptoms and the physical findings associated with ovarian cancer represent an advanced cancer of the ovary. An abdominal mass, distension, or both are prime diagnostic features. However, ovarian cancers seldom produce symptoms until they grow to 15 cm, and they cannot be palpated abdominally until they attain this size. Pain in the early stage is associated with a complication, such as torsion or rupture. Later, pain occurs when there is infiltration of adjacent organs or nerve sheaths by tumor. Menstrual disorders may be seen with endocrine-producing tumors. Vaginal bleeding may occur in the menopausal patient and has been attributed to the functioning stroma in the tumor. Ascites with positive cells is a sign of advanced disease, and 5-year survival is reported in fewer than 8% of these patients.

Pelvic Examination

Routine pelvic examination detects only one cancer for every 10,000 examinations of asymptomatic women. Ovarian tumors cannot be palpated abdominally until they reach 15 cm in size. Pelvic findings are often minimal and not helpful for making a diagnosis, even in patients with advanced disease.

However, combined with a high index of suspicion, they may help alert the physician to the diagnosis. There are nine pelvic signs.

1. Mass in the ovarian area
2. Relative immobility due to fixation and adhesions
3. Irregularity of the tumor
4. Shotty consistency with increased firmness
5. Tumors in the cul-de-sac described as a handful of knuckles
6. Relative insensitivity of the mass
8. Increasing size under observation
8. Bilaterality (70% for ovarian carcinoma versus 5% for benign cases)
9. With late disease; common findings of nodular hepatomegaly, ascites, and palpation of the omental cake
10. Areas that are soft, some cystic, some rubbery, and some hard due to unequal growth of the blood vessels in the ovarian cancer

Preoperative Evaluation

The diagnostic procedures include the Papanicolaou smear, which has been reported to be positive in 40% of patients with advanced disease, and a 90% incidence of positive cells on cul-de-sac taps. My results are poor compared to these figures. The roles of sonography, computed tomography, and magnetic resonance imaging are discussed in Chapter 8.

The value of laparoscopy remains to be determined. It has proved useful for staging lesions preoperatively, particularly those in the area between the liver and the diaphragm and extending down to the posterior peritoneum. It has limited value for monitoring tumors during prolonged chemotherapy regimens. If the examination proves positive, it has meaning; but if there is no evidence of disease on laparoscopic examination, it has not ruled out the possibility that ovarian cancer is present in the retroperitoneal area.

A complete workup in suspected cases should include the following.

1. Careful history
2. Complete physical examination, including careful rectal and pelvic examinations
3. Papanicolaou smear

4. Proctoscopy as deemed indicated
5. Complete blood count and urinalysis
6. SMA-12
7. Chest roentgenogram
8. Intravenous pyelogram
9. Gastrointestinal series ⎫
10. Barium enema ⎬ optional
11. Colonoscopy examination ⎭
12. Optional paracentesis, laparoscopy, and lymphangiogram
13. CEA, CA 125, LASA-P, NB/70K

This workup helps document the extent of disease and indeed may determine whether the cancer is primary or metastatic to the ovary. About 5 to 10% of ovarian cancers are metastatic. A complete diagnostic evaluation is outlined in Chapter 8.

Gusberg and Frick's indications for an exploratory laparotomy are listed below, with a slight modification (item 6).

1. Any pelvic mass that has appeared after menopause, particularly if it is an adnexal mass
2. Adnexal mass that progressively enlarges beyond 5 cm while under observation in a woman of any age
3. Appearance or persistence of an ovarian mass while the patient is on the combined contraceptive pill
4. Any adnexal mass 10 cm or larger
5. Inability to determine accurately whether the mass is a fibroid or an ovarian tumor
6. Palpation of what would have appeared to be a normal-sized ovary in a premenopausal woman but is found in a patient 3 to 5 years postmenopausal (indicative of an ovarian tumor)

Summary

The symptoms, signs, and diagnosis must be based on knowledge of the natural history of ovarian cancer.

Natural History of Ovarian Cancer

Because our ability to diagnose ovarian cancer early is limited, we must resort to the knowledge of its natural history when trying to identify the patient at high risk. We do know some facts, however, and we should be alert to them: Most ovarian cancers (epithelial) occur after age 35, most commonly after age 40. The diagnosis of ovarian cancer, as with all other malignancies, is most beneficial to the patient when it is made while the tumor is still localized. For ovarian carcinoma, this means identifying it when the only physical finding is an enlarged ovary.

It is also possible that the diagnosis can be based on hormonal activity of the ovarian tumor, but this parameter is much less specific. Unfortunately, most ovarian carcinoma is diagnosed only after the patient develops symptoms due to the spread of tumor. When a woman after age 40 appears with vague gastrointestinal symptoms that are difficult to diagnose, consider that the problem may be ovarian. The late English gynecologist Stanley Way said that most ovarian cancers are nurtured in a sea of sodium bicarbonate or antacids for months before the diagnosis is established.

Diagnosis

Early diagnosis has been more a matter of chance than scientific approach, so we must begin to use any clues available. An enlarged ovary should always be evaluated regardless of the patient's age, because when ovarian cancers are found in this way cure rates are high. On the other hand, when disease has already spread throughout the abdomen before the diagnosis—as it has in 70% of ovarian cancer patients—the 5-year survival rate is less than 20%. The chances of improving these dismal figures would be immeasurably better if we could find ways to make an early diagnosis or uncover borderline or potentially malignant cases.

Cytology

Some investigators claim good results in detecting ovarian cancer by means of vaginal and cervical cytology, but our own experience has not been encouraging. Cytology is also used to diagnose cells obtained from the posterior cul-de-sac by way of culdocentesis, but we have found this method to be of little benefit. Not only do patients find the procedure painful, but in our hands the results have not been reliable. Moreover, by the time an ovarian cancer has spilled malignant cells that can be identified in cytologic smears, it may no longer be in an early stage of growth. Also, if an inflamed mesothelial cell appears in the smear, it may resemble a malignant cell, in which case surgery is almost mandatory.

I find cytologic diagnosis to be of value in elderly, poor-risk patients in whom there is evidence of advanced ovarian cancer, including pelvic and abdominal masses and ascites, and in whom laparotomy would be too dangerous. In these patients a presumptive diagnosis of cancer may be made on the basis of cells obtained by paracentesis. Nonsurgical treatment can then be started.

Clinical Clues

A pattern suggestive of ovarian carcinoma may warn of difficulty. Although symptoms are certainly not specific, the following gastrointestinal complaints are not uncommon.

Loss of appetite
Indigestion
"Gas"—with concomitant distension

Furthermore, do not neglect gynecologic or hormonal disorders. Ovarian carcinoma patients often have a long history of heavy periods, premenstrual tension, dysmenorrhea, breast swelling, and miscarriages. It seems that the ovary is like a cam running off center—never completely normal.

The following triad of findings should arouse the suspicion of ovarian cancer.

1. Woman in the high-risk age group (> age 40)
2. History of ovarian dysfunction
3. Vague gastrointestinal symptoms such as dyspepsia, indigestion, gas with concomitant distension

Bibliography

Barber HRK: Ovarian cancer: still an enigma. *Dr* 1:17, 1975.
Barber HRK, Graber EA: Surgical aspects of

ovarian tumors. In: *Selected Topics of Cancer Current Concepts*. Symposia Specialists, Miami, 1974, p. 163.

Barber HRK, Graber EA, Kwon T: *Ovarian Cancer*. American Cancer Society, Atlanta, 1975.

Barr W: Current problems in diagnosis and management. *Ovarian Cancer Adv Biosci* 26:1, 1980.

DiSaia PJ, Morrow CP, Townsend DE: *Synopsis of Gynecologic Oncology*. Wiley, New York, 1975.

Griffiths CT: The ovary. In Kistner RW (ed): *Gynecology Principles and Practice*. Year Book, Chicago, 1975, p. 335.

Gusberg SB, Frick HC II: Corscaden's Gynecologic Cancer. Williams & Wilkins, Baltimore, 1970.

McGowan L: Peritoneal Fluid Profiles: Symposium on Ovarian Carcinoma. *Nat Cancer Inst Monogr* 42:75, 1975.

Rutledge F, Boronow RC, Wharton JT: *Gynecologic Oncology*. Wiley, New York, 1976.

Way S: *Malignant Disease of the Female Genital Tract*. Blakiston, Philadelphia, 1951, p. 183.

8

Diagnostic Evaluation and Preoperative Work-up

Cancer of the ovary is the leading cause of death from gynecologic cancer. Early diagnosis is a matter of chance rather than a scientific approach. The inability to diagnose ovarian cancer is evident from reports showing that 60 to 70% of these lesions are in stages III and IV at the time of diagnosis. The physician must have a high index of suspicion, use any and all clues, and evaluate an enlarged ovary regardless of the patient's age. Our chances for improving the low 5-year survival would be immeasurably better if we could find ways to make an early diagnosis or diagnose the borderline or potentially malignant cases. The means for diagnosis are nonspecific but are reviewed.

Cytology

Some investigators claim good results in detecting ovarian cancer by means of vaginal and cervical cytology, but my experience with cytology has not been good. McGowan reported that cytology is also used to diagnose cells taken from the posterior cul-de-sac by culdocentesis, but this method also has been found to be of little benefit. Not only do patients find the procedure painful, but in my hands the results have not been reliable. By the time an ovarian cancer has spilled malignant cells that can be identified in cytologic smears, it may no longer be in an early stage of growth. Also, if an inflamed mesothelial cell appears in the smear, it may resemble a malignant cell, in which case surgery is almost mandatory. Posi-

tive cells from cul-de-sac taps have been reported in 90% of patients with ovarian cancer, but my results have been poor compared to these figures.

Cytologic diagnosis has limited application. It is valuable in the elderly, poor-risk patient in whom there is every evidence of advanced ovarian cancer, including pelvic and abdominal masses and ascites and in whom laparotomy would be considered too dangerous. In these patients a presumptive diagnosis of ovarian cancer may be made based on the cells collected by paracentesis. Treatment can then begin.

Chemistries

Although carcinoembryonic antigens (CEA), alpha-fetoprotein (AFP), lactic dehydrogenase (LDH, CA 125, NB/70K and LASA-P) do not help to make the diagnosis, if elevated they serve to monitor the patient's response to therapy. Some investigators have raised the possibility that LDH elevation may be valuable as a screening test. In a prospective study I did not find it useful as a preoperative screening test. Total serum LDH is moderately elevated in most cancer patients with extensive hepatic metastases. The increase is usually associated with minor changes in the isoenzyme pattern, particularly an increase in LDH-3 and LDH-5 (the faster-moving isoenzymes). The LDH titer is higher in pleural and peritoneal effusions with malignant cells than it is in the serum. When the association of LDH and advanced ovarian cancer was examined, a review of our data failed to confirm correlation of the LDH level with the extent of disease.

Our laboratory has routinely performed CEA tests with ovarian cancer patients, but we have not confirmed the reports that CEA has been identified in the plasma of 35% of these patients. I believe that more cases and more time are required before a definite statement can be made about the relation between CEA and ovarian cancer. In a study from our laboratory, neither the heterologous nor the homologous antibody against the common epithelial tumors cross-reacted with CEA. In view of our clinical findings and the laboratory data, I doubt that CEA will play a significant role as a prognostic screening test. However, in certain patients it may serve to monitor progress during treatment of the cancer.

Serum AFP assays have currently gained an important place in the diagnosis of hepatocellular and testicular tumors as well as the endodermal sinus tumors. The observation that AFP may be elevated before tumors are detected by other means has important implications. In addition, successful therapy is associated with a decline in AFP levels to normal and a subsequent rise when the tumor recurs. AFP is known to be a product of the human fetal liver, gastrointestinal tract, and yolk sac. It has been shown that the endodermal sinus tumor, which is of vitelline origin, invariably gives a positive test for AFP.

Investigators from the National Cancer Institute have shown that malignancies other than trophoblastic disease produce elevated chorionic gonadotropin titers. Significantly, 30% of common epithelial tumors and up to 90% or more of embryonal ovarian carcinomas are associated with measurable amounts of this hormone. Although the findings of these substances do not identify the kind of malignancy —or in some cases whether the patient has a malignancy at all—it certainly indicates high risk and warrants investigation.

Additional markers for ovarian cancer are discussed in Chapter 25. They include CA 125, LASA-P, NB/70K.

Changes in the levels of humoral immunoglobulin in blood serum of patients with ovarian cancer have been recorded and used to monitor progress with chemotherapy. The levels of immunoglobulins (Ig) G, A, and M were regularly examined in 18 patients with ovarian carcinoma during the time of chemotherapy. The IgG level dropped at least 10% in ten patients, and the IgA and IgM levels dropped in nine patients. During long-term chemotherapy the IgG and IgA levels were more markedly changed than the IgM level.

Melnick and Barber studied the cellular immunologic responsiveness to extracts of ovarian epithelial tumors. The leukocyte migration inhibition assay was employed in an attempt to detect cellular immunologic responsiveness to a solubilized extract of pooled, epithelially derived ovarian carcinomas. In six of seven patients with cystadenocarcinomas of the ovary, leukocyte migration inhibition was noted in the presence of the ovarian tumor extract in their tissue culture system when compared to the migration test of leukocytes that were not exposed to the ovarian extract. Compared to control leukocytes, those from patients with nonepithelial ovarian cancers, benign ovarian neoplasms, and other genital tract cancers showed no inhibition of migratory behavior when exposed to the ovarian tumor extract. Cells from normal pregnant and nonpregnant females, as well as male subjects, also showed no inhibitory response when incubated with the ovarian tumor extract. Although the exact nature of the antigenic specificities uniquely associated with common epithelial ovarian carcinomas is unknown, their data suggest that cellular immune mechanisms may be involved in the host response to cells bearing tumor-specific antigens.

McGowan and coworkers have studied peritoneal fluids and have established profiles. They found the peritoneal fluid to be sensitive to many physiologic and pathologic gynecologic and obstetric conditions. They reported that peritoneal fluids from women with ovarian cancer had significantly higher indexes for the following biochemical parameters than did the fluids from women with benign ovarian tumors: calcium, inorganic phosphorus, urea nitrogen, uric acid, cholesterol, total protein (not albumin), total bilirubin, LDH, and glutamic oxaloacetic acid transaminase (G-OT). In normal patients the pH of the peritoneal fluid was 7.81, whereas in patients with ovarian carcinoma it was 7.43. McGowan and associates believed that these biochemical tests are affected by the amount of tumor present, but there appears to be no critical amount of disease needed, other than invasive cancer, for them to reflect change from normal and to form a biochemical pattern for ovarian cancer. Serial peritoneal fluid profiles may serve to monitor the patient undergoing surgical, radiation, or chemical therapy. However, it is not an easy or specific method for monitoring the patient.

In terms of function it must be emphasized that a variety of paraendocrine effects (e.g., hypercalcemia, hypoglycemia, and Cushing syndrome) and hemolytic anemia may rarely be related to the presence of an ovarian tumor.

Pelvic Evaluation

Routine pelvic examination detects few asymptomatic ovarian cancers. It is estimated that only one ovarian cancer is found among 10,000 examinations of asymptomatic women. In addition, because tumors cannot be palpated abdominally until they reach 15 cm in size, pelvic findings are often minimal or uncertain even in patients with advanced disease. As ovarian cancer enlarges and presses against the uterus, the pelvic examination often gives a false impression of a midline mass that is mistaken for a fibroid uterus. Consideration must be given to surgery in those patients suspected of having a fibroid but in whom the ovaries cannot be felt. Unfortunately, the ovarian cancer may be deep in the pelvis; the patient may be obese, heavily muscled, uncooperative, or aged; and the vagina may be inelastic and conical, all of which make palpation difficult if not impossible. Detection of a truly early ovarian cancer is not possible by pelvic examination. The smallest tumor that can be detected clinically or by any test is usually about 1 cm³ (1/16 in³) in size and weighs about 1 g (1/30 oz). A tumor of this size contains at least a billion (10⁹) cells and has the capacity for spreading.

This information is included to highlight the difficulty of early diagnosis by clinical means.

Although pelvic findings have limited value in diagnosis, the physician must be alert to:

1. Mass in the ovary
2. Relative immobility due to fixation and adhesions
3. Irregularity of the tumor
4. Shotty consistency with increased firmness
5. Tumors in the cul-de-sac described as "a handful of knuckles"
6. Relative insensitivity of the mass
7. Solid or semisolid consistency
8. Increasing size under observation
9. Bilaterality (70% in ovarian carcinoma versus 5% in benign lesions)
10. Ovarian malignancies of the common epithelial variety often showing a variegated consistency that on pelvic examination are revealed to be areas that are soft, some cystic, others rubbery, and often hard and knobby areas
11. Common findings of omental cake, nodular hepatomegaly, and ascites in advanced disease

The most important diagnostic procedure in any case of suspected or confirmed ovarian carcinoma is exploratory laparotomy. The indications suggested by Gusberg and Frick with additions and modifications are as follows.

1. Any mass that has appeared after the menopause, particularly an adnexal mass
2. Adnexal mass in a woman of any age that progressively enlarges beyond 5 cm while under observation
3. Appearance or persistence of an ovarian mass while the patient is on the combined contraceptive pill
4. Adnexal mass 10 cm or larger
5. Mass that cannot be definitely diagnosed as either a fibroid or a carcinoma (The pelvic mass must be considered an ovarian cancer until both ovaries are felt on palpation.)
6. Palpation of an ovary that in the premenopausal woman would be considered normal sized but is found in the postmenopausal woman (representing an ovarian tumor)

Ultrasonography

Ultrasonography is being used in many hospitals and physicians' offices to aid in the detection of ovarian neoplasia and other pelvic pathology. Donald preferred the term "sonor" for "electrosonic diagnostic echography." He repeatedly emphasized that sonor cannot supplant good, clinical examination but may help materially to reinforce or modify the clinician's findings. The information provided indicates macroscopic appearance only and is concerned with tissue density and outlines, their distribution, and fluid content. Donald stressed that the pictures must therefore be interpreted in the light of clinical knowledge and common sense. Sonor is no substitute for laparotomy and biopsy in a suspected tumor.

"Ultrasound" is the name given to a sound with a frequency over 20,000 cycles per second, the upper limit of the human ear. A simple explanation of the ultrasound is included for orientation purposes.

Ultrasound is basically a wave. The source of these waves is called a pulse generator, an apparatus that passes high-voltage current through a crystal, causes it to vibrate at high frequencies, and emits ultrasonic pulses at rates between 200 and 1000 per second. These pulses are formed into a beam that is directed into the abdomen and reflected back to the crystal (transducer) whenever it meets two apposed surfaces of different density (an interface). This reflected wave or echo is converted by the transducer into electrical energy and is represented on a cathode ray tube, either by a vertical deflection of a horizontal line (known as A-scanning) or by a bright spot (B-scanning). A third modality of ultrasound diagnosis involves the Doppler shift, a relative change in the frequency of a reflected echo when the wave strikes a moving object. Separate receiving and transmitting crystals are used. The receiving crystal processes frequency shifts caused by motion. The frequency differences can also be heard.

An additional technique, a gray scale of the intermediate shades between black and white, was developed to permit greater discrimination and more precise evaluation. Some have questioned the additional diagnostic value of the gray scale. Transmission imaging is an innovation that, unlike the gray scale, is still unavailable to most clinicians. Ultrasound pulsation is passed directly through the tissues, then recorded in optical form for interpretation. The resultant soft tissue image is analogous to a roentgenogram in that it is isomorphic with its real-life model.

The real-time scanner has greatly increased the scope of information available from ultrasound examinations. The modality has been applied to numerous areas of the body. The main advantages of real-time scanning are the rapidity with which the examination can be completed and the ability to observe motion. Real-time scanners usually employ either a rotating transducer or a linear array of transducers. The real-time scanner has added another modality to be used for the diagnosis of pelvic pathology. It has not helped significantly to make an early diagnosis but has had a place in the monitoring of patients who are undergoing therapy for their ovarian cancer.

The ultrasound examination of the pelvis employs the B-mode two-dimensional scans, A-mode deflection patterns, and real-time scanning. The only specific preparation for examination is the drinking of four 8-oz glasses of fluid to distend the urinary bladder. The distended bladder serves as a window through which the pelvic structures are evaluated.

The normal ovaries are ordinarily not identified with certainty because of their variability in position, the superimposition of air-filled small bowel, and the difficulty of differentiating the ultrasonic pattern of ovaries from the adjacent bowel pattern.

In most instances it is possible to differentiate ovarian cysts, both malignant and benign, from solid masses. A mass separate from the uterus associated with disorganized internal echoes at normal sensitivity suggests ovarian cancer. Ascitic fluid loculations may add to the confusion when evaluating suspected masses. Implants in the omentum may be interpreted as masses, especially in serial studies. It is accepted that the efficacy of preoperative evaluation of the primary mass has been adequately documented. More correlation is needed to establish the role that ultrasonography can play in the diagnosis and management of the patient with disseminated ovarian carcinoma.

Ultrasonography is the premier gynecologic imaging method. It has many advantageous characteristics, including relatively low cost, a wide availability, noninvasiveness, multiplanar imaging, and digital format. In the female pelvis it is currently unexcelled, particularly in obstetrics, where avoidance of radiation is required. The ability of ultrasonography to characterize tissue as solid or cystic and to portray structures rapidly on axial, coronal, and sagittal planes remains attractive.

The superior contrast and spatial resolution of computed tomography (CT), however, makes it clearly the procedure of choice in many applications. Doppler applications, including color, now permit noninvasive evaluation of blood flow in many organs.

Transvaginal Ultrasonography and Color Flow Doppler Studies

The development and introduction of the transvaginal curvilinear transducer has been a major advancement and has added a new dimension to the ultrasound examination. The transducer offers an added advantage in the field of gynecology by being able to directly target small structures such as the ovary or fallopian tube. The patient is also spared the discomfort of drinking four 8-oz glasses of water to distend the urinary bladder. A distended bladder serving as a window through which pelvic structures are evaluated is not required for transvaginal sonography.

The color flow Doppler display has added another dimension to ultrasonography. The Doppler method adds color to the study of moving targets (e.g., blood), providing directional information concerning the object field. Doppler imaging has been particularly helpful in obstetrics but also has contributed to identifying gynecologic problems. Color Doppler sonography serves to detect ovarian tumors,

anteriovenous malformations and thromboses within gonadal and parauterine veins. It has also helped in the detection of vascular uterine tumors.

Transvaginal color flow imaging is used to identify areas of neovascularization in the ovary. Preliminary reports indicate that areas of neovascularization in the ovary may indicate early tumorigenesis. More work and improved technology are required to determine if this technique has value for screening to detect early ovarian cancer.

A full discussion of female pelvic disease detected with ultrasonography is well beyond the scope of this text. Some common conditions of the ovaries can be well evaluated with ultrasonography. For example, physiologic cysts can be differentiated from solid malignant processes. Cystic malignancies, however, can be difficult to differentiate from benign complex tumors.

Ultrasonography has some limitations. Bowel gas interferes with ultrasonographically generated echoes. Often postoperative patients have numerous gas-filled loops in the bowel or pelvis that obscure pelvic anatomy. Ultrasonography is limited in terms of detecting the spread of tumor to the pelvic walls and therefore is less versatile than CT for staging cancer or for assessing a patient for possible recurrence.

The advantage of ultrasonography over CT are a lack of radiation exposure, no possibility of a reaction to contrast material, and the superiority of differentiating cystic and the more frequently malignant solid ovarian tumors; moreover, it is less expensive. There are no pathognomonic ultrasonographic findings. However, as the percentage of echogenic (solid) material increases on the ultrasonogram, the more likely it is that the tumor is malignant. Conversely, the more anechogenic it is, the more likely it is that the tumor is benign. Vaginal ultrasonography has proved to be more sensitive and better able to identify lesions in the pelvis than abdominal ultrasonography.

Fine-needle ovarian aspiration biopsy is not advocated for the diagnosis of ovarian cancer because it ruptures the mechanical barrier (the capsule), which allows the spread of cancer cells, and it is associated with a high, false-negative rate; moreover, even with benign ovarian neoplasms the tumor must be removed. Whenever the capsule is pierced and cells escape into the peritoneal cavity, the clinical stage becomes more advanced.

Computed Tomography

Computed tomography has revolutionized the neurosciences and has altered the way physicians evaluate a variety of clinical problems in the chest and abdomen. The last-generation scanners are capable of demonstrating the nature and extent of lesions to a degree not previously possible.

Computed tomography is a method of utilizing x-rays to image cross sections of the body with a degree of contrast resolution that is approximately 500 times that of plain film radiography. X-rays are collimated to a thin beam that sweeps across the patient. The beam is received by sensitive photoelectric crystals or gas tubes (similar to those used in nuclear medicine), which are much more sensitive than film. The data from the receptors is transmitted to a computer, which mathematically reconstructs an image of the body. Because diagnostic information is digitized, the image can be manipulated to optimize contrast. Also, computed reconstructions can be done in planes at a variety of angles to the original plane of screening.

The skin area transversed by each scan slice is exposed to approximately 1 to 3 rem. The dose is not overlapping and thus is not additive for successive slices. Multiple slices can be taken without undue exposure to the patient. The last generation of CT scans enables acquisition of up to 20 images or slices per second.

Major CT artifacts are caused by motion, metallic objects, beam hardening, and partial volume averaging. Patient motion degrades the image of all scanners. Beam hardening occurs when the x-ray beam first passes through the dense media such as bone. Black streaks re-

sults, and adjacent soft tissue is measured falsely as having lower attenuation.

Water-soluble iodiated contrast agents are frequently used with CT. The average dose is 100 ml of a 60% iodinated contrast agent. With contrast, vascular structures can be better identified, kidney function grossly estimated, the extent of tumor or abnormal tissues better defined, avascular tissue detected, and dynamics of cine-CT images obtained.

Abdominal CT is used for organ assessment. Precontrast and postcontrast scans are routinely obtained. Postcontrast scans are obtained to rule out nodes, tumor, and abscess. All scans are performed with optimal oral contrast opacification: 1 oz of Gastrografin is given the night before and at least two cups of oral contrast medium before the scan. Rapid bowel opacification may be achieved with administration of large amounts of dilute oral contrast medium given via a nasogastric tube.

Computed tomography is useful for gynecologic pelvic imaging. Benign masses can be detected and characterized (fat and a teratoma), and malignancies of the pelvis (rectum, uterus, cervix, vagina, vulva, fallopian tubes, and ovaries) can be staged. When malignancies are staged, CT examination in the abdomen is usually included.

It demonstrates retroperitoneal and pelvic nodes and assesses their degree of local invasion of adjacent structures. On occasion CT is crucial for delineating a mass not fully demonstrated by ultrasonography.

Magnetic Resonance Imaging

Magnetic resonance imaging (MRI) is a relatively new technique that involves the use of radiofrequency waves in varying magnetic fields to produce cross-sectional images of the body. The image depends on the number of hydrogen nuclei in the tissue and the extent to which the hydrogen is bound within each organ molecule. MRI is noninvasive, avoids ionizing radiation, and poses no observable hazard. One of its greatest assets is that the images can easily be obtained in direct coronal, sagittal, and routine transverse planes. The pelvis is particularly well suited to MRI scanning because of the abundant natural contrast produced by pelvic fat, urine in the bladder, gas within the bowels, and the absence of respiratory motion. MRI is potentially a promising modality for characterizing pelvic masses or staging of pelvic malignancies. The main disadvantages of MRI scanning are its long scanning time and high cost of equipment and performance of examinations.

Motion degrades the quality of images obtained with MRI. Therefore sedating the agitated patient is of prime importance. No other specific preparation is necessary. Pacemakers and cerebral aneurysm clips represent absolute contraindications to MRI scanning. The magnetic field destroys credit cards and bank cards (erasing their magnetic code on the black strip) and may permanently damage watches of any kind. Critically ill patients cannot be properly monitored in most MRI units, and conventional respirators should not be brought into the scanning area. Also, motion severely degrades an MRI image.

The MRI scans can demonstrate local spread of malignancy, ascites, and adenopathy, but CT is much more sensitive for the detection of mesenteric and serosal implants and abdominal adenopathy. As a result, at this point in time, CT is more accurate than MRI for staging ovarian carcinoma.

Gallium Imaging

Gallium 67 citrate accumulates in liver, spleen, bone marrow, lobes, adrenals, urinary tract, kidneys, salivary glands, breast, genitals, nasopharynx, and colon. Because of the long half-life, gallium imaging can be performed for 48 to 72 hours after injection or longer if required.

Gallium accumulates at sites of active infection and in a variety of neoplasms. It also accumulates in sites of abdominal infection (peritonitis, Crohn's disease, diverticulitis, pancreatic infections or abscess, cholecystitis), active skeletal infections, thyroiditis, and certain malignancies.

It has been useful for the detection and localization of occult abscesses and the determination of active osteomyelitis and the activity of chest disease when plain films and clinical evaluation are inconclusive. Occasionally, it helps to detect or stage occult neoplasms, although it is more commonly used to follow patients with known disease.

Gallium scanning has limitations that make it secondary to other modalities for the detection of occult neoplasms or abscesses. Spatial resolution with gallium is poor. Although the sensitivity of gallium scanning is high, abdominal imaging with CT for occult abscesses or tumor is faster and more specific.

Laparoscopy

Laparoscopy, or peritoneoscopy, has been found to be useful for staging suspected ovarian cancer patients and for the follow-up of these patients. It has had limited value as a diagnostic modality in patients with ovarian cancer.

Laparoscopy has been employed as a tool for a second look in ovarian cancer and has been performed in patients who have achieved clinical remission with chemotherapy. Its value can be summarized by saying that a positive finding with biopsy is conclusive, but a negative laparoscopy must be followed by an exploratory laparotomy before chemotherapy can be terminated. The role of laparoscopy or peritoneoscopy remains to be evaluated.

It has been reported that although patients appear at exploratory laparotomy to have disease localized to the pelvis nearly 50% of these women die within 5 years with recurrent tumor after what should have been curative surgical and radiotherapeutic treatment. Bagley and coworkers demonstrated the high frequency of unsuspected diaphragmatic metastases in patients with stages I and II ovarian cancer. Rosenoff and colleagues evaluated a group of patients who had been explored, staged, and then referred to the National Cancer Institute for further treatment, usually chemotherapy. Sixteen of their tumors had been previously staged as I or II; but at the time of laparoscopy prior to treatment, 7 (44%) were found to have metastatic disease to the diaphragm and were restaged as III.

Summary

Unfortunately, there is no one test or profile that helps make an early diagnosis of ovarian cancer. The physician must have a high index of suspicion and must use any and all means, including exploratory laparotomy, to arrive at the diagnosis.

Although there is hope that work being carried out in the field of immunology will provide a serologic test for early diagnosis, time is required to bring it to fruition. Until it is possible to utilize the unusual discriminatory powers of the immunologic system, which can detect a difference of a few molecules, ovarian cancer will remain a problem that can be diagnosed only by clinical means. Moreover, because 10% of ovarian cancers are metastatic from the bowel, breast, or thyroid, thorough workup is imperative before treatment is started.

Bibliography

Abelev GI: Alpha fetoprotein in oncogenesis and its association with malignant tumors. *Adv Cancer Res* 14:295, 1971.

Alexander P: Fetal "antigens" in cancer. *Nature* 235:137, 1972.

Alpert ME, Uriel J, DeNechaud B: Alpha fetoglobulin in the diagnosis of human hepatoma. *N Engl J Med* 278:964, 1966.

Bagley CM Jr, Young RC, Schein PS, et al: Ovarian carcinoma metastatic to the diaphragm—frequently undiagnosed at laparotomy: a preliminary report. *Am J Obstet Gynecol* 116:397, 1973.

Bagley CM Jr, Young RC, Canelos GP, et al: Treatment of ovarian cancer: possibilities for progress. *N Engl J Med* 287:856, 1972.

Baldwin RW: Tumor-specific antigens associated with chemically induced tumors. *Rev Eur Etud Clin Biol* 25:593, 1970.

Baldwin RW, Erubleton MJ: Demonstration by colony inhibition methods of cellular and humoral immune reactions to tumor-specific antigens associated with aminoazo-dye-induced rat hepatomas. *Int J Cancer* 7:17, 1971.

Barber HRK: A new test for ovarian cancer? *Female Patient* 15:11, 1990.

Barber HRK (ed): *Immunobiology for the Clinician.* Wiley, New York, 1977.

Barber HRK: Surgical management of ovarian cancer. *Curr Obstet Gynecol Tech* 1:6, 1975.

Barber HRK, Graber EA: Surgical aspects of ovarian tumors. In: *Selected Topics of Cancer Current Concepts.* Symposia Specialists, Miami, 1974, p. 161.

Barber HRK, Graber EA, Kwon T: *Ovarian Cancer.* Professional Education Publication. American Cancer Society, Atlanta, 1974, p. 2.

Coligan JE, Eagan ML, Todd CW: Detection of carcinoembryonic antigen by radioimmune assay. *Natl Cancer Inst Monogr* 35:427, 1972.

Collins WP: Transvaginal color flow imaging: a possible new screening technique for ovarian cancer. *Br Med J* 299:1367, 1989.

Donald I: Diagnostic uses of sonar in obstetrics and gynecology. *J Obstet Gynecol Br Commonw* 72:907, 1965.

Donald I: New problems in sonar diagnosis in obstetrics and gynecology. *Am J Obstet Gynecol* 118:299, 1974.

Donald I, MacVicar J, Brown TG: Investigation of abdominal masses by pulsal ultrasound. *Lancet* 1:1188, 1958.

Edynak EM, Hirshant Y, Old LJ, Trempe GL: Antigens of human breast cancer. *Proc Am Assoc Cancer Res* 12:75, 1971.

Fleischer AC, Zaleski WM, Kepple DM: Abdominal and pelvic applications of color Doppler sonography. *Toshiba Med Rev* 30:37, 1989.

Fleischer AC, Rao BK, Kepple DM: Transvaginal color doppler sonography: preliminary experiences. *Dynamic Cardiovascular Imaging* 3:52, 1990.

Gaylord GM, Davis LP, Baker SR: *Diagnostic and Interventional Radiology: A Clinical Manual.* Saunders, Philadelphia, 1989.

Graber EA: Early diagnosis of ovarian malignancy. *Clin Obstet Gynecol* 12:958, 1969.

Gusberg SB, Frick HC II: *Corscaden's Gynecologic Cancer.* Williams & Wilkins, Baltimore, 1970.

Haber E: *Radioimmunoassay—Principles and Practical Applications.* Little, Brown, Boston, 1974.

Hassani SN (ed): *Ultrasound in Gynecology and Obstetrics* (in collaboration with Bard RL). Springer-Verlag, New York, 1978, p. 12.

Ioachim HL, Dorsett BH, Sabbath M, et al: Antigenic and morphologic properties of ovarian carcinoma. *Gynecol Oncol* 1:130, 1973.

Kobayashi T, Osamutakantani HN: Echographic evaluation of abdominal tumor regressing during antineoplastic treatment. *J Clin Ultrasound* 2:131, 1974.

Kremkau FW: Doppler instruments. In: *Diagnostic Ultrasound.* Saunders, Philadelphia, 1988, pp. 177–197.

Laurence DJR, Munro N: Fetal antigens and their role in diagnosis and clinical management of human neoplasms: a review. *Br J Cancer* 26:335, 1972.

Laurora J, Jandora A, Skoda A, et al: Verhalten des Immunoglobulinspiegels in Blutserum ber Patientinsan mit Carcinoma Ovarii. *Zentralbl Gynakol* 97:540, 1975.

Leopold GR, Asher WM: Ultrasound in obstetrics and gynecology. *Radiol Clin North Am* 12:127, 1974.

LoGerfo P, Krupey J, Hansen HJ: Demonstration of antigen common to several varieties of neoplasia. *N Engl J Med* 283:138, 1971.

McGowan L: Peritoneal fluid profiles: symposium on ovarian carcinoma. *Natl Cancer Inst Monogr* 42:75, 1975.

McGowan L, Stein DB, Miller W: Cul-de-sac aspiration for diagnostic cytologic study. *Am J Obstet Gynecol* 96:413, 1966.

Melnick H, Barber HRK: Cellular immunologic responsiveness to extracts of ovarian epithelial tumors. *Gynecol Oncol* 3:77, 1975.

Meyers MA: The spread and localization of acute intraperitoneal effusions. *Radiology* 95:547, 1970.

Mitchison NA: Immunologic approaches to cancer. *Transplant Proc* 2:92, 1970.

Richart RM, Fenoglio CM: Principles of diagnosis. In Gusberg SB, Frick HC II (eds): *Corscaden's Gynecologic Cancer*. 5th Ed. Williams & Wilkins, Baltimore, 1978, p. 24.

Rosenoff SH, DeVita VT Jr, Hubbard S, Young RC: Peritoneoscopy in the staging and followup of ovarian cancer. *Semin Oncol* 2:223, 1975.

Rosenoff SH, Young RC, Anderson T, et al: Peritoneoscopy: a valuable tool for the initial staging and "second look" in ovarian carcinoma. *Ann Intern Med* 83:37, 1975.

Samuels BI: Usefulness of ultrasound in patients with ovarian cancer. *Semin Oncol* 2:229, 1975.

Shuster J: Immunologic diagnosis of human cancers. *Am J Clin Pathol* 62:243, 1974.

Stolbach LL, Krant MJ, Fishman WH: Ectopic production of an alkaline phosphatase isoenzyme in patients with cancer. *N Engl J Med* 281:757, 1969.

Straub WH (ed): *Manual of Diagnostic Surgery*. Little, Brown, Boston, 1989.

Thaler I, Bruck A, Bar-Yann Y: The vaginal probe—physical considerations. In Timor-Tritsch IE, Rottem S (eds): *Transvaginal Sonography*. Elsevier, New York, 1988, pp. 1–15.

Updated guide to diagnostic ultrasound. *Contemp Obstet Gynecol* 3:105, 1974.

Van Nagell JR, Meeker WR, Parker JC Jr, Harralson JD: Carcinoembryonic antigen in patients with gynecologic malignancy. *Cancer* 35:1372, 1975.

Young RC, Hubbard SP, DeVita VT: The chemotherapy of ovarian cancer. *Cancer Treat Rev* 1:99, 1974.

Zemlyn S: Comparison of pelvic ultrasonography and pneumography for ovarian size. *Clin Ultrasound* 2:331, 1974.

9

Preoperative and Postoperative Management

Cancer of the ovary raises many challenges during the preoperative, operative, and postoperative periods. It is not only the site of origin of a variety of tumors but a target for metastases from many other organs (i.e., thyroid, breast, stomach, colon, and the opposite ovary). Therefore it is important to rule out the ovarian tumor as a metastatic lesion before exploratory laparotomy. To be forewarned is indeed to be forearmed. The diagnostic evaluation has been covered in Chapter 8.

The management of ovarian cancer has come full circle since the early 1950s. At that time extended surgery was carried out, including the ultraradical surgery of pelvic exenteration. It became obvious that ovarian cancer was a surface spreader and often involved the upper abdomen with small metastases that were difficult to detect by methods then available. Despite aggressive surgery, most patients succumbed to recurrent cancer if they survived the postoperative period.

Now, with modern methods of management with chemotherapy, the patient has an opportunity for extended survival, particularly if the disease has been debulked. The more liberal use of hyperalimentation has permitted more aggressive management without compromising the survival of the patient who develops a complication, especially those involving the gastrointestinal tract. This development has led to an extension of the standard ovarian cancer extirpation techniques. Improvements in preoperative and postoperative care have been equally important. Even the most superior technical skill does not obviate the need for excellence in preoperative and postoperative management.

The patient or the family may ask about the particular risks involved. It is important for the gynecologist to discuss in detail the options, risks and complications associated with the surgery. The gynecologist must give reasons for the procedure and answer questions. The consent form must outline the operation in terms that a lay person understands (not salpingo-oophorectomy, but removal of tubes and ovaries). The consent form must outline the complications of the operation and that options have been presented to the patient.

The operative risk is influenced by age, associated medical disorders (cardiovascular, respiratory, metabolic), the familiarity of the surgeon with the natural history of the disease and the planned procedures, the experience of the anesthetist, the equipment and physical facilities necessary for the surgical procedure, the duration of the anesthesia or operation, the staff of the recovery room, and the team for managing the postoperative care of the patient.

It is important to evaluate the operative risk, and the surgeon and anesthetist must institute appropriate corrective measures during the preoperative period to establish optimal conditions before the surgical procedure. Training the patient preoperatively in the use of proper ventilation and use of the breathing equipment is important, particularly for patients who smoke or have any chronic lung problem. The average patient with ovarian cancer is over age 40 and in general is a fairly good operative risk.

Among patients with suspected ovarian cancer the diagnostic workup and preoperative care can be carried out simultaneously. The workup is best accomplished at least 2 days before surgery.

It is the responsibility of the surgeon (shared with the surgical team) to evaluate the patient properly and to institute measures that prepare the patient for surgery. These measures must include a general evaluation of her physical status and a detailed medical history.

The preoperative regimen should start before admission to the hospital with a complete explanation of the workup to be carried out and the anticipated surgery. It is important to reassure the patient and to prepare her psychologically. If the patient smokes, she should be advised to stop before admission to the hospital. A well-balanced diet is advised, and iron and vitamins should be prescribed.

The patient admitted to the hospital for treatment of cancer is subject to a general evaluation of her physical status. A complete history is obtained, and specific answers regarding the following items are essential: duration of present symptoms, history of weight change, previous neoplastic disease, if she is a twin, menstrual history, abortions, history of her pregnancies, treatment with hormones, and previous operations. The history should be carefully reviewed for sensitivity to medications and anesthetic agents. It should be determined if the patient is taking any long-term medication that might be a factor during anesthesia or for operative or postoperative complications. Antihypertensive drugs, diuretics, and tranquilizers are among the agents that might have such an influence.

With the routine physical examination, pelvic and rectal examinations should be carefully carried out and recorded. Papanicolaou smears should be prepared and, if feasible, smears or biopsy specimens of the endometrium obtained. In addition to measuring the hemoglobin level, white blood cell count and differential, and the red blood cell count, routine urinalysis and the following blood coagulation studies should be done: bleeding time, clotting time, tourniquet test, prothrombin time, prothrombin consumption time, clot retraction time, partial thromboplastin time, and platelet count. An electrocardiogram, chest roentgenogram, and intravenous pyelogram are essential.

Because 10% or more of all pelvic cancers are metastatic from another organ, additional radiographic studies should be performed as indicated. Such studies include mammography, a gastrointestinal series, and a barium enema, as well as bone and liver scans as judged necessary. If barium studies are carried out, a flat plate of the abdomen should be obtained before surgery to make certain there is no residual barium in the bowel.

A patient who has cancer generally suspects the nature of her illness, or often she has been told the diagnosis or that such a diagnosis cannot be ruled out. Therefore when entering the hospital she is apprehensive, regardless of appearance. A well-organized admission routine can be reassuring. The house officer and nurse should refrain from general discussion of neoplastic disease, methods of treatment, specific diagnosis of her case, and prognosis. The terms tumor or growth should be used in relation to her condition—not the word cancer. On admission, medication should be prescribed to allay apprehension, ensure sleep, and control pain.

Special Preoperative Orders for Surgery of Ovarian Cancer

The general principles of preparation for laparotomy and major pelvic surgery are followed for ovarian cancer surgery, with the addition of the procedures noted below. Upon return of laboratory reports, any abnormal values are rectified by appropriate measures, i.e., blood transfusions for anemia and hypoproteinemia and indicated parenteral fluids for chloride, potassium, or sodium deficiencies. Because patients with advanced ovarian cancer are frequently debilitated and emaciated, hyperalimentation is being used more often in these patients (discussed later).

In debilitated patients, preoperative blood volume studies may be carried out and blood replacement performed as needed. Ordinarily such studies are not indicated. Among patients with clinical evidence of a depleted blood volume, transfusions can be given and the patient's response monitored with serial hematocrit levels. A rise in the hematocrit of 2 to 3% after a transfusion of 500 ml of whole blood usually indicates that the blood volume deficit has been corrected.

Lower abdominal surgery is followed by clinically detectable pulmonary mechanical malfunction in nearly 30% of patients, which contributes significantly to postoperative morbidity. This problem is particularly common in the patient with abdominal distension secondary to ovarian cancer and ascites. Unlike the internist, who is interested primarily in the diagnosis and treatment, the anesthetist is mainly concerned with the pulmonary reserve of the patient and whether this reserve, if low, can be improved prior to administering anesthesia to the patient.

Screening tests are mandatory in all patients suspected of having pulmonary abnormalities because effective preoperative treatment of airway disease reduces the frequency of postoperative complications. It has been shown that 70% of patients with chronic obstructive pulmonary disease develop postoperative pulmonary complications, whereas 3% of patients who are negative symptomatically had an abnormal pulmonary function test. Evaluating the pulmonary status of a patient prior to surgery does not require a battery of expensive, time-consuming tests.

The history is important. Particularly important are the past illnesses and exposure to contagious diseases, a knowledge of the patient's type of work, her tolerance of physical activity, and her smoking habits, which are essential for determining the patient's ventilatory reserve. It is important to question the patient about cough characteristics.

Because exercise leads to increased oxygen consumption, CO_2 production, and lactic acid output, ventilatory reserve can be roughly estimated by having the patient walk briskly or climb one or two flights of stairs. If this exercise can be accomplished without dyspnea, respiratory reserve is obviously not seriously compromised, and the following simple test for pulmonary function suffices.

The "match test" establishes the ability to blow out a match 3 inches from the patient's widely open mouth without pursing the lips and correlates well with the maximum breathing capacity of more than 4 liters per minute and a mid-expiratory flow rate of more than 0.06 liters per second. It is important that the patient not purse her lips because an increased linear velocity due to flow through a narrow orifice may alter the results. It has been noted that 85% of patients with a forced expiratory volume over the first second (FEB <1.6 liters could not extinguish the match. Thus the match test, requiring no sophisticated equipment, can select those patients for whom further evaluation is indicated.

Another test measures how long the patient can hold her breath. If she is unable to hold it for more than 10 seconds, she is considered to have a markedly reduced respiratory reserve.

Additional information concerning ventilatory function, as it is affected by muscular strength or bronchial caliber, can be gained by measuring the maximum voluntary ventilation. This parameter is the greatest volume of air a subject can move by rapid, deep breaths within a given period (12 seconds); it is expressed in liters per minute.

When an obstructive element is present (as in asthma), a marked delay in expiration is seen. If a patient can exhale completely in 4 seconds, there is little obstruction present. To perform this maneuver, place a stethoscope on the patient's chest and have her take a deep breath and blow it out as hard and as fast as possible. If the patient requires longer than 4 seconds to exhale, further studies should be performed before elective surgery.

If one should find, in the office or bedside, that the patient has abnormal pulmonary functions, two valuable procedures that may be ordered from the pulmonary function laboratory are barometry and measurement of flow rates. A conclusive determination of ventilatory insufficiency can only be established by arterial blood gas measurements.

A thorough preoperative bowel preparation is important in patients suspected of having ovarian cancer. Although the mechanical bowel preparation is the most important part, the addition of a sulfa preparation or an antibiotic has proved helpful. The bowel can be cleaned out and flattened by administration of 60 ml of 50% magnesium sulfate solution for 2 days, followed by 45 ml of castor oil on the afternoon before surgery. The question of preoperative antibiotics has not been resolved but is included in this protocol. If time permits, one of the sulfa preparations in doses up to 10 g per day for 5 to 7 days is given, or a short course of neomycin is instituted in a 1-g dose every hour for six doses on the day before surgery. The vagina is prepared with an antibiotic suppository or one of the sulfa vaginal creams for 2 or 3 days before surgery. The night before surgery, the patient takes a shower using PhisoHex. At the time of examination in the operating room povidone-iodine (Betadine) is instilled into the rectum.

The evening before surgery an infusion of glucose and water is started with 1000 units of heparin in the infusion. This infusion runs through the night, during surgery, and during the postoperative period.

Preoperative medication is given 30 to 45 minutes before the patient is taken to the operating room. Although the medication and dose are selected for each patient depending on size, debilitation, and age, the average is usually 100 mg of secobarbital (Seconal) plus 0.4 mg of atropine by hypodermic, 50 mg of hydroxyzine (Vistaril) plus 0.4 mg of atropine, or 50 mg of meperidine (Demerol) plus 0.4 mg of atropine by hypodermic.

Aggressive surgery, chemotherapy, or both for the treatment of ovarian cancer has given rise to many complications. Among them are bowel fistulas and debilitation of the patient, which carried a high mortality before the use of hyperalimentation. Parenteral hyperalimentation was originally used therapeutically, but more and more it is being used prophylactically to prepare patients for their anticipated treatment or for patients who have had a weight loss of 10% or more.

Hyperalimentation is a unique form of intravenous therapy that, parenterally, provides all of the daily nutritional requirements. Par-enteral hyperalimentation, or total parenteral nutrition, is the technique of providing enough calories, amino acids, and other nutrients to promote growth, weight gain, and normal healing. This technique has had a tremendous impact on the critically ill patient who faces slow starvation because of the inability to provide oral alimentation. If adequate nutrition is not available, the body turns to itself for a source for the energy necessary to remain alive. Rapid deterioration of lean tissue, muscle, and fat ensues.

In the fasting state the body breaks down approximately 75 g of protein per day (12 g of nitrogen). Liver glycogen stores are depleted within 24 hours. The catabolism of protein to glucogenic amino acids and finally to glucose is responsible for the maintenance of serum glucose during starvation. The body turns to stores of lean tissue and muscle for a source of glucose, rather than to fat stores. Therefore a protein deficiency rapidly develops. As a result, secondary deficiencies develop in tissue synthesis, blood proteins, leukocytes, enzymes, hormones, and antibodies with consequent delay in healing and susceptibility to infection. The significance of supplying adequate nutrition to the seriously ill patient is evident. Severe injury, sepsis secondary to surgery, or other trauma may cause an increased breakdown of body protein-nitrogen of up to 50%. Thus when hyperalimentation is considered, the daily metabolic requirements should also be calculated as 50% greater than normal. Hyperalimentation should be used with extreme caution in patients with (1) impaired renal function, (2) hepatic insufficiency, or (3) diabetes.

The technique of catheter placement is not discussed, nor is a detailed plan of management described. The purpose here is to emphasize the importance of hyperalimentation for managing the debilitated cancer patient.

There are typical formulas for parenteral hyperalimentation, such as the protein hydrolysate solutions and free amino acid mixtures. Electrolytes, vitamins, and minerals should be added as needed. Heparin should be added to each infusion and insulin given as needed.

Basic guidelines for safe intravenous feeding include daily measurement of body weight and water balance. Serum electrolytes, blood sugar, and blood urea nitrogen should be measured daily until they are stabilized and then measured every 2 to 3 days. The urine glucose concentration should be measured every 6 hours. Liver and kidney function should be evaluated initially and then every 2 to 3 weeks. Periodic measurements of arterial and central venous pressure, blood acidity, and dissolved gases may be indicated for the management of patients with heart, kidney, lung, or metabolic disorders. It is a cardinal rule, however, that whenever an infection caused by a catheter is suspected the catheter should be removed immediately and cultured. Blood cultures should also be taken.

It is important to avoid hyperosmolar, hyperglycemic, nonketotic diabetic coma. Adequate fluid intake must always be maintained and the urine carefully monitored for sugar and acetone. Insulin must be given as needed. Rapidly developing hyperglycemia syndrome may follow a too rapid infusion of glucose. The patient complains of frontal headaches followed shortly by convulsions. Insufficient insulin and hyperglycemic complications can be avoided by preventing hyperglycemia by not allowing the blood glucose level to rise over 200 mg/dl.

The surgical technique is described in Chapter 16 and is not reviewed here. Two points are discussed briefly: removal of a great volume of ascitic fluid and the start of oozing or bleeding during the operation. The removal of 2 liters of ascites fluid or more may lead to an unstable vasomotor system, which may result in shock. Therefore enough plasma and fluids and electrolytes should be given to correct the imbalance. It is important to remove the ascitic fluid slowly, which allows stabilization of the cardiovascular system.

The second point concerns the diagnosis and therapy of hemorrhagic disorders that occur during surgery. Acute, unexpected bleeding during or shortly after operation in the absence of an accountable surgical source is a vexing problem that may catch the surgeon unprepared with a definite plan for management. In such an emergency there is usually little time to run a battery of time-consuming hematologic tests. The discussion that follows is based on the assumption that bleeding is not from a vessel but is related to a hemorrhagic disorder.

The plan of action suggested for the management of these patients is based on three features: (1) clinical judgment; (2) rapid blood tests; and (3) selective therapy. Clinical judgment is founded on a careful workup before operation. Preexisting disorders, congenital or acquired, would presumably be exposed by a thorough history, careful physical examination, and necessary preoperative tests. When preexisting hematologic defects have been ruled out, the causes of unexpected bleeding may be narrowed down to (1) bleeding from a surgical source, (2) fibrinolysis, (3) defibrination, (4) thrombocytopenia due to massive blood bank transfusions, (5) anticoagulants and their antagonists, and (6) mixed clotting problems.

Hemostasis involves an interdependence of the blood platelets, the coagulation mechanism, and the blood vessels. The least understood and least studied factor in hemostasis is that involving the blood vessels. In summary, clotting consists in platelet aggregation, consolidation, formation of the fibrin clot, clot retraction, and, in pathologic states, fibrinolysis. It can be assumed that blood loss sufficient to require almost constant transfusion to maintain blood pressure is attributable to a surgical cause until proved otherwise.

The circumstances before and at the time of bleeding may help to determine the cause. The onset of abnormal bleeding after massive blood transfusions is probably due to thrombocytopenia associated with five or more units of banked blood. A platelet count or estimation of the platelet count may confirm that platelet deficiency is the cause of the bleeding. Bleeding that follows one transfusion may be due to mismatched blood and favors hemolysis and intravascular coagulation.

Rapid blood tests should be available within 10 to 15 minutes. Test tubes containing a 3.8% sodium citrate solution should be ready in the operating rooms at all times. There are five tests that can be done in all hospitals:

1. *Partial thromboplastin time* (PTT) is a sensitive test for identifying undiagnosed hemophilia, a variety of coagulation defects, and circulating anticoagulants.
2. *Rapid estimation of platelets* has helped to identify the etiology of the bleeding. Platelet counts considerably below 100,000/μl may point to massive bank blood transfusion as a source of bleeding.
3. *Bleeding time* helps identify the reason for the bleeding. In patients in whom the bleeding is prolonged beyond 4 minutes, attention must be directed to a platelet abnormality or vascular hemophilia (von Willebrand's disease). Bleeding time is normal in hemophilia.
4. *Prothrombin time* that is abnormal may indicate intravascular coagulation, fibrinolysis, or liver dysfunction.
5. *Thrombin time* that is prolonged indicates overheparinization, defibrination, or fibrinolysis.

Selective treatment depends on identification of all factors that contribute to the bleeding state. Because the emergency therapy available is rather limited, it is perhaps best to approach the diagnosis by selective treatment. When using this approach one assumes that hemophilia or other severe, lifelong bleeding disorder would probably have been diagnosed preoperatively. There are indeed few therapeutic modalities available clinically at this time: (1) Fresh frozen plasma can be used to replace any plasma coagulation factor deficiency, as can antihemophilic plasma. (2) Platelet concentrates (or a poor second choice of fresh whole blood) can be used to replace platelets deficient in number or function. (3) ϵ-Aminocaproic acid, used to arrest fibrinolysis, probably acts by competitive inhibition of plasminogen activators.

The triad of thrombocytopenia, hypofibrinogenemia, and lysis of a blood clot within 2 hours points to the probability of disseminated intravascular coagulation (DIC). Heparin may rapidly restore the platelet count and fibrinogen level and thus attenuate the bleeding. After heparin has been given, the consumed clotting factors such as platelets and fibrinogen may have to be replaced in the form of plasma, platelet concentrates, or fresh blood. While the DIC is being treated, therapy for the precipitating cause (hypovolemic shock) should be carried out. In fact, DIC of short duration can be treated without heparin therapy by removing the precipitating cause. Only with profound, long-standing shock and DIC is heparin therapy necessary. Heparin should be considered an adjunct to treatment but not a panacea for the patient in hypovolemic shock who needs a massive transfusion of blood.

Special Postoperative Orders for Ovarian Cancer Surgery

Immediately after operation the vital signs—blood pressure, pulse, and respirations—are noted at 15-minute intervals until sensoria are fully recovered. Urine output per catheter is recorded at hourly intervals. The normal rate is about 50 ml/hr. The urine output is a simple, reliable guide for the administration of fluids.

Sedation for pain is gauged to maintain comfort and at the same time to avoid respiratory distress. Fasting (including fluids) is continued until the bowel sounds are normal. Antibiotics are used as deemed necessary by the surgeon. Cephaloridin and gentamicin are the two usually chosen. However, in the presence of known *Bacteroides* infection, cleomycin should be given. Nasogastric suction is used as needed.

The following schedule for fluids, electrolytes, and plasma should be instituted: 1000 ml 5% glucose and water; 1000 ml Ringer's lactate; 1000 ml 5% glucose and water; 1000 units heparin added to each bottle. Plasma is added as needed to stabilize the blood pressure and to improve urinary output. After day 1, additional plasma, saline, and potassium are required. The losses from the nasogastric tube must be added to this baseline. Hemoglobin and hematocrit should be recorded twice a day for 2 days.

After surgery for ovarian cancer, any of the complications that are associated with major surgery may occur. A few of the more common ones are noted and discussed briefly. Postoperative intestinal problems are not infrequent and include ileus, intestinal obstruction, peritonitis, and fistula formation. Postoperative infections are not unusual, particularly infections of the wound, and dehiscence is more common among these patients than among those operated on for benign disease. Thromboembolic disease and pulmonary embolization occur more frequently among cancer patients.

Ileus

Ileus is one of the most frequent complications during the postoperative period, following surgery for ovarian cancer. It may vary in severity from mild distension to a full-blown picture of paralytic ileus, with its accompanying electrolyte, water, and acid-base imbalance. It is important to make certain that the problem is indeed paralytic ileus and not mechanical small bowel obstruction. Although the fluid and electrolyte replacement may be the same, the definitive approach to the underlying problem is different.

Ileus is most often preceded by a diminution in urine volume. Fluids and electrolytes collect in the intestines. The abdomen becomes distended and pushes the diaphragm up, which often gives rise to atelectasis and predisposes to respiratory acidosis. The extracellular fluid is therefore decreased, which in turn leads to a decrease in glomerular filtration with a drop in the urinary output. The clinical picture includes the following features.

1. Vomiting and distension occur on the second or third day after surgery.
2. Vomitus is first mucus, then bile, and later altered blood.
3. Constipation is the rule.
4. Abdomen rapidly distends with gas.
5. Peristalsis is absent.
6. Bowel sounds are absent.
7. Pain is usually absent, but if present it is colicky.
8. Patient becomes dehydrated.
9. Pulse becomes rapid.
10. Respiratory rate, temperature, and leukocyte count rise.
11. Urinary output drops despite good intake.
12. Patient becomes toxic.
13. Flat plate of the abdomen shows (1) a gas-distended loop and multiple fluid levels in the small bowel, and (2) sometimes a little gas in the cecum and pelvic colon.

Paralytic ileus must be differentiated from a mechanical obstruction. Four cardinal symptoms of mechanical intestinal obstruction are (1) colicky abdominal pain that is intermittent, comes on suddenly, reaches a peak, then subsides. (Auscultation at the time of pain reveals loud, metallic, high-pitched peristaltic rushes. This point is the most important difference between obstruction and ileus.); (2) frequent and copious vomiting; (3) distension; and (4) obstipation.

The signs and findings that are most helpful for judging whether the patient is improving or deteriorating are the (1) pulse; (2) respiratory rate, temperature, and white blood cell count; (3) urine output; and (4) follow-up flat plate of the abdomen.

Peritonitis

Peritonitis is an inflammation of the peritoneum, a condition marked by exudation of serum and by fibrin, cells, and pus in the peritoneum. Diagnosis of the full-blown disease is easy, but early diagnosis may be elusive. The following signs and symptoms may help in the diagnosis.

1. Initial stages depend on the mode of infection.
2. Temperature is elevated.
3. Most important sign of pelvic peritonitis after operation is a pulse that is more rapid than would be expected from the temperature elevation.
4. Once peritonitis is established, the picture is characteristic.
5. Pain distribution follows the spread of infection.
6. Vomiting is usual.
7. Constipation is more common than diarrhea.
8. Patient lies motionless and supine, most often with legs drawn up.
9. Patient's expression is anxious, and the face is drawn and gaunt.

10. Abdominal muscles over the inflamed site are slightly contracted.
11. With diffuse peritonitis, the whole abdomen is rigid, ligneous, and motionless. There is no movement of the abdomen during respiration.

Management of the fluid, electrolytes, and plasma imbalance is not discussed here. However, peritonitis manifests similar to a 15- to 30-degree body burn, and the basic principles suggested by Barber for fluid and plasma protein replacement is followed.

Thromboembolic Disease

Thrombophlebitis is not uncommon with general gynecologic surgery and is more frequent when the operation is carried out for treatment of a malignancy. It usually develops between days 5 and 10 postoperatively. Most reports state that the phlebitis probably starts in the operating room. Thromboembolic disease may have an insidious onset with few if any clinical signs or symptoms until pulmonary embolization occurs. Superficial phlebitis is not dangerous, and fatalities result only from deep venous thrombi.

Pulmonary embolism may be the first and only sign that thrombophlebitis is present. Other signs of phlebothrombosis and thrombophlebitis include (1) tenderness of the foot, particularly on the medial side; (2) painful dorsiflexion of the foot (Homan's sign)—an unreliable sign and one that is difficult to evaluate; (3) an ascending stepladder pulse associated with temperature elevation and increased respiration; and (4) pain and swelling of the affected leg.

Cranley has developed phleborheography as an accurate method for diagnosing thrombophlebitis. Phleborheography, defined as the tracing of moving currents within a vein, has been considered an accurate term to designate a plethysmographic technique for diagnosing deep venous thrombosis of the lower extremity. The technique is practical and highly accurate, and it has become a standard clinical test. It is noninvasive and accurate for diagnosing deep venous thrombosis of the lower extremity. Phleborheography can be performed by a technician in the laboratory, at the bedside, or in the office. It has taken the guesswork out of diagnosing deep vein thrombosis. Therapy consists in anticoagulation, bed rest, elevation of the extremity, and a pneumatic pad. The rationale for the use of anticoagulants is to prevent embolization, control additional clot formation, and interrupt the local pain and swelling.

During the past few years, prophylactic heparinization has been established as a method of treatment on our service and it has proved most rewarding. The minidose heparin (1000 units of heparin in 1000 ml of infusion to run over 8 hours) is started the evening before surgery and is continued during surgery and during the first 3 to 4 postoperative days. It has been reported to be more effective by this plan of administration than if it were started in the operating room or during the immediate postoperative period.

Pulmonary Embolization

Pulmonary embolization is a feared complication following pelvic surgery for a malignant condition. It occurs most frequently after coughing and squeezing on bed pans when the glottis closes followed by a sudden release of pressure. The embolization may be sudden and dramatic, resulting in death, or it may progress from minor symptoms. The patient may faint and have an acute pain in the chest followed by cyanosis and respiratory distress, or she may have an unexplained tachycardia for a few days with a slight elevation of temperature.

A high index of suspicion is most important for making the diagnosis. The triad of elevated levels of serum glutamic oxalic transaminase, bilirubin, and serum LDH are helpful, as is the evaluation of arterial blood gases. Lung scans have some value, but the most specific test in this diagnosis is pulmonary angiography.

Immediate therapy is indicated for a suspected case of acute pulmonary embolism. The patient should be given heparin 15,000 units IV as an initial dose. The clotting time should be checked every 2 hours after the initial dose. If the clotting time 2 hours after the initial dose is

25 minutes or longer, the heparin response is satisfactory; continue heparin 15,000 units IV every 6 hours the first day and give 10,000 units IV every 6 hours thereafter. If the clotting time 2 hours after the initial dose is shorter than 25 minutes, the patient has an increased requirement for heparin; increase the subsequent heparin dose and recheck with clotting times until a satisfactory response is obtained. The administration of oxygen to increase blood PO_2 and reduce pulmonary artery pressure is essential.

Sepsis and Septic (Bacteremic) Shock

Septic shock is defined as that condition seen in a patient with an apparent infection that includes a temperature either elevated above or depressed below normal, thready pulse (110 or more per minute), hypotension (systolic usually 80 mm Hg or below), and a decrease in urinary output (below 20 ml/hr).

Shock is defined as that state in which capillary profusion is inadequate to sustain life. Vital cells starve for lack of oxygen, and other nutrients and metabolic products are not removed from tissues because capillary flow is slow or does not exist. Shock is an emergency situation, whether it is caused by severe injury with blood loss or severe infection, heart failure, or other causes. The situation must be dealt with immediately or cellular injury and death soon progress to organ failure and death of the patient.

Bacteremic shock is one of the true emergencies of medicine. The gram-negative organisms most frequently causing this disorder are *Escherichia* (most common), *Proteus mirabilis*, *Pseudomonas aeruginosa*, and *Aerobacter aerogenes*. Among the most frequently cultured gram-positive bacteria are enterococci, anaerobic streptococci, *Bacteroides*, and *Clostridium perfringens*. Infections caused by *Bacteroides* are being reported with increasing frequency. Bacteremic shock carries a mortality rate of 80%, and it is higher when *P. mirabilis* or *C. perfringens* are the infecting organism.

Shock is noted especially in conjunction with infected abortion, premature rupture of the membranes (chorioamnionitis), pyelonephritis (especially during pregnancy), and diffuse peritonitis. It may be associated with gynecologic cancer or may follow extensive radical surgery. Sepsis and septic shock may follow chemotherapy for pelvic malignancy or gestational trophoblastic disease.

Although the entire mechanism has not been elucidated, most physicians accept the theory that the basic physiopathology is generalized intravascular clotting, initiated by the release of endotoxins (mainly lipopolysaccharides) by the previously named gram-negative bacteria.

Two mechanisms, selective vasospasm and DIC, are used to explain the findings in endotoxic shock. Pathophysiology can be attributed to both of these mechanisms and to the patient's reduced myocardial response to sympathetic stimuli.

Clostridium perfringens secretes exotoxins, and it is probably the most serious of all infections. Soon after the exotoxins are liberated from the infecting organisms, they become irreversibly bound to tissue. Because the toxin is fixed to tissue, specific antitoxins are of questionable value. The exotoxins contain the enzyme lecithinase, which causes necrosis of tissue as well as rapid lysis of red and white blood cells and collagenase (a proteolytic enzyme that causes necrosis of muscle tissue). There is a lack of oxygen to vital organs because of compensatory generalized vasoconstriction that impairs tissue profusion.

The clinical syndrome is characterized by (1) a change in the sensoria; (2) the sudden drop in blood pressure to below 70 mm Hg systolic; (3) a weak, thready pulse; (4) respiratory disturbance that is initially a respiratory alkalosis; and (5) electrolyte deficit and urine suppression. The usual laboratory findings are a rise in the hematocrit, serum transaminases (SGOT and SGPT), LDH, catecholamines, blood urea nitrogen (BUN), blood amylase, and blood glucose levels. Metabolic acidosis occurs later. The importance to early diagnosis of the triad of hyperventilation, mental confusion, and fever cannot be overemphasized.

A conventional vasopressor agent is used for management of gram-negative sepsis to increase urinary output and coronary profusion pressure. However, such an agent also has sig-

nificant hemodynamic advantages and is unlikely to improve survival. Routine use is dis-
couraged. Volume repletion is an important
part of therapy for gram-negative sepsis.

Disseminated Intravascular Coagulation Syndrome

Two forms of the DIC syndrome are recognized. The acute form, which is often associated with spontaneous hemorrhage and shock,
frequently requires therapy. With the chronic
or subacute form, hemorrhagic manifestations
rarely occur unless the patient's hemostatic
defense mechanism is stressed by surgery or
trauma. This form rarely requires specific therapy. Thus the DIC syndrome is not a defined
disease entity but, rather, an intermediary
mechanism in a host of totally unrelated disease states. Therapy of DIC should therefore
be directed toward treatment of the underlying
disorder whenever possible. A useful coagulation profile for DIC includes the tests in Table
9.1.

Because fibrin degradation products interfere with either fibrin polarization or the action
of thrombin, the thrombin time can serve as a
rapid screening test for gross elevations of fibrinogen degradation products. The fibrinogen
time, however, is relatively insensitive, and
valid results can be obtained only if the fibrinogen level is higher than 75 mg/dl. More
sensitive and specific methods are available for
detecting fibrin degradation products. The best
one of these methods at present is the tan red
blood cell hemagglutination inhibition immunoassay, which is sensitive to both early and
late split products. The "Fi odd" and the
staphylococcal clumping tests are relatively insensitive to late products (i.e., fragments D
and E). The euglobulin clot lysis time, an index
of plasma fibrinolysis, is relatively insensitive
and difficult to perform.

The preferred antibiotic for gram-negative
infection is usually gentamicin. When a diagnosis of *Pseudomonas* septicemia is made, I use a
combination of gentamicin and carbenicillin.
Clindamycin is the preferred drug for the treatment of *Bacteroides* infections. Rarely, *Salmonella* is a cause of gram-negative bac-

TABLE 9.1. Tests for differential diagnosis of DIC

Test	Acute DIC	Subacute DIC
Prothrombin time (PT)	Prolonged	Variable
Partial thromboplastin time (APTT)	Prolonged	Variable
Thrombin or reptilase time	Prolonged	Prolonged
Fibrinogen level	Decreased	Decreased
Degradation products (FDP)	Increased	Increased
Platelet count	Decreased	Variable

teremia, and when present chloramphenicol is
the preferred treatment. When gentamicin is
used, it should be given as 1.5 mg/kg body
weight IV over a 3-minute period every 8
hours. Volume replacement is an important
part of therapy of the gram-negative sepsis.

There are two indications for using a conventional vasopressor agent for managing gram-
negative sepsis: to increase urinary output and
to increase coronary profusion pressure. These
agents have significant hemodynamic advantages and are likely to improve survival. Their
routine use is not encouraged, but there are
specific indications for their use. Dopamine has
been considered to be one of the best of the
catecholamine drugs to use for shock. Dopamine is essentially three drugs in one, depending on the dose used and the patient's response. Small doses (2–5 µg/kg/min) produce
dopaminergic response, that is, specific dilation of gut and kidney vessels to increase blood
flow to essential viscera. Moderate doses (5–30
µg/kg/min) have, in addition, an ionotropic
effect (increased heart force) and increase the
cardiac output. High doses (>30 µg/kg/min)
cause vasoconstriction that is just as powerful as that caused by norepinephrine or
epinephrine. In other words, high doses of
dopamine have the same pressor effects as
norepinephrine. Isoproterenol is used in patients with inappropriately slow pulses and, in
small doses (1–2 µg), for patients with bronchospasm. Dopamine does not cause bronchial
dilatation, whereas isoproterenol does; and
when bronchospasm accompanies shock, dopamine should be used with isoproterenol.

Fibrinogen is no longer dispensed because

of the likelihood of hepatitis B, as each lot is prepared commercially from plasma from thousands of donors. Cryoprecipitate from relatively few donors supplies fibrinogen with much less risk of hepatitis. Cryoprecipitate is an available source of fibrinogen and factor VIII (AFH). Its potential utility of fibrinogen replacement was one of several strong arguments favoring the withdrawal of commercial fibrinogen concentrates; the high risk of hepatitis transmission with the concentrates and the rarity of patients who require only fibrinogen replacement were other prime considerations.

Despite the awareness that fibrinogen is concentrated in cryoprecipitate, little has been published to date to indicate the quantity of fibrinogen present. To supply 4 g of fibrinogen, 15 to 20 bags of cryoprecipitate, each from an individual donor, is required. There is considerable variability among the data published. The estimates range from 100 to 300 mg of fibrinogen per bag of cryoprecipitate. Dosage recommendations vary in major hematology texts from two to four bags of cryoprecipitate per 10 kg body weight; the variation is probably due in large part to the lack of reliable information about the fibrinogen content of cryoprecipitate.

Heparin is being used with decreasing frequency. The infusion of heparin to try to block DIC associated with placental abruption has been abandoned. Heparin is a potent anticoagulant that can be predicted to aggravate hemorrhage when there has been gross disruption of the vasculature.

Shock Lung Syndrome

Shock lung syndrome has three distinguishing characteristics: gross intrapulmonary shunting and relative or absolute hypoxemia, reduced pulmonary compliance, and diffused bilateral pulmonary edema. It occurs as a result of shock due to hemorrhage or sepsis and develops 18 to 48 hours after the profound hypotensive episode.

The syndrome must be differentiated from acute respiratory distress syndrome (ARDS), which includes many heterogeneous clinical entities that result in acute respiratory insufficiency (e.g., thermal lung injuries, aspiration of noxious gases or gastric fluid, near-drowning in fresh or salt water, pulmonary fat emboli, acute pancreatitis, oxygen toxicity, fluid overload, and viral lung infection). Patients with ARDS have intrapulmonary shunting, decreased pulmonary compliance, and radiographic findings consistent with pulmonary edema. In contrast, shock lung syndrome is not associated with any of these causes and is always preceded by hemorrhagic or septic shock. Also, therapy directed to shock lung syndrome may not be beneficial in conditions that comprise ARDS. Shock lung syndrome, which is always preceded by hemorrhagic or septic shock, is seen more commonly now because of the modern resuscitation methods permitting management of the acute episode. Death due to respiratory failure often supervenes 24 to 48 hours later despite therapy with a combination of mechanical ventilation with or without positive end-expiratory pressure (PEEP), antibiotics when indicated, diuretics, cardiac glycosides, and a single pharmacologic dose of cortisone. Mortality despite these therapeutic measures is variously reported to be 60 to 90%.

The shock lung has often been confused with such pathologic diagnoses as bronchopneumonia, patchy atelectasis, and agonal changes. In the acute state the lung grossly shows edema, congestion, hemorrhage, heaviness, and relative airlessness. The lungs are liver-like, consolidated, and markedly saturated with fluid, literally oozing fluids onto their surface. Microscopically, the same characteristics are evident with patchy atelectasis, intraalveolar edema, congestion, and hemorrhage with or without microthrombi.

The clinical picture is characterized by apprehension, tachypnea, air hunger, and sepsis. Cyanosis, however, may not be present in the early stages. Expiratory wheezes are almost pathognomonic of impending shock lung, but bronchial rales and signs of consolidation may not be present early in the disease. Three conditions that commonly lead to shock lung are systemic sepsis, massive fluid replacement, and a period of hypotension. A roentgenographic study of the lungs may show no evidence of impending shock changes until

36 to 48 hours postoperatively. At this time a characteristic "snowfield" patchy pneumonitis and pulmonary haziness may be present.

Blood gases and tidal volumes, especially serial measurements, are diagnostic and prognostic. The changes in the arterial blood gases are diminished PaO_2 and $PaCO_2$; and in late stages of septic shock $PaCO_2$ may be elevated. These changes are secondary to severe shunting and hyperventilation. Early in the development of shock lung, the serum PO_2 ranges from 50 to 60 mm Hg and the serum PCO_2 from 20 to 30 mm Hg. The pH is often alkalotic. During the initial alkalotic phase, the PO_2 may be maintained by increasing the inspired concentration of oxygen and by hyperventilating the patient. Later in the untreated patient the PO_2 declines further, but the PCO_2 rises or remains normal and the pH becomes acidotic. These measurements give an indication of the ability of the lung to utilize oxygen and show the degree of arteriovenous shunting. Arterial $PaCO_2$ that remains low after the patient has inspired 100% oxygen for 30 minutes indicates a high degree of shunting, and the chance for survival is thus poor. Prognosis is also poor when lung compliance is low and decreases progressively. In the latter instance, functional residual capacity decreases as minute volume increases.

Treatment must be aggressive and must be started early. Treatment should include maintenance of PEEP, large amounts of steroids, infusion of albumin and diuretics, administration of broad-spectrum antibiotics, restriction of fluids to levels that can be handled by the compromised cardiopulmonary system without difficulty, and careful filtration of all fluids given to decrease the chance of particles forming microemboli in the lungs. If carried out in a carefully controlled manner, these measures may greatly decrease the incidence of death due to this disease. Serum salt albumin (50 g over 1 hour) or low-molecular-weight dextran enhances the colloidal osmotic pressure of the pulmonary perfusate. This treatment helps prevent pulmonary edema. Fluid therapy is monitored by urinary output, which gives some indications of tissue perfusion. The end-

expiratory pressure is first set at 3 cm H_2O and is gradually increased to 18 to 20 cm H_2O, a level that maintains arterial PO_2 at the desired level of 60 to 90 mm Hg on minimal percentage inspired oxygen. PEEP should be maintained in patients with shock lung until all signs of disease have disappeared.

Central venous pressure (CVP) is not an infallible indicator of mild cardiac insufficiency. Its use should be accompanied by frequent auscultation of the lungs to determine the presence of moist rales and auscultation of the heart to determine the presence of protodiastolic gallop sounds. CVP monitoring measures only the function of the right side of the heart. Pulmonary arterial pressure and pulmonary wedge pressure (PWP) monitoring by means of a Swan-Ganz catheter gives an index of left ventricular competence.

In the critically ill patient, the auscultation of blood pressure by the cuff measure is inaccurate, and it is better to cannulate a peripheral artery and to connect it to a strain gauge transducer measuring device. Cuff pressures may be regarded as minimal pressures. If the actual mean arterial pressure with an arterial needle is measured, the mean arterial pressure in shock should be raised to 10 mm Hg less than the patient's usual level (i.e., about 80 mm Hg). If the patient has coronary artery disease, it is best to raise it only to 20 mm Hg less than the usual (i.e., 70 mm Hg). The cuff measure may read 60 mm Hg palpable when the actual blood pressure is 240/100 mm Hg with a mean arterial pressure of 100 mm Hg, so it is necessary to be careful when treating patients using the cuff blood pressure as a guide and always to palpate central pulses to confirm the cuff readings. Cuff pressures are usually too low by 10 to 20 mm Hg. Consequently, the responsible physician does not attempt to raise the cuff pressure to normal.

Fluid replacement is adequate when either urinary output returns to adequate levels (>40 ml/hr) or the CVP or PWP rise rapidly. If urinary output is not reestablished by fluid loading, furosemide (Lasix) 80 mg or ethacrynic acid 100 mg is given. In most patients, arterial blood pressure (CVP and PWP), urinary output, and pulse pressure are restored to normal or near-normal levels with these measures alone. If urinary output does not return to adequate levels, however, indicating adequate perfusion, the patient should rapidly receive a digitalis preparation.

For patients with gram-negative or endotoxic shock it has been recommended that methylprednisolone at a dose of 30 mg/kg body weight be given once or twice. This drug has been used for the treatment of shock lung at the same dose either as a single dose or repeated after 2 to 4 hours. However, if methylprednisolone is used to improve pulmonary blood flow, stabilize the endothelium of the small pulmonary vessels, and slow the leakage of protein-containing fluid, adequate tissue levels of the agent must be continued long enough to maintain these effects, not merely initiate them. The doses that Lillehei et al. indicated may be beneficial for the pure shock states are probably adequate to maintain the hypothesized therapeutic action of the steroid on the lung when repeated every 6 hours.

It therefore seems reasonable to give patients with shock lung syndrome early treatment with methylprednisolone 30 mg/kg every 6 hours for 48 hours after the onset of the syndrome and then attempt to determine if this therapy can improve arterial oxygenation and resolve the pulmonary edema. Of course, the agent must always be used as an adjunct to therapy directed at the cause of shock, as its only action is on the damaged lungs; it does not correct the shock.

Mortality due to shock lung ranges up to 80%. The condition is supposedly reversible if support can be continued for a sufficient period, and for this reason many investigators have attempted long-term support with membrane oxygenators and partial right heart bypass in cases where ventilatory failure is imminent despite conventional modes of therapy. Reported series are small, but some successes have been noted.

Awareness of potential pulmonary complications combined with adequate therapy contributes to the preservation of life in cases that just a few years ago were considered hopeless.

Summary

Aggressive surgery can be carried out in cases of ovarian cancer because of a better understanding of the pathophysiology relating to sepsis, blood loss, and shock lung. In addition, it is possible now to improve the patient's nutrition and maintain her in good balance by the liberal use of hyperalimentation. The use of hyperalimentation, the Swan-Ganz catheter, more potent antibiotics, and an overall better understanding of preoperative and postoperative care has opened up the field of aggressive surgery for managing the patient with ovarian cancer.

A well-planned, well-coordinated workup may alert the physician to a diagnosis of metastatic, rather than primary, ovarian cancer. In addition, it may reveal a physiologic imbalance that could result in morbidity or mortality unless corrected. A detailed diagnostic workup may be outlined as follows.

1. Complete history and physical examinations, including pelvic and rectal examinations
2. Careful palpation of the thyroid
3. Hemogram
4. Urinalysis
5. Blood chemistry profile
6. Serum electrolyte profile
7. Anteroposterior and lateral chest roentgenograms
8. Electrocardiogram
9. VDRL
10. Intravenous pyelogram
11. Mammography
12. Cystoscopy
13. Proctoscopy
14. Barium enema
15. Gastrointestinal series
16. Skeletal survey
17. Lymphangiogram
18. Liver scan
19. Ultrasonography

Note: Prior to an exploratory laparotomy, the patient should have an examination under anesthesia and fractional curettage. Laparoscopy or peritoneoscopy for staging the ovarian cancer is optional.

Bibliography

Barber HRK: Fluid, electrolyte and nutritional management of the gynecologic patient. Part I. In Goldstein DP, Leventhal J (eds): *Current Problems in Obstetrics and Gynecology*. Year Book, Chicago, 1979.

Barber HRK: Fluid, electrolyte and nutritional management of the gynecologic patient. Part II. In Goldstein DP, Leventhal J (eds): *Current Problems in Obstetrics and Gynecology*. Year Book, Chicago, 1979.

Barber, HRK (ed): *Manual of Gynecologic Oncology*. Lippincott, Philadelphia, 1980, p. 68.

Barber HRK: Fluid and Electrolyte Problems. In Barber HRK, Fields DH, Kaufman SA (eds): *Quick Reference to Ob/Gyn Procedures*. Third Ed. Lippincott Philadelphia, 1990, p 343.

Beran DR: Perioperative care: intraoperative fluid balance. *Br J Hosp Med* 19:445, 1978.

Cranley JJ: Phleborheography: new noninvasive method of diagnosing deep venous thrombosis of lower extremity is highly accurate. *RI Med J* 58:111, 1975.

Cranley JJ, Gay AY, Grass AM, et al: A plethysmographic technique for the diagnosis of deep venous thrombosis of the lower extremities. *Surg Gynecol Obstet*. 136:385, 1973.

Dudrick SJ, Copeland EM III, MacFayden BV Jr: Long-term parenteral nutrition. *Hosp Pract* 10:47, 1975.

Dudrick SJ, Rhoads JE: Total intravenous feeding. *Sci Am* 226:73, 1972.

Hammond WP, Dale DC: Infections in the compromised host. *Hosp Med* 15(May):87, 1978.

Hull RL: Physiochemical considerations in intravenous hyperalimentation. *Am J Hosp Pharm* 31:236, 1975.

Kinnaird DW, Aldrete A: Preoperative care. In Preston FW, Davis WC (eds): *General Surgery*. Harper & Row, Hagerstown, ch. 12, 1975.

Kinnaird DW, Aldrete A: Postoperative care. In Preston FW, Davis WC (eds): *General Surgery*. Harper & Row, Hagerstown, ch. 13, 1975.

Laufman H, Lalezari P: A plan for management of unexpected bleeding problems related to surgery. *Pacific Med Surg* 75:362, 1967.

Lillehei RC, Dietzman RH, Morsas S: Treatment of septic shock. *Mod Treat* 4:321, 1967.

Maki DG: Infection control in intravenous therapy. *Ann Intern Med* 79:867, 1973.

Miller RD: Complications of massive transfusions. *Anesthesiology* 39:82, 1973.

Ryan GM, Howland WS: The diagnosis and therapy of hemorrhagic disorders occurring during surgery. *Surg Dig* 3:29, 1968.

Weil MH: Therapy of septic shock. *Surg Infect Semin* (Schering Corp.) 13, 1977.

Winslow EBJ: *The Role of Catecholamines in Patients with Septic Shock*. Arnar-Stone Laboratories, Education Program Developed by SKM Ltd., Northfield, Il, 1977.

10

Diagnosing and Managing the Adnexal Mass

Age is an important consideration in the management of a patient with an adnexal mass. For the following discussion, I have divided patients into three age groups: birth to 20 years, 20 to 40 years, and over 40 years. Occurrence during pregnancy is considered separately, later in the chapter.

A mass in the very young and the very old is presumed to be *abnormal*. The best management consists in a careful workup and exploratory laparotomy. There is no time or place for observation and procrastination with patients in these age groups. Management of the adnexal mass diagnosed during pregnancy or in patients between 20 and 40 may arouse controversy. This topic is presented in depth later in the chapter.

Birth to Age 20

Any palpable adnexal mass in the newborn and the prepubertal patient is suspect, and a new growth must be ruled out. Although ovarian tumors account for about 1% of new growths in children under age 16, they remain the most frequent genital neoplasm of childhood and adolescence. The problems related to diagnosis are surpassed only by the problems and confusion related to therapy. It is difficult for many of those involved with patients in this group to accept the possibility of ovarian malignancy and even more difficult for the physician to deprive a child of her reproductive potential.

Ovarian neoplasms may occur at any age during childhood or adolescence, but they tend to be most common at puberty (between 10 and 14 years). This fact had led to conjecture that some control mechanism may be activated or that pituitary stimulation of a latent ovarian factor may be the triggering mechanism. A graph drawn for ovarian tumors presenting in this age group would project a bell shape, with the peak at puberty.

The most common malignant ovarian tumor in infants and young children is the dysgerminoma. Although it is rare to diagnose a malignancy in this age group, dysgerminomas have been found soon after birth or later. Multiple retention cysts and luteal cysts are also occasionally seen in the newborn. If the tumors are not complicated by torsion, rupture, or infection, observation for a couple of weeks is acceptable; during this time there should be marked regression.

Ovarian tumors in children may produce few symptoms. The symptomatology is related to the rapidity of growth, position, degree of malignancy, and the tumor's ability to secrete hormones. The complications associated with tumors, such as twisting, rupture, infection, and hemorrhage, focus attention on them.

When symptoms occur, a general physical examination that includes the pelvic, rectal, and rectovaginal areas should be carefully carried out. It is almost universally impossible to palpate normal ovaries in children; therefore it can be assumed that a palpable ovary is abnormal. The size determines whether it can be felt abdominally or by rectoabdominal palpation. In the prepubertal girl the ovary is an abdominal organ; it does not migrate into the pelvis until puberty.

Diagnostic procedures should include a blood count, urinalysis, chest roentgenogram, intravenous pyelogram, and, if indicated, radiographic studies of the gastrointestinal tract. In patients suspected of having a hormone-producing tumor, hormone assays may have some value, but radiographic studies of bone age may be even more helpful. The role of ultrasound studies and laparoscopy in this age group remains to be clarified. Alpha-fetoprotein (AFP) and carcinoembryonic antigen (CEA) levels may be significantly elevated. Elevation of AFP has been found to be associated with endodermal sinus tumor and certain embryonal carcinomas. An elevated chorionic gonadotropin titer may be present in embryonal tumors, especially when chorionic elements are found in the tumor.

The key to treatment is conservatism. However, any spread beyond the ovary demands a more aggressive approach. Treatment is outlined here by groups of tumors within a given classification. Although common epithelial ovarian tumors are rare in this age group, the physician must occasionally manage a mucinous or serous cystadenocarcinoma. If the tumor is unilateral and encapsulated, if there is negative pelvic cytology, and if the opposite ovary is negative on biopsy, unilateral salpingo-oophorectomy is acceptable therapy. With any evidence of spread of disease beyond the ovary, however, total abdominal hysterectomy (TAH), bilateral salpingo-oophorectomy (BSO), and omentectomy (if an omentum has developed) are indicated, along with the instillation of 10 mCi of radioactive phosphorus (^{32}P) if the responsible physician believes it is indicated. The management of low potential malignancy (borderline) tumors is presented in Chapter 15.

Germ cell tumors vary a great deal in their response to treatment. The dysgerminoma is a highly radiosensitive tumor that occurs bilaterally in up to 10% of the patients. The treatment of choice, although controversial, is unilateral salpingo-oophorectomy, based on the assumption that no positive cells are present in the pelvis. (The value of pelvic cytologic studies of this tumor has not been established.) The opposite ovary and the paraaortic nodes must be free of tumor on biopsy. If there is spread beyond the ovary in which the tumor occurs, TAH-BSO is required. X-irradiation should be employed if the disease spreads to the pelvis or upper abdomen. The need for mediastinal and supraclavicular node therapy with x-irradiation for this age group has not been determined.

Embryonal carcinomas and extraembryonal carcinomas (endodermal sinus tumor, polyvesicular vitelline tumor, and choriocarcinoma) are highly malignant. If unilateral and encapsulated, however, they are treated just as well by unilateral oophorectomy as by more radical surgery. Radiation therapy offers little help because these tumors are relatively radioresistant. Multiple chemotherapy, however, has been producing encouraging results, and some improvement in survival rates is being reported. There is controversy over whether the uterus and remaining tube and ovary should be removed before instituting triple chemotherapy. Only time will provide the answer, but a conservative surgical approach is currently recommended if there is no evidence of spread.

Gonadal stromal tumors (formerly referred to as sex-cord tumors) include tumors that have the potential to produce either an estrogenizing or a masculinizing effect, although they do so in only 25% of patients. Of the female cell type, the only important malignant tumor is the granulosa cell tumor. It is usually unilateral and exhibits late recurrence, often beyond 5 years. Typically, spread is local, and recurrence is confined to the pelvis. Because the tumor is of low-grade malignancy and is seldom bilateral, unilateral oophorectomy is indicated when the tumor is encapsulated and the other ovary is normal.

Among tumors of the male cell type, the Sertoli-Leydig cell tumor (formerly called arrhenoblastoma) is the most important. If it secretes a hormone, the resulting clinical picture is defeminization followed by masculinization. When it is malignant, the natural history is similar to that of granulosa cell carcinoma, and treatment is the same for both. Once the patient has completed her family, hysterectomy and removal of the other ovary are indicated in patients who have had either a granulosa cell tumor or a Sertoli-Leydig cell tumor.

Gonadoblastoma is composed of germ cells and gonadal stromal cells in nearly equal proportion. Its malignant potential is determined by the type of germ cell present. The gonadoblastoma is usually found in the intersexual patient, and therefore the accepted treatment is bilateral oophorectomy.

Metastatic ovarian cancer in this age group is treated as in adults. As much tumor as possible is removed, including the primary cancer.

Age 20 to 40

In the 20- to 40-year age group, as the patient's age moves toward 40 there is little controversy about management of an adnexal mass. An aggressive approach is usually adopted as far as diagnosis and therapy are concerned. Management in the over 40 age group is TAH-BSO, even though the tumor may be low grade. In the group age 20 to 30 years, controversy often arises over the best management. Like the childhood and adolescent group, the most common lesion seen in this age group is the germ cell tumor followed by the gonadal stromal tumor. There has also been an increased number of common epithelial ovarian tumors diagnosed.

If the patient is in her twenties and the mass is cystic, smooth, movable, and less than 6 cm, it is good medical practice to reevaluate after a menstrual period. Functional cysts start to regress following the period. Some investigators have advocated the use of a combined estrogen-progesterone pill to inhibit pituitary stimulation of the ovary. If it is a functional cyst, it should promptly begin to regress. Even a short period of observation is not justified if the patient is taking oral contraceptive pills.

At the time of laparotomy, management of the adnexal mass in the patient in her twenties is similar to that described for management of tumors in children. It is important to individualize treatment not only according to histogenetic classification but also according to

stage of disease. In general, a conservative approach is justified if the tumor is unilateral and encapsulated and there is negative cytology with a normal opposite ovary. Among dysgerminomas it is important also to evaluate the paraaortic area. There is usually less concern about conservative management if the patient has already had several children.

A careful history is of prime importance, followed by a thorough pelvic examination to include the vaginal, rectal, and rectovaginal areas. The ideal time to examine the patient is after she has been given an enema. There are causes for the presence of an adnexal mass other than ovarian pathology. Certain diagnoses are more likely to be made at a given age; for example, diverticulitis is more common after age 40, whereas an ectopic pregnancy is more common when the patient is in her twenties. The differential diagnosis should include myomas (pedunculated); retroperitoneal tumors; pelvic-kidney, tuboovarian, or appendiceal abscesses; diverticulitis; adhesions; anterior sacral meningocele; ectopic pregnancy; and neoplasms of the large bowel.

The preoperative workup must be thorough so the primary site of a metastatic tumor is not overlooked. It should include blood counts and chemistries as well as urinalysis. Chest roentgenograms and intravenous pyelography are helpful, and sonography is optional. Whether mammograms and roentgenograms of the intestinal tract are indicated depends on the symptomatology and age of the patient. Biologic markers such as CEA, AFP, chorionic gonadotropin titers, and lactic dehydrogenase (LDH) levels have value only if they are elevated. They can then serve to monitor the response to therapy. The value of laparoscopy has not proved valuable for making an early diagnosis but has a role in the staging of the ovarian cancer. It has a limited place in monitoring treatment because a positive finding is significant, whereas a laparoscopic examination that is negative for disease requires a laparotomy to be certain no disease is present in the retroperitoneal space.

If the patient is in her twenties and the mass is cystic, smooth, and movable, it is good medical practice to reevaluate after one or two menstrual periods. A functional cyst should start to regress during this time. It is important to explain to the patient the reason for re-evaluating after a period. It should be carefully recorded on the chart that she has been instructed to return after her period. This practice offers medicolegal protection if the patient does not return. She is then guilty of contributory negligence. Some investigators have advocated the use of a combined estrogen-progesterone pill to inhibit pituitary stimulation of the ovary. The question of whether the triphasic oral contraceptive pill is associated with an increase in the incidence of functional cysts of the ovary has been raised. However, carefully followed control groups in a significant series has not confirmed this suspicion. If it is a functional cyst, it should promptly begin to regress. Even a short period of observation is not justified if the patient is already taking oral contraceptives.

At the time of laparotomy, management of the adnexal mass in the patient in her twenties is similar to that described for tumors in children. It is important to individualize treatment not only according to histogenetic classification but also according to stage of disease. In general, the conservative approach is justified if the tumor is unilateral and encapsulated. Also, there should be negative cytology, and the tumor should be well differentiated, particularly if it is a dysgerminoma or a gonadal stromal type. The patient should be of low parity or nulliparous, and there should be a negative biopsy of the opposite ovary as well as negative omental or pelvic and paraaortic node biopsies.

There is an increase in the number of common epithelial ovarian cancers being reported in the younger age group. Most of these cancers are serous cystadenocarcinomas and mucinous cystadenocarcinomas. Endometrioid and clear-cell carcinomas appear in the older age group. The mucinous cystadenocarcinoma is bilateral in about 5% of patients. Because it is rarely bilateral and is less aggressive than serous tumors, it can be managed with unilateral salpingo-oophorectomy. Serous cystadenocarcinoma that is unilateral, encapsulated, and freely movable with no pathology in the opposite ovary or positive cytology can be managed conservatively, but in both instances the patient and her family must know that she is at risk.

Any evidence of spread demands maximal surgical treatment, including TAH-BSO, omentectomy, and appendectomy. Although patients between age 20 and 40 become subjects of the greatest degree of controversy when an adnexal mass is found, there is no dispute over treatment if the mass is bilateral, larger than 10 cm, or irregular in outline with cystic and solid areas present, or if it continues to grow under observation. TAH-BSO, omentectomy, appendectomy, and ^{32}P instillation may be used at the discretion of the clinician.

Adnexal Mass During Pregnancy

The adnexal mass during pregnancy is always cause for concern. Approximately 1 in 1000 pregnancies is complicated by an ovarian tumor. During pregnancy most ovarian masses represent a normal cystic corpus luteum, which may become as large as 10 cm. Corpus luteum cysts are usually unilateral and freely movable. The differential diagnosis of an adnexal mass in the pregnancy patient is the same as that in the nonpregnant patient in the same age group.

The incidence of malignancy in ovarian tumors diagnosed during pregnancy is variously reported between 2.5% and 5.0%. Fortunately, most malignancies during pregnancy are discovered at stage I because the patient seeks examination early. The survival rate of pregnant patients with ovarian cancer is the same as that of nonpregnant patients. The type of tumor and its anatomic spread determine the 5-year cure rate. Pregnancy has no effect on the tumor. Only aggressive, early exploration can save the patient. Interruption of pregnancy has no beneficial effect on the future of this disease. If the tumor is diagnosed during the third trimester, surgery can be delayed until the fetus has become viable. Delay beyond that point is not justified.

Management of an ovarian mass during pregnancy depends to a certain extent on the trimester of the pregnancy and on whether torsion or hemorrhage occurs as a complication. A freely movable, encapsulated, unilateral adnexal mass can be observed until the second trimester. A corpus luteum cyst regresses during the second trimester. If the mass persists or increases in size, surgical intervention is indicated. When an ovarian tumor is found during pregnancy, it is usually either a dermoid or a cystadenoma. Both of these tumors can be managed by conservative therapy at the time of exploratory laparotomy.

However, if the mass is knobby, fixed, or bilateral with any signs of fluid or with differences of consistency throughout the tumor and is larger than 10 cm, surgery is indicated without delay despite the trimester of pregnancy. Management depends on the stage of the disease and the histology of the tumor.

Age 40 and Older

Patients 40 years of age and older comprise the high-risk group because they are either perimenopausal or postmenopausal. The same diagnostic workup and differential diagnosis are followed as in the 20 to 40-year age group. Metastatic cancers of the ovary are probably more common in this high-risk age group. Because chances of malignancy are higher than in the younger age group, there is no indication for observation, especially if the mass is larger than 5 cm or is adherent and gives the impression of having different areas of consistency throughout.

Treatment should consist of TAH-BSO, appendectomy, and omentectomy; instillation of ^{32}P may be used at the discretion of the clinician. The epithelial ovarian tumor is the most commonly encountered ovarian tumor. About 8% occur before age 40, and the incidence peaks at age 77 years.

What is considered a normal-sized ovary in the premenopausal woman is an ovarian tumor in the patient who is more than 2 years postmenopausal. There is no such thing as physiologic cysts in this age group. The contrast between the premenopausal and postmenopausal ovary is striking. Whereas the normal

ovary measures $3.5 \times 2.0 \times 1.5$ cm, the ovary in the patient who is 2 years or more postmenopausal may be as small as $1.50 \times 0.75 \times 0.50$ cm. These patients should not be followed and reevaluated; the presence or absence of a tumor must be substantiated immediately. To wait until a solid tumor mass of up to 5 cm can be felt and then to expect a cure is an exercise in futility.

The tumors reviewed in this chapter are discussed in greater detail in other chapters.

Summary

Age is an important consideration to the management of a patient with an adnexal mass. Between birth and age 20, germ cell tumors are the most common. Except for the embryonal and extraembryonal tumors, germ cell tumors are associated with a respectable survival rate. Often it is possible to be conservative with management of the ovarian tumor without compromising the survival of the patient. In the 20- to 40-year age group, a variety of ovarian tumors are encountered. Those patients who fall into the 20- to 30-year group usually have germ cell or gonadal stromal tumors, and a conservative approach is acceptable if the findings indicate that the patient's prognosis will not be jeopardized. Patients 40 years or older usually have a common epithelial ovarian tumor. The decision on management is not difficult because more aggressive therapy is the management chosen in this age group. The ovarian tumor during pregnancy may be followed until the end of the first trimester if it is unilateral, freely movable, and does not increase in size. However, if it is bilateral, fixed, hard, and knobby with areas that are rubbery or cystic, the patient should be explored without a period of observation.

The common epithelial ovarian cancer is starting to appear at a younger age. The two types most commonly seen are the serous cystadenocarcinoma and the mucinous cystadenocarcinoma. If they are unilateral, freely movable, have negative cytology, and the opposite ovary is negative, conservative management is acceptable. However, the patient and her family must be informed that the patient is at risk.

Bibliography

Barber HRK, Graber EA: The PMPO syndrome (postmenopausal palpable ovary syndrome). *Obstet Gynecol.* 38:921, 1971.

Barber HRK, Graber EA: Gynecologic tumors in childhood and adolescence. *Obstet Gynecol Surv* 28:357, 1973.

Barber HRK, Graber EA: Surgical aspects of ovarian tumors. In Charyulu KKN, Sudarsanam A (eds): *Selected Topics of Cancer—Current Concepts.* Intercontinental Medical Book Corp, New York, 1974, pp. 161–183.

Hilaris BS, Clark DGC: The value of postoperative intraperitoneal injection of radiocolloids in early cancer of the ovary. *Am J Roentgenol Radium Ther Nucl Med* 112:749, 1971.

Munnell EW: Is conservative therapy ever justified in stage I cancer of the ovary? *Am J Obstet Gynecol* 103:641, 1969.

Novak ER, Long JH: Arrhenoblastoma of the ovary. *Am J Obstet Gynecol* 92:1082, 1965.

Scully RE: Recent progress in ovarian cancer. *Hum Pathol* 1:73, 1970.

Sjstedt D, Wahlen T: Prognosis of granulosa cell tumors. *Acta Obstet Gynecol Scand* 6:40, 1961.

Teilum G: Tumors of germinal origin. In: *Ovarian Cancer. International Union Against Cancer Monograph Series.* Vol. 2. Springer-Verlag, New York, 1948, p. 58.

11

Staging Ovarian Cancer

Ovarian cancer is becoming a common malignancy. It has been considered a family of malignancies arising within the ovary rather than a single entity. The ovary is complex in its embryology, histology, steroidogenesis, and potential for malignancy. It is made up of germ cells, gonadal stromal cells, and cells of the mesenchymal tissue, each with its own potential to form a tumor. Although sex is determined genetically at fertilization, the ovary passes through its early phases as an indifferent organ with parallel development that could allow it to become an ovary or a testis. Alterations or imbalances during these steps of development may provide the setting for the later cellular malfunctioning that produces endocrine imbalances as well as malignancy. The ovary is unique in that it not only gives rise to a great variety of malignancies but itself is a favorite site for metastases from many other organs.

Therapeutic statistics on ovarian cancer are of limited value if attention is not paid to the histologic type of the growth. However, experience has shown that there is no clear correlation between clinical and histologic malignancy in ovarian tumors in all instances. This point holds true for various neoplasms, but especially for epithelial tumors, granulosa cell tumors, and virilizing tumors.

Until 1971 there were as many classifications for staging ovarian cancer as there were hospitals in the United States, and there were as many subdivisions as there were physicians practicing in those hospitals. A common language for staging ovarian cancer was provided by the International Federation of Gynecology and Obstetrics (FIGO) in 1971 that provided a more accurate method for evaluating results among hospitals.

In a review of the material at Lenox Hill Hospital, the conclusion reached was that staging and histologic type are both important and should be used to establish therapy. It is obvious that they are not competitive but, rather, complementary. The importance of grading (histologic, nuclear, and stromal) in endometrial and cervical cancers has been established and accepted. It remains for a universal grading system to be adopted for ovarian cancer. This study showed that the grade was important for predicting prognosis in the early stages of ovarian cancer but was a less reliable guide for the more advanced cancers. *In general, stage of disease has proved to be more important than histologic or nuclear grades.*

Within each stage there is a great deal of variation, making it difficult to compare results among institutions. Because there are varying degrees of malignancy in groups of a particular stage, it is important to examine tumor tissues microscopically to determine their grade or degree of malignancy according to the histologic and nuclear grade as well as the stromal reaction. *Staging* is determined clinically and estimates the extent of disease and the size of the tumor, whereas histologic type and grading provide its microscopic character. It has been determined that in any stage there is considerable variation, and it is suggested that there are certain tumors more potent than others within a given stage. If these findings are accepted, *treatment should be tailored to the cancer rather than to the stage of disease.*

Unlike other gynecologic malignancies, ovarian cancer is staged at the time of exploratory laparotomy or after a complete microscopic examination of the primary specimen, and biopsy specimens are obtained from the abdominal cavity. All other gynecologic malignancies are staged before the start of therapy; and no matter what new findings are uncovered during treatment, the original and initial staging stands. It is not so with ovarian cancer.

With ovarian tumors it is desirable to have a clinical stage grouping before definitive therapy is begun. Sometimes it is impossible to come to a final diagnosis by inspection or palpation or by any other method recommended for clinically staging carcinoma of the ovary. Therefore the Cancer Committee of FIGO has recommended that the clinical staging of ovarian cancer be based on clinical examination as well as on findings at laparotomy and the microscopic findings postoperatively.

Rules for Staging Primary Carcinoma of the Ovary

Anatomy

Primary Site

Ovaries (ICD-0183.0) are a pair of solid bodies—flattened ovoids 2 to 4 cm in diameter—that are connected by a peritoneal fold to the broad ligament and by the infundibulopelvic ligament to the lateral wall of the pelvis. The peritoneum, including the omentum, pelvic and abdominal viscera, and diaphragm, are common sites for seeding.

Regional Lymph Nodes

The lymphatic drainage occurs by the uterine-ovarian and round ligament trunks and the external iliac accessory route into the following regional nodes: external iliac, common iliac,

hypogastric, laterosacral, and paraaortic nodes and rarely to inguinal nodes.

Metastatic Sites

Peritoneum, including the omentum and pelvic and abdominal viscera, are common sites for seeding. Diaphragmatic involvement and metastasis to the surface of the liver are common. Pulmonary and pleural involvement may also occur.

Only rarely is it possible to come to a final diagnosis of ovarian carcinoma by inspection or palpation or by any of the other means recommended for clinical staging of carcinoma of the uterus and vagina. Therefore the Committee on Gynecologic Oncology of FIGO recommends that the clinical staging of primary carcinoma of the ovary should be based on findings by laparoscopy or laparotomy, as well as the usual clinical examination and roentgenographic studies.

Thus laparotomy and resection of ovarian masses, as well as hysterectomy, are used for staging. Biopsies of all suspicious sites, such as the omentum, mesentery, liver, diaphragm, and pelvic and paraaortic nodes, are required.

The final histologic findings after surgery (and cytologic studies when available) are to be considered during the staging. Clinical studies, if carcinoma of the ovary is diagnosed, include routine roentgenographic studies of the chest. Computed tomography (CT) may be helpful for both initial staging and follow-up of the tumors.

Definitions of the Stages in Primary Carcinoma of the Ovary

The following are correlations of the FIGO, International Union Against Cancer (UICC), and the American Joint Committee on Cancer (AJCC) nomenclatures. *Staging is based on findings at clinical examination and surgical exploration.*

Stage I	Growth limited to the ovaries
Ia	Growth limited to one ovary; no ascites
	No tumor on the external surface; capsule intact

Ib   Growth limited to both ovaries; no ascites

No tumor on the external surfaces; capsules intact

Ic* Tumor either stage Ia or Ib but with tumor on surface of one or both ovaries; or with capsule ruptured; or with ascites present containing malignant cells or with positive peritoneal washings

Stage II   Growth involving one or both ovaries with pelvic extension

IIa Extension and/or metastases to the uterus and/or tubes

IIb Extension to other pelvic tissues

IIc* Tumor either stage IIa or IIb but with tumor on surface of one or both ovaries; or with capsule(s) ruptured; or with ascites present containing malignant cells or with positive peritoneal washings

Stage III   Tumor involving one or both ovaries with peritoneal implants outside the pelvis and/or positive retroperitoneal or inguinal nodes

Superficial liver metastasis equals stage III

Tumor limited to the true pelvis but with histologically proved malignant extension to small bowel or omentum

IIIa Tumor grossly limited to the true pelvis with negative nodes but with histologically confirmed microscopic seeding of abdominal peritoneal surfaces

IIIb Tumor involving one or both ovaries with histologically confirmed implants of abdominal peritoneal surfaces none exceeding 2 cm in diameter; nodes negative

IIIc Abdominal implants more than 2 cm in diameter and/or positive retroperitoneal or inguinal nodes

Stage IV   Growth involving one or both ovaries with distant metastases; if pleural effusion present, there must be positive cytology to allot a case to stage IV

Parenchymal liver metastasis equals stage IV

*To evaluate the impact prognosis of the different criteria for allotting cases to stage Ic or IIc it would be of value to know:

1. If the source of malignant cells detected was
   a. Peritoneal washings *or*
   b. Ascites
2. If rupture of the capsule was
   a. Spontaneous *or*
   b. Caused by the surgeon

Stage Grouping for Primary Carcinoma of the Ovary

The stage grouping categories are based on findings at clinical examination, at surgical exploration, or both. Histologic characteristics are to be considered in the staging, as are results of cytologic testing so far as effusions are concerned. It is desirable that a biopsy be performed on suspicious areas outside the pelvis.

Stage I epithelial ovarian carcinoma is a disease limited to one or both ovaries. Stage Ia is limited to one ovary and stage Ib to both ovaries. Stage Ic is tumor that is either stage Ia or Ib but with tumor on the surface of one or both ovaries; or with the capsule ruptured; or with ascites present containing malignant cells or with positive peritoneal washings (Fig. 11.1).

Stage II indicates growth involving one or both ovaries with pelvic extension of the tumor. Stage IIa is extension and/or metastases to the uterus and/or tubes; stage IIb extension to other pelvic tissues, and stage IIc is tumor of either stage IIa or IIb, each with the tumor on the surface of one or both ovaries; or with capsule(s) ruptured; or with ascites present containing malignant cells or with positive peritoneal washings (Fig. 11.1).

To evaluate the impact on prognosis of the different criteria for allotting cases to Ic or IIc, it is of value to know (1) if rupture of the capsule was spontaneous or caused by the surgeon and (2) if the source of malignant cells detected was peritoneal washings or ascites.

STAGE I   Growth limited to the ovaries.

Stage IA

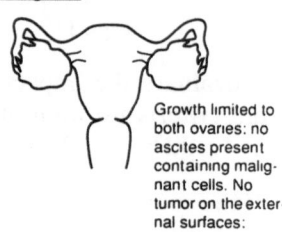

Growth limited to the ovary: no ascites present containing malignant cells. No tumor on the external surface; capsule intact.

Stage IB

Growth limited to both ovaries: no ascites present containing malignant cells. No tumor on the external surfaces: capsules intact.

Stage IC

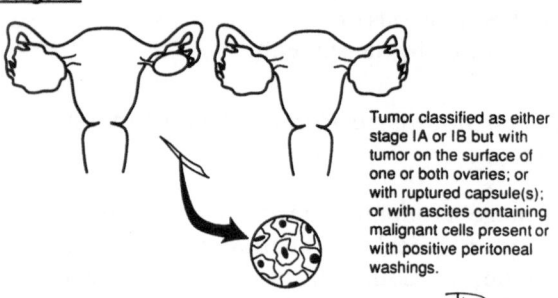

Tumor classified as either stage IA or IB but with tumor on the surface of one or both ovaries; or with ruptured capsule(s); or with ascites containing malignant cells present or with positive peritoneal washings.

STAGE II   Growth involving one or both ovaries, with pelvic extension.

Stage IIA

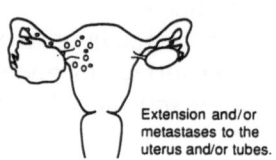

Extension and/or metastases to the uterus and/or tubes.

Stage IIB

Extension to other pelvic tissues.

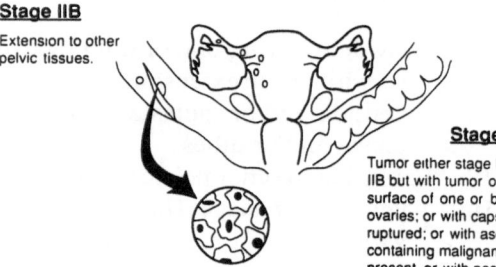

Stage IIC

Tumor either stage IIA or IIB but with tumor on the surface of one or both ovaries; or with capsule(s) ruptured; or with ascites containing malignant cells present or with positive peritoneal washings.

STAGE III   Tumor involving one or both ovaries with peritoneal implants outside the pelvis and/or positive retroperitoneal or inguinal nodes. Superficial liver metastasis equals stage III. Tumor is limited to true pelvis but with histologically proven malignant extension to small bowel or omentum.

Stage IIIA

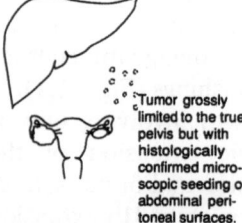

Tumor grossly limited to the true pelvis but with histologically confirmed microscopic seeding of abdominal peritoneal surfaces.

Stage IIIB

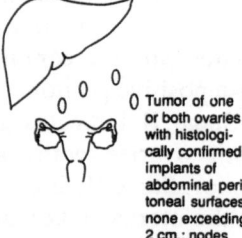

Tumor of one or both ovaries with histologically confirmed implants of abdominal peritoneal surfaces none exceeding 2 cm.; nodes negative.

Stage IIIC

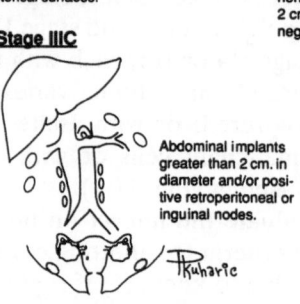

Abdominal implants greater than 2 cm. in diameter and/or positive retroperitoneal or inguinal nodes.

STAGE IV

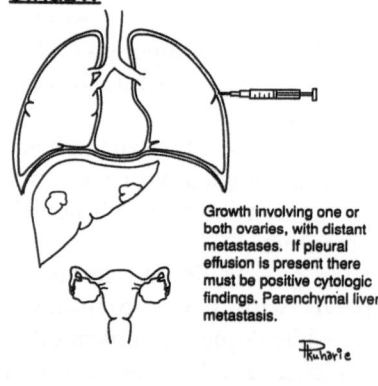

Growth involving one or both ovaries, with distant metastases. If pleural effusion is present there must be positive cytologic findings. Parenchymal liver metastasis.

FIGURE 11.1. Clinical staging of common epithelial ovarian cancers. Staging is based on findings at clinical examinations and surgical exploration, as approved by the General Assembly of the International Federal of Gynecology and Obstetrics.

Stage III is tumor involving one or both ovaries with peritoneal implants outside the pelvis and/or positive retroperitoneal or inguinal nodes. Superficial liver metastases equals stage III. Tumor is limited to the true pelvis but with histologically verified malignant extension to small bowel or omentum. Stage IIIa is tumor grossly limited to the true pelvis with negative nodes but with histologically confirmed microscopic seeding of the abdominal peritoneal surfaces; stage IIIb is tumor of one or both ovaries with histologically confirmed implants of abdominal peritoneal surfaces, not exceeding 2 cm in diameter. The nodes are negative in stage IIIb; stage IIIc has abdominal implants larger than 2 cm in diameter and/or positive retroperitoneal or inguinal nodes (Fig. 11.1).

Stage IV is growth involving one or both ovaries with distant metastases. If pleural effusion is present, there must be positive cytologic tests results to allot a case to stage IV. Parenchymal liver metastases equals stage IV disease (Fig. 11.1).

Stage I and II spell out specifically the amount of disease, but stages III and IV, which in previous classifications were not so specific, have now been better documented in the updated staging. It is important for operating gynecologists to record the volume of tumor to the best of their ability because tumor volume has an important relation to therapy and prognosis.

Staging and detailed histologic studies serve as a guide to understanding the natural history of the disease. Both are important when selecting a therapeutic regimen. Although there are many deficiencies in this classification, it has focused attention on evaluating the extent of the disease. In summary, the stage of disease is the most reliable guide to therapy and prognosis.

TNM System

The AJCC in cooperation with the TNM Committee of the UICC brings together all currently available information on staging of cancer at various anatomic sites. All of the schemes included here are uniform between the two organizations. AJCC has worked closely with FIGO in the classification of cancer of gynecologic sites. Staging of malignant tumors is essentially the same, and stages are comparable by the two systems.

This classification is included because the recommendations of the AJCC with the TNM Committee of the UICC are to be used in the cancer programs approved by the Commission on Cancer of the American College of Surgeons. Also future reports by the Surveillance Epidemiology and End Results Program (SEER) of the National Cancer Institute (NCI) are based on the classifications recommended by the AJCC.

The definitions of the T (primary tumor) categories correspond to the several stages accepted by FIGO. Both systems are included for comparison.

Primary Tumor (T)

TNM	FIGO	Definition
TX		Primary tumor cannot be assessed
T0		No evidence of primary tumor
T1	I	Tumor limited to ovaries
T1a	Ia	Tumor limited to one ovary; capsule intact, no tumor on ovarian surface
T1b	Ib	Tumor limited to both ovaries; capsules intact, no tumor on ovarian surface
T1c	Ic	Tumor limited to one or both ovaries with any of the following: capsule ruptured, tumor on ovarian surface, malignant cells in ascites, or peritoneal washing
T2	II	Tumor involves one or both ovaries with pelvic extension
T2a	IIa	Extension and/or implants on uterus and/or tube(s)
T2b	IIb	Extension to other pelvic tissues
T2c	IIc	Pelvic extension (T2a or T2b) with malignant cells in ascites or peritoneal washing
T3	III	Tumor involves one or both ovaries with microscopically

confirmed peritoneal metastasis outside the pelvis and/or regional lymph node metastasis

T3a   IIIa   Microscopic peritoneal metastasis beyond pelvis

T3b   IIIb   Macroscopic peritoneal metastasis beyond pelvis 2 cm or less in greatest dimension

T3c   IIIc   Peritoneal metastasis beyond pelvis and/or N1 more than 2 cm in greatest dimension and/or regional lymph node metastasis

M1   IV   Distant metastasis (excludes peritoneal metastasis)

Note: Liver capsule metastasis is T3/stage III, liver parenchymal metastasis is M1/stage IV. Pleural effusion must have positive cytology for M1/stage IV.

Regional Lymph Nodes (N)

Regional lymph nodes include the hypogastric (obturator), common iliac, external iliac, internal iliac, lateral sacral, paraaortic, and inguinal nodes.

NX   Regional lymph nodes cannot be assessed

N0   No regional lymph node metastasis

N1   Regional lymph node metastasis

Distant Metastasis (M)

TNM	FIGO	Definition
MX		Presence of distant metastasis cannot be assessed
M0		No distant metastasis
M1	IV	Distant metastasis (excludes peritoneal metastasis)

Note: The presence of nonmalignant ascites is not classified. The presence of ascites does not affect staging unless malignant cells are present.

pTNM Pathologic Classification

The pT, pN, and pM categories correspond to the T, N, and M categories.

Stage grouping	T	N	M
IA	T1a	N0	M0
IB	T1b	N0	M0
IC	T1c	N0	M0
IIA	T2a	N0	M0
IIB	T2b	N0	M0
IIC	T2c	N0	M0
IIIA	T3a	N0	M0
IIIB	T3b	N0	M0
IIIC	T3c	N0	M0
	Any T	N1	M0
IV	Any T	Any N	M1

Specific sites according to the following notations:

Pulmonary	PUL
Osseous	OSS
Hepatic	HEP
Brain	BRA
Lymph nodes	LYM
Bone marrow	MAR
Pleura	PLE
Skin	SKI
Eye	EYE
Other	OTH

Postsurgical Residual Tumor (R)

The absence or presence of residual tumor after treatment is described by the symbol R:

RX   Presence of residual tumor at the primary site cannot be assessed

R0   No residual tumor
R1   Microscopic residual tumor
R2   Macroscopic residual tumor
          Specify

Histopathology

Ovarian carcinoma is a common malignant tumor, but because of its many histologic variations it cannot be regarded as a single entity. Therapeutic statistics on ovarian cancer are of limited value if attention is not paid to the histologic type of growth.

Histologic Classification of the Common Primary Epithelial Tumors of the Ovary

1. Serous cystomas
   a. Serous benign cystadenomas
   b. Serous cystadenomas with proliferating activity of the epithelial cells and nuclear abnormalities, but with no infiltrative destructive growth (borderline cases; low potential malignancy)
   c. Serous cystadenocarcinomas
2. Mucinous cystomas
   a. Mucinous benign cystadenomas
   b. Mucinous cystadenomas with proliferating activity of the epithelial cells and nuclear abnormalities but with no infiltrative destructive growth (borderline cases; low potential malignancy)
   c. Mucinous cystadenocarcinomas
3. Endometrioid tumors (similar to adenocarcinoma in the endometrium)
   a. Endometrioid benign cysts
   b. Endometrioid tumors with proliferating activity of the epithelial cells and nuclear abnormalities but with no infiltrative destructive growth (borderline cases; low potential malignancy)
   c. Endometrioid adenocarcinomas
4. Clear-cell tumors (mesonephroid tumors)
   a. Benign mesonephroid tumors
   b. Mesonephroid tumors with proliferating activity of the epithelial cells and nuclear abnormalities but with no infiltrative destructive growth (borderline cases; low potential malignancy)
   c. Mesonephroid cystadenocarcinomas
5. Undifferentiated carcinoma
   A malignant tumor of epithelial structure that is too poorly differentiated to be placed in any of types 1 to 4 or type 6
6. Mixed epithelial tumors
   Tumors composed of a mixture of two or more of the malignant types 1c, 2c, 3c, or 4c described above and where none is predominant. Thus a case should be listed as "mixed epithelial tumor" only if it is not possible to decide the predominant structure. The pathologist should always try to determine the leading structure and classify the tumor according to that element.
7. No histology or unclassifiable
   Cases where explorative surgery has shown that obvious ovarian epithelial malignant tumor is present but where no biopsy has been taken, or where the specimen is unclassifiable because of, for instance, necrosis.

The recommendations above are to be used in the cancer programs approved by the Commission on Cancer of the American College of Surgeons. Also, reports of the Surveillance Epidemiology and End Results Program of the National Cancer Institute are based on the classifications recommended by the AJCC; the form may be found in the *Manual for Staging of Cancer*, Third Edition (American Joint Committee on Cancer, 1988, p. 167).

Summary

The clinical stage or extent of tumor growth at the time of diagnosis is generally considered the best indicator of prognosis. Unlike other gynecologic cancers, ovarian carcinoma is staged at the time of exploratory laparotomy or when the final histologic findings are reported.

FIGO revised their 1971 classification in 1974 and then again in January 1987. Although the original staging included only the common epithelial ovarian tumors, the others, including germ cell and gonadal stromal tumors, are now staged according to this method.

The new classification for ovarian cancer created additional subgroups. It has been designed to evaluate the impact on prognosis of the criteria for allocating cases to stages Ic to IIc. It would be of value to know (1) if rupture of the capsule was spontaneous or caused by the surgeon, and (2) if the source of malignant cells detected was peritoneal washings or ascites.

Although it is important to stage the ovarian carcinomas, it is also important to remember that potency of tumors varies within a given stage, and that treatment should be tailored to the cancer rather than merely to the stage of disease. The concept of how to stage ovarian cancer is not always correctly interpreted. It must therefore be restated that ovarian cancer is staged at the time of exploratory laparotomy or when the final histologic findings are reported. Despite this criterion, Knapp and Friedman reported on aortic lymph node metastasis of early ovarian cancer, and their report is widely quoted regarding the incidence of aortic nodes and stage I ovarian cancer. They reported that aortic node biopsies performed in 26 patients with stage I ovarian cancer revealed five with metastases. The lesion should not have been classified as stage I but, rather, by definition should have been included as stage III ovarian cancer. The conclusion to be drawn is not that there are 19% positive aortic nodes in stage I ovarian cancer but, rather, that *these patients were incorrectly staged*.

Proper classification and staging of ovarian cancer allow the physician to determine treatment more appropriately, to evaluate results of management more reliably, and to compare worldwide statistics reported from various institutions on a local, regional, and national basis more confidently.

Staging of cancer is not a fixed science. As new information becomes available about etiology and various methods of diagnosis and treatment, the classification and staging of cancer change. Periodically, revisions are made to reflect the changing knowledge, but revision occurs at reasonable periods. At the present time, the anatomic extent of disease is the primary basis for staging; the extent of differentiation of the tumor and age of the patient are also factors in some tumors. In the future, biologic markers and other factors may play a part.

Bibliography

American Joint Committee for Cancer Staging and End Results Reporting Task Force on Gynecologic Sites, Staging System for Cancer at Gynecologic Sites 1979. AJCC, Chicago.

Averette HE, Haskins WJ, Dudan RC, Nordqvist SRB: The ovary. In Nealon TF Jr (ed): *Management of the Patient With Cancer*. Saunders, Philadelphia, 1976, p. 618.

Barber HRK: Ovarian cancer. Part I. *CA* 29:341, 1979.

Barber HRK: Ovarian cancer. Part II. *CA* 30:2, 1980.

Barber HRK, Kwon T: Current status of the treatment of gynecologic cancer by site—ovary. *Cancer* 38:610, 1976.

Barber HRK, Sommers SC, Snyder R, Kwon T: Histologic and nuclear grading and stromal reactions as indices for prognosis in ovarian cancer. *Am J* Obstet 121 (no. 6):795, 1975.

Knapp RC, Friedman EA: Aortic lymph node metastases in early ovarian cancer. *Am J Obstet Gynecol* 119:1013, 1974.

Kolstad P: Prognostic indicators and staging: ovarian cancer. *Adv Biosci* 26:67, 1980.

Report presented by the Cancer Committee to the General Assembly of FIGO: New York, April 1970. *Int J Gynecol Obstet* 9:172, 1971.

12

Treatment of the Common Epithelial Cancers

Tumors that originate in the surface epithelium and ovarian stroma constitute 75 to 90% of primary ovarian cancers. Only about 8% of these cancers occur in women under the age of 35, but figures indicate that this number may be increasing. Most common epithelial cancers develop in patients between 40 and 60. Nevertheless, the patient is at risk throughout her entire life to develop cancer of the ovary. Conservative surgery is not indicated in this group, nor should it be considered. Treatment consists in an exploratory laparotomy, washings for cytology, scraping biopsy of the diaphragm, total abdominal hysterectomy (TAH), bilateral salpingo-oophorectomy (BSO), omentectomy, appendectomy, sampling of paraaortic and pelvic lymph nodes, and instillation of ^{32}P if it is thought to be indicated. Chemotherapy has been added to the protocol for prophylaxis of stages I and II where the disease has been macroscopically removed and as definitive therapy for stages II and IV.

The treatment for common epithelial tumors is presented by stage of disease, providing a framework for management, though it is impossible to assert rigid criteria for the management of each and every problem that may arise. Armed with the general principles to be outlined, physicians caring for women with ovarian cancer should be able to modify this protocol as they deem necessary and are in a better position to make proper decisions on the management of these patients.

The suggested management of the patient with truly invasive common epithelial cancers includes the following measures.

1. Examination under anesthesia
2. Exploratory laparotomy
3. Washings of pelvis and upper abdomen for cytologic evaluation
4. Scraping biopsy of the diaphragm
5. Total abdominal hysterectomy
6. Bilateral salpingo-oophorectomy
7. Appendectomy
8. Omentectomy
9. Sampling of paraaortic and pelvic lymph nodes
10. Insertion of tubes for administration of ^{32}P, if indicated (used only if all macroscopic disease has been removed and only free-floating cells are found on cytology)

Treatment Plan by Stages

Stages IA, IB, IC

Examination under anesthesia, exploratory laparotomy, aspiration of cells or washings for cytologic examination, scraping or biopsies of the diaphragm, TAH-BSO, omentectomy, and instillation of ^{32}P if it is thought to be indicated. Ideally, paraaortic and pelvic lymph node sampling is indicated for all stages of ovarian cancer. All patients should have any free fluid aspirated before surgical exploration; if none is present, the pelvis should be irrigated with saline and the fluid submitted for cytology according to the Papanicolaou technique.

There is considerable controversy over the value of omentectomy. Occasionally, islands of tumor cells are found in the omentum, advancing the stage from I to III. In addition, the presence of the omentum interferes with the even distribution of ^{32}P and should be removed if the use of ^{32}P is contemplated. Metastatic disease may be found in the opposite, normal-appearing ovary. Reports in the literature indicate that approximately 10% of patients with seemingly stage I ovarian cancer have metastatic cancer between the liver and the diaphragm along the posterior wall of the abdominal cavity, advancing the disease to stage III. In view of this finding, the author's protocol has been revised to include prophylactic chemotherapy in stage I cancer of the ovary.

Stages IIA and IIB

Treatment for stages IIA and IIB is the same as that recommended for stages IA, IB, and IC; all adhesions surrounding the ovarian carcinoma should be biopsied to document the extent of disease. Chemotherapy is applied to all stage II carcinomas of the ovary, and ^{32}P may be considered if all the macroscopic disease has been removed.

Stage III

The treatment recommended for stages I and II is also appropriate for stage III. Total abdominal irradiation is no longer employed as a definitive method of treatment particularly as adjuvant therapy, because of ethical reasons. This change in protocol has come about because it is necessary to shield the kidneys and the liver, and it was thought that cancer on or adjacent to these organs would not be adequately treated. Therefore these patients would be selected for failure by the treatment method chosen. Chemotherapy as a definitive, adjunctive treatment is given for stage III carcinoma of the ovary.

Stage IV

The ideal management for stage IV ovarian cancer consists in removing as much cancer as possible; hopefully, then, the disease can be treated as for stages I, II, and III. Chemotherapy is given as definitive adjunctive therapy, and radiation is reserved for controlling the disease in the supraclavicular, inguinal, and localized areas of the pelvic side wall.

Although it is occasionally necessary to resect isolated segments of bowel, I do not favor exenterative or ultraradical surgery for management of ovarian carcinoma because of the type of spread of this neoplasm. Ovarian carcinoma is a surface spreader and moves swiftly over all organ surfaces and to the upper abdomen.

I perform an appendectomy in these women because the appendix is often the site of clinically undetectable disease. Findings of tumor on the appendix may require a change in the staging of diseases particularly for therapy. I also remove the omentum because it helps to stage the disease accurately. Contrary to the fears of some gynecologists, it has not resulted in any increased morbidity if the surgery is carried out according to sound surgical principles. Unfortunately, many gynecologists do not have extensive training in upper abdominal surgery and therefore are reluctant to excise the omentum. The height of professional integrity is to ask for consultation if it is indicated.

How Much Is Too Much?

Not everyone agrees on the amount of tumor that can be excised safely. We try to remove as much as we think we can without running a risk of a gastrointestinal or genitourinary fistula. Success of subsequent chemotherapy, irradiation, or both is inversely proportional to the amount of tumor left in the abdomen after surgery. Therefore aggressive surgery is indicated because it may be curative and it potentiates other forms of treatment. If it is true that the patient is immunized by her own tumors, this self-immunization can be more effective when the bulk of tumor has been decreased. Removal of a volume of tumor may decrease the possibility of acquired tolerance and, by decreasing the number of antigen-antibody complexes, reduce the change of immunologic enhancement. Debulking helps improve metabolic and symptomatic status. By reducing the volume of the tumor, the growth rate of the remaining tumor is increased which helps get a higher concentration of chemotherapy to the tumor. By debulking, the blood supply to the remaining tumor is improved which results in more chemotherapy getting to the remaining tumor.

The aggressive management of ovarian cancer has evolved through a full cycle. During the early 1950s an aggressive surgical program was carried out but was complicated by high morbidity and increased mortality. If the patient survived the postoperative period, the cancer recurred despite the debulking operation. The poor results were followed by less radical management of the patient with ovarian cancer. Currently, the increased use of hyperalimentation and better management with use of the Swan-Ganz catheter and more potent broad-spectrum antibodies have lowered the morbidity. The philosophy at present is to be aggressive regarding the diagnosis and treatment of ovarian cancer without creating inordinate morbidity and mortality.

Higher cure rates are now reported among stage I patients (90+% survival). There is a dramatic difference between the survival rates of the various stages of cancer. It is significant that there is a marked decrease in survival between stages IIA and IIB, similar to cancer of the cervix. Although several explanations have been suggested, it appears that stage IIA represents geographic spread of the ovarian cancer, whereas stage IIB represents biologic spread. There is a drop-off in survival beyond stage IIA. The increased volume of tumor in stages IIB, III, and IV overwhelms the host's protective mechanisms and probably accounts for the precipitous drop in survival.

External radiation therapy has been phased out of the treatment protocol for common epithelial cancer except in select instances where a small volume of tumor remains on the side wall or the cul-de-sac which can be outlined at surgery with radio-opaque clips permitting a cancerocidal dose of radiation to be delivered to a small area. This development is discussed in Chapter 21.

Chemotherapy has assumed a more signif-icant role in the prophylaxis and therapeutic management of ovarian cancer. It is given prophylactically for stages I and II when all gross disease has been eliminated and for stage III when the gross disease can be excised by omentectomy. It is given therapeutically for stages IIB, III, and IV when gross disease has been left behind. The plan of therapy with chemotherapy is reviewed in Chapter 20.

Radioactive isotopes, particularly ^{32}P, if indicated, are given only when all gross disease has been removed. ^{32}P has been effective in those patients who have only free-floating carcinoma cells left. Therefore for stages I and II, as well as in a limited number of patients with stage III in whom the gross disease can be completely removed, the use of ^{32}P may be considered. It should not be used in the presence of gross disease or even in patients with nodules larger than 2 cm.

Summary

The acceptance and use of clinical staging and histologic classification established by the World Health Organization and the International Federation of Gynecology and Obstetrics has helped compare therapeutic results among institutions around the world. It has led to a greater insight into the natural history of ovarian cancer, resulting in a more rational approach to therapy with anticipated improved results.

The philosophy of ovarian cancer management has evolved into an aggressive surgical and chemotherapeutic approach. The use of hyperalimentation, better control of the patient's management through the use of the Swan-Ganz catheter, and more potent antibiotics have resulted in a decrease in morbidity. The judicious and more skillful use of chemotherapeutic agents to control the carcinoma have contributed immensely to the current concepts of the management of ovarian cancer.

Bibliography

Barber HRK: Ovarian cancer: still an enigma. *Dr* 1:17, 1975.

Barber HRK, Kwon T: Current status of the treatment of gynecologic cancer—by site. *Cancer* 38:610, 1976.

Brady LW: Radiation therapy in gynecologic cancer: future prospects. *Clin Obstet Gynecol* 18:125, 1975.

Buchsbaum HJ, Keetel WC, Latourette HB: The use of radioisotopes as adjunct therapy of localized ovarian cancer. *Semin Oncol* 2:247, 1975.

Changes in definitions of clinical staging for carcinoma of the cervix and ovary: International Federation of Gynecology and Obstetrics. *Am J Obstet Gynecol* 156(1):263, 1987.

Clark DGC, Hilaris BS, Ochra M Jr: Treatment of cancer of the ovary. *Clin Obstet Gynecol* 3:159, 1976.

Frick HC II: An overall evaluation of chemotherapy for ovarian cancer. *Clin Obstet Gynecol* 12:1003, 1969.

Fuks Z: External radiotherapy of ovarian cancer: standard approaches and new frontiers. *Semin Oncol* 2:253, 1975.

Manual for Staging of Cancer. 3rd Ed. American Joint Committee on Cancer. Lippincott, Philadelphia, 1988.

Smith JP: Chemotherapy in gynecologic cancer. *Clin Obstet Gynecol* 18:109, 1975.

Young R: Chemotherapy of ovarian cancer: past and present. *Semin Oncol* 2:267, 1975.

13

Managing Ovarian Tumors of Childhood and Adolescence

The term *childhood* or *adolescent gynecologic tumor* is used to indicate any new growth (benign or malignant) that develops between birth and age 16. It implies the growth of newly formed cells derived from normal body cells or that preceding the developmental cells of origin. Benign neoplasm indicates a tumor that does not itself destroy the host, whereas a malignant neoplasm, if left untreated, does destroy the host.

Cancer Facts and Figures, published by the American Cancer Society in 1992, reported that cancer is second only to accidents as the cause of death among children under 15 years of age. Childhood cancer accounts for 1 of 28 deaths compared to 1 of 6 among adults. However, since 1950, death rates for all sites have declined somewhat. It seems to be partly a result of the decreasing death rates for leukemia, kidney cancer, and lymphomas. The actual number of deaths has also decreased during this period.

There is an estimated 6,600 new cases anticipated for 1992, making malignancy rare as a childhood disease. Common sites include the blood and bone marrow, bone, lymph nodes, nervous system, kidneys, and soft tissue.

There was an estimated 1800 deaths in 1990, about half of them from leukemia. Despite its rarity, cancer is the chief cause of death by disease in children between the ages of 3 and 14. Mortality has declined from 8.3 per 100,000 in 1950 to 3.5 per 100,000 in 1989.

Cancers in children often are difficult to recognize. Parents should see that their children have regular medical checkups and be alert to any unusual symptoms that persist. Such symptoms include an unusual mass or swelling; unexpected illness and loss of energy; sudden tendency to bruise; persistent, localized pain or limping; prolonged, unexplained fever or illness; frequent headaches, often with vomiting; sudden vision changes; and excessive, rapid weight loss.

About 3% of malignancies during childhood and adolescence are related to the gynecologic system. Even busy gynecologists, unless specializing in pediatric gynecology, see relatively few tumors of the genital tract in children in their practice. Because average pediatricians' exposure to pediatric gynecologic oncology is markedly limited, they should refer any case in which the diagnosis is in doubt or therapy beyond their capabilities to a qualified specialist or clinic. It must be emphasized that in some cases time is the critical factor between localized and widespread disease. Procrastinating and hoping that time will take care of the disease are fraught with danger for the patient; and from the physician's standpoint, they expose him or her not only to the disappointment, frustration, and emotional turmoil of having missed an important diagnosis but also to the threat of a large malpractice award to the patient. If in doubt, consult!

Etiology

All tissues in the body are liable to undergo malignant change, and all cells have an inherent potential for the development of cancer. The origin may be unicentric or multicentric.

All of the known carcinogenic factors associated with cancer in the adult (i.e., viruses, chemical factors, ionizing energy, and genetic factors) are found also in the child. The theory of misplaced blastomeres may take on added significance in this age group.

Natural History

When dealing with the wide variety of tumors found in the female reproductive system, it is obvious that each system and indeed each tumor within a given system has a natural history that is unique unto itself. As an example, the ovary is complex in its embryology, histology, steroidogenesis, and potential for malignancy. It is made up of a variety of cells; and rather than giving rise to a single type of malignancy, the ovary produces a family of cancers. However, it can be reported that cancer originating in the reproductive system in this age group is characterized by rapid growth, early spread, and frequently a fatal outcome.

Basic Differences from Adult Pelvic Cancer

1. The space available for tumor expansion is more limited in children.
2. The effect of therapy (especially radical surgery or irradiation) on the further development of the patient must be given greater consideration.
3. The high degree of malignancy in cancer of the young must be taken into account.
4. The most common neoplasms are a special group of ovarian tumors and a specific type of uterovaginal sarcoma, which are discussed later in the chapter.
5. The immunologic surveillance mechanism is inefficient during childhood.

Embryology

A complete understanding of gynecologic neoplasms in children requires at least a brief review of the embryology of the female genitourinary tract. The urogenital organs include two systems with wholly different functions, but they are so closely related embryologically

and anatomically that it is impossible to study one while ignoring the other. Although mesoderm is the major component in the development of the urogenital system, the entoderm and ectoderm also make important contributions.

The urogenital fold, or mesonephric ridge, is a large, important body occupying the posterior or dorsal portion of the primitive peritoneal cavity. This structure lies on each side of the midline and runs the entire length of the fetus. From this urogenital fold arise the ovaries, kidneys, fallopian tubes, uterus, and parts of the vagina. Even during the later development of the fetus, the distance between the structures is measured in millimeters. The urogenital fold serves to explain the interrelation between these structures, as well as the possibility for congenital rests between organ systems.

The steps in normal embryologic development are outlined briefly below.

Müllerian Ducts

The müllerian duct (paramesonephric duct) develops as a groove in the mesonephric ridge, and by a process of folding (in front of the mesonephros and the gonadal area) it fuses in its distal portion to form the uterus, cervix, and possibly the upper part of the vagina. The female duct (müllerian or paramesonephric duct) has an abdominal opening through the fimbriated end of the tubes. Although the mesonephric tubules and ducts degenerate, a few may remain near the ovary and are known as the epoöphoron and paraoöphoron. The mesonephric duct may persist as a Gartner duct and runs along the uterus, cervix, and vagina. In some instances these structures develop cysts that require surgery.

Gonads

The gonads appear as a swelling on the medial surface of the urogenital fold close to the mesonephros and mesonephric duct and run parallel to it. The gonad is relatively short, so the mesonephros extends beyond it at both ends. The ovary and testis have a similar embryonic origin; and up to a certain point they cannot be distinguished from each other. The coelomic epithelium covering the gonad is thickened to form the germinal epithelium. The sex cords grow into the mesenchyme from the coelomic epithelium. Oogonia probably come from the entoderm of the yolk sac and migrate by ameboid movement via the gut mesentery to the ovary. These cells, called primordial germ cells, develop into ova, each surrounded by a group of follicular cells to form a primary follicle.

Kidneys

The three kidneys arise from the mesonephric area in succession: the pronephros, the mesonephros (wolffian body), and the metanephros (the permanent kidney). The metanephros has a double origin. The ureter, pelvis, calyces, and collecting tubules arise from an outgrowing of the wolffian duct, whereas the secreting parts of the tubules are formed directly from the posterior end of the intermediate cell mass.

Adrenal (Suprarenal) Gland

Although the adrenal gland is not a part of the urogenital system, its proximity, overlapping function, and propensity for producing aberrant rests in the reproductive system proper make it appropriate to include a brief outline here.

The adrenal gland is formed by a combination of mesodermal elements that develop into the cortex and an ectodermal portion that forms the medulla. Mesothelial cells located between the root of the mesentery and the developing gonad begin to proliferate during the fifth week of development and penetrate the underlying mesenchyme. Here they differentiate into formation of the fetal or primitive cortex. Shortly thereafter a second wave of cells from the mesothelium penetrates the mesenchyme and forms the definitive cortex of the gland. During the time the cortex is developing, cells originating in the sympathetic system (ectoderm) invade its medial aspect and be-

come arranged in cords and clusters, forming the medulla.

Progression of Genitourinary Embryologic Development

1. Genetic sex (time of fertilization), determined by sperm
   a. Each ovum contains one X chromosome.
   b. Approximately half of all spermatozoa contain an X chromosome and the other half a Y chromosome.
2. Undifferentiated gonad (1–6 weeks)
   Undifferentiated ("sexless") gonads come into existence when primordial germ cells migrate into primitive gonadal folds.
3. Differentiation of the gonad (week 7)
   A still unidentified factor (evocator) stimulates the primitive gonad to develop in a direction corresponding to the genetic sex and, depending on which sex predominates, an ovary or testis develops. In the male the wolffian system becomes dominant during the development of the genital system, and the müllerian system atrophies. In the female the opposite occurs. Any upset in this mechanism causes variations with mixtures. (1) The cortex basically forms an ovary. (2) The medulla basically forms a testis.
4. Development of the internal genital system (8–12 weeks)
   a. Müllerian ducts originate from the lateral aspect of the urogenital fold.
   b. Wolffian ducts originate from the mesonephros.
   c. It has been shown that castration of the embryo before any sexual development has begun results in development of the female internal and external genital system.
5. Development of the external genital system (13 weeks to birth)
   Differentiation of external genitalia involves changes in the urogenital sinus and genital tubercle, the anlage of which are already present at week 5.
6. Birth to puberty
   There is little change until puberty, when

the reproductive system matures toward the adult form.

Ovarian Neoplasms: Origins and Concepts

From the time the ovary differentiates as a modified portion of coelomic epithelium after the menopause, it is a constantly changing organ. The primitive germ cells migrate in the dorsal mesentery from the primitive hindgut to the genital ridges, and from these cells the primordial follicles are stimulated to grow. The stroma of the ovary arises from the same cells as do the follicle cells, and no new germ cells are formed after the early postnatal period.

The ovary is made up of germ cells, cells of the sex cord, and cells from the mesenchymal tissue, each with its own potential to form a tumor. It is generally agreed that at least 10% of all ovarian neoplasms in children are malignant and that the germ cell tumors comprise the greatest number. Papillary serous and mucinous cystadenocarcinomas are relatively rare during childhood. The most common benign tumor of childhood and adolescence is the cystic teratoma, or dermoid, which comprises approximately 30% of all ovarian tumors in this age group.

A major conceptual advance in cancer research was achieved when it was established that cancers do arouse a specific immune response in the organism within which they appear. In fact, antigenic differences represent the first known qualitative distinctions between cancer cells and their normal counterparts. Following Gold's work on the carcinoembryonic antigen (CEA), a great number of tumors have been subjected to immunologic study. Although the CEA is related to endodermal structures, a carcinoembryonic-like antigen has been found in many other systems. Closely related to the endodermal CEA, it may come from the same chromosomal group. Lawrence reported that plasma CEA levels were elevated in 7 of 20 ovarian cancer patients (35%), whereas none of four patients with a benign tumor showed an elevation. Presenting one case to support his hypotheses, Ballas reported that teratoid neoplasms containing a significant vitelline component are most likely to give rise to alpha-fetoprotein in the serum. The significance of these studies in relation to diagnostic technique is yet to be proved, but so far the findings appear promising.

Ectopic production of human chorionic gonadotropin (hCG) by neoplasms has received a great deal of attention. Teratocarcinomas containing chorionic elements, as well as choriocarcinomas of the ovary, give positive results. Currently, the β-subunit component of hCG, a specific test for gonadotropins produced by the placenta, is being evaluated. Studies suggest a positive hCG titer in 30 to 40% of adenocarcinomas of the ovary and a much higher incidence in embryonal cancers.

Alpha-1-fetoprotein (AFP) is a serum protein synthesized in the fetus by perivascular hepatic parenchymal cells and found in a high percentage of patients with hepatomas and malignant teratomas, especially of the endodermal sinus type. It is present in concentrations up to 400 mg/dl during early fetal life, diminishing to less than 3 mg/dl in adults. Increased levels may be detected in the serum of adults with hepatoma (80% positive) or malignant teratoma (40% percent positive) and may be used to follow the progress of the disease.

Because AFP is produced in the yolk sac of the placenta during the first trimester and is not normally present at birth, it provides a specific tumor marker for endodermal sinus tumors of the ovary, embryonal carcinomas of the ovary, and ovarian teratomas with either of these tumors. It is not elevated in epithelial ovarian carcinomas. It is elevated in those patients with endodermal sinus tumor of the ovary, decreases with response to therapy, and increases with recurrence, making it an almost perfect tumor marker for this disease. Other markers are discussed in Chapter 25.

Most tumors are now classified according to histogenesis, behavior, and functional attributes. Advances in finding tumor-specific antigens on the tumor surfaces may promote a new field in diagnostic pathology that would provide answers to etiology as well as predict behavior patterns and prognosis. Furthermore, such techniques offer promise as a means of monitoring the effects of treatment.

Tumors of the Ovary

Among the common epithelial cancers, about 8% occur under the age of 35, and of this number few occur among the pediatric and adolescent groups. The ovarian cancers that are found during childhood almost always arise from the germ cell or sex cord (mesenchymomas or gonadal stromal) cells. The malignant germ cell tumors are generally encountered during childhood or among young adults. However, malignant changes (2% of cystic adult teratomas) are encountered in dermoid cysts.

When ovarian cancer is diagnosed, the question of management is raised, and rightfully so in view of the young age of the patient. To help formulate a plan of therapy, each tumor type in the germ cell and sex cord groups is reviewed individually. The tumor types are classified below. According to the International Federation of Gynecology and Obstetrics (FIGO) classification, only the tumors of epithelial and stromal origin are usually discussed. However, during childhood the germ cell tumors are encountered most commonly and the gonadal-stromal tumors less so. Therefore the classification has been modified according to World Health Organization (WHO) classification to emphasize this difference.

Classification of Ovarian Neoplasms

I. Tumors of epithelial and stromal origin
    A. Serous
    B. Mucinous
    C. Endometrioid
    D. Clear cell (mesonephric)
II. Germ cell tumors
    A. Dysgerminoma
    B. Tumors in teratoma group
       1. Extraembryonal forms
          a. Endodermal sinus tumor (mesoblastoma vitellium yolk sac carcinoma, extraembryonic membrane tumor)
          b. Choriocarcinoma
       2. Embryonal teratomas, solid and cystic
       3. Adult teratomas

a. Solid
b. Cystic (dermoid cyst)
   i. Benign
   ii. With malignant change
       4. Struma ovarii
       5. Carcinoid
    C. Mixed forms of the above
III. Gonadoblastoma
    A. With germinoma
    B. Without germinoma
IV. Gonadal stromal tumors (sex cord mesenchymal tumors)
    A. Female cell types
       1. Granulosa cell tumor
       2. Thecoma-fibroma type
    B. Male cell types
       1. Sertoli-Leydig cell tumor (arrhenoblastoma, androblastoma)
       2. Sertoli cell tumor (androblastoma tubulare)
       3. Hilus (Leydig) cell tumor
    C. Mixed cell types (gynandroblastoma)
    D. Indeterminate cell types
V. Tumors not specific for ovary
    A. Lymphoma
    B. Burkitt's lymphoma
VI. Miscellaneous
    A. Sarcomas
    B. Fibromas
VII. Metastatic tumors
    A. Krükenberg
    B. Choriocarcinoma

The stage grouping for primary common epithelial cancer is presented in Chapter 11. Although FIGO's clinical staging of ovarian cancer was designed to include only the common epithelial ovarian tumors, it has been used as a guide to judge the extent of disease for germ cell tumors and gonadal stromal tumors.

Wollner and coworkers proposed a new grouping to define the extent of disease. They considered the new approach more useful for planning therapy; it is also applicable to the extent and location of disease found at the time of disease recurrence, which is the time when most of these patients are seen for the first time at the Comprehensive Cancer Centers. The grouping is presented in Table 13.1.

In the Wollner study, grouping or staging of

TABLE 13.1. Proposed grouping for malignant ovarian tumors during childhood

Group	Extent of disease
I	Disease limited to one ovary. Negative peritoneal washing.
II	Disease limited to one ovary and ipsilateral para-aortic nodes. Bilateral primary ovarian tumors without pelvic extension, with or without para-aortic node involvement. Negative peritoneal washing.
III	Disease spread to pelvis, mesenteric and paraaortic nodes, abdominal wall, peritoneum, diaphragm, liver, and other organs in the peritoneal cavity.
IV	Distant metastases (lungs, bone, brain, peripheral nodes).

the extent of disease at the time of diagnosis seemed to contribute little to determining the patient's prognosis. If, however, some means of indicating the extent of disease must be utilized for documentation or future comparative studies, Wollner believed that this new grouping system is better able to chart the course of these tumors in children.

It has been shown that there is no correlation between clinical and histologic malignancy in ovarian tumors. It holds true also for various types of neoplasm, but especially for epithelial tumors, granulosa cell tumors, and virilizing tumors. The committee recommended that cases of germ cell tumors, hormone-producing neoplasms, and metastatic carcinomas should be excluded from therapeutic statistics on ovarian epithelial tumors. However, a clinical plan for staging ovarian cancer does focus attention for carefully evaluating the extent of all ovarian cancers.

There are five primary points that should be emphasized concerning ovarian tumors during childhood: (1) The ovary is the most common site of new growths involving the gynecologic organs that appear during childhood. (2) The ovary in a child is essentially an abdominal organ, and tumors are abdominal rather than pelvic. (3) Ovarian tumors during childhood are especially susceptible to torsion because of a longer ovarian suspensory ligament. (4)

About one in ten ovarian neoplasms are malignant; therefore the odds are generally good that the tumor is benign. Panic is not justified, but judicious concern is indicated. (5) The evolution of ovarian tumors in children is more rapid because of contracted spatial relations. Large tumors produce relatively greater pressure symptoms and dyspnea. Cachexia and ascites are increased.

Incidence

Ovarian tumors comprise about 1% of all new growths in children who are less than 16 years of age. However, they are the most frequent genital neoplasms during childhood and adolescence. The problem of diagnosis is surpassed only by the confusion related to therapy. It is difficult to accept psychologically the possibility of ovarian malignancy in this age group and even more difficult for the physician to deprive a child of her reproductive potential. In general, although certain ovarian tumors are more common in children, almost any tumor found in the adult may also be found in the child.

Age

Analysis of age distribution shows that although ovarian neoplasms may occur at any age during childhood or adolescence they tend to be most frequent at puberty, between the ages of 10 and 14. This fact permits the conjecture that some control mechanism is released or that pituitary stimulation of some latent factor in the ovary is the triggering mechanism.

The most common tumors in infants and young children are cystic teratomas (dermoid tumors) and teratosarcoma. These lesions may be found soon after birth or later. Multiple retention cysts and giant follicle cysts at birth have also been described. Occasionally, theca lutein and corpus luteum cysts are found in neonates. In adolescents the most frequent tumors, in order of frequency, are cystic teratoma, mucinous cystadenoma, serous cystadenoma, corpus luteum cysts, paraovarian cysts, and endometrioma. To this list we can add the more infrequent embryonal teratoma, granulosa cell tumors, dysgerminoma, endodermal sinus tumor, and carcinoma.

Diagnosis

Symptoms and Signs

Ovarian new growth in children may produce minimal symptoms in its early state of development. The degree of symptomatology and the physical signs relate directly to the rapidity of growth, position, degree of malignancy, potential to produce hormones, and possible accidents associated with these neoplasms (e.g., torsion, rupture, hemorrhage, and infection in children). Because ovarian tumors are frequently abdominal and have their embryologic origin from the level of T10, it is not surprising that abdominal pain and abdominal tumors are common. Pain may be related to the relatively small pelvic and abdominal cavity, which causes the new growth to stretch the peritoneum and produce pressure on adjacent organs. Rectal examination often reveals that the pelvis is free of tumor, but a negative rectal examination does not rule out an ovarian neoplasm because frequently it presents only as an abdominal mass during childhood.

The hormone-producing tumor, though rare, produces the clinical picture related to the type of hormone being secreted.

The clinical history should be carefully assessed for symptoms not related to the abdominal contents, such as persistent and unexplained headaches for possible space-occupying lesions in the brain, pain in the back related to specific vertebral bodies, symptoms related to the extremities or control of sphincters, and cough, chest pains, or bone pain.

Physical Findings

A general physical examination including pelvic and rectal examinations should be carried out. In most instances it is impossible to palpate normal ovaries in children because they are an abdominal organ until puberty, at which time they descend into the pelvis. Therefore it can be assumed that if an ovary is enlarged on palpation, it is abnormal. The size determines whether it can be felt abdominally or by recto-abdominal palpation.

Diagnostic Procedures

Baseline blood counts should be determined and urinalysis and blood chemistry studies performed. A flat plate of the abdomen may help determine if a dermoid cyst is present. Intravenous pyelograms and roentgenographic studies of the gastrointestinal tract are indicated if time permits. In those patients suspected of having a hormone-producing tumor, radiographic studies of bone age may be helpful. A hormone assay profile sometimes documents the type of tumor. Pneumoperitoneum has been used to outline small tumors, and ultrasound methods have been introduced. The role of laparoscopy in the study of abdominal and pelvic problems in this age group remains to be clarified. Levels of AFP and CEA should be determined for follow-up of tumor activity and regression. Urinary levels of chorionic and pituitary gonadotropins should be measured and, if abnormal, may serve as baselines for evaluation of therapy.

Special studies include scans of the brain (with ^{99m}Tc pertechnetate scans), soft tissue (with gallium ^{67}Ga citrate form), and liver (with ^{99m}Tc sulfur colloid), as well as lymphangiography.

Differential Diagnosis

The clinical picture and physical findings usually point to the diagnosis. However, the differential diagnosis should include appendiceal abscess, intussusception, obstruction, salpingitis, hematometra, and pyelonephritis.

Origin

Tumors of the ovary during childhood and adolescence may be derived from any of a number of cellular elements: coelomic epithelium or its derivatives (mesotheliomas), including serous, mucinous, endometrioid, and clear-cell tumors; and gonadal stromal tumors, including granulosa cell, thecal cell, Sertoli-Leydig, Sertoli, and germ cell tumors (dysgerminomas and embryonal teratomas).

Common Epithelial Tumors

Ninety percent of ovarian tumors in adults originate in the ovarian surface epithelium and stroma. In premenarchal girls, about 90% of ovarian tumors are of germ cell origin. On the other hand, in patients between 13 and 20 years of age, 40% of ovarian neoplasms are of nongerminal origin. Tumors of epithelial origin include the serous and mucinous types. No endometrioid tumors have been reported in this age group, although after puberty serous and mucinous tumors are occasionally diagnosed.

Primary epithelial tumors occur during the postpubertal period; almost all are unilateral, and most are on the right. The malignancy rate (7.5%) is less than that among older patients. Most investigators believe that these tumors arise from invagination of the surface coelomic epithelium of the ovary or its derivatives. Because these tumors occur almost exclusively after puberty, the question of hormonal stimulation has been raised, but no correlation has been established.

Therapy must be tailored to the patient's needs and to the extent of the disease. A frozen section is carried out to determine whether the tumor is benign or malignant. Benign disease is treated by extirpation of the tumor, leaving as much normal ovary as possible. If the tumor is malignant, the most important considerations of therapy and prognosis are the *stage* and *grade* of the neoplasm. A malignancy that has spread beyond the ovary should receive radical extirpative therapy including total abdominal hysterectomy (TAH), bilateral salpingo-oophorectomy (BSO), omentectomy (the omentum is usually small in the child), appendectomy, and the instillation of radioactive ^{32}P if indicated.

If there is any doubt about the type of tumor or if a malignancy is present, and if the tumor has an intact capsule and is freely movable, it is better to perform a salpingo-oophorectomy on the side of the tumor. If the tumor proves to be highly malignant on permanent section examination, the abdomen may be opened and the remaining reproductive organs excised if it appears to be the best course.

X-irradiation has been practically phased out for the treatment of common epithelial ovarian cancer and is used only rarely for any childhood pelvic tumor. Chemotherapy has been chosen as the adjunctive treatment for the common epithelial ovarian carcinomas. With certain low grade malignancies the previously performed treatment may be considered sufficient to ensure a cure. Low malignant potential (borderline) tumors are relatively benign; their 5-year survival rate is between 90 and 95%.

Germ Cell Tumors

Germ cell tumors are almost always found in children or adolescents. Knowledge of the natural history of these tumors can be used as a guide for avoiding undertreatment or overtreatment of these patients.

Teilum has reported the scheme shown in Figure 13.1 to illustrate the histogenesis and interrelation of ovarian and testicular tumors of germ cell origin. With this classification Teilum reported that the term *embryonal carcinoma* is restricted to tumors composed of undifferentiated neoplastic embryonal cells representing the undifferentiated forms of extraembryonic as well as embryonic types. This relation is demonstrated in Figure 13.1.

Dysgerminomas (Germinomas)

Dysgerminomas are ovarian tumors of an embryonal type resembling the sexually undifferentiated germ cells of the early gonad. Hughesdon reported that the origin of this tumor, composed of germ cells and undifferentiated stromal cells, is probably linked to the continuing proliferation of unencapsulated germ cells and to the associated stimulation of the surrounding stromal or ovarian mesenchymal cells.

Certain patients with these tumors show subnormal gonadal development and coincidental abnormal secondary sex characteristics (pseudohermaphroditism); the ambiguous sex status is not reversed after removal of the tumor.

Dysgerminoma is characteristically smooth or lobulated and surrounded by a dense capsule. It has a doughy or rubbery consistency

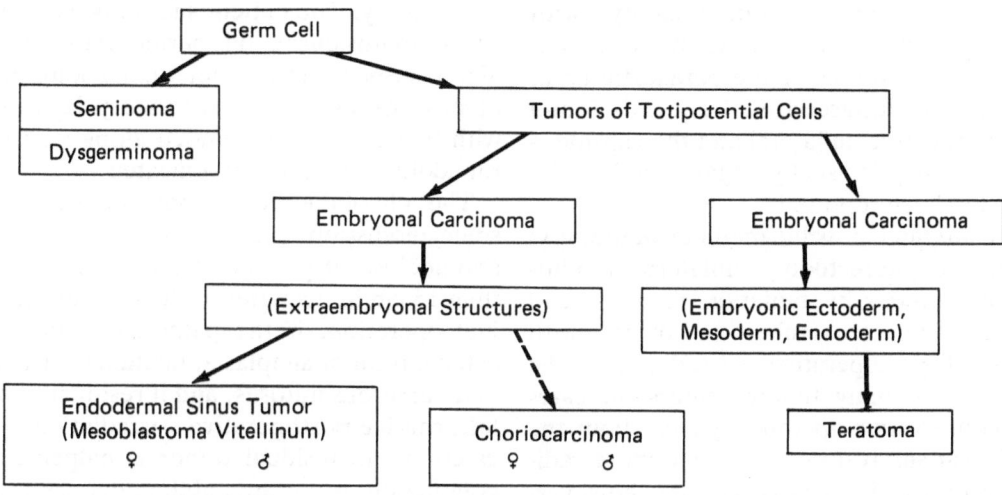

FIGURE 13.1. Interrelation of ovarian and testicular tumors of germ cell origin.

and may vary in size from a few centimeters in diameter to a mass large enough to fill the pelvis and abdomen.

Histologically, the tumor is characterized by large, round cells with dark-stained nuclei and by stroma that divides the tumor into nests of cells. The septa are heavily infiltrated with lymphocytes and symplasmic giant cells. These lymphocytes may be associated with a cell-mediated immunity, which perhaps explains the good prognosis (70–90% survival at 5 years) for patients with pure dysgerminoma. The survival rate with bilateral ovarian involvement ranges from 5 to 12%.

The germinomas have the same nuclear sex as their host (sex chromatin-positive in the dysgerminomas of the female; sex chromatin-negative in the male seminomas). Presumably these neoplasms are derived from diploid germ cells prior to haploid reduction division.

In the broad controversy about the treatment of dysgerminoma, most disagreement is related to incorrect diagnosis. It is important to distinguish pure germinomas (dysgerminoma) from those intermingled with teratoid elements. The latter may be of widely varying types, such as endodermal sinus tissue, embryonal forms of cancer (Schiller's mesonephroma), or choriocarcinoma (dysgerminoma with choriocarcinoma elements) that may produce a positive pregnancy test. Pure dysger-

minomas are not associated with hormone activity. However, the diagnostic problem here is that with hemagglutination inhibition tests, and even with radioimmunoassay, hCG cross-reacts with luteinizing hormone (LH). A newly developed test for the β-subunit of hCG uses an antiserum that can differentiate between tumor LH and hCG. Incidentally, some mixed dysgerminomas also produce human placental lactogen.

Although dysgerminomas are highly radiosensitive, tumors possessing other teratoid elements (e.g., endodermal sinus and choriocarcinoma) are relatively insensitive to radiation therapy and are particularly deadly. Thus an accurate histologic diagnosis is crucial.

In the pediatric and adolescent group the question is raised, and rightfully so, about the type of treatment to be followed. The cure rate for unilateral pure germinoma ranges between 80 and 90%, even greater than the general cure rate previously cited. On the other hand, if the tumor is bilateral or shows local extension, the chance of 5-year cure drops to 20 to 30%.

Ascites or the discovery of a mixed teratoma or choriocarcinoma elements within the tumor, or rupture through the capsule, are indicative of a poor outcome and require aggressive therapy.

When the neoplasm is unilateral, encapsulated, and freely movable, it should be treated by unilateral salpingo-oophorectomy with wedge resection of the opposite ovary and exploration and biopsies of the paraaortic area. Microscopic metastases are infrequently found when the tumor is unilateral and the capsule is intact. Cytology is usually negative unless the capsule has been ruptured.

There are three possible methods of therapy: unilateral oophorectomy; unilateral oophorectomy followed by radiation therapy; and excision of the uterus, tubes, and ovaries with or without postoperative x-irradiation. The experience at many tumor centers indicates that a conservative operation yields about the same 5-year survival rate as do the more radical procedures; the recurrence rate, however, is higher following the more conservative operation. Fortunately, these recurrent tumors are highly sensitive to radiation therapy, and an appreciable number can be cured.

At the time of exploration the paraaortic area should be carefully explored and biopsy specimens obtained of any enlarged nodes. This step is an important part of management, as dysgerminomas, like seminomas, metastasize to the retroperitoneal paraaortic nodes.

When disease invades pelvic structures and is outside the reproductive tract or cannot be encompassed by conservative surgery because of the extent of disease, a more radical approach is indicated: The uterus, tubes, ovaries, omentum, and appendix should be removed. The use of radiation therapy to the pelvis and paraaortic nodes, rather than the use of combination chemotherapy, should be carried out at the discretion of the responsible physician. Neither a planned, definitive pelvic lymphadenectomy nor paraaortic lymphadenectomy should be performed for dysgerminomas, but rather a sampling of the nodes is indicated; this tumor drains to the mid or upper abdomen, and these cases can best be treated with irradiation or chemotherapy. If the spread is within the abdomen, total abdominal hysterectomy is indicated; and the decision about radiation therapy versus chemotherapy should then be made.

The greatest incidence of recurrence (25–40%) occurs within the first 3 years after the initial therapy. The patient should be seen every 3 to 4 months during this period. Any change is highly suspect; and rather than a long period of observation, early exploratory laparotomy with biopsy is recommended along with plans for additional therapy if indicated.

The role of the second-look operation merits some discussion, particularly in the pediatric and adolescent patient. If the mass was larger than 15 cm in diameter at the time of the original operation, if the pathology report indicated a triad of anaplasia, medullary structure, and numerous mitoses, and if residual tumor is left, routine postoperative x-irradiation is indicated. If no residual tumor is palpable after completion of therapy, abdominal exploration is indicated at 8 months. The author's experience suggests that 6 months is too early to detect early growth, and that 12 months is too late to treat a recurrence adequately. At the time of the second look, any recurrent or residual tumor is removed in toto. As a general rule, however, a second look is useless with a palpable tumor. Dr. Howard Jones, formerly of The Johns Hopkins Hospital, stated that these tumors exhibit the troublesome clinical and pathologic phenomena of late recurrence in the opposite ovary. Therefore it is prudent to remove the intact ovary after the patient's reproductive destiny has been fulfilled.

General considerations of *dysgerminomas* include the following.

1. It is a disease of young women (median age 22 years).
2. Ten percent are bilateral.
3. Three-fourths are stage I (86% of these lesions are stage Ia).
4. It spreads via the lymphatics.
5. The tumor is highly radiosensitive.
6. It may be associated with other germ cell or stromal elements.
7. Most common germ cell tumors are associated with gonadoblastoma and dysgenetic gonads.
8. Pure tumor has no detectable hormonal activity.
9. Prognosis deteriorates with increase in size, i.e., larger than 10 cm.

10. Five-year survival rate drops from 96% to 63% when disease spreads beyond the ovaries.

Teratoma Group

Five basic types comprise the category of germ cell tumors called teratomas. The first is the extraembryonal form, of which there are two subtypes: endodermal sinus tumor and choriocarcinoma.

Endodermal Sinus Tumors

The endodermal sinus tumors are known by many names, such as membrane tumor, embryonal carcinoma, yolk-sac carcinoma, extraembryonic (endomesodermal) membrane tumor, mesonephroma ovarii (Schiller), and endodermal sinuses of Duval, or Teilum's tumor. This mesometanephric rest tumor was so designated to cover both müllerian and mesonephric origins, but this term is no longer used. On the basis of his research, Scully believed that this tumor has a müllerian origin. Although the tubular structures resemble renal tubules and the masses of clear cells suggest renal carcinoma (hypernephroma) and Growitz tumor, neither term is now accepted, and all have been included as endodermal sinus tumors.

Endodermal sinus tumors are highly malignant neoplasms characterized by an overgrowth of extraembryonic mesoblast associated with yolk-sac endoderm. They have been interpreted by Teilum as recapitulating a yolk-sac structure. The microscopic picture is similar to that found in the placenta of a rat. These tumors may contain a great number of blastocyst-like yolk-sac (endoblast) vesicles and are referred to as polyembryonic, whereas the polyvesicular vitelline tumor has a typical histologic pattern occasionally found as a predominant characteristic of vitelline tumors in the ovary.

The endodermal sinus tumor and its related group occur in young patients and are not sensitive to radiation. Cure rates after conservative surgery do not differ from those after radical surgery. Only an occasional 5-year survival is reported, and these tumors, whose incidence is less than 1% of all ovarian cancers, are almost 100% fatal within 5 years.

Some reports indicate tumor response following triple therapy with methotrexate/ dactinomycin/chlorambucil. Although the dosages must be calculated for each individual according to age, weight, and general health, certain guidelines can be stated: Initially, methotrexate 5 mg daily is given simultaneously with chlorambucil. Both agents are administered orally. This regimen is continued for 16 to 25 days. In addition, 0.5 mg (500 μg) of dactinomycin is given intravenously for 5 days, starting on the 3rd, 12th, and 21st days after methotrexate; and chlorambucil therapy is initiated on day 21. A repeat course, started 2 weeks after completion of the initial treatment if blood count and chemistries are normal, consists of 5 mg methotrexate and 10 mg chlorambucil given orally as a single dose daily for 5 days, with 0.5 mg (500 μg) of dactinomycin begun intravenously on the third day and repeated daily for 5 days. Subsequent repeat courses are given 2 to 3 weeks after completion of the previous course—provided blood count and chemistry values remain within normal limits—and are repeated at 2- and 3-week intervals until there is no evidence of disease. An alternate plan, which is simpler and appears to be equally effective, is a 5-day regimen that includes 200 mg cyclophosphamide (Cytoxan)/ 0.5 mg actinomycin D/1mg vincristine/50 mg adriamycin on day 1; on days 2, 3, 4, and 5 only cyclophosphamide and actinomycin D are given. All drugs are given intravenously. The patient is carefully monitored by daily blood counts and blood chemistries. The electrocardiogram is checked before adriamycin is given, and the drug is stopped if there is any change in the rhythm or voltage. The total dose of adriamycin never exceeds 450 mg/m^2. Currently, cis-platinum, vinblastine, and bleomycin have been given as treatments. Because it is difficult to accumulate a large series of endodermal sinus tumors the responsible physician should work out a chemotherapeutic regimen and administer it, watching for the development of any signs of toxicity.

An exploratory laparotomy as a second-look procedure should be carried out to make sure that all tumor has been eradicated before the therapy is stopped. Blood counts and blood chemistries, including AFP assays, should be done at least every 2 to 3 weeks during treatment, and a bone marrow biopsy is done as indicated.

General considerations of the *endodermal sinus tumor* are as follows.

1. Median age of the patients is 19 years (range 14 months to 45 years).
2. They constitute 22% of malignant germ cell tumors.
3. They are almost always unilateral.
4. Tumor growth is probably the fastest of any malignancy.
5. Thirty percent have obvious spread at operation; and of apparent stage IA tumors, 84% have occult metastases. About one-fourth rupture before or during surgery.
6. Most patients require adjuvant therapy.
7. These tumors are chemosensitive (80% five-year survival); prior to chemotherapy nearly all patients were dead within 2 years.
8. They are relatively radioresistant.
9. All (100%) of these tumors are AFP producers (i.e., AFP is an accurate tumor marker), so the AFP assay should be repeated weekly after surgery.
10. Pure endodermal sinus tumors do not produce hCG.

Choriocarcinoma

In children, choriocarcinoma is a rare, highly malignant tumor composed of trophoblasts. Although it is placed in the broad category with extraembryonic germ cell tumors, it may arise from a teratoma, from an ovarian cancer, or as a metastasis from a primary teratoma originating elsewhere. Postpubertal ovarian choriocarcinoma is more likely to be associated with an ovarian pregnancy than it is to be a primary germ cell tumor.

The gross picture of choriocarcinoma, identical to that in an adult, is characterized by extensive hemorrhage, ulceration, and necrosis, which convert it to a brittle, spongy, friable, red mass. The tumor may attain huge proportions and has a propensity for invading blood vessels.

Histologically, this tumor is characterized by columns or alveoli of trophoblastic cells with nests of Langhans' cells enveloped by syncytiotrophoblast. The cell masses are usually separated by spaces filled with clotted blood. Extensive necrosis often makes tumor diagnosis difficult.

Choriocarcinoma may be associated with rapidly developing sexual precocity. In part, this syndrome is triggered by ovarian estrogen production induced by chorionic gonadotropin elaborated by the tumor. The titers of estrogen and chorionic gonadotropins, which may be markedly elevated, drop when the tumor is entirely removed and rise if the tumor recurs.

Tumor growth is rapid, filling the pelvis and abdomen and becoming fixed to surrounding tissue, with early metastases, particularly to the lungs. The child becomes rapidly cachectic. If the tumor is discovered early, the uninvolved ovary may be markedly enlarged with multiple cysts of both follicular and lutein types and exhibits a pseudodecidual reaction.

As stated above, the tumor is not radiosensitive. Radical excision has no advantage over conservative surgery if the neoplasm is unilateral and encapsulated. However, if the neoplasm has spread outside the ovary, TAH-BSO, appendectomy, and omentectomy should be carried out. The role of radioactive phosphorus has not been established, but the isotope can control ascites if there is not a large volume of tumor. Although these tumors have not responded as well to chemotherapy as those arising from an intrauterine pregnancy, some success has been achieved with a 3- or 4-day regimen, as outlined above. Gestational trophoblastic neoplasm is folic acid-dependent, whereas nongestational trophoblastic tumors are folic acid-independent.

General considerations of *choriocarcinoma (nongestational)* are as follows.

1. The tumors may be primary or metastatic.
2. The primary is a rare tumor (40 cases in the literature).

a. Pure tumor arises in an ovarian ectopic pregnancy or de novo.

b. Mixed germ cell tumors are the most common primary form.

3. Choriocarcinomas may be metastatic from the uterus (or tube), which is the primary site (gestational).

Most primary choriocarcinomas of the ovary are combined with other malignant germ cell elements and are best placed in the category of mixed germ cell tumors. Most ovarian lesions are, however, secondary to the gestational uterine disease. To be unequivocally derived from germ cells, the tumor must occur in a child who has not reached puberty. It must be emphasized that pure, nongestational choriocarcinoma is thus rare.

The chemotherapeutic agents are not nearly as effective for the teratomatous choriocarcinoma as they are for the gestational choriocarcinoma of the uterus, possibly due to the fact that there are often other germ cell elements present and the teratomatous choriocarcinoma is folic acid-independent.

Embryonal Teratoma

The second tumor type in the teratoma group is the embryonal teratoma. In premenarchal girls the most frequent germ cell tumors (90%) are either dysgerminomas or embryonal teratomas; the remainder are mixed germ cell neoplasms. Embryonal (i.e., immature) teratomas are usually solid but may also contain small cystic areas that rarely take the form of a single large cyst. Their degree of malignancy can be determined only by microscopic examination, but these tumors are rarely benign, and most are highly malignant and rapidly fatal. They contain a mixture of embryonal and mature tissue derived from all three embryonic layers, whereas the solid, adult teratoma (discussed below) is composed of adult (i.e., mature) tissue from all three layers. Survival is directly related to the pathology rather than to the mode of therapy.

The embryonal teratoma has a poor prognosis, with fewer than 5% of patients surviving 5 years, whereas the solid, adult teratoma is benign. However, the cystic adult teratoma has a 2% malignancy rate. The degree of maturity or lack of it is best judged by histologic examination and provides a more logical basis for nomenclature than does the gross appearance.

According to Tielum, the term "embryonal carcinoma" should be restricted to tumors composed of undifferentiated neoplastic cells. Embryonal teratomas often show histologic evidence of other types of germ cell tumor. Consequently, some investigators have used the terms "malignant embryonal teratoma" and "embryonal carcinoma" interchangeably, and the result has been some confusion. The prognosis for patients with embryonal carcinoma depends on the predominant type of cell present; malignant neural tissue or malignant struma ovarii has a much better prognosis than does a tumor containing choriocarcinoma or endodermal sinus components, for example. Other combinations are melanoepithelioma, adenocarcinoma, spindle-cell sarcoma, fibrosarcoma, rhabdosarcoma, chondrosarcoma, and osteogenic sarcoma.

In approximately 10% of patients, involvement is bilateral. When the tumor is unilateral and encapsulated, radical surgery has shown no advantage over unilateral oophorectomy. However, if the tumor has spread, excision of the uterus, tubes, ovaries, appendix, and omentum is advocated. Unfortunately, the extent of the surgical procedure has little effect on the outcome; practically all patients with tumor spread die within 14 months. These tumors are radioresistant, and there are insufficient positive data to support the use of prophylactic chemotherapy. Data do support treating recurrence with a regimen of three or four drugs such as those outlined above for endodermal sinus tumors.

General considerations regarding the *immature (malignant) teratoma* are as follows.

1. Median age of the patients is 19 years (range 14 months to 40 years).
2. They constitute 15 to 20% of malignant germ cell tumors.
3. They almost always are unilateral.
4. More hormonal activity is present in pure tumor (i.e., AFP and hCG would be found to be within the normal range).

5. A variety of immature tissue in varying grades of maturity is seen histologically; neural tissues are most common and are easiest to grade.
6. Tumors are graded histologically 0 to 3 by (1) degree of immaturity and (2) the amount of neuroepithelium.
7. Five-year survival is as follows: grade 1, 81%; grade 2, 60%; grade 3, 30%.

Adult Teratoma

The third basic type of teratoma is the adult (i.e., mature) teratoma, or cystic teratoma (dermoid cyst). More than one-third of ovarian tumors in children are benign cystic teratomas, which are composed of all three germinal layers, although ectodermal structures predominate.

Nuclear sex chromatin in ovarian teratomas uniformly shows a female pattern, and XX sex chromosomes have been confirmed by chromosome studies. Nuclear sex chromatin also suggests that these cells are diploid rather than haploid. Interestingly, a significant portion of teratomas in the male have shown the sex chromatin pattern of females; this discrepancy may be explained by the fact that teratomas in males are derived from haploid germ cells by autofertilization or fusion of adjacent haploid cells. The result would be a diploid with either XX or XY chromosomes. The same process in the female could result only in XX diploid cells. Because some teratomas in the male have shown a mosaic pattern with sex chromatin-positive and sex chromatin-negative cells, it has been suggested that their origin is multicentric rather than from a single germ cell.

The cystic (dermoid) teratoma reveals a round, doughy, nontender, smooth, heavy, mobile mass more likely to be present in older children than in the young child. In small children the mass is usually above the true pelvis, and roentgenographic studies of the abdomen demonstrate teeth or calcification in about 40% of the cases.

Microscopic examination may reveal all types of mature ectoderm, mesoderm, and endodermal elements. It is not uncommon to find gastrointestinal mucosa, stratified squamous epithelium, hair follicles, sebaceous glands, cartilage, and nerve and respiratory tract elements. Giant cells and pseudoxanthoma cells are often seen. Occasionally, an overgrowth of thyroid tissue results in a functioning struma ovarii.

The first sign may be a mass in the abdomen, although often it is a complication from the cyst—twisting, hemorrhage, rupture, infection, or malignancy—that brings the patient to the physician's office.

Although 2% of all dermoids are complicated by malignancy, the incidence of malignancy among children is lower. In adults the malignant change is usually confined to one ovary, and squamous carcinoma within the cyst is associated with a much higher survival rate than are the other forms of malignancy (sarcoma, carcinoids, and adenocarcinoma). No comparable studies have been reported for children.

Torsion of the cyst occurs in about 16% of reported cases; 1.3% are said to rupture spontaneously, producing a clinical picture that suggests chronic granulomatous peritonitis, tuberculosis, or carcinomatosis. These possibilities should be ruled out by biopsies and frozen section studies.

When a dermoid cyst is suspected, the pelvis should be well walled off by laparotomy pads at surgery. If spillage occurs, a thorough saline wash should be carried out to prevent the chemical peritonitis that may result from the oily component of the cyst fluid. Dermoid cyst is best managed by dissecting the cyst from the ovary with preservation of the ovary, although occasionally the ovary is damaged beyond salvage due to torsion, hemorrhage, or infection; unilateral oophorectomy is then indicated. Because the bilaterality rate ranges from 5 to 12%, wedge biopsy should be carried out on the opposite ovary.

Struma Ovarii

The fourth type of teratoma is the struma ovarii, a dermoid tumor with thyroid tissue as its main or sole teratoid element. Few of these tumors prove to be malignant. About 10% of the patients with these tumors show evidence of thyrotoxicosis.

Carcinoid Tumors

Carcinoid tumors (argentaffinomas) of the ovary, the last category of teratoma, may arise in the wall of a dermoid cyst from either intestinal or bronchial epithelium; occasionally they metastasize. The syndrome resulting from this tumor includes intermittent flushing, cyanosis, diarrhea, and asthma attacks. The clinical manifestations are attributed to the production of excessive quantities of 5-hydroxytryptamine (serotonin) by the argentaffin cells of the tumor. Argentaffin granules can be identified with silver nitrate stain. Although dermoid cysts in children may contain thyroid or argentaffinoma tissue, they rarely grow large enough to cause the typical symptoms.

Gonadoblastoma

The gonadoblastoma is found almost exclusively in patients with androgen-insensitive tumors (testicular feminizing syndrome), Turner syndrome, pure gonadal dysgenesis, mixed gonadal dysgenesis, or hermaphroditism. Bilateral involvement occurs in about one-third of the patients. The coincidence of gonadoblastoma mixed with choriocarcinoma is 1 in 75 cases.

Composed of a mixture of germ cells (dysgerminoma) and sex cord cells (granulosa-Sertoli), the tumor had previously been reported only in intersex individuals and was called "dysgenetic gonadoma." In most cases in which sex chromatic studies have been done, the nuclear pattern has been negative in the patient (46,XY) or has shown a sex chromosome mosaicism (XO/XY). Most patients with a gonadoblastoma are intersexual with a phenotype female habitus, amenorrhea, and perhaps virilization.

Grossly, the tumor ranges from a solid mass of gray to cream-colored fleshy tissue resembling a dysgerminoma to a firm, fibrous mass. A characteristic feature is calcification, which may be evident on roentgenographic examination of the pelvis. Microscopic examination reveals masses of large germ cells that wrap themselves around immature granulosalike cells. Between the nests of these cells are large numbers of other cell types suggestive of Leydig cells.

The malignant potential of pure gonadoblastoma has not been established. Some investigators consider it an in situ carcinoma because its germ cells commonly progress to invasive germinoma. However, the possibility of malignant behavior may well depend on the mixture of gonadoblastoma with other germ cell elements, such as dysgerminoma or endodermal sinus tumor. Because these patients often reveal eunuchoidal features, sterility, or signs of Turner syndrome, and because the tumor has a potential for malignancy, removal of both gonads is indicated. In fact, late recurrence in the remaining gonad mandates bilateral extirpation. All streaks should be removed as well.

Estrogen and progesterone should be prescribed for these girls when they reach the age of puberty. The prognosis after removal of these tumors is usually good. Neither recurrence nor metastasis has been reported after removal. However, if the tumor is extensive or only partially removed, subsequent difficulty may ensue.

General considerations of *gonadoblastomas* (mixed germ cell and gonadal stromal tumors) are as follows.

1. They are rare tumors: Probably fewer than 75 cases are recorded in the literature.
2. The age range of the patients is 1 to 38 years.
3. The phenotype is female in more than 80% of cases.
4. The patients are chromatin-negative.
5. The karyotype is 46,XY, 46,XO/XY, 47,XXX/XO, rarely 46,XX.
6. Ninety percent of all patients have a Y chromosome.
7. Secondary sex characteristics are depressed, sometimes virilized with amenorrhea or masculinization, or precocious puberty.
8. Gonadoblastoma is the most common

malignancy occurring in dysgenetic gonads and arises almost exclusively in them.

9. Eighteen percent occur in dysgenetic testes, and most are seen in abnormal gonads of dysgenetic type.
10. Thirty percent are bilateral.
11. Twenty-two percent occur in streaked gonads.
12. Malignancy supervenes in 75%.
13. Malignant change is usually in germ cell elements (dysgerminoma, teratoma, choriocarcinoma, or endodermal sinus tumor).
14. Granulosa or Sertoli-Leydig elements may also be present.

Gonadal Stromal Tumors (Sex Cord Mesenchymal Tumors)

The fourth major tumor group is composed of neoplasms derived from ovarian mesenchyme. There are three basic categories: gonadal stromal tumors of (1) the female cell type (granulosa and granulosa-thecoma tumors); (2) the male cell type (Sertoli-Leydig cell tumors, i.e., arrhenoblastoma or adrenoblastoma), Sertoli, and hilus (Leydig) cell tumors; and (3) mixed cell types (gynandroblastoma). Tumors in this group are not as common as the germ cell tumors, nor are they as malignant. The first subcategory includes granulosa cell tumors, which are infrequent during childhood. Although approximately 100 have been reported in children, only three have proved to be malignant. From 5 to 10% of the tumors occur before the patient reaches the age of puberty and feminize an occasional patient. For example, they may produce a feminine habitus, maturation of the genitalia, and enlargement of the breasts, but with scant pubic hair. Vaginal bleeding may occur.

Although precocious puberty is usually constitutional and only rarely results from an ovarian tumor, it must be remembered that it may also result from gonadotropin production (by such tumors as teratoma and choriocarcinoma), which in turn triggers estrogen production. Also, precocious heterosexual puberty may result from masculinizing tumors or lipoid cell tumors. Of 225 cases of female sexual precocity reported in the literature, six were due to ovarian tumors.

Usually the diagnosis is made after an abdominal or pelvic mass is discovered. Exploratory laparotomy shows that the tumor is rounded or lobulated with a smooth surface. A thin capsule covers the tumor, and the bulk is either solid or marked with numerous cystic spaces that may be filled with clotted blood. If these cysts rupture, acute abdomen may result from hemoperitoneum. These cysts are bilateral in about 5% of patients.

Treatment for the unilateral, encapsulated, freely movable tumor is unilateral oophorectomy with wedge resection of the opposite ovary. For extension beyond the ovary to pelvic structures, TAH-BSO should be carried out. The decision on whether to use adjunctive combination chemotherapy or postoperative x-irradiation therapy is at the discretion of the responsible physician. The tumor carries a good prognosis, depending on its degree of anaplasia and the stage of the disease. The malignancy rate, about 20% in adults, is much lower in children, ranging from 3 to 6%.

Malignant granulosa cell tumors have the capacity to produce estrogens from androstenedione, dehydroepiandrosterone, progesterone, and testosterone. Recurrences are usually local, and distant metastases are rare. Recurrences often take many years to develop, although they may occur at any time. The histologic appearance of a tumor of this group offers no index to its final behavior. If the tumor is primarily a thecoma, its potential for malignancy is less than 1%. It can be classified as malignant only if there is metastasis.

These tumors are sensitive to x-rays as well as combination chemotherapy, and the decision should be left to the treating physician. Classifying these tumors separately into granulosa cell and theca cell groups has been abandoned because most tumors are mixtures and both cell types have identical origins. Some researchers disagree with this concept, stating that pure granulosa cell tumors tend to be more malignant, either initially or after many years, whereas granulosa cell/theca cell mixtures or thecomas are more benign.

It is important to follow children with these tumors for life. Vaginal cytology in the premenarchal child reveals increasing estrogen stimulation if recurrence is developing. Late recurrence is a well-documented characteristic of granulosa cell tumors. The remaining ovary should be removed after childbearing is completed.

General considerations of *granulosa cell tumors* are as follows.

1. They are a disease of any age but are most commonly seen in older women (mean age 53 years).
2. Tumors are unilateral in 95% of cases.
3. Many fewer than half of the patients have symptoms suggestive of an endocrine disorder (i.e., precocious puberty, postmenopausal bleeding).
4. Associated endometrial hyperplasia and adenocarcinoma are found more frequently than would be expected if the tumor was not present.
5. Granulosa cell tumors occasionally cause virilization, especially during pregnancy.
6. Malignancy is relatively low. The overall 5-year survival is 81% ranging from 95% for stage I to 20% for stage III.
7. Time to recurrence may be long. The mean duration is 8.9 years (range 1–22 years).
8. Histologic grade and mitotic index (mitoses per 10 high-power fields) are important prognostic factors.
9. Plasma follicle-stimulating hormone level plus estriol estimation may be used as markers.
10. The tumor is generally radiosensitive.
11. It is difficult to assess the merits of chemotherapy at this time.

General considerations of *theca cell tumors* (theca-fibroma group) are as follows.

1. They constitute 1% of all ovarian neoplasms.
2. Most are benign.
3. Two-thirds of the patients are postmenopausal.
4. Symptoms and signs are similar to those produced by granulosa cell tumors.
5. High association exists with endometrial hyperplasia and carcinoma.
6. Benign thecomas are cured by simple oophorectomy. Malignant thecomas are treated with more aggressive treatments: exploratory laparotomy, removal of the uterus, tubes, and ovaries, or biopsies followed by combination chemotherapy.

The term "Sertoli-Leydig cell tumor" is used instead of the more familiar "arrhenoblastoma" because many of these tumors are nonfunctioning or have estrogenic physiologic effects rather than masculinizing tendencies. The more immature the tumor cells, the greater their potential for producing hormones.

Tumors with a predominance of functioning Sertoli cells may have the effect of a feminizing neoplasm. However, if the Leydig cells are predominant and functional, the patient is first defeminized (atrophy of breasts, loss of female contour, amenorrhea) and then masculinized (hirsutism, hypertrophy of clitoris, voice changes). Androgens suppress normal ovarian functions and cause the signs of virilization, and it is a high level of testosterone that mediates the masculinization resulting from this tumor.

The tumor usually affects women of childbearing age and is rare during childhood. Malignant behavior, seen in 3 to 20% of the patients, is usually manifested by intraabdominal spread rather than by distant metastasis. The tumor is bilateral in 5% of the patients. The plan of management outlined for the granulosa cell tumor can be applied to this tumor, and a wedge resection of the opposite ovary is indicated if unilateral oophorectomy is elected.

Signs and symptoms regress after tumor excision; however, the patient may be left with permanent hirsutism and voice changes. Because these tumors have a history of late recurrence, the question is raised about the validity of reexploration after the patient has completed her reproductive life. Some clinicians suggest that hysterectomy with oophorectomy may be carried out. Unfortunately, this question cannot be resolved at this time.

Whenever a child develops virilization, virilizing adrenal tumors must be considered. Dexamethasone is not able to suppress an adrenal tumor. Endocrinologists have utilized hCG stimulation (10,000 IU intramuscularly daily) while continuing the high dose of dexamethasone for adrenal suppression. An increase (twofold) in 17-ketosteroid secretion following gonadotropic stimulation of the ovary is thought to delineate an ovarian source for excess androgens. It is now thought that this response is highly variable, frequently difficult to interpret, and almost always unnecessary. When a high degree of clinical indication exists for the presence of an ovarian androgen-producing tumor, laparotomy is the only definitive diagnostic approach.

Included among the gonadal stromal tumors is a mixed type, gynandroblastoma. Gynandroblastomas should contain typical aggregates of granulosa cell with Call-Exner bodies and hollow tubules of Leydig cells containing crystalloids of Reinke. There are no reports of this tumor in children, but there is no reason to believe that it would differ in behavior from granulosa cell or Sertoli-Leydig cell tumors, depending on which group of cells predominates. The malignancy of gynandroblastomas is undocumented.

General considerations of *Sertoli-Leydig cell tumors* (arrhenoblastoma) are as follows.

1. Most common patient age range is 11 to 45 years.
2. Pure Sertoli cell tumors (which tend to be estrogen-secreting) and pure Leydig cell tumors (which tend to be androgen-secreting) are always benign.
3. Defeminization and virilization occur with 70% of all differentiated Sertoli-Leydig cell tumors and with 90% of less well differentiated tumors.
4. Plasma testosterone and urinary oxysteroids are usually markedly elevated.
5. Prognosis is difficult to define, but the outlook is generally good.
6. Mortality in various series varies from 3% to 34%.

Nonspecific Ovarian Tumors

The ovary may be involved as part of disseminated Hodgkin's disease. Although these tumors are usually found almost exclusively among the adult population, ovarian involvement has been reported in children suffering from Burkitt's tumor. It is interesting that the first virus to be suspected of causing a human cancer was isolated as a result of epidemiologic observations made in populations of tropical Africa, particularly in those with Burkitt's tumor. The particular distribution of the tumor from the geographic and ecologic standpoint, as well as its age distribution, typical of an infectious disease, has led to the suspicion that Burkitt's tumor may be caused by an infectious agent. A concerted effort has in fact resulted in isolation of a virus (Epstein-Barr virus) from Burkitt's tumor cells. Cyclophosphamide (Cytoxan) is effective in treating these tumors, but a large tumor causing symptoms should be excised.

Miscellaneous Tumors

The miscellaneous category includes *fibroma* and *sarcoma*. Ovarian fibromas are more common in adults than in children; these tumors are benign and should be removed when their size makes the diagnosis obvious or complications cause symptoms.

On the other hand, ovarian sarcomas occur more frequently in children than in adults. Grossly, these tumors are solid, lobulated, or soft growths that rapidly fill the abdomen. The cut surfaces of the cellular sarcomas are soft and fleshy, whereas the more fibrous ones are firm and somewhat granular when sectioned. Azoury and Woodruff, reporting on 47 primary sarcomas of the ovary, noted that the most common symptoms were abdominal pain and swelling.

Regardless of the types of therapy employed, survival is poor. In patients with unilateral encapsulated disease, unilateral oophorectomy is as efficacious as more radical surgery. The most common type of sarcoma in this age group is teratoid (90%), and the tumor is undifferentiated; the prognosis is uniformly poor.

Ovarian sarcomas include sarcomas arising in teratomas, mixed müllerian tumors (carcinosarcoma), and fibroleiomyosarcomas. Sarcoma can also secondarily involve the ovary (i.e., lymphoma, retroperitoneal sarcoma). These rare tumors are treated in similar fashion to malignant epithelial tumors.

Metastatic Cancer

The final major tumor type that can affect the ovary in children is metastatic cancer. Metastatic ovarian tumor must be considered whenever a primary malignancy of any other pelvic structure or abdominal organ, or of the thyroid gland, is found. The diagnosis can be made only with a high index of suspicion. Involved ovaries are usually smooth, firm, and freely movable; and involvement is bilateral in approximately 55% of the patients. Twenty percent of involved ovaries are of normal size, although many have a bizarre histologic pattern. The main lesion reflects the characteristics of the primary tumor.

Krükenberg tumor, for example, usually arises in the gastrointestinal tract and metastasizes to the ovary, although this tumor may occur primarily in the ovary as well. Probably arising in germinal epithelium having müllerian potentialities, it is often bilateral and typically solid, and the ovary retains its normal shape. A few cases have been reported in children. Krükenberg tumors are characterized histologically by large, swollen, signet-ring-like cells that lie in clumps within areas of mucoid degeneration, scattered through an edematous stoma-like matrix. Only tumors meeting these criteria should be so designated. Ovarian metastases should be removed whenever feasible.

Summary

Some additional comments must be made about ovarian cancer in children. There are certain characteristics that distinguish the picture from that in adults.

1. Limited space for tumor expansion
2. High degree of virulence in cancer
3. Less effective immunologic response
4. Possibility that therapy may affect future physical and emotional development

Thus the picture is usually one of rapid progression once the tumor has expanded beyond its original site. When dealing with advanced cancer, the physician must strike a balance between doing too little and too much. Therapy should be aimed at relieving symptoms with palliative measures to keep the patient comfortable for as long as possible. This approach should include surgery for relief of intestinal obstruction, drainage of abscesses, or repair of fistulas. If liver, bone marrow, and kidney functions are adequate, chemotherapy may be valuable in selected cases, and when indicated judicious use of irradiation is helpful.

Ovarian tumors in children trigger excessive emotionalism in the child, her parents, and her physician. Parents may first tend to deny the threat to their child's life. If a diagnosis of cancer is made, they tend to become utterly panic-stricken and seem to lose the ability to think clearly. Physicians must be pillars of strength in this situation and assume broad responsibilities. They must guide the parents and soothe the child. Above all else, they must control their own feelings of pity and avoid projecting themselves into the picture as a surrogate parent, lest emotion cloud clinical decisions.

When dealing with ovarian tumors in children, the gynecologist must use the same principles of assessing operability as those used for adults. This approach offers the maximum opportunity for successful treatment. The ancient medical philosophy of not inflicting harm if one cannot achieve good is especially applicable to children with ovarian cancer. It is better for a child to die at home in the loving care of her parents than alone in a cold, forbidding hospital room.

However, the greatest tranquilizer for all concerned is to emphasize that most ovarian tumors in children are nonmalignant. In all likelihood the child can be hospitalized and cured in a few short days. These young patients heal quickly and recuperate at a remarkably rapid rate; most can be sent home in 4 or 5 days. Even for malignant tumors that are encapsulated and free of adjacent tissue, cure rates are high, depending of course on the type of tumor. This positive philosophy should pervade our discussions whenever ovarian tumors in children are evaluated.

Bibliography

Anstey A, Gowers L, Vass A, Robson AO: Ovarian dysgerminoma presenting with hypercalcaemia: case report and review of the literature. *Br J Obstet Gynaecol* 97:641, 1990.

Averette HE, Hoskins WJ, Dudan RC, Nordqvist SRB: The ovary. In Nealon TF Jr (ed): *Management of the Patient with Cancer*. Saunders, Philadelphia, 1976, p. 618.

Azoury RS, Woodruff JD: Primary ovarian sarcoma: report of 47 cases from the Emil Novak ovarian tumor registry. *Obstet Gynecol* 37:920, 1971.

Ballas M: Yolk sac carcinoma of the ovary with alpha fetoprotein in serum and ascitic fluid demonstrated by immuno-osmophoresis. *Am J Clin Pathol* 57:511, 1972.

Barber HRK: A guide to ovarian tumors in children. *Consultant* 15:83, 1975.

Barber HRK: Ovarian cancer. *CA*. 36(3):149, 1986.

Barber HRK, Graber EA: Gynecological tumors in childhood and adolescence. *Obstet Gynecol Surv* 28:369, 1973.

Barber HRK, Graber EA: Managing ovarian tumors of childhood and adolescence. *Contemp Obstet Gynecol* 3:123, 1974.

Boles ET, Hardacre JM, Newton WA: Ovarian tumors and cysts in children. *Arch Surg* 83:112, 1961.

Breen JL, Maxson WS: Ovarian tumors in children in adolescence. *Clin Obstet Gynecol* 20:607, 1977.

Brownstein GD, Vaitukaitis JL, Carbone PP, et al: Ectopic production of human chorionic gonadotropin. *Ann Intern Med* 78:39, 1973.

Butt JA: Ovarian tumors in children. *Obstet Gynecol* 69:833, 1955.

Cancer Facts and Figures, 1991. American Cancer Society, Atlanta.

Cangir A: Malignant genital tract tumors in children. *Curr Probl Cancer* 10:301, 1986.

Cangir A, Smith J, VanEys J: Improved prognosis in children with ovarian cancer following modified VAC (vincristine sulphate, actinomycin, and cyclophosphamide) chemotherapy. *Cancer* 42:1234, 1978.

Chambers JT, Merino MJ, Kohorn EI, Schwartz PE: Borderline ovarian tumors. *Am J Obstet Gynecol* 159:1088, 1988.

Devi NS: Mesodermal mixed tumors of the female generative tract. Presented at the 6th International Congress on Obstetrics and Gynecology, New York, 1970.

Dicker D, Dekel A, Feldberg D, et al: Bilateral Sertoli-Leydig cell tumor with heterologous elements: report of an unusual case and review of the literature. *Eur J Obstet Gynecol Reprod Biol* 22(3):175, 1986.

Einhorn LH, Williams SD: Current concepts in cancer: the role of cisplatinum in solid tumor therapy. *N Engl J Med* 300:289, 1979.

Gargano G, DeLeonardis A, Perrotti P, et al: Ovarian bilateral cystic teratomas: diagnosis and therapy in a young woman. *Clin Exp Obstet Gynecol* 17:37, 1990.

Gershenson DM, Silva EG: Serous ovarian tumors of low malignant potential with peritoneal implants. *Cancer* 65:578, 1990.

Gold P, Freeman SO: Demonstration of tumor-specific antigens in human colonic carcinoma by immunological tolerance and absorption technique. *J Exp Med* 121:439, 1965.

Govan AD: Ovarian tumors: clinical and pathologic features. *Clin Obstet Gynecol* 3:89, 1976.

Grosfeld JL, Valentine TVN, Lowe D, Baehner RL: Benign and malignant teratomas in children: analysis of 85 patients. *Surgery* 80:297, 1976.

Gynaecological Oncology. Protocols of Management. 2nd Ed. King George V. Hospital, Royal Prince Albert Hospital, Sydney, 1989.

Hays DM: Malignant solid tumors of childhood. *Curr Probl Surg* 23:161, 1986.

Heald FO, McCraig J, Ming P-ML: Ovarian tumors in adolescents: types and presenting feature. *Clin Pediatr Phila* 6:401, 1967.

Herman RJ, Norris HJ: Malignant germ cell tumors of the ovary. *Hum Pathol* 8:551, 1977.

Hughesdon PE: Structure, origin and histological relations of dysgerminoma. *J Obstet Gynaecol Br Commonw* 66:566, 1959.

Huffman JW: *Gynecology of Childhood and Adolescence*. Saunders, Philadelphia, 1968, p. 286.

Jereb B, Golough R, Havlicek S: Ovarian cancer in children in adolescence, a review of 15 cases. *Med Pediatr Oncol* 3:339, 1977.

Kaufman RH, Gardner HL: Benign mesodermal tumors. *Clin Obstet Gynecol* 8:953, 1961.

Knox JM, Freeman RG: Epidermal tumors. *Clin Obstet Gynecol* 8:925, 1965.

LaPolla JP, Fiorica JV, Turnquist D, et al: Successful therapy of metastatic embryonal carcinoma coexisting with gonadoblastoma in a patient with 46,XY pure gonadal dysgenesis (Swyer's syndrome). *Gynecol Oncol* 37:471, 1990.

Lauer ME, Camitta BM: Home care for dying children: a nursing model. *J Pediatr* 97:1032, 1980.

Lawrence DJR, Neville MA: Fetal antigens and

their role in the diagnosis and clinical management of human neoplasms: a review. *Br J Cancer* 26:335, 1972.

Lucraft H, Mann JR, Pearson D: Malignant ovarian tumors in children. *Ovarian Cancer Adv Biosci* 26:97, 1980.

Luisi, A.: Metastatic ovarian tumors. In: *Ovarian Cancer. International Union Against Cancer. Monograph Series*. Vol. 2. Springer-Verlag, Berlin, 1968, p. 87.

Mann JR, Lakin GE, Leonard JC, et al: Clinical application of serum CEA and AFP levels in children with solid tumors. *Arch Dis Child* 53:366, 1978.

Miller OJ: Sex chromosome abnormality. *Am J Obstet Gynecol* 90:1078, 1964.

Miser A, Miser J: The treatment of cancer pain in children. *Pediatr Clin North Am* 36:979, 1989.

Moore JG, Schrifrin BS, Erez S: Ovarian tumors in childhood and adolescence. *Am J Obstet Gynecol* 99:913, 1967.

Morris J, McLean O, Scully RE: *Endocrine Pathology of the Ovary*. Mosby, St. Louis, 1969, pp. 65–95.

Nielsen SN, Gaffey TA, Malkasian GD Jr: Immature ovarian teratoma: a review of 14 cases. *Mayo Clin Proc* 61(2):110, 1986.

Orr PS, Gibson A, Young DG: Ovarian tumors in childhood: a 27 year review. *Br J Surg* 63:367, 1976.

Parson L, Sommers SC (eds): *Gynecology*. Saunders, Philadelphia, 1963.

Pepus M, Hutchison JB, Ruffolo EH, et al: Ovarian neoplasm and sexual precocity. *Obstet Gynecol* 29:828, 1967.

Raafat F, Klys H, Rylance G: Juvenile granulosa cell tumor. *Pediatr Pathol* 10:617, 1990.

Radman HM, Koman W: Ovarian tumors in children. *Am J Obstet Gynecol* 79:989, 1960.

Scheelhaus HF, Trujillo JM, Rutledge FN, et al: Germ cell tumors associated with XY gonadal dysgenesis. *Am J Obstet Gynecol* 109:1197, 1971.

Scully RE: Ovarian tumors: a review. *Am J Pathol* 87:686, 1977.

Scully RE: Recent progress in ovarian cancer. *Hum Pathol* 1:73, 1970.

Scully RE: Sex cord-mesenchyme tumors. In: *Ovarian Cancer. International Union Against Cancer Monograph Series*. Vol. 2. Springer-Verlag, Berlin, 1968, p. 40.

Shakfeh SM, Woodruff JD: Primary ovarian sarcomas: report of 46 cases and review of the literature. *Obstet Gynecol Surv* 42:331, 1987.

Shebib S, Sabbah RS, Sackey K, et al: Endodermal sinus (yolk sac) tumor in infants and children; a clinical and pathologic study: an 11 year review. *Am J Pediatr Hematol Oncol* 11:36, 1989.

Southam AL: Disorder of menstruation in adolescents. *Clin Obstet Gynecol* 9:779, 1966.

Susnerwala SS, Pande SC, Shrivastava SK, Dinshaw KA: Dysgerminoma of the ovary: review of 27 cases. *J Surg Oncol* 46:43, 1991.

Taylor ES: Editorial comment: virilizing adrenal tumors. *Obstet Gynecol Surv* 23:981, 1968.

Teilum G: Tumors of germinal origin. In: *Ovarian Cancer. International Union Against Cancer Monograph Series*. Vol. 2. Springer-Verlag, Berlin, 1948, p. 58.

Vergote IB, Abeler VM, Kjrstad KE, Trope C: Management of malignant ovarian immature teratoma: role of adriamycin. *Cancer* 66:882, 1990.

Wallach EE: Female isosexual pseudoprecocious puberty. *Clin Obstet Gynecol* 11:795, 1968.

Wollner N, Exelby P, Woodruff JM, et al: Malignant ovarian tumors in childhood. *Cancer* 37:1953, 1976.

Young RH, Scully RE: Ovarian sex cord-stromal tumors: recent advances and current status. *Clin Obstet Gynecol* 11:93, 1984.

14

Ovarian Cancer Complicating Pregnancy

An estimated 21,000 new cases of ovarian cancer in the United States were anticipated in 1991 and 13,000 deaths due to this lesion. It is estimated that about 1 of every 70 newborn girls (1.4%) will develop ovarian cancer during their lifetime. This neoplasm accounts for 4% of all cancers among women and 27% of the cancers of the female reproductive system. Although ovarian cancer ranks second in incidence among gynecologic cancers, it causes more deaths than any other cancer of the female reproductive system.

Deaths from this disease have slowly increased over the years and the rate is now 2.5 times that of the 1960 rate. Cancer of the ovary is the leading cause of death from gynecologic cancer. Common epithelial ovarian cancer is usually seen in women over age 40, but there is an increasing number seen in younger women as well. Germ cell tumors of the ovary are seen most commonly from birth to age 20. Gonadal stromal tumors are usually seen during the child-bearing years. Germ cell and gonadal stromal tumors are more often unilateral than are common epithelial ovarian cancers; therefore if the tumor is confined to the ovary, unilateral salpingo-oophorectomy may be an acceptable treatment.

Ovarian tumors have been reported to occur once in every 1000 pregnancies: 1 in 10 of them are normal physiologic corpus luteum cysts. Ovarian cancer occurs in about 1 in every 18,000 pregnancies. In the nonpregnant state about 20% of ovarian tumors are malignant, whereas pregnancy may protect against the development of ovarian tumors, suggested by the fact that ovarian cancers are rare in populations that do not practice birth control. Therefore incessant ovulation is considered an etiologic factor.

Chung and Birnbaum found that fewer than 40 cases of ovarian cancer complicating pregnancy had been reported between 1963 and 1972 and added an additional 10 cases during and after pregnancy. Beisher and colleagues recorded 164 ovarian tumors that were diagnosed during pregnancy or the puerperium at the Royal Women's Hospital in Melbourne during the years 1947 until 1969. More than 50% were either adult cystic teratomas or mucinous cystadenomas, and 4 (2.4%) were malignant. Beisher commented on the difficulty of establishing a definitive diagnosis during pregnancy and concluded that the size of the tumor was not a reliable criterion of malignancy. The various favorable pathologic types (adult cystic teratoma, mucinous cystadenoma) reflected an overall 5-year survival rate for ovarian neoplasia during pregnancy of 76% compared to a general figure for all age groups of 25%.

Novak and colleagues reported on 100 cases of malignant ovarian neoplasia associated with gestation. There were 45 common epithelial ovarian tumors, 14 gonadal stromal tumors, 33 germ cell tumors, 2 sarcomas, 2 metastatic Krükenberg type tumors, and 4 metastases of which two were unclassifiable. The absolute 5-year survival among these 100 cases was 76%. The excellent salvage is a reflection of the favorable prognosis with these tumors.

The signs and symptoms of ovarian neoplasm are not basically different than those seen in the nonpregnant state. The presenting symptoms, such as torsion, rupture, hemorrhage, or infection, may be a complication of the tumor.

The pelvic findings are an important part in the decision of whether to operate immediately or to observe the patient until the second trimester. The unilateral, seemingly well-encapsulated, freely movable mass of uniform consistency that is less than 10 cm in diameter can be kept under observation until the second trimester. If the mass decreases in size, presumably it represents a corpus luteum cyst. However, progressive growth requires exploration without further delay. On the other hand, a hard, knobby, fixed mass of variegated consistency, bilateral masses, and signs of ascitic fluid are indications for surgical intervention regardless of the trimester of pregnancy.

Fortunately, most malignancies during pregnancy are diagnosed at an early stage (stage I) because the patient seeks medical advice prior to the occurrence of symptoms related to the tumor and is examined at her antepartum visit. The survival rate, which is much the same as for the nonpregnant patient, is determined by the stage and type of tumor. If the tumor is diagnosed during the third trimester, surgery may be delayed until the fetus is viable, but to delay beyond that point cannot be justified.

There is little difference between a 1-inch incision for laparoscopy and a 5- to 6-inch incision, which permits thorough evaluation of the tumor, thorough inspection of all the other abdominal viscera, and removal of affected organs. Diagnostic workup should include a Papanicolaou smear, proctosigmoidoscopy, pelvic and recto-vaginal examination, and a careful search for extrapelvic metastasis. If there is an omental cake, hepatomegaly, or gross ascites, the outlook for long survival is grim. Only about 8% of patients with ascites live 5 years. The toll of cancer will be lowered only if physicians begin to suspect cancer in every persistently enlarged ovary.

The presenting symptom may be a complication of ovarian tumor, such as torsion, rupture, hemorrhage, or infection. This symptom may be accompanied by acute abdominal pain with vomiting and possible shock. Surgical intervention is indicated immediately. In other instances the cysts or tumor should be removed to eliminate the need for cesarean section, to remove the danger of the complications listed above, and to eliminate the danger of malignancy. Cesarean section can then be reserved for the usual obstetric indications.

Therapy of Ovarian Cancer During Pregnancy

If surgeons find an ovarian tumor, cyst, or malignancy during abdominal exploration, their first obligation is to stage the disease, collect peritoneal fluid for cytologic and cell block examination, and remove the lesion for immediate frozen section in order to obtain definitive diagnosis and documentation. This procedure is followed by whatever other surgery is indicated, depending on the type of tumor, its histologic grading, and the degree of anatomic spread. Biopsies of omentum, peritoneum, or any other intraabdominal area where one suspects tumors are indicated. The information may prove helpful for selecting the appropriate therapy and for future follow-up examinations and studies.

Papillary serous cystadenocarcinoma, the most common type of ovarian malignancy, is probably an advanced stage of a benign serous cystadenoma. If it is contained so papillary processes are within an intact capsule, the prognosis is reasonably good. Once there is extension through the capsule with papillation on the exterior of the tumor, extension to the surrounding organs appears promptly, with a great diminution in the chance of 5-year survival. General abdominal carcinomatosis soon follows with death. The treatment is total abdominal hysterectomy (TAH), bilateral salpingo-oophorectomy (BSO), appendectomy, omentectomy, and sampling of pelvic and paraaortic nodes. Currently, combination chemotherapy is the favored adjuvant treatment. Therapy must be tailored to the patient and the extent of disease. When there is doubt about the type of tumor or that a malignancy is present, if the tumor has an intact capsule and is freely movable, especially in a patient under age 30, it is better to perform a salpingo-oophorectomy on the side of the tumor. The pelvis should be aspirated prior to the excision and sent for a cell block examination. If the tumor proves to be highly malignant or the cell block results are positive, the abdomen may be opened and the remaining reproductive organs excised as outlined above, if it appears to be the best course. With certain low-grade malignancies the previously performed treatment may be considered sufficient to ensure a cure.

Papillary mucinous cystadenocarcinoma is the next most common type of ovarian cancer. About one in four is bilateral. The clinical picture and operative findings again depend on whether the tissue is contained in an intact capsule. The spread of this tumor is fortunately slower than the spread of the papillary serous variety, so the prognosis is better. Treatment is the same as that for serous cystadenocarcinoma.

Solid Adenocarcinoma

The solid adenocarcinoma is a common epithelial ovarian carcinoma with the same cells as those found in papillary serous or mucinous carcinoma of the ovary. These tumors are solid and highly undifferentiated, and they have a great potential to spread and metastasize. They are bilateral in more than 50% of patients, and the prognosis is poor. Treatment is similar to that outlined above.

Dysgerminoma

Dysgerminoma is not aggressively malignant in young patients, and in fact pure dysgerminoma has a surprisingly high 5-year survival rate. If the tumor is unilateral and still encapsulated, unilateral oophorectomy may be carried out if (1) the remaining ovary is negative on biopsy; (2) the peritoneal fluid is negative; and (3) the external, common, and paraaortic nodes are negative as well. Dysgerminomas in patients over age 35 and surely in those over age 40 should undergo more aggressive attack. If the tumor is bilateral or the capsule is perforated, TAH-BSO, omentectomy, appendectomy, and postoperative x-ray therapy must be carried out in any age group.

Other germ cell tumors, both extraembryonal and embryonic carcinomas, are highly malignant. The treatment is generally excision of the uterus, tubes, ovaries, appendix, and omentum. Combination chemotherapeutic agents should be given at monthly intervals for 6 to 8 months and consideration given to a second-look operation. As a group these tumors are relatively radioresistant.

Gonadal Stromal Tumors

The gonadal stromal tumors (granulosa cell, Sertoli-Leydig) are rarely associated with pregnancy. However, if they are unilateral and encapsulated, with a negative opposite ovary on biopsy, negative cytology, and no evidence of spread, unilateral salpingo-oophorectomy is usually adequate therapy. If there is any evidence of spread or if the tumor is bilateral, it should be managed as outlined above. These tumors are characterized by local, late recurrence and are radiosensitive.

Sarcoma

Sarcoma of the ovary, either primary or metastatic, is highly malignant and spreads quickly by local invasion and blood vessel and lymphatic extension. It is usually found before childbearing age. Prompt therapy should be complete removal of the pelvic gynecologic organs. Combination chemotherapeutic agents should be given for 6 to 8 months and a decision then made whether to reexplore the patient or to continue therapy for a longer period.

Metastatic Carcinoma

Metastatic carcinoma of the ovaries from the uterus, breasts, thyroid, stomach, or colon may occur, although it is rare. There is confusion over whether all or only certain secondary cancers are properly but eponymically designated Krükenberg tumors. The signet-ring cell type of carcinoma described by Krükenberg is most often metastatic to the ovary from the pyloric end of the stomach. The ultimate prognosis is poor, but removal of the uterus, ovary, and tubes may permanently control the pelvic manifestations of the problem. Bilateral tumors are the rule. Of course, removal of the original focus of the disease probably will not result in cure at this date, but at least adequate palliation might be accomplished. Some Krükenberg tumors that appear during pregnancy are hormonally active. Reports of androgenicity as well as estrogen secretion affecting even the fetus can be found in the literature.

It should be noted that ovaries at the end of pregnancy are "resting" and are comparatively small. They often have shaggy, eosinophilic, wispy material on their surfaces that is decidua. *Any enlargement of the ovaries in a term pregnancy should be suspect*, and it is in the best interest of the patient for the operating surgeon to obtain biopsy specimens and frozen sections as a guide to additional therapy.

Nonmalignant ovarian tumors may be encountered during pregnancy. After they are diagnosed as benign, the question of their management is raised. A brief discussion is included to serve as a guide to management.

Therapy for Nonmalignant Ovarian Tumors

There are eight basic principles of therapy for the nonmalignant ovarian tumor.

1. If the tumor is cystic, less than 6 to 8 cm in diameter, and steadily diminishes in size as the pregnancy continues, it can simply be observed. Operation is not indicated unless there is torsion or rupture. If the tumor becomes enlarged, however, operative intervention is mandatory. When cystic tumors do not regress, the ideal time for operation is during the early part of the second trimester (12–14 weeks). By this time the corpus luteum of pregnancy is no longer important for maintaining the pregnancy. In most instances, after the 60th day of pregnancy removal of the corpus luteum does not materially affect the outcome. If the tumor is benign on frozen section, the cyst should be resected and as much of the normal portion of the ovary as possible left.

2. Solid or suspicious tumors should be removed at once regardless of the trimester of pregnancy. With evidence of torsion, hemorrhage, or necrosis, prompt surgery is mandatory.

3. The uterus should be handled as little and as carefully as possible during the early months. Excessive manipulation contributes to an increased abortion rate. Although some advise prophylactic progesterone therapy postoperatively, it is generally unnecessary. The results do not justify the means.

4. After the 18th week it may be more difficult to remove a tumor because of the enlarged uterus. It can be done, but there are technical problems. Also, the closer the patient is to term, the greater is the stress on the healing abdominal wound by the enlarging uterus, with possible weakening and herniation. The earlier the surgery is done, the greater is the time remaining for proper healing.

5. During the last trimester of pregnancy the main problem is a known or unsuspected tumor that may be blocking delivery. The fetal and maternal complications make operation mandatory. If the diagnosis is made before the onset of labor, surgical intervention is indicated about 1 week before the anticipated delivery date or, if the date is unreliable, during early labor. The operation consists in low flap cesarean section and either ovarian resection or oophorectomy.

If the exit of the child is not blocked and the tumor lies above the inlet, the child should be delivered vaginally and the tumor removed abdominally as soon as the patient's condition permits, which usually is within the first 48 hours postpartum. During the interval between delivery and operation, one must watch for acute torsion because, as mentioned previously, torsion during the puerperium is a likely complication.

6. A tumor above the inlet and evidence of pain, tenderness, or peritoneal reaction while the patient is in labor probably indicates torsion or rupture. Prompt surgery is indicated. Cesarean section plus oophorectomy is the surgery of choice.

7. If a tumor blocking the pelvis is first diagnosed when the patient is in advanced labor and fully dilated, the abdomen can be opened, the tumor dislodged, and the baby delivered vaginally by an assistant. The tumor is then removed, and the abdomen closed. This maneuver is spectacular, but most obstetricians do

not see one case of this type in a lifetime. It is really an indictment of the patient's medical care. At the very least, the diagnosis should have been made during early labor. In this litigious environment most obstetricians would perform a cesarean section and then tailor the operation to fit the needs of the patient and the extent of the tumor.

8. If the tumor is diagnosed during the puerperium, operation within 48 hours is indicated. With torsion, immediate surgery is mandatory.

Summary

The management of ovarian cancer during pregnancy is simple. Be aware of the condition, have a high index of suspicion, make the diagnosis early, and tailor the treatment to the needs of the patient and the extent of the disease. One of the main reasons for difficulty is that the patient resists abdominal exploration during pregnancy because she fears abortion or possible damage to her fetus. She should be assured that this argument against operation is not valid. The potential danger to the mother far exceeds the imagined danger to the child. The extra time spent gaining the patient's confidence, a consultation when necessary to reinforce one's advice, and a steadfast stand on the need for operation are important. Most of the tumors seen with ovarian tumors are sins of omission, rather than commission. If patients do not follow the advice of their physicians, the physicians must withdraw from the case, relieving themselves of the responsibility of future difficulty. The mortality due to ovarian cancer can never be lowered with the present state of our diagnostic armamentarium unless the tumor is attacked early and completely.

If surgeons find an ovarian malignancy during the abdominal exploration, their first obligation is to stage the disease, collect peritoneal fluid for cell block diagnosis, and remove the lesion for immediate frozen section to enable definitive diagnosis and documentation. This procedure is followed by whatever further surgery is indicated, depending on the type of tumor, its histologic grading, and the degree of anatomic spread. Biopsies of omentum, peritoneum, or any other intraabdominal area where one suspects tumors are indicated.

If the tumor is unilateral, is well encapsulated, shows no anatomic evidence of spread, and is reported as one of those listed with a comparatively low degree of malignancy, and if the peritoneal fluid contains no malignant cells, it is permissible to perform a unilateral oophorectomy and to permit the pregnancy to continue. The other ovary, however, should be split and biopsied to ensure its freedom from disease. This procedure is permissible with a histologically low-grade mucinous cystadenocarcinoma, dysgerminoma, granulosa-thecal cell tumor, arrhenoblastoma, gynandroblastoma, and possibly a low-grade papillary tumor when it is unclear whether it is a cystadenoma or a cystadenocarcinoma. The patient is then delivered vaginally at term. Six weeks after delivery of the child, the patient is reexplored and TAH-BSO are done. If the patient wishes to take a calculated risk, she can undertake another pregnancy; but she must be carefully observed and surgery must follow the next delivery. If, on the other hand, the tumor is any other than those enumerated, the therapy must be immediate TAH-BSO (and omentectomy when indicated). Chemotherapy is instituted promptly. If the entire tumor cannot be removed, the pregnancy should be terminated, as much tumor as possible removed surgically, and chemotherapy instituted as soon as feasible. The pregnancy is a secondary consideration.

The primary responsibility of the physician is to treat the mother. If the baby can be saved, it is a dividend. Before undertaking surgery in the pregnant patient with possible ovarian cancer it is mandatory that the problem be completely disclosed to the patient and informed consent be obtain to allow the surgeon to proceed in any manner deemed necessary.

In most reported series about one-third of the cases are stage III or IV at surgery, and one must be prepared for this contingency. The most aggressive lesions, in terms of early spread, are the solid adenocarcinomas and serous cystadenocarcinomas.

The survival of pregnant patients with ovarian cancer is no different from survival in the nonpregnant group. The type of tumor and its anatomic spread determine the 5-year cure rate. Pregnancy has no effect on the tumor.

Only aggressive early exploration can save the patient. Interruption of pregnancy has no beneficial effect on the future course of this disease.

With cancer of the ovary metastatic from the stomach, colon, liver, or breast, decisions about therapy must be made on an individual basis. Certainly nobody would quarrel with a decision to "shoot the works" and clean out the entire pelvis. In certain instances the expectant parents, aware of the poor prognosis for the mother, may elect to have the baby for whatever joy it may bring to the remaining time of the mother's life and to the father in the future. Under these circumstances, vaginal delivery (if there is no tumor blocking the pelvic canal) followed by pelvic surgery after the birth of the child might well be the most compassionate procedure. Cesarean section is performed if indicated for obstetric reasons, and the uterus and tumors are removed at this time.

The basic principles regarding cancer of the ovary during pregnancy can be summarized as follows.

1. It occurs in 1 of 18,000 pregnancies, including abortions.
2. The malignancy rate of ovarian tumors complicating pregnancy is 2 to 5%, in contrast to an 18 to 20% malignancy rate in the nonpregnant state.
3. The signs and symptoms are not basically different from those of the nonpregnant state.
4. Usually an adnexal mass is found at the time of the first antepartum visit.
   a. If it regresses on follow-up, the diagnosis is functional cyst.
   b. If it is more than 10 cm and persists, laparotomy is indicated at the beginning of the second trimester.
   c. If it is hard, knobby, fixed, or bilateral or has areas of varied consistency scattered throughout the tumor, surgery is indicated without a period of observation.
5. Rarely is the ovarian tumor bilateral.
6. The presenting symptom may be a complication of the ovarian tumor (e.g., torsion, rupture, hemorrhage, or infection). There may be sudden acute abdominal pain with vomiting and possibly shock.

The management depends on the findings, but a general plan can be described.

1. Treat the cancer as it would be treated in a nonpregnant patient.
2. If it is a low-grade malignancy confined to one ovary, unilateral oophorectomy and bisection of the opposite ovary are recommended. When the peritoneal cavity is opened, prior to exploration the abdomen and pelvis should be aspirated for cytologic examination. The pregnancy is then allowed to go to term.
3. If the ovarian cancer has extended beyond the ovary from which it arose, TAH-BSO, omentectomy, appendectomy, and postoperative chemotherapy are recommended.
4. At all cesarean sections, routine inspection of the tubes and ovaries is mandatory.

Bibliography

Atar E, Dgani R, Shoham Z, Bornstein R: Malignant ovarian tumors in pregnancy. *Harefuah* 119:146, 1990.

Barber HRK: Ovarian cancer. *CA* 36:149, 1986.

Barber HRK: Gynecologic cancer complicating pregnancy. In *Gynecologic Oncology*. Excerpta Medica, Amsterdam, 1970, pp. 283–288.

Barber HRK: Editorial comment. In Barber HRK, Graber EA (eds): *Surgical Disease in Pregnancy*. Saunders, Philadelphia, 1974.

Barber HRK, Brunschwig A: Gynecologic cancer complicating pregnancy. *Am J Obstet Gynecol* 85:156, 1963.

Barber HRK, Graber EA: Surgical aspects of ovarian tumors. In *Selected Topics of Cancer—Current Concepts*. Symposia Specialists, Miami, 1974.

Beischer NA, Buttery BW, Fortune DW, Macafee CA, Jr: Growth and malignancy of ovarian tumors in pregnancy. *Aust NZ J Obstet Gynaecol* 11:208, 1971.

Benavides-Ledezma RR, Barboza-Quintana O, Barboza-Quintana A, Saldivar D: Primary Burkitt-type undifferentiated lymphoma in the ovary and pregnancy. *Ginecol Obstet Mex* 56:293, 1988.

Betson JR, Golden ML: Primary carcinoma of the ovary coexisting for pregnancy. *Obstet Gynecol* 12:589, 1958.

Betson JR, Golden ML: Cancer and pregnancy. *Am J Obstet Gynecol* 81:718, 1961.

Boughton RS, Hughmanick S, Marin-Padilla M:

Malignant melanoma arising in an ovarian cystic teratoma in pregnancy. *J Am Acad Dermatol* 17:871, 1987.

Chung A, Birnbaum SJ: Ovarian cancer associated with pregnancy. *Obstet Gynecol* 41:211, 1972.

Creasman WT, Rutledge F, Smith JC: Carcinoma of the ovary associated with pregnancy. *Obstet Gynecol* 38:111, 1971.

Farahmand SM, Marchetti DL, Asirwatham JE, Dewey MR: Ovarian endodermal sinus tumor associated with pregnancy: review of the literature. *Gynecol Oncol* 41:156, 1991.

Firket C: Pregnancy and ovarian tumors. *Rev Med Liege* 44:263, 1989.

Fox LP, Stamm WJ: Krükenberg tumor complicating pregnancy. *Am J Obstet Gynecol* 92:702, 1965.

Frymire LJ: Arrhenoblastoma with two subsequent pregnancies. *Obstet Gynecol* 17:248, 1961.

Gillibrand PN: Granulosa-theca cell tumors of the ovary associated with pregnancy: case report and review of the literature. *Am J Obstet Gynecol* 94:1108, 1966.

Graber EA: Ovarian tumors in pregnancy. In Barber HRK, Graber EA (eds): *Surgical Disease in Pregnancy*. Saunders, Philadelphia, 1974, pp. 428–437.

Green WL, Jones EH: Coexistent pseudomucinous cystadenocarcinoma and pregnancy. *Obstet Gynecol* 13:349, 1959.

Greene GG, Smith AE, McClelland T: A malignant granulosa cell tumor associated with pregnancy. *Am J Obstet Gynecol* 60:686, 1956.

Jolles CJ: Gynecologic cancer associated with pregnancy. *Semin Oncol* 16:417, 1989.

Jubb ED: Primary ovarian carcinoma in pregnancy. *J Obstet Gynecol* 85:345, 1963.

King LA, Nevin PC, Williams PP, Carson LF:

Treatment of advanced epithelial ovarian carcinoma in pregnancy with cisplatin-based chemotherapy. *Gynecol Oncol* 41:78, 1991.

Lawrence WD, Larson PN, Hange ET: Primary Krükenberg tumor of the ovary in pregnancy. *Obstet Gynecol* 10:84, 1957.

McGowan L: *Cancer in pregnancy. American Lecture Series*. Charles C Thomas, Springfield, IL, 1967.

Metz SA, Day TG, Pursell SH: Adjuvant chemotherapy in a pregnant patient with endodermal sinus tumor of the ovary. *Gynecol Oncol* 32:381, 1989.

Novak ER, Lanbron, Woodruff JD: Ovarian tumors in pregnancy, an ovarian tumor registry review. *Obstet Gynecol* 46:401, 1975.

Phelan JT: Cancer and pregnancy. *NY State J Med* 68:3011, 1968.

Sawada M, Yamasaki M, Urabe T, et al: A case of ovarian cystadenocarcinoma associated with pregnancy. *Jpn J Clin Oncol* 20:199, 1990.

Smith AH, Ward SV: Dysgerminoma in pregnancy. *Obstet Gynecol* 28:502, 1966.

Spadoni LR, Lindberg MC, Mottet NK, Herrman WL: Virilization coexisting with Krükenberg tumor during pregnancy. *Am J Obstet Gynecol* 92:981, 1965.

Taylor ES: Ovarian tumors in pregnancy. *Obstet Gynecol Surv* 27:43, 1972.

Tweeddale DN, Dockerty MB, Pratt JH, Hranilovich GT: Pregnancy with recurrent granulosa cell tumor. *Am J Obstet Gynecol* 70:1039, 1955.

Van Dessel T, Hameeteman TM, Wagenaar SS: Mucinous cystadenocarcinoma in pregnancy: case report. *Br J Obstet Gynaecol* 95:527, 1988.

White HC: Ovarian tumors in pregnancy. *Am J Obstet Gynecol* 116:544, 1973.

15

Low Malignant Potential Ovarian Tumors: Borderline Ovarian Tumors

A Committee of the International Federation of Gynecology and Obstetrics (FIGO) proposed a classification of common epithelial ovarian tumors as well as the clinical staging of these tumors. The classification and clinical staging, adopted in 1971, were the result of approximately 10 years of work by the Committee. The clinical staging has been revised on two occasions, the last being in 1987. Until that time there were as many classifications as there were hospitals in the country and as many subdivisions of these classifications as there were physicians in practice. Until the profession and scientists started to talk this common language, chaos reigned. It was impossible prior to establishment of the FIGO classification to compare results between centers and almost impossible to structure protocols for workup, management, and follow-up of patients with these tumors. The FIGO classification established histologic typing only for the common epithelial ovarian cancer. The World Health Organization (WHO) expanded the classification and included gonadal stromal tumors, germ cell tumors, the gonadoblastomas, and metastatic tumors.

The ovarian tumors are classified according to their most differentiated portion and graded from their least differentiated parts. The accumulated experience showed that between obviously benign and obviously malignant neoplasms there exists a group of tumors that, in their clinical behavior, resemble true carcinomas inasmuch as they give rise to implantation—metastases and ascites—but have a different course. It is this group of ovarian cancers of low malignant potential that is reviewed in this chapter.

The FIGO classification is based primarily on the microscopic characteristics of the tumor and thus reflects the nature of morphologically identifiable cell types and patterns. The WHO reported that borderline cancer can be defined as tumor that has some, but not all, of the morphologic features of cancer, including, in varying combinations: (1) epithelial cell stratification; (2) apparent detachment of cellular clusters from sites of origin; and (3) mitotic activity and nuclear abnormalities intermediate between those of clearly benign and those of questionably malignant tumors of similar cell type. Obvious invasion of the adjacent stroma is lacking. Tumors with epithelial cell proliferation or atypicality of minor degree should be considered in the benign category.

It must be emphasized that unless the epithelial layer invades the stroma the tumor cannot be truly identified as invasive cancer. Formerly, because the mucinous tumor is often parvilocular and multilocular with nests of cells within the stroma, invasion was diagnosed if the tumor was composed of at least four cells in height. This criterion has been changed, and the only criterion currently used for making a diagnosis of invasive cancer for mucinous tumors is invasion through the basement membrane. Therefore lack of destructive invasion of the underlying stroma places the tumor in the low malignant potential (borderline) category. Benign, borderline, and malignant forms of any of the neoplastic types may coexist in any one tumor. It is most important that multiple sections be taken before a tumor is designated a low malignant potential (borderline) lesion.

Surface papillomas are included as a separate entity, as increasing evidence suggests that they are more prone to spread than the completely encapsulated tumor. Both are in the same clinical stage, however.

General Considerations

Low malignant potential (LMP) tumors, or borderline tumors, are now well recognized as a clinical entity. Histologically, they are intermediate between the truly benign tumors and those with invasive characteristics; and they constitute approximately 10 to 20% of all ovarian epithelial tumors. Metastatic lesions (or multiple primary sites) are present in approximately 20% of these cases and are found in the usual sites for ovarian carcinoma metastases. These so-called secondary lesions may in fact be of an invasive nature.

Clinical staging of the LMP tumors is similar to that of invasive tumors. Eighty percent of these tumors are reported to be limited to the ovaries (i.e., stage I), although adequate staging procedures may well reduce this figure in the future.

Provided the lesion is limited to the ovaries, the prognosis is excellent. The 5-year survival rate reported in the 20th volume of the *Annual Report on the Results of Treatment in Gynecological Cancer* is 87.3% in stage Ia and 86.3% in stage Ib; and among 128 patients with stage III disease, 65.6% were still alive after 5 years.

The 21st volume of the *Annual Report* presents a summary of low potential malignancy from Volume 15 through Volume 21. The figures show an improvement in results from the beginning of the 1970's. Thereafter, the results are unchanged. The 5-year actuarial survival for stages Ia through IV reported in the 21st volume is 89.1%.

The dominating histopathologic classes are serous and mucinous tumors, and it seems that the outcome for stage Ia disease is somewhat better for the serous tumors than the mucinous tumors. A conservative approach is therefore

possible with stage I disease. Provided the disease is limited to one ovary (after a full staging procedure) unilateral salpingo-oophorectomy may be considered in a young woman requiring childbearing function. Once the disease has spread from the ovary, survival rates fall but not as rapidly as with invasive cancer. The survival rates from the *Annual Report* are as follows: stage II, 62%, stage III, 48%; and stage IV, 33%. These patients should be treated as though they have invasive cancer.

Decisions on Management

Although the choice of a conservative operation in a young woman with a unilateral, encapsulated, though potentially malignant tumor may be justified statistically, there is always the possibility that a more aggressive tumor may be present in a single, minute section. Benign, borderline, and malignant forms of any of the neoplastic types of common epithelial ovarian carcinoma may coexist in any one tumor. It is therefore essential that multiple and representative sections of the tumor be studied before the tumor is identified as low malignant potential or borderline. To demonstrate the absence of even focal areas of stromal invasion necessitates adequate tumor sampling by the pathologist. At least one tissue section for every 1 cm of maximal tumor diameter should be obtained for microscopic examination. Therefore an ovarian tumor measuring 10×12 cm should have at least 12 samples for adequate histologic evaluation.

The most difficult management decision arises when the ovary presents with excrescences on the surface. If positive cells are present in the pelvis on cytologic examination, the decision can be more readily made and more aggressive treatment carried out. Patients who have excrescences on the surface combined with a histologic picture of low potential malignancy present a situation in which the decision is difficult.

In these patients it is essential to study the histology carefully, examine the opposite ovary, and obtain washings from the upper abdomen and the pelvis. If these tests all prove negative, the decision must be based on the age of the patient and her desire (and that of her family) to continue to menstruate and to have the opportunity to reproduce. In general, when the ovary contains a tumor of low potential malignancy and no positive cytology is evident in the pelvis, a conservative approach may be undertaken despite the fact that excrescences are visible on the tumor surface. It is important to exercise careful clinical judgment, and it is one of the times that the art of medicine may rule the science of medicine.

Management According to Age Group

The management of ovarian tumors is related to the age group in which they occur. From birth to age 20, the most frequently observed ovarian tumors are the germ cell types, although occasionally a gonadal stromal tumor is seen. Common epithelial ovarian carcinomas are rarely diagnosed in this age group.

From ages 20 to 30, the most common ovarian tumor is the germ cell tumor. Gonadal stromal tumors occur more frequently than those reported in the younger age group. Until recent years, the common epithelial ovarian cancer was rarely seen in this age group; now it is being diagnosed with increasing frequency. The reasons are not clear, but its incidence parallels the increased diagnoses of common epithelial ovarian carcinomas in all the highly industrialized nations. The possible cause may be change in life style, including an increase in cholesterol and fatty acids in the diet.

Women aged 30 to 40 show an increase in the number of common epithelial ovarian cancers that are diagnosed and a decrease in germ cell and gonadal stromal tumors. Management of these tumors is discussed later in the chapter.

Low Malignant Potential (Borderline) Tumors

The LMP (borderline) tumors are now well recognized as a clinical entity. Histologically, they are intermediate between truly benign tumors and those with invasive characteristics; and they constitute about 15% of all ovarian epithelial carcinomas. About 3000 new cases are diagnosed yearly in the United States. These tumors occur in women at a younger age

than do invasive ovarian epithelial tumors. In addition, they usually have an earlier stage of disease and have a much better prognosis than those with truly invasive ovarian epithelial cancer.

As with invasive ovarian epithelial carcinoma, there are few symptoms associated with small ovarian LMP tumors. Patients with early LMP disease are often asymptomatic, although they occasionally have a host of vague intestinal complaints, symptoms related to compression due to a pelvic mass (e.g., urinary frequency), or acute pain should the ovarian tumor become twisted. With large tumors confined to the ovary or with disseminated intraperitoneal disease, the patient may exhibit an obvious increase in abdominal girth and complain of tight-fitting clothing. Increased gastrointestinal symptoms, including early fullness after eating or even symptoms of partial bowel obstruction, are not uncommon. Respiratory distress due to tumors elevating the diaphragm or to pleural effusion may also occur, although these problems are relatively uncommon.

About 66% of the LMP tumors are stage I, 12% stage II, 20% stage III, and 1% stage IV. This situation is different from that in patients with invasive epithelial cancer, where the figures show that 20% are stage I, 10% stage II, 65% stage III, and 5% stage IV.

Patients with ovarian epithelial carcinoma of low malignant potential have an excellent prognosis. The 5-year survival rate for all stages combined is about 95%, with a 10-year survival of 87%. These figures compare well with the overall 5-year survival of 30% for patients with invasive carcinoma and 60% survival for stage I and stage II patients combined.

There are five histologic types of ovarian epithelial carcinoma of low malignant potential: mucinous tumors, serous tumors, endometrioid tumors, clear-cell tumors, and Brenner tumors. Although there are features common to all five types, each category has its own specific characteristics.

Mucinous Tumors

The mucinous tumors, although considered an apparently single entity within the broad grouping of common epithelial ovarian tumors, are not in fact a homogeneous group. In most cases the epithelium is of the endocervical type on both light and electron microscopy. This substantial group of neoplasms contain epithelium that is of the enteric type and that contains argyrophilic, argentaffinic, and even Paneth cells. Because they contain these cells they are often found in association with cystic teratoma, and the question has been raised if they should rightfully be classified under the germ cell tumors. In addition, they have an excellent prognosis, similar to that found with the germ cell tumors. More specifically, it has been shown that 20% of mucinous tumors have gastric or intestinal rather than endocervical-type epithelium, and 5% are associated with dermoid cysts. Fenoglio et al., studying the ultrastructure of these tumors, classified them as the common epithelial ovarian tumors. These authors concluded that the presence of an intestinal type of epithelium in some of these tumors reflects metaplasia of the surface epithelium as it undergoes neoplastic change.

Mucinous tumors of low malignant potential are lined by stratified atypical epithelial cells. Secondary cysts and short papillary infolding usually occur. The papillae are usually smaller than those in serous tumors. Cellular exfoliation from short papillary processes is common. True intraglandular ridging is uncommon; patterns in which the bridges seem unsupported are usually due to tangential sections, which obscure foreign vascular supporting septae. In LMP tumors, the mucinous epithelial cells are irregular, nuclei are hyperchromatic with large nucleoli, and atypia is mild to moderate, although marked atypia may occur. Two or more mitotic figures per 10 high power fields are often seen.

Two features can be used to differentiate a mucinous tumor of low malignant potential from mucinous carcinoma. Stromal invasion, of course, is seen only with carcinoma. Small secondary cysts are common in mucinous tumors, so invasion may be difficult to identify. If the periphery of the tumor has individual cells, cords, or nests of cells penetrating the stroma, it may be considered an indication of invasion. Solid sheaths of atypical epithelium exceeding half of a low power field (having a

radius of 2.1 mm), with or without glandular differentiation, may also be regarded as invasion, although this definition is arbitrary and requires general acceptance. Dissection of mucin through supporting stroma of the ovary (pseudomyxoma ovarii) occurs in nearly half of the cases, and it is not a form of invasion.

The mucinous tumors have a low rate of bilaterality and malignancy. In the presence of a unilateral, encapsulated tumor (determined with the aid of cytology) and a negative opposite ovary (determined on biopsy), it is acceptable to manage such tumors in women under age 35 by performing a unilateral salpingo-oophorectomy. If there is any evidence of spread beyond the ovary (rare among the histologically LMP group), total abdominal hysterectomy (TAH) and bilateral salpingo-oophorectomy (BSO) (if an omentum has been developed) should be performed. Use of ^{32}P is optional, but it should not be instilled if adhesions are present or if there is evidence of an inflammatory response. Because the LMP tumors appear similar to normal tissue, there is a small margin of safety in the use of chemotherapeutic drugs. However, in selected cases combination chemotherapy is probably indicated. When common epithelial ovarian cancer occurs in the younger age group, many reports indicate that the serous tumor is more frequent, but in my experience the cancers are usually of the mucinous type (Figure 15.1).

Serous Tumors

Serous tumors are composed of epithelium resembling that of the fallopian tube or the surface epithelium of the ovaries; ciliated cells are found almost always in the benign serous tumors, usually in those of low malignancy potential (borderline) malignancy and rarely in the carcinomatous forms.

Although the management of serous tumors is similar to that for mucinous tumors, it poses a more difficult management decision. The serous tumor is more inclined to be bilateral than the mucinous tumor; it sheds cells more frequently; and it has a higher recurrence rate. On the other hand, it is usually easier to distinguish the LMP serous tumor from the truly invasive tumor on histologic examination. No

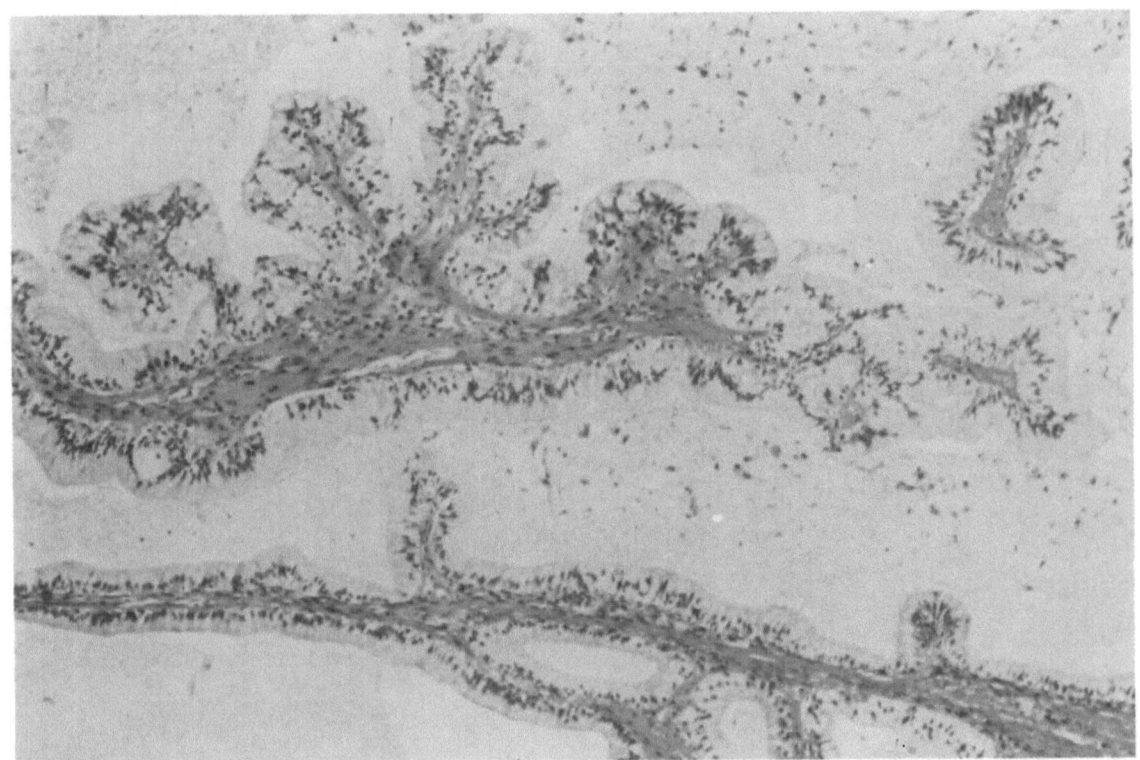

FIGURE 15.1. Mucinous tumor. Epithelium is of the endocervical type.

matter how disorganized the epithelium looks, unless it invades the stroma the tumors are considered of low malignant potential (borderline).

In serous tumors of low malignant potential there is no stromal invasion, but the epithelium forms complex, branching papillary fronds. The fronds are lined by stratified layers of cells forming tufts from the piling up of cells into a bud of four or more cells without stalk. Mild to moderate cellular atypia is present owing to hyperchromatism, nuclear enlargement, and enlarged and prominent nucleoli. Increased mitotic figures in cellular pleomorphism occur, along with epithelial disorganization reflected by the loss of polarity of the cells lining basement membranes. Papillary excrescences, usually located along the inner cyst wall, are a hallmark of these tumors. Focal or extensive necrosis, stromal inflammation, psammoma bodies, and surface bridges are found in the serous tumor of low malignant potential and yet do not indicate carcinoma. The extent of

tufting and papillary formation, the extent of cribriform change, and the degree of mitotic activity and necrosis within a serous LMP neoplasm are considerably less than in serous carcinoma. Although the above morphologic features are useful for identifying the serous tumors of low malignant potential, no single feature correlates with the prognosis. More evidence is needed to prove the contention that mitotic activity alone is related to the prognosis and can identify truly malignant serous tumors.

By definition, serous LMP tumors lack stromal invasion. Cribriform glands within the stroma do not reflect stromal invasion. Although nests of epithelial cells can be identified within the fibrovascular cores of papillary fronds, the absence of reactive stromal fibrosis (desmoplasia) precludes the diagnosis of stromal invasion. Stratification of the epithelium aligning into four or more cells in depth has no known significance. Serous LMP tumors must be distinguished from cystadenomas with atypia. The latter have some cellular prolifer-

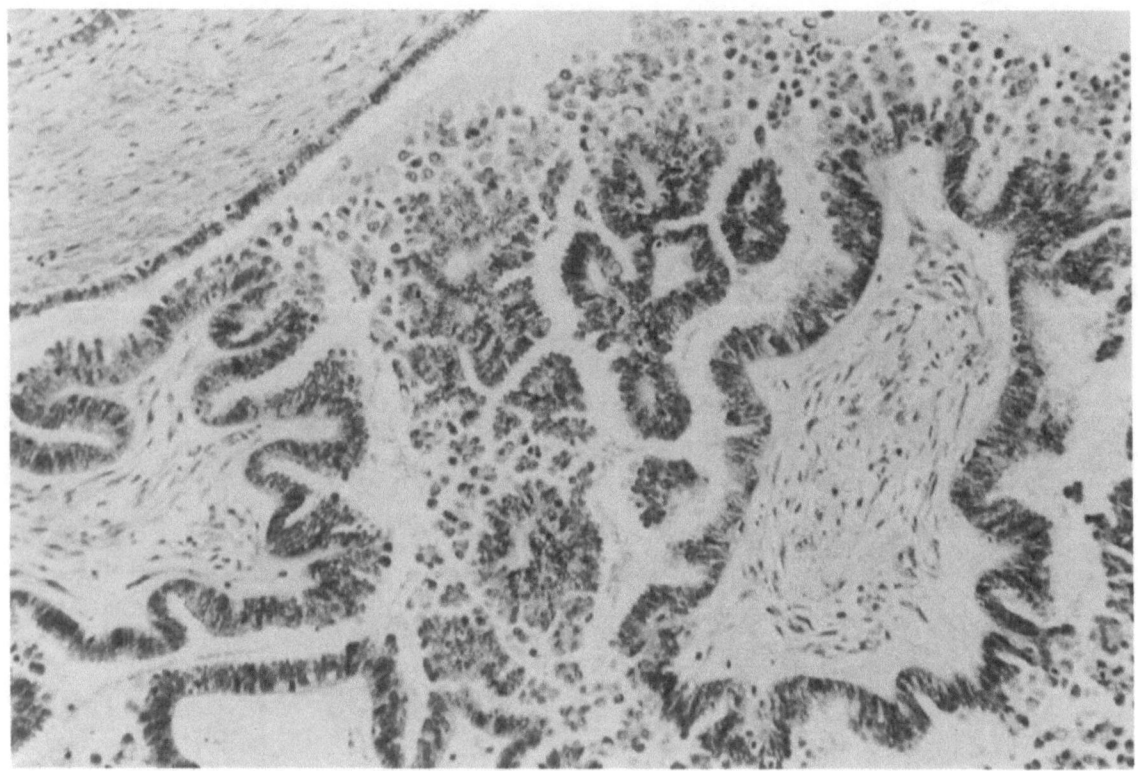

FIGURE 15.2. Serous tumor. Epithelium resembles that of the fallopian tube or the surface epithelium of the ovary.

ation and atypia, but they lack the papillary budding of stratified atypical cells and a detachment of atypical cell groups that characterize the serous LMP tumor.

If the tumor is encapsulated, is unilateral, and exhibits negative cytology, and the opposite ovary is negative on biopsy, a unilateral salpingo-oophorectomy can be carried out in the young age group. However, if there is any evidence of spread beyond the ovary, management similar to that described for mucinous tumors that have spread must be undertaken. Unlike the patient with the mucinous tumor, those with a serous cystadenocarcinoma of the low malignancy type must be told that they are at risk, and although the danger is probably small it is always present. In most instances, I recommend that these women have children if they wish and, on completing their family, undergo removal of the other ovary and the uterus. Although this decision is arbitrary and subject to challenge, it probably represents the

method that provides the patient maximum protection against the development of a neoplasm in the opposite ovary or a metastatic lesion (Fig. 15.2).

Advanced LMP (Borderline) Serous Tumors

Advanced LMP (borderline) serous tumors have been reported by Scully's group, who found that the histologic features of the peritoneal implants were related to prognosis. They identified invasion, cytologic atypia, mitotic activity, and the presence of residual tumor as adverse prognostic factors and calculated that patients with at least one of these factors had a 56% chance of being dead of tumor at 10 years. It is possible that this information will permit selection of a high-risk group of patients with advanced borderline tumors who can most benefit from additional treatment. The relative rarity of advanced borderline tumors, however, makes prospective trials difficult indeed.

Endometrioid Tumors

Endometrioid tumors of low malignant potential are uncommon. They are predominantly solid with some cystic areas. At least three types have been identified. One form has a major fibrous component and appears to be related to and possibly to arise from an endometrioid adenofibroma. The second type is basically epithelial in nature, with only a minor fibrous supporting stroma. The epithelium in both types is like that of the endometrium, forming crowded, irregular glands with complex epithelial processes resembling endometrial or atypical hyperplasia. With both forms, the atypia is usually mild and the mitotic activity low. About half of the endometrioid tumors of low malignancy potential undergo squamous metaplasia. The epithelium at the periphery is circumscribed around it, reflecting expansive growth.

With adenofibromatous forms, supporting stroma is fibrous and extensive, so at least half of the tumor is visibly solid. It has complex epithelium of an endometrial type with squamous metaplasia that lies within dense fibrous stroma. Despite the bland cytologic features, the prominence of the epithelium within the stroma in the adenofibromatous form reflects obvious proliferation. There is no destructive infiltrative growth, however. Endometriosis is more often associated with endometrioid tumors than with the other ovarian epithelial tumors. About one-fourth to one-half of the endometrioid tumors of low malignancy potential are associated with pelvic endometriosis and 10% with endometrial carcinoma of the uterus. The endometriosis may occur in the same ovary or elsewhere in the pelvis.

The second type of LMP endometrioid tumor has epithelium that lines delicate connective tissue columns and papillary processes as in a complex endometrial hyperplasia. The third pattern is a mixture of the adenofibroma and papillary patterns.

Benign and LMP endometrioid tumors comprise a small proportion of all endometrioid tumors, as most endometrioid neoplasms are carcinomas. Endometrioid tumors of low malignancy potential constitute only 2 to 10% of all LMP tumors. The rarity of these tumors has hindered delineation of their microscopic characteristics and behavior.

Mitosis is generally low in LMP endometrioid tumors. Stromal invasion is absent.

Clear-Cell Tumors

Clear-cell tumors are characterized by the presence of tubular and cystic structures set in a fibrous stroma, papillary formations that are frequently of a complex pattern, and often relatively large sheets of clear cells. Electron microscopic studies have suggested that these neoplasms bear a considerable resemblance to mesothelioma. It is important to differentiate this tumor from the endodermal sinus tumor. The clear-cell tumor usually occurs in the older age group, whereas the endodermal sinus tumor occurs usually before age 20. Reports indicate that the clear-cell carcinoma of the ovary is usually invasive and not of the LMP class (Fig. 15.3).

This rare tumor has not been well documented. Some believe that clear-cell carcinoma of the ovary is an endometrioid tumor. It frequently coexists with endometriosis and shares some ultrastructure features with endometrioid carcinoma. Regardless of this view, the cell type is sufficiently distinct that clear-cell tumors merit an category of their own. The natural history of the LMP clear-cell tumors is uncertain.

Proliferative Brenner Tumors

A Brenner tumor with proliferative characteristics is intermediate between a benign Brenner tumor and its fully malignant counterpart, the malignant Brenner tumor. Generally accepted as an intermediate form of Brenner tumor, none of the proliferative Brenner tumors has demonstrated metastatic ability or produced a fatality, so an LMP designation may be inappropriate. Until malignancy is proved, the preferred term for this intermediate Brenner tumor is "proliferative Brenner tumor."

The proliferative Brenner tumor has gross and microscopic characteristics distinctive from

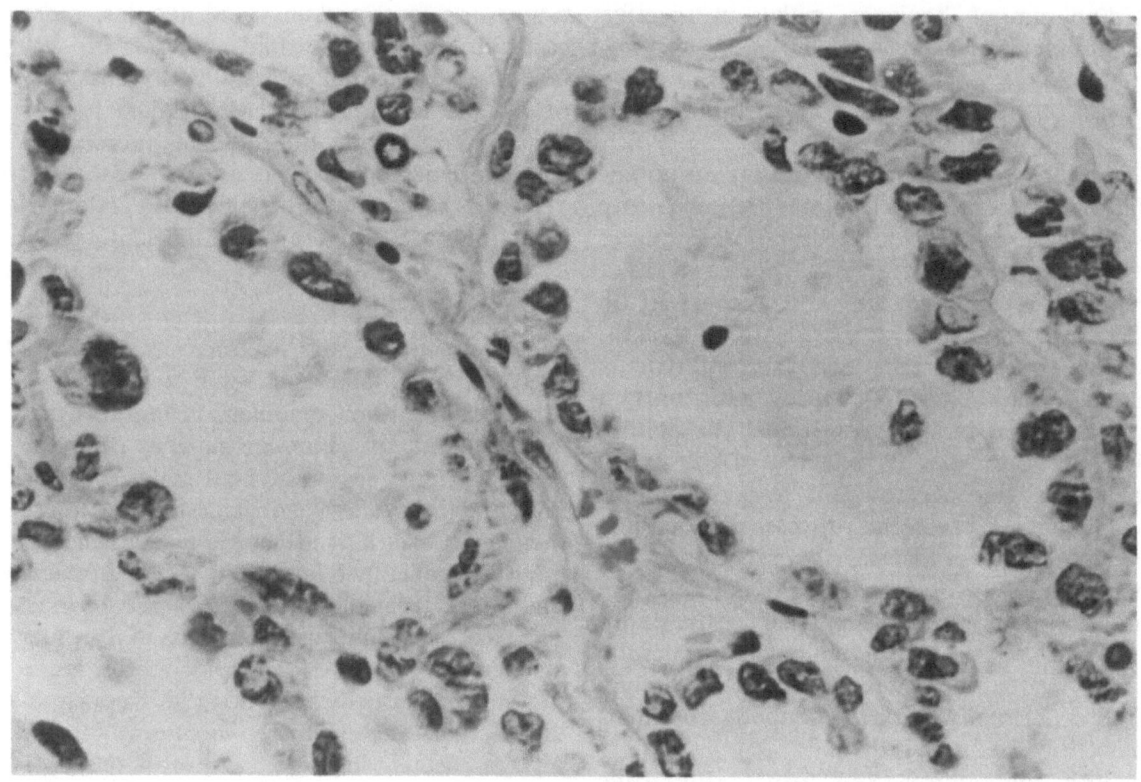

FIGURE 15.3. Clear-cell tumor. It is characterized by the presence of tubular and cystic structures set in a fibrous stroma with large sheets of clear cells.

its benign counterpart, and it is usually large and partly cystic or multicystic. Papillary processes lined by transitional cell epithelium protrude from the inner wall of the cyst and appear in the stroma in sheaths and nests. The transitional cell epithelium is clearly proliferating because it may have cellular stratification of 20 cells or more and moderate mitotic activity. Mild to moderate cytologic atypia is usually present. The transitional epithelium is common in proliferative Brenner tumors. A proliferative Brenner tumor has a striking resemblance to a low-grade papillary transitional cell carcinoma of the bladder. However, metastasis to the ovary from urinary tract carcinoma is a rare event, and only about 1% of bladder carcinomas metastasize to the ovary. The demonstration of transition from a benign Brenner nest can exclude the possibility of a metastasis. If a benign Brenner tumor coexists with a proliferating Brenner tumor, it is good evidence

that the primary site is in the ovary. No destructive stromal invasion is identified.

A proliferative Brenner tumor can be distinguished from a malignant Brenner tumor by the absence of marked cytologic atypia and confinement to the ovary. Malignant Brenner tumors are identified by one of three features: (1) metastasis; (2) high-grade cytologic features; or (3) destructive stromal invasion. Unequivocal invasion of the stroma by highly atypical cells arranged singly or in groups and sheaths is often difficult to recognize in a tumor with accompanying fibrous stroma such as the Brenner tumor. Therefore high-grade cytologic features or metastatic deposits are the main distinguishing feature. Differentiation to mucinous and squamous adenocarcinomas also occurs in some malignant Brenner tumors. The malignant Brenner tumor is less likely to be cystic and usually lacks the broad papillary processes of the proliferative Brenner tumor. The latter has never been reported to be bilateral. Unilateral salpingo-oophorectomy is adequate therapy for this tumor, but because they occur in older women TAH-BSO is the treatment usually chosen.

Cystadenofibromas with Atypia and Low Malignant Potential

Cystadenofibromas and adenofibromas containing varying degrees of epithelial atypia have been described. Some have mild to moderate epithelial atypia, whereas others exhibit more advanced cellular atypia, cellular stratification, papillary processes, epithelial tufting, and detachment of atypical cell clusters as seen in tumors of low malignancy potential. Because these tumors have not shown any aggressive behavior, it is best to designate them cystofibroma with epithelial atypia. The epithelium of the adenofibroma with atypia is usually serous, but endometrioid, mucinous, and clear-cell differentiation occur in pure and mixed forms. The rare occurrence of a malignant adenofibroma (adenocarcinoma arising in an adenofibroma) may occur but is rare.

Cystadenofibromas with epithelial atypia comprise fewer than 10% of cystadenofibromas. The median age of patients who have cystadenofibromas with atypia is 10 years older than patients with the usual cystadenofibroma, suggesting that these tumors may arise from an ordinary cystadenofibroma. If the cystadenofibroma with atypia proves benign on follow-up, it may be because cystadenofibroma has less epithelial surface area and greater envelopment of the epithelium by connective tissue than do the serous tumors of low malignancy potential.

Nonepithelial Ovarian Tumors

Although the germ cell and gonadal stromal tumors are usually not included in a study devoted to low malignant potential, there are undoubtedly some tumors in these two categories that qualify for inclusion.

Germ Cell Tumors

Dysgerminoma, a tumor of uniform appearance, is composed of large, rounded, clear cells that resemble primordial germ cells morphologically and histochemically (Fig. 15.4). The pure dysgerminoma occurs principally between the ages of 10 and 30 years of age and is formed of cells that resemble primordial germ cells not only at the histologic level but electron microscopically as well. Dysgerminomas are identical in all aspects to the seminoma of the testis and to the primary germinomas of the anterior mediastinum and perineal region.

Dysgerminomas almost always occur in children or adolescents rather than adults. Knowledge of their natural history provides guidelines for the physician. Dysgerminomas occur bilaterally in 5 to 10% of patients. It is difficult histologically to identify a dysgerminoma as an LMP tumor, but patients have a much better survival rate than previously reported. The dysgerminoma, like most germ cells lesions, rarely sheds cells and does so only if the capsule is perforated. Therefore in young patients with a unilateral, encapsulated tumor, negative ovary on biopsy, and particularly negative paraaortic area and lymph node area, a unilateral salpingo-oophorectomy is the treatment of choice. These patients should be followed every 2 months for the first 2 years with pelvic examinations and frequent chest roentgenograms. If there is any evidence of spread at initial surgery, TAH-BSO is the treatment of choice. These tumors are highly radiosensitive, and administration of postoperative x-ray therapy is determined on an individual basis; it should not be used if conservative surgery is carried out. Because these patients are young, the responsible physician is reluctant to subject them to external irradiation if alternate therapy is available.

Gonadal Stromal Tumors

Some gonadal stromal tumors have the potential to produce either an estrogenizing or masculinizing effect. It must be pointed out that only 25% of these tumors are functioning and produce hormones. The only important malignant tumor of the female cell type is the granulosa cell cancer, which is usually unilateral and recurs after 5 years when it does recur; metastases are typically limited to the pelvis. Because the tumor has a low grade of malignancy,

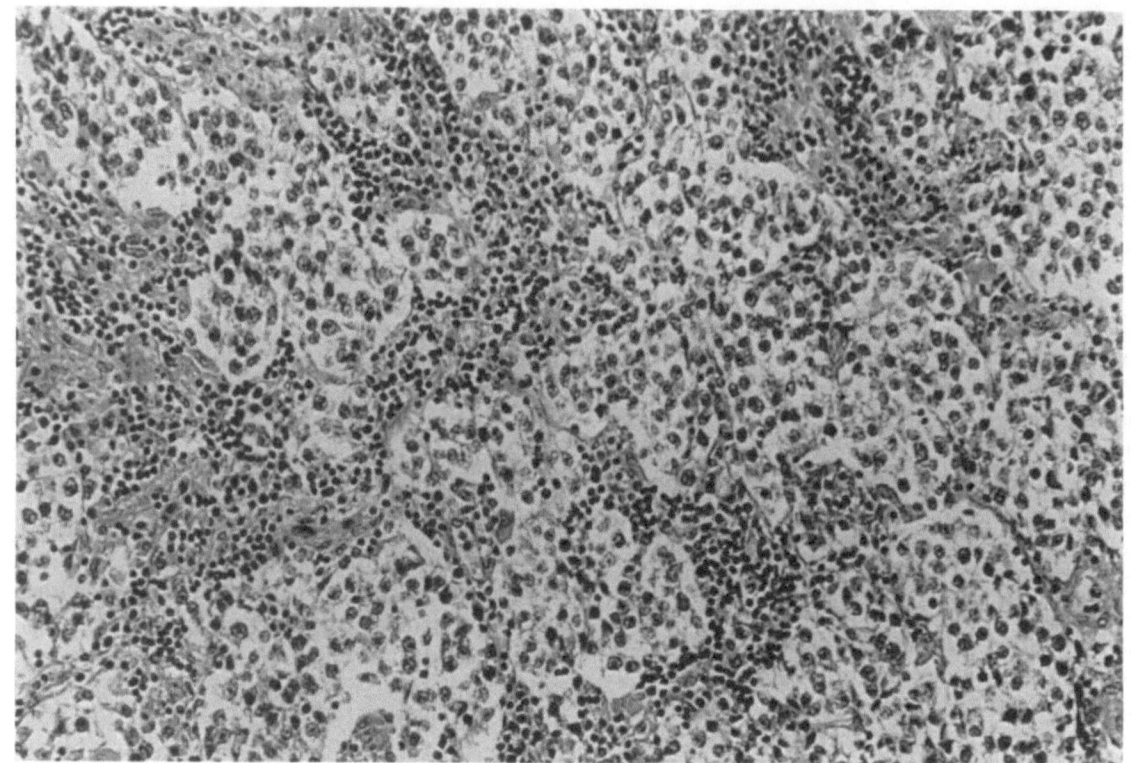

FIGURE 15.4. Dysgerminoma. It of uniform appearance, composed of large, rounded cells that resemble primordial germ cells. The stroma is usually infiltrated with lymphocytes.

conservative surgery is indicated in the young person in the form of unilateral oophorectomy when the tumor is unilateral and encapsulated.

One pattern of granulosa cell tumor is sometimes seen in young girls. Known as the granulosa cell tumor of juvenile type, it is characterized by nodules of neoplastic granulosa cells and a diffuse pattern of growth often with extensive luteinization, hyperchromatic nuclei (Fig. 15.5), and atypical mitotic figures—features that give it a somewhat malignant appearance, which is not supported by its generally benign pattern of clinical behavior. The usual granulosa cell tumor is of low grade malignancy. There are a few histologic features that enable the pathologist to determine when a particular granulosa cell tumor is likely to behave in a more malignant fashion than another; certainly the so-called sarcomatoid, or diffuse, histologic pattern is of no prognostic significance. Pleomorphism and mitotic activity

within the tumor are of only limited prognostic significance. Probably the most significant features indicative of a poor prognosis are the age of the patient (those over age 40 at the time of diagnosis have a poor prognosis) and the size of the neoplasm at the time of initial diagnosis (those measuring more than 15 cm in diameter are associated with a gloomy outlook). It must be stressed that the follow-up of patients with granulosa cell tumors has to be long term, as a high proportion of recurrences or metastases occur after 10, 15, or even 20 years.

Among the male cell types, the Sertoli-Leydig cell tumors (arrhenoblastomas) are the most significant (Fig. 15.6). They generally occur in women of childbearing age. The term "androblastoma" is now preferred to "arrhenoblastoma" largely because the latter implies an invariable virilizing effect, which is not the case. The term "androblastoma" is more applicable partly because it does not carry any

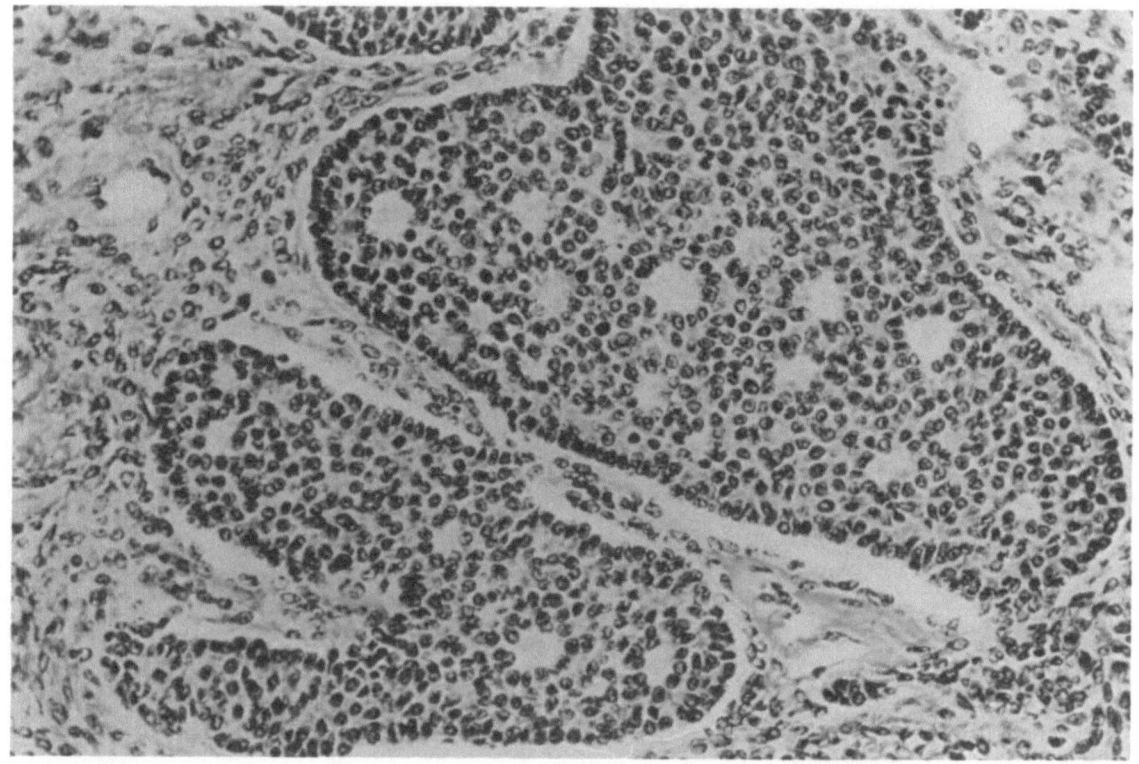

FIGURE 15.5. Granulosa cell tumor. It may be macrofollicular or diffuse, often with luteinization and hyperchromatic nuclei.

connotation of specific endocrine activity and partly because it conveys the sense that these tumors tend to recapitulate phases of the embryologic development of the testis.

When functioning endocrinologically, these tumors defeminize and then masculinize the patient. The first change is the cessation of menstruation; the patient then loses her feminine body contour, and her breasts become smaller. This phase is followed by increased hair growth and an increase in the size of the clitoris; if permitted to go on long enough, there is a voice change. All of these alterations are reversible after treatment except the voice, which retains its masculine quality.

Like the granulosa cell tumor, the Sertoli-Leydig cell has a low malignancy rate. The malignant type usually spreads within the pelvis, rarely to distant organs. Indications for conservative surgery are the same as for the granulosa cell tumors.

Mixed Gonadal Stromal Tumors

Gynandroblastomas, comprising about 10% of gonadal stromal tumors, are composed of cells from male and female cell type in about equal proportion. They are rare tumors and can be diagnosed only if mature granulosa cells coexist with either clearly and separately demonstrable tubules lined by Sertoli cells with definite Leydig cells. In the past the term has been wrongly interpreted as having only an endocrinologic significance and has been indiscriminately applied to sex cord tumors with paradoxical endocrine activity, such as estrogenic androblastomas or androgenic granulosa cell tumors. The diagnosis, however, should be made on purely morphologic grounds and irrespective of the nature of any associated endocrine activity. The management of these tumors is the same as for the granulosa cell and Sertoli-Leydig cell tumors.

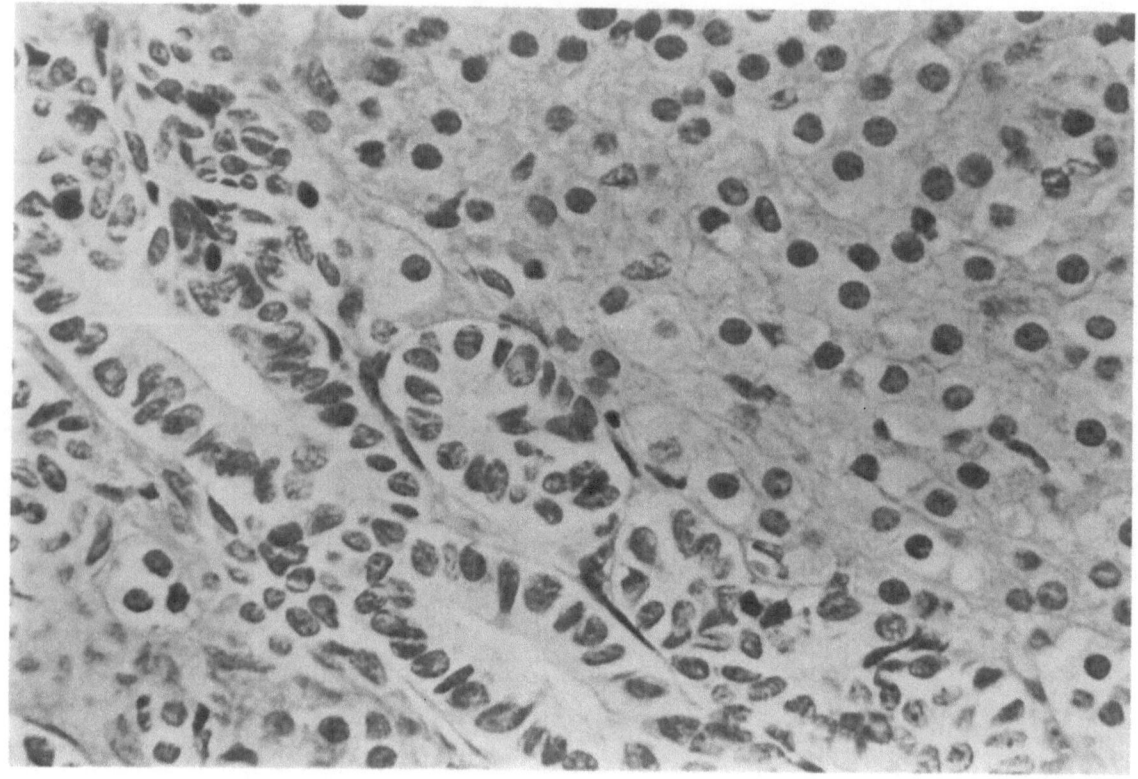

FIGURE 15.6. Sertoli-Leydig cell tumor. It is composed of Sertoli cells, which form glands, and eosinophilic Leydig cells.

Gonadoblastomas

Gonadoblastomas are composed of both germ cells and gonadal stromal cells (Fig. 15.7). Patients in whom gonadoblastomas are diagnosed are intersexual and have primary amenorrhea. Approximately 90% of the patients are chromatin-negative. The most frequently encountered karyotypes are 46,XY, 45,XO, and 46,XY. Typically, hyaline bodies that stimulate Call-Exner bodies are usually present, and foci of calcification are common. Calcifications may be demonstrated by roentgenographic studies of the pelvis and abdomen. Malignant potential is determined by the germ cell present. Approximately half the gonadoblastomas are associated with dysgerminoma and are therefore relatively benign. Occasionally, endodermal sinus tumors, choriocarcinomas, and embryonal carcinomas represent the germ cell type present in the tumor, and the malignancy

rate is then increased. Because these tumors are commonly found in the intersexual patient, bilateral oophorectomy is indicated.

Current Research

The Gynecologic Oncology Group has designed a study to assess the natural history of untreated borderline tumors and their response to single alkylating agent melphalan (Alkeran) and *cis*-platinum (Platinol), but many more years of accrual and follow-up are required before any conclusions can be drawn. However, for those who fail melphalan therapy, *cis*-platinum is administered. This study will determine the effectiveness of adjuvant chemotherapy for those patients with an ovarian epithelial carcinoma of low malignant potential who have a suboptimally resectable tumor at the time of diagnosis or whose tumors show clinically observable proliferative activ-

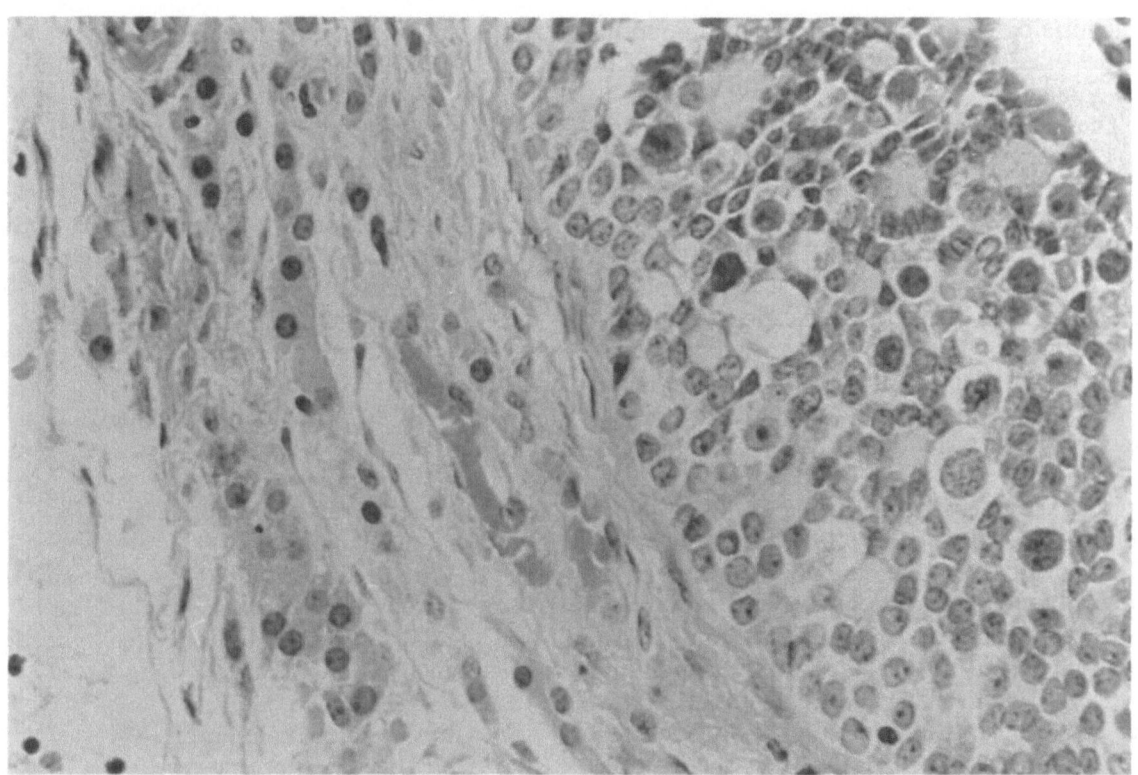

FIGURE 15.7. Gonadoblastoma. It is composed of both germ cells and gonadal stromal cells.

Summary

ity. Some arms of the research protocol include a second look laparotomy.

At an international meeting on the ovary, one of the speakers stated that there are no borderline tumors, just borderline pathologists—because if you treat borderline tumors with borderline treatment you get borderline deaths. The other participants disagreed strongly with this view. I quoted this statement to emphasize the fact that almost everybody is in agreement that there is a group of low malignancy potential or borderline tumors. It is most important that we identify these tumors because they can be managed differently in the young age group, and their prognosis is entirely different from the truly invasive ovarian cancer.

It must be reemphasized that benign, borderline, and invasive areas may be present in the same tumor. It is therefore important to obtain multiple sections before classifying a tumor as of low malignant potential or borderline. It has been shown that stage II and III borderline serous tumors do almost as well as those with stage I neoplasia. Julian and Woodruff reported 65 cases of papillary serous tumors that were borderline. They showed that conservative surgery is indicated when the disease is limited to a single ovary. The absolute 5-year survival was 83% and the relative 5-year survival 92%. They pointed out that multiple sections of the tumor are required to define the cellular uniformity of the lesion.

In conclusion it may be said that ovarian tumors of low potential malignancy or borderline malignancy: (1) have a high survival rate; (2) follow a typical and indolent course when they behave in a malignant fashion; (3) are associated with occasional spontaneous regression of peritoneal implants; (4) are fatal in only a small percentage of cases; (5) must have the diagnosis based exclusively on an examination of the ovarian tumor without considering if it has spread.

These tumors represent a specific classification of tumors, and the classification does not mean that the pathologist is undecided. It means simply that the pathologist has made up his or her mind clearly and positively and is making a diagnosis of a tumor showing epithelial abnormalities and proliferation but without stromal invasion. It is a positive diagnosis and does not imply indecision. It has been repeatedly reported that the grade of these tumors offers a good indication of the prognosis. Those tumors in which the degree of epithelial atypia is slight and there is no invasion of the stroma behave in a benign fashion. Fox reported that the carcinoembryonic antigen (CEA) concentrations in these tumors of borderline malignancy are different, and he divided them into two groups: Those containing a high CEA titer have a more aggressive natural history than the others. This work is preliminary but may be helpful when deciding on the management of these tumors if indeed they can be classified by the CEA titer.

The nonepithelial tumors (germ cell and gonadal-stromal tumors) do not lend themselves to a diagnosis of low potential malignancy as well as do the common epithelial tumors. However, a protocol for their identification and management is included.

The prognosis for the individual patient is difficult to predict on histologic and clinical grounds. DNA analysis has shown that aneuploid tumors are more likely to progress. Morphometric analysis is also an accurate predictor of clinical behavior when it is available.

Classification of Ovarian Neoplasms

I. Tumors of epithelial origin
  A. Serous
  B. Mucinous
  C. Endometrioid
  D. Clear cell (mesonephric)
II. Germ cell tumors
  A. Dysgerminoma
  B. Tumors in teratoma group

1. Extraembryonal forms
  a. Endodermal sinus tumor (mesoblastoma vitellium, yolk sac carcinoma, extraembryonic membrane tumor)
  b. Choriocarcinoma
2. Embryonal teratomas, solid and cystic
3. Adult teratomas
  a. Solid
  b. Cystic (dermoid cyst)
    i. Solid
    ii. With malignant change
4. Struma ovarii
5. Carcinoid
  C. Mixed forms of the above
III. Gonadoblastoma
  A. With germinoma
III. B. Without germinoma
IV. Gonadal stromal tumors (sex cord mesenchymal tumors)
  A. Female cell types
    1. Granulosa cell tumor
    2. Thecoma-fibroma type
  B. Male cell types
    1. Sertoli-Leydig cell tumor (arrhenoblastoma, androblastoma
    2. Sertoli cell tumor (androblastoma tubulare)
    3. Hilus (Leydig) cell tumor
  C. Mixed cell types (gynandroblastoma)
  D. Indeterminate cell types
V. Tumors not specific for ovary
  A. Lymphoma
  B. Burkitt's lymphoma
VI. Miscellaneous tumors
  A. Sarcomas
  B. Fibromas
VII. Metastatic tumors
  A. Krükenberg
  B. Choriocarcinoma

Bibliography

Agrofo JO, Blancha A, Gibbs ACC, Langley FA: Histological discrimination of malignancy in mucinous ovarian tumors. *Histopathology* 1:431, 1977.
Annual Report on the Results of Treatment in Gynecological Cancer. 20th Vol. *Int J Obstet Gynecol* Pettersson F (ed) Elsevier, Stockholm, FIGO, 1986.

Annual Report on the Results of Treatment in Gynecological Cancer. 21th Vol. *Int J Obstet Gynecol* Pettersson F (ed) Elsevier, Stockholm, FIGO, 1990.

Barber HRK: Ovarian cancer Part I. *CA* 29:341, 1979; Part II. *CA* 30:2, 1980.

Barber HRK, Sommers SC, Snyder R Kwon TH: Histologic and nuclear grading and stromal reaction as indices for prognosis in ovarian cancer. *Am J Obstet Gynecol* 121:795, 1975.

Barnhill DR, O'Connor D: Management of ovarian neoplasms of low malignant potential. *Oncology* 5(1):21, 1991.

Bell DA, Weinstock MA, Scully RL: Peritoneal implants of ovarian serous borderline tumors: histologic features and prognosis. *Cancer* 62:2212, 1988.

Burrmeister RE, Heckner RE, Franklin RR: Endosalpingiosis of the peritoneum. *Obstet Gynecol* 34:310, 1969.

Colgan T, Norris H: Ovarian epithelial tumors of low malignant potential: a review. *Int J Gynecol Pathol* 1:367, 1983.

Copeland LJ: Review of article on management of ovarian neoplasms of low malignant potential. *Oncology* 5(4):31, 1991.

Decker DG, Melkasian GD Jr, Taylor WF: The prognostic importance of histologic grading in ovarian cancer. *Natl Cancer Inst Monogr* 42:9, 1975.

Fenoglio CM, Frenczi A, Richart RM: Mucinous tumors of the ovary: ultrastructural studies of mucinous cystadenomas with histogenetic considerations. *Cancer* 36:1709, 1975.

Fox H: Advantage in the histopathology in ovarian tumors: ovarian cancer. *Adv Biosci* 26:9, 1980.

Fox H, Langley FA: *Tumors of the Ovary.* Heinemann, London, 1976.

Fox H, Agrawall K, Langley FA: A clinical pathologic study of 92 cases of granulosa cell tumors of the ovary, with special references to the factors influencing prognosis. *Cancer* 35:231, 1975.

Friedlander ML, Russell P, Taylor IW, et al: Flow cytometric analyses of cellular DNA content as an adjunct to the diagnosis of borderline malignancy. *Pathology* 16:301, 1984.

Gershenson DM, Silva EG: Serous ovarian tumors of low malignant potential with peritoneal implants. *Cancer* 65:578, 1990.

Gondoz B: Electron microscopic studies of papillary serous tumors of the ovary. *Cancer* 27:1455, 1971.

Hart WR: Ovarian epithelial tumors of borderline malignancy (carcinomas of low malignant potential). *Hum Pathol* 8:541, 1977.

Hart WR, Norris HJ: Borderline and malignant mucinous tumors of the ovary: histologic criteria and clinical behavior. *Cancer* 31:1031, 1973.

Herman RJ, Norris HJ: Germ cell tumors of the ovary. *Pathol Annu* 13:291, 1978.

Julian CJ, Woodruff JD: The biologic behavior of low grade papillary serous carcinoma of the ovary. *Obstet Gynecol* 40:860, 1972.

Katzenstein AL, Azor MT, Morgan TE, et al: Proliferative serous tumors of the ovary: histologic features and prognosis. *Am J Surg Pathol* 2:339, 1978.

Lim-Tan SK, Cajigas HE, Scully RE: Ovarian cystectomy for serous borderline tumors: a follow-up study of 35 cases. *Obstet Gynecol* 72:775, 1988.

Marchand A, Fenoglio CM, Pasqual R, et al: Carcinoembryonic antigens in human ovarian neoplasm. *Cancer Res* 5:3807, 1975.

Roth L, Dallenbach-Hellweg G, Czernobrisky B: Ovarian Brenner tumors. *Cancer* 56:582, 1985.

Roth L, Langley F, Fox H, et al: Ovarian clear cell adenofibromatous tumors. *Cancer* 53:1156, 1984.

Rubin SC: Review of article on management of ovarian neoplasms of low malignant potential. *Oncology* 5(4):26, 1991.

Russell P: Borderline epithelial tumors of the ovary: a conceptual dilemma. *Clin Obstet Gynecol* 11:259, 1984.

Sampson JA: Endometrial carcinoma of the ovary, arising in endometrial tissue in that organ. *Arch Surg* 10:1, 1925.

Scully RE: Gonadoblastoma: a review of 74 cases. *Cancer* 25:1340, 1970.

Scully RE: Recent progress in ovarian cancer. *Hum Pathol* 1:73, 1970.

Scully RE: Ovarian tumors: a review. *Am J Pathol* 87:686, 1977.

Serov SF, Scully RE: *Histologic Typing of Ovarian Tumors.* World Health Organization, Geneva, 1973.

Snyder R, Norris H, Tavassoli F: Endometrioid proliferative and low malignant potential tumors of the ovary. *Am J Surg Pathol* 12:661, 1988.

Woodruff JD: The pathogenesis of ovarian neoplasia. *Johns Hopkins Med J* 144:117, 1979.

Wynen JA, Rosenshein MB: Surgery in ovarian cancer. *Arch Surg* 115:863, 1980.

16

Postmenopausal Palpable Ovary Syndrome

The time has come to reevaluate our clinical approach to ovarian pathology. Although carcinoma of the endometrium is still the most prevalent cancer of the female reproductive system, ovarian carcinoma has become the leading killer of women who die from gynecologic malignancy. With the present state of diagnostic development, diagnosis of an ovarian tumor is a matter of chance rather than a scientific discovery. By the time it is diagnosed, ovarian cancer in more than 70 to 80% of the patients has spread beyond the ovary. The hard fact remains that a pelvic mass found during a pelvic examination is the only practical and consistent clinical method available to us to detect an ovarian tumor. Certain functional or dysontogenetic tumors with hormone activity are the exception. However, there are only a few such tumors compared to the number of epithelial tumors, which comprise the main group of killers.

We euphemistically state that women are protected if they have a pelvic examination every 6 months. However, it has been reported that the chance of detecting an ovarian neoplasm during routine pelvic examination in an asymptomatic woman is 1 in 10,000.

The insidious onset of ovarian cancer needs no elaboration. Many competent gynecologists have had the devastating experience of finding widespread disease in a patient who had a negative pelvic examination 6 months before. Pelvic examination itself has many limitations because of the difficulties inherent in evaluating the pelvic contents in the presence of obes-

ity, a long conical inelastic vagina with contracted fornices, vaginal atrophy, or lack of cooperation from an apprehensive or defensive patient. Among patients who survive, it is serendipitous that she was seen at a time when the tumor was still localized and could be removed intact. In many, the tumor is found accidentally or incidentally. By the time a patient complains of a mass, abdominal enlargement, or pain, the tumor has usually involved the surrounding organs with disease or adhesions; indeed, in a high percentage of such patients, the regional lymph nodes are already affected. It follows that because it is not usually possible to diagnose ovarian cancer in its early stages it is not possible to treat it with any predictable degree of certainty for cure.

It is an accepted axiom that the ovary may be too old to function but never too old to form tumors. Because the peak incidence of ovarian tumors occurs after age 40, especially careful evaluation (combined with constant suspicion) should be carried out in this high-risk group. It is important to look at the ovarian cancer incidence rates and distribution of cases by age. The incidence of ovarian cancer starts to rise at age 40 with an annual rate of 10 per 100,000 women and peaks at about age 77 when the rate is about 52 per 100,000; it then drops at age 80 to a rate of about 45 per 100,000. The rate plateaus at this point and remains steady for the remainder of life. It is essential that these figures and the distribution of this curve be kept in mind when making the decision whether to retain ovaries at the time of hysterectomy in women over age 40. Because the incidence of ovarian cancer is on the increase in the highly industrialized nations, an effort must be made to achieve earlier diagnosis than in the past or to practice prophylaxis by removing the ovaries at the time of surgery in women over age 40. Currently, more than 800,000 hysterectomies are being done each year, most of them in women over age 40, providing an opportunity to practice prophylaxis. It is the height of professional integrity to explain to the patient that ovarian cancer is the leading cause of death from gynecologic cancer and that it is on the increase. It should also be emphasized that it is almost impossible to make an early diagnosis, as 70 to 80% are in stages III and IV when they present for treatment and the overall survival for truly invasive ovarian cancer is between 15 and 25%. If the patient then elects to keep her ovaries, she should be asked to sign a document stating that she has been thoroughly informed about being at risk for ovarian cancer.

Background

Recognizing that there is no method for early diagnosis and that early diagnosis is a matter of chance rather than science, I have been exploring the potential for a serologic diagnosis, using immunologic techniques that take advantage of the extraordinary power of discrimination of the immune defense mechanism itself. However, the realization of this method is far in the future, and the means available for diagnosis and prophylaxis must be utilized now if women are to be protected from the scourge of advanced ovarian cancer.

In early 1971 one of the postmenopausal patients whom I had been following for routine checkups came in for a pelvic examination. I palpated what appeared to be a normal premenopausal ovary and was struck by the fact that it had not been present on previous examinations. The patient was advised to return in 1 week for another pelvic examination (having taken an enema the night before). The same findings were present on the second examination. The patient was admitted to the hospital, examined under anesthesia, and ex-

plored. I found a normal premenopausal-sized ovary that had been replaced by ovarian cancer. In this patient, during the incidental appendectomy at the time of total abdominal hysterectomy and bilateral salpingo-oophorectomy (TAH-BSO) clumps of tumor cells were found within the lymphatics of the appendix. Within the next several months, I operated on three other patients with similar pelvic findings, and each had an early cancer of the ovary.

The literature suggests that a pelvic examination should be done every 6 months. This routine should help to detect early changes in the ovary. Despite the protocol for regular examinations, the chance of detecting an ovarian neoplasm during routine pelvic examination in an asymptomatic woman is 1 in 10,000 examinations. It is obvious that the detection rate is low. In most instances, doctors judge any ovarian enlargement under 5 cm as of little significance. This concept must be challenged, especially in the postmenopausal woman.

Although we may accept the axiom that the ovary may be too old to function but never too old to form tumors, we are lulled into a sense of false security if the mass has not reached the size of 5 cm. Until recently, it was thought that the common epithelial ovarian carcinoma practically never occurred before age 40 and its incidence peaked by age 60. However, more recent figures show that at age 25 there is an annual rate of 3 per 100,000 women and at age 60 there are 40 per 100,000 women. The rate then continues to climb and reaches a peak at age 77. If the premise is accepted that a cancer starts as a derangement within the cell and progresses from atypia to dysplasia to in situ carcinoma to invasive carcinoma, there is a greater possibility of making an early diagnosis when any change is detected in the ovary. Early cancer is not a tumor in the sense that a mass is present. The volume of tumor must be present before a mass can be detected. As a matter of fact, the earliest a tumor can be detected by any means is when it reaches 1 cm^3; by that time, the cancer contains 10^9 (one billion) cells with the potential to metastasize and to kill. Therefore even though it is small, it is not truly an early cancer.

Diagnostic Signs

One diagnostic sign of early cancer in the ovary of postmenopausal patients has proved to be both valuable and consistent in our hands. It is simply that palpation of *what is interpreted as a normal-sized ovary in the premenopausal woman represents an ovarian tumor in the postmenopausal woman.* This suggestion may appear to be insignificant in terms of the total problem, but it has been my experience that all such palpable findings proved to be a new growth; they were not all necessarily malignant, but none was functional or dysfunctional. It is my opinion that the postmenopausal palpable ovary is a significant finding, and it is hoped that this observation will alert the gynecologist to its importance. The postmenopausal palpable ovary (PMPO) syndrome does not include a cyst. It is related only to the size and consistency of a normal premenopausal ovary.

The designation postmenopausal palpable ovary syndrome is a misnomer, and it is unfortunate that a more descriptive term had not been chosen. It does not mean that anything palpated in the adnexa is abnormal. Every gynecologist has been able to feel an ovary that measures 2 cm in a thin, relaxed patient with an elastic and distensible vagina. It must be reemphasized that the PMPO syndrome is defined simply as palpation, in the postmenopausal woman, of what would be interpreted as a normal-sized ovary in the premenopausal woman, here representing an ovarian tumor. Figure 16.1 shows the normal ovary and the ovary during early and late menopause drawn to scale. Note the dramatic difference in size between the normal premenopausal ovary and the ovary during the late menopausal period.

Several points can be enumerated to support this thesis. There is no such thing as physiologic enlargement of the postmenopausal ovary. Physiologic cysts can only arise from nonrupture of a graafian follicle (follicular cysts) or from cystic degeneration of a corpus luteum (lutein cysts). There are no follicular or lutein cysts in a postmenopausal ovary simply because there are no follicles or corpora lutea.

The contrast between the premenopausal and postmenopausal ovary is striking. Whereas

Premenopausal
3.5 × 2 × 1.5 cm

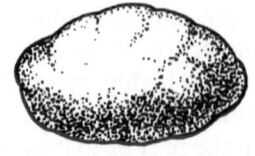

Early menopause
(1 – 2 years)
2 × 1.5 × 0.5 cm

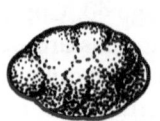

Late menopause
(2 – years)
1.5 × 0.75 × 0.5 cm

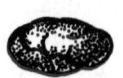

FIGURE 16.1. Relative sizes of premenopausal, menopausal, and late menopausal normal ovaries.

the normal ovary measures $3.5 \times 2.0 \times 1.5$ cm, the menopausal ovary tends to atrophy and shrink when the graafian follicles and ova disappear. The tunica albuginea becomes dense and causes the surface of the ovary to become scarred and shrunken. The cortex is marked with increased thinning as well as numerous corpora fibrosa and corpora albuginea with areas of dense fibrosis and hyalinization. The ovary shows varying degrees of avascularity. Eventually the ovary becomes an inert residue that consists of connective tissue, and it clings to the posterior leaf of the broad ligament. Its pink color becomes pure white. It shrinks to $2.0 \times 1.5 \times 0.5$ cm, and in some it may be as small as $1.50 \times 0.75 \times 0.50$ cm. Its wrinkled surface resembles the gyri and sulci of the cerebrum. At this point it cannot be palpated. The postmenopausal palpable ovary is not a normal ovary for this stage of life.

Traditionally, a woman who is amenorrheic is clinically considered menopausal. However, chemically and anatomically, the changes described above occur over a period of time. Although they are rapid, it takes approximately 3 to 5 years for the final histologic changes to occur. The conclusion must then be drawn that if an ovary is palpated 3 to 5 years after the clinical menopause it is a pathologic ovary until proved otherwise, regardless of its size in centimeters. It is my recommendation that the patient (without delay for observation) should have the benefit of an expedited examination under anesthesia, and if the previous impression is verified she should undergo laparotomy. A careful abdominal exploration followed by TAH-BSO should be the treatment chosen. Although splitting and biopsying the ovary may be justified for detecting early cancer in the premenopausal patient, the ovaries should be removed without biopsy in the postmenopausal group.

Misinterpreting the Meaning of the PMPO Syndrome

The 1971 article that I coauthored with Dr. Edward A. Graber on the PMPO syndrome has been misquoted and misinterpreted. Although few physicians have read the original publication, many have quoted it and misrepresented its content. Unfortunately, many of these critics are among the leading gynecologic oncologists in the United States. Simply, the article stated that "palpation of what is interpreted as a normal-sized ovary in the premenopausal patient represents an ovarian tumor in the patient that is at least three years postmenopausal." This statement *does not mean that anything that is palpated in the adnexa is abnormal.* Furthermore, the observation does not apply to patients who are under anesthesia but to those who are having a regular pelvic examination, as it is merely a clinical diagnosis that depends on the size and consistency of the ovary and the time during the postmenopausal period that the diagnosis is made. It does not apply to a small, 1 cm cyst discovered on ultrasound examination. Hopefully, this section will clear up the misunderstanding and misinterpretation of this syndrome, and energies can now be directed toward providing optimal care for patients.

The contrast between the premenopausal and postmenopausal ovary is striking. As already noted, whereas the premenopausal ovary measures $3.5 \times 2.0 \times 1.5$ cm the menopausal ovary tends to shrink, and within 3 to 5 years after the last menstrual period it reaches $1.50 \times 0.75 \times 0.50$ cm. In addition, the ovary in the advanced menopausal patient is often found as a flattened structure against the pelvic wall. It would be almost impossible to palpate such an ovary even in a thin, relaxed patient. Based on these observations, the physician must be cognizant that ovaries deemed normal for their size in the premenopausal woman during the late postmenopausal years are not a normal finding and require investigation and treatment.

The menopause should not be confused with the climacteric. Menopause is merely the patient's last menstrual period. The menopause may be due to the decreased sensitivity of the hypothalamus to steroid feedback and alteration of ovarian sensitivity to follicle-stimulating and luteinizing hormones or simply to the absence of primordial cells in the ovary. It is possible that all three phenomena play a role.

Ultrastructure data indicate that an occasional primordial follicle appears in a postmenopausal ovary. Although there is a great increase in the number of atretic follicles in postmenopausal ovaries, normal-appearing follicles are occasionally found; the granulosa cells, however, are smaller. Any observed corpus luteum is usually undergoing atresia (corpus atretica or fibrotica). Although differentiating ovarian follicles are rare, these follicles and oocytes usually appear to be normal but are unresponsive to pituitary stimulation.

Occasionally ovarian follicles are found in a resting state during the postmenopausal period. Generally, the advanced follicles identified in postmenopausal ovaries are undergoing atretic changes but may contain small, cystic structures. Any observed corpus luteum has also undergone atresia (corpora albicans). Sometimes a small cyst is present in the so-called burned-out corpus luteum or corpus albicans. However, either the follicle or the corpus luteum that may persist in patients in this age group is in a resting stage. It is impossible for the hypothalamic-pituitary axis to stimulate the follicles in this ovary. A small cyst may merely represent what would have been the last period if it had occurred, but for some reason or other the small cyst is held in suspended animation.

With the advent of more sensitive ultrasound equipment and use of the vaginal probe, the presence of small cysts on the ovary is being reported more frequently than ever before. This finding may cause a great deal of concern because those who have never studied the ovary expect it to be fibrous tissue during the postmenopausal years. This finding is generally so, but in some cases there is persistence of a small cyst or cysts that appear to be held in suspended animation. The sonographer may report these small cysts as an unusual finding in women of this age. It creates a problem if the physician interprets it as an abnormal finding. Here a second opinion usually results in the diagnosis of a postmenopausal palpable ovary (which it is not) with the recommendation that it be removed. This practice is poor.

When a report of this type is received from a sonographic examination, the gynecologist should direct the patient to return to the office for reexamination after taking an enema. If the physician cannot palpate a structure in adnexa that resembles a premenopausal-sized ovary, the patient should be reevaluated within 6 weeks to 2 months with another pelvic examination and a sonogram. If these findings remain the same (and almost certainly they will be), the patient does not require an exploratory laparotomy with removal of the uterus, tubes, and ovaries. However, the patient should be directed to return in 6 weeks to 2 months for a repeat examination and sonogram. If the findings are again the same, the patient can be followed at 4- to 6-month intervals.

With the increased incidence of carcinoma of the ovary and the poor 5-year survival rate, most physicians believe that the report of an abnormal finding by the sonographer places them in an ethically untenable position. It would be in the best interest of the patient that sonographers report their findings and not make any suggestions beyond this report.

It is becoming increasingly important in the present consumer–provider climate that the gynecologic surgeon demand a second opinion by a designated knowledgeable gynecologist before permitting surgery to proceed for the so-called PMPO syndrome. In order to show good will and establish confidence among patients and public, this consultation service should be offered free of charge.

The time is fast approaching when geriatric gynecology will become a subspecialty within the division of obstetrics and gynecology. As transvaginal sonography becomes the state of the art, more of these cases will be reported after a sonogram of the pelvis. Often physicians working in other specialties request routine sonography of the pelvis and abdomen; and when these small, 1 cm, cysts are reported the patient is referred to the gynecologist. It often leads to a problem for the gynecologist because of the strong wording of the sonography report. It is important for the gynecologist to exercise prudent judgment. The morbidity and mortality caused by removal of these healthy ovaries (which have been reported as abnormal) outweigh any good contributed by the concept of the PMPO syndrome.

It is important for gynecologists to familiarize themselves with the normal findings of the postmenopausal ovary. It is the height of professional integrity for a gynecologist to make a judgment based on the findings rather than on an attempt to please a colleague. When judging how to manage the postmenopausal patient with a sonographic finding of a small cyst, the gynecologist must follow the rule of "do no harm." The gynecologist should bear in mind that a small, 0.5- to 1.0-cm cyst in the postmenopausal ovary does not represent "the PMPO syndrome."

Summary

On the basis of the Third National Cancer Survey data, about 1 of every 70 newborn girls (1.4%) develops cancer of the ovary during her life. Cancers of the ovary account for roughly 5% of all cancers in women, according to statistics reported by both the State of Connecticut and the Third National Cancer Survey.

The age-specific incidence rates for ovarian cancer rise steadily up to age 80 and then drop off slightly in the older age groups. The greatest number of cases is found among women age 50–54 years and 55–59 years. The mean age is 62.3 and the median age 59.0. The trends in age-standardized death rates for major sites show that the rate for the ovary is increasing.

The observed median survival times by age for white women are as follows: 1.6 years for all ages; more than 5 years for those under age 45; 1.9 years for age 45–54; 1.5 years for age 55–64; 0.9 year for age 65–74; and 0.6 year for patients 75 years and older. The observed median survival time by age for black women are as follows: 0.9 year for all ages; more than 5 years for those under age 45; 2.0 years for age 45–54; 0.7 year for age 55–64; 0.5 year for age 65–74; and 0.4 year for those 75 years and older.

If we are to save more women and diminish the mortality rate from ovarian cancer, we must become more liberal in our indications for operation. I suggest that the palpation of what appears to be a normal-sized ovary in a patient who is 3 to 5 years postmenopausal is indicative of an ovarian tumor and should be investigated promptly. These patients should not be followed and reevaluated but, rather, subjected to examinations to obtain proof of the presence or absence of an ovarian tumor. To wait until one feels a solid tumor mass of up to 5 cm and then to expect a cure is an exercise in fancy and futility.

When a small, 0.5- to 1.0-cm, clear cyst is reported in the adnexal area in the postmenopausal woman after a sonographic examination, the patient should be reevaluated within 6 weeks to 2 months with another pelvic examination and a sonogram. If these findings remain the same (and almost certainly they will) the patient should not be explored with removal of the uterus, tubes, and ovaries; rather, she should be reexamined in another 6 weeks to 2 months, and if the findings are the same she can be followed at 6-month intervals. It must be repeated that the PMPO syndrome represents the "palpation of what is interpreted as a normal-sized ovary in the premenopausal woman and does not mean anything that is palpated is abnormal." The PMPO syndrome is strictly a clinical diagnosis established by palpation, and the patient must be more than 2 years postmenopausal.

Bibliography

Barber HRK: The postmenopausal palpable ovary syndrome. *Compr Ther* 5(9):58, 1979.

Barber HRK, Graber EA: The PMPO syndrome (postmenopausal palpable ovary syndrome). *Obstet Gynecol* 38:921, 1971.

Kistner RW: *Gynecology, Principles and Practice*. 2nd Ed. Year Book Medical Publishers, Chicago, 1971.

Piel G: The treason of the clerks. *Proc Am Philos Soc* 109:259, 1965.

Rutledge F, Boronow RC, Warden JT: *Gynecologic Oncology*. John Wiley & Sons, New York, 1976.

Silverberg E: *Gynecologic Cancer. Statistical and Epidemiological Information*. Professional Education Publication. American Cancer Society, Atlanta, 1975, 1980.

U.S. Department of Health, Education, and Welfare: *End Results in Cancer*. Report No. 4. U.S. Public Health Service, National Institutes of Health, Bethesda, 1972, p. 113.

U.S. Department of Health, Education and Welfare: *End Results in Cancer*. Report No. 5. U.S. Public Health Service, National Institutes of Health, Bethesda, 1976.

17

Surgical Treatment of Cancer of the Ovary: Technique

Ovarian carcinoma is the most frustrating problem in gynecology. The inability to diagnose it is reflected in the figures reporting that 70 to 80% of the patients have stage III and IV lesions when they present for treatment. With well-structured treatment protocols, the survival rate for the truly invasive ovarian cancers ranges between 15 and 25%. When the ovarian cancer presents in the form of widespread millet seed or pinhead-sized nodules covering all peritoneal surfaces, including the bowel, liver, and kidney areas, it is no longer a surgical disease. However, surgery is the backbone of therapy, and every attempt must be made to excise all tumor; failing with this optimal approach, it is important to remove as much tumor as possible. Debulking and significant reductive surgery can in many instances convert a patient from the poor prognosis group to a more favorable group. The size of the largest residual tumor mass remaining after surgery is the most important prognostic factor when determining the survival of patients with common epithelial ovarian cancer. It is probably related to the biology rather than to the volume of tumor.

Surgical excision of ovarian cancer should be approached with a planned, methodical technique. The goal of ovarian cancer surgery is to excise as much tumor as possible and at the same time avoid the possibility of hemorrhage or fistula complication. Granted that ovarian cancer may be a surprising finding, these early, well-encapsulated ovarian cancers can be managed without difficulty. However, 60 to 80% of all ovarian cancers present in stages III and IV. Proper surgery for ovarian cancer patients then requires relatively sophisticated techniques, not always available in every hospital. Add to this fact the requirements for chemotherapy, irradiation, accurate pathology reports, and the fluid and electrolyte management that almost invariably follows abdominal surgery, and it is not difficult to make a case for a large medical center as the optimal place for ovarian cancer care. The extensive dissection required to debulk the disease adequately often compromises the patient to the extent that hyperalimentation is needed. With this disease, we must assume the worst and be ready for any emergency or complication.

The gynecologic oncologist has come full cycle from a radical surgical attack to a conservative approach, back to a supraaggressive surgical attack. Why has this cycle come about? During the late 1940s and early 1950s, after carrying out a radical surgical operation, oncologists did not have enough knowledge of chemotherapy to control the residual disease; thus recurrence or continued growth of persistent disease was usual. With the improved knowledge of fluids and electrolytes, as well as the increased use of hyperalimentation and the technology available through the Swan-Ganz catheter to monitor these patients, the morbidity associated with management of these patients has been reduced.

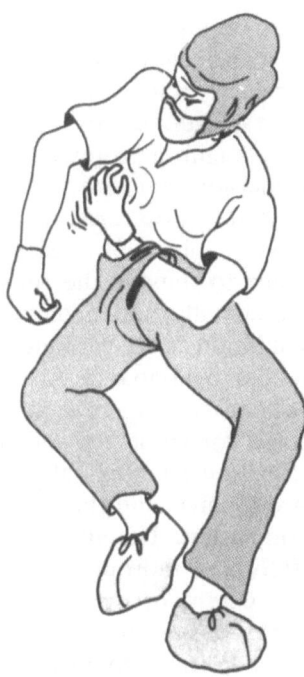

FIGURE 17.1. Pfannenstiel and low transverse incision has no place in the management of ovarian cancer. Denis Cavanagh said it is like scratching your axilla through your fly.

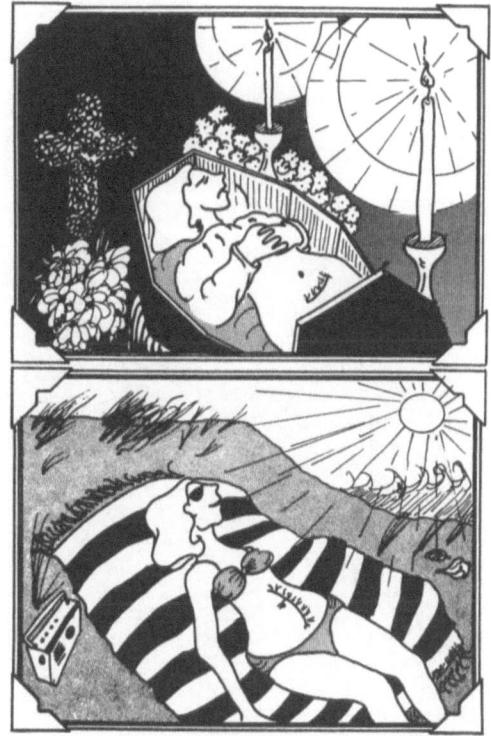

FIGURE 17.2. (Top) An aesthetic corpse is pleasing only to a mortician. (Bottom) Beauty is in the eye of the beholder. Life can be beautiful.

Incision

There is no place for the management of common epithelial ovarian cancer using a Pfannenstiel incision. Figure 17.1 displays the problem when the Pfannenstiel incision is used. It is impossible to explore the patient adequately through a Pfannenstiel incision because it is not possible to palpate between the liver and the diaphragm on the posterior peritoneum where millet seed or pinhead areas of cancer may be present. When the common epithelial ovarian cancer is understaged it is undertreated. Reports indicate that only about 20% of patients with common epithelial ovarian cancer have an appropriate incision at the time of their original treatment. When a patient is referred to me for additional treatment for common epithelial ovarian cancer and if a Pfannenstiel incision has been done, the patient is considered to be a fresh case and undergoes reexploration with proper staging and possibly more appropriate

surgery. Use of the Pfannenstiel incision during management of the common epithelial ovarian cancer is perverse and represents malpractice. The argument that it is cosmetically more attractive and has been requested by the patient violates the rules of professional integrity. The patient looks to a gynecologist for advice, suggestions, and recommendations. It should be carefully explained to the patient why it is necessary to use a vertical incision. She should be told about the consequences of understaging or rupturing the tumor by trying to deliver it through an inadequate incision and how it converts the stage of cancer to a less favorable prognostic group. The incision must be as ruthless as the cancer itself. An aesthetic corpse is of little interest and pleasing to no one except a mortician (Figs. 17.2 and 17.3). The patient and her family would much prefer to have her alive and able to carry out her social and eco-

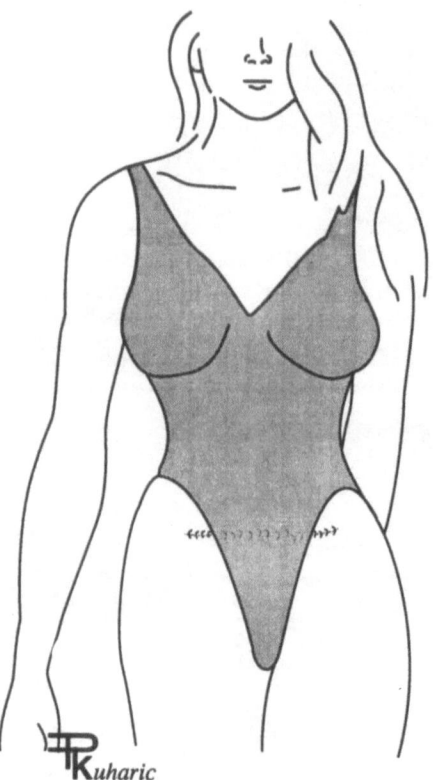

FIGURE 17.3. Bathing suit styles, rather than good surgical judgment, may determine the type of incision.

rupture of the tumor, converting it from a lesser stage to a stage with spill, compromising the chance for cure. In many instances a Pfannenstiel incision selects patients for therapeutic failure. It is the height of professional integrity to choose an incision that extends beyond the upper limits of the gross disease and allows adequate, easy exploration, providing the optimum chance to remove the tumor intact. Morally, professionally, and medicolegally, the Pfannenstiel incision is to be condemned for management of an ovarian tumor.

When the abdomen is opened, any fluid present is collected for cytology; and in the absence of fluid, about 50 ml of saline should be instilled into the pelvis and then aspirated for cytologic examination. The abdomen and pelvis are carefully and thoroughly evaluated to determine the extent of disease. If tissue is readily available for easy biopsy, a frozen section diagnosis is desirable to document the site and type of primary lesion. It is especially important to evaluate the area on the posterior abdominal wall between the liver and the diaphragm. Stage I cancer of the ovary has been found here in about 10 to 15% of cases.

nomic responsibilities for herself, her family, and the community even though the incision rules out wearing a bikini. This situation is certainly better than being a corpse with a small transverse incision.

Technique

To minimize the possibility of hemorrhage or hold blood loss to a minimum, a methodical and planned approach should be used when operating on patients with ovarian cancer. The abdomen must be opened by a vertical incision that extends beyond the upper limits of the mass and is adequate to explore the posterior area between the liver and the diaphragm. Unless this step is properly carried out it is impossible to stage accurately the amount of ovarian cancer present. In addition, a small incision such as a Pfannenstiel may result in

When one has determined the extent of disease, it is desirable to incise the posterior peritoneum lateral to and just above the pelvic brim, as carried out at the start of a radical hysterectomy (Figs. 17.4 and 17.5). This approach exposes the infundibular ligament and, by clamping it, decreases the blood loss that occurs when ovarian cancer is excised. This procedure permits identification of the ureter, which can be isolated and left attached to the medial peritoneal flap. The ovarian vessels running in the infundibular ligament can be isolated, clamped, cut, tied, and doubly ligated in toto. As soon as a similar procedure is carried out on the opposite side, a considerable amount of blood is diverted from the ovarian cancer.

With the ureter protected from injury, it is possible by blunt and sharp dissection to incise the peritoneum down to the round ligament and, after it is clamped and ligated, to continue the incision of the peritoneum lateral to the bladder. If the bladder flap of peritoneum is involved with cancer, the incision in the peri-

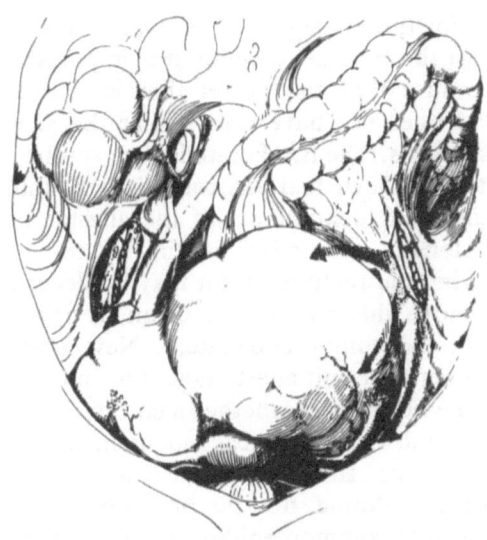

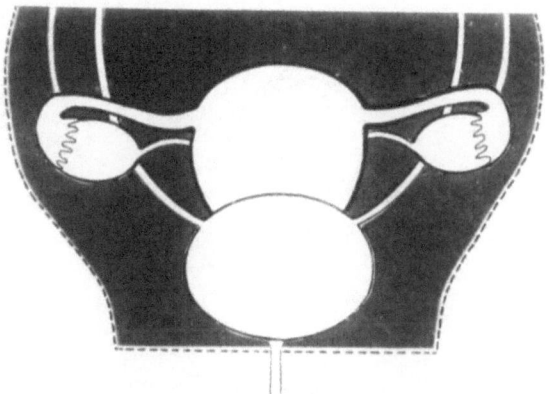

FIGURE 17.6. Shaded area represents the extent of the peritoneum removed in a radical operation for a fixed ovarian tumor. Front view.

FIGURE 17.4. On opening the peritoneal cavity, it is important to identify all landmarks. The cecum is mobilized on the right and the sigmoid on the left for identification of the ureter and high ligation of the infundibulopelvic ligament. The ureter is shown here in relation to all of the vessels in the infundibulopelvic ligament. (From Barber HRK: Surgical management of ovarian cancer. *Current Ob/Gyn Techniques* 1:6, 1975. Copyright © Surgical Communications Inc. All rights reserved. By permission.)

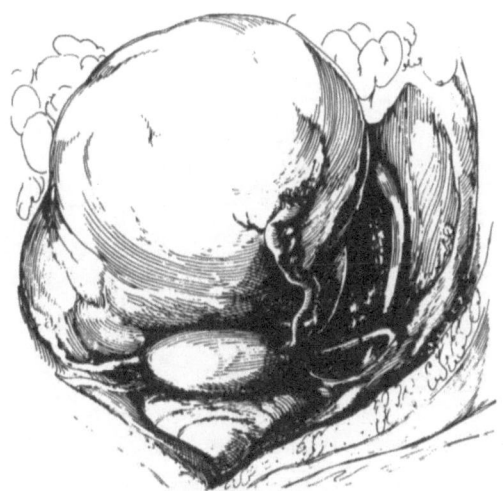

FIGURE 17.5. Round ligament, uterus, and a large pelvic mass. (From Barber HRK: Surgical management of ovarian cancer. *Current Ob/Gyn Techniques* 1:6, 1975. Copyright © Surgical Communications Inc. All rights reserved. By permission.)

toneum should be continued to the pubis (Fig. 17.6). The lateral side of the peritoneum over the bladder can be elevated and dissected by sharp, blunt dissection from the bladder, which is then left denuded. The flap of peritoneum is dissected off the dome of the bladder and left attached to the lower uterine segment; it is removed as an en bloc dissection with the uterus. Posteriorly, with the ureter under direct vision, the peritoneum medial to the ureter is incised down over the rectum. This maneuver frees up the cul-de-sac from the bowel and leaves it attached to the back part of the uterus (Fig. 17.7). The entire specimen can be removed as the hysterectomy is carried out.

With this technique it is possible to remove a large bulk of cancer without inordinate blood loss. If the tumor involves the rectum, which would constitute the only place where macroscopic disease would be left behind, a decision must be made about whether the bowel should be resected to encompass the disease. When this step is accomplished, the omentum should be removed at the level of the transverse colon. It is important to use suture ligatures to protect against possible postoperative bleeding. Because the appendix is often involved in the tumor mass and because it is the site of metastases, its removal is recommended.

The operating surgeon should be prepared to resect the small or large bowel if only a segment is involved. Multiple resections are not of

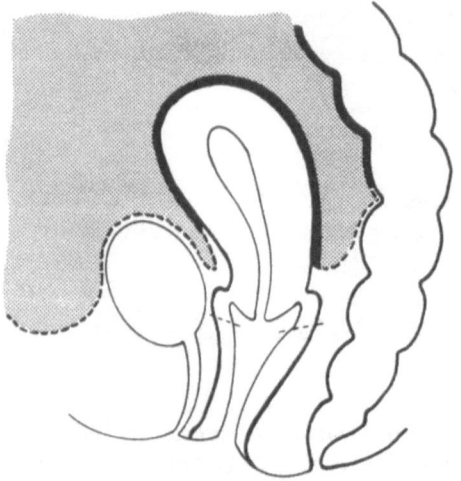

FIGURE 17.7. Shaded area represents the extent of the peritoneum removed in a radical operation for a fixed ovarian tumor. Side view.

value for the management of ovarian carcinoma. At the time of resection it is important to make sure that the bowel that is reanastomosed does not have tumor near the site of anastomosis. The fistula rate is high among patients who have had anastomosis with tumor within a few centimeters of the anastomosis. Occasionally, tumor is found in the cul-de-sac involving the rectum, and it may be necessary to remove this part of the colon in order to debulk the tumor adequately. New stapling instruments permit anastomosis low in the pelvis. The decision of whether a colostomy is indicated must be a clinical judgment made by the operator. In most instances a permanent colostomy should not be performed in the presence of common epithelial ovarian cancer. Griffiths and Fuller have reported improved results employing intensive surgical and chemo-

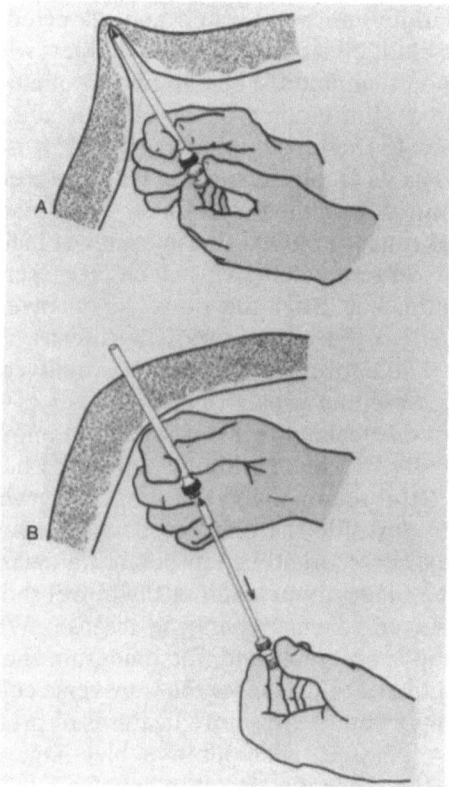

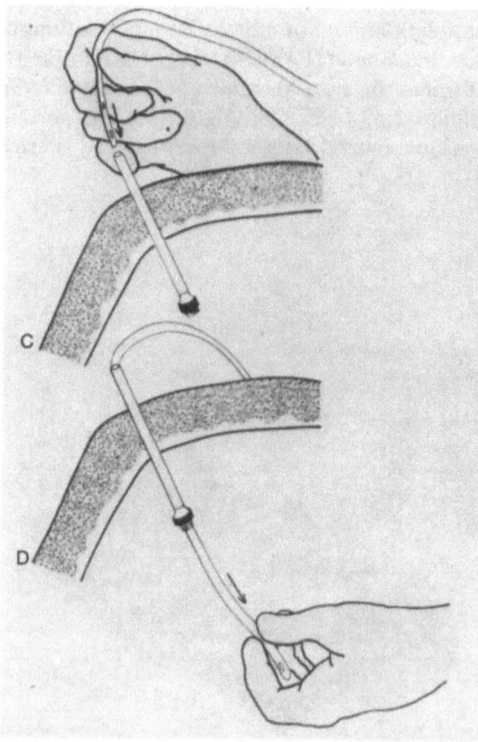

FIGURE 17.8. (A) Before inserting the tubes for postoperative ^{32}P instillation, a trocar is inserted through the abdominal wall from inside the abdomen by raising the skin just above the inguinal ligament. (B) Trocar is now through the abdominal wall, and the stylet is being removed. (C) Small catheter (a baby feeding tube) is being threaded through the trocar. (D) Threading the catheter is now advanced, after which the trocar is removed.

therapeutic management of advanced ovarian cancer.

If ^{32}P tubes are to be used, they should be placed in the abdomen through trocars, which are pushed through the abdominal wall from inside the abdomen to the skin in each lower quadrant (Fig. 17.8). The trocars are directed lateral to the epigastric vessels. Small baby-feeding tubes with extra holes cut in them are then threaded into the trocar, and the trocar is withdrawn into the pelvic cavity with the tube. The ends of the tubes remain sealed so that when the ^{32}P is instilled it has a watering-can effect (Fig. 17.9). The trocar is removed, and the tube is placed along the lateral gutter as high as the diaphragm on the right side and to the liver on the left side. The tubes are secured in place with black silk sutures. One suture is placed in the opening made by the trocar and left long so it can be tied in place when the ^{32}P tube is removed following instillation of the

radioactive phosphorus. Phosphorus is instilled within 24 to 48 hours after completion of the surgery. ^{32}P is instilled only if all macroscopic disease has been removed.

The abdomen and pelvis are carefully washed with saline, and the peritoneum is closed with a running Maxon no. 0 or 1 or PDS no. 1 suture, which is interrupted at the half-way mark; another similar suture is used to complete the closure. The abdomen is closed without drains. It is important to close the peritoneum carefully so there is no leakage from instillation of the radioactive material. The fascia is closed with Maxon no. 0 or 1 suture or a PDS no. 1, which is placed as a running suture and interrupted at the halfway mark, then continued to the upper part of the fascial incision. Approximately six to eight nylon retention sutures are used as well. The retention sutures are placed through the skin and fascia about 1 cm from the incision and continue to the opposite side, where they secure just the edge of fascia. They continue under the fascia on the opposite side to about 1 cm from the incision, where they are brought through the fascia and skin. When these sutures are tied in place, they close the subcutaneous spaces and give good support. Black silk sutures are used to close the skin. A dry, sterile dressing is placed on the incision. The tubes are taped to the abdomen, and the opening made by the trocar is covered with dry, sterile dressings.

How Much Is Too Much?

Gynecologic oncologists do not always agree on the amount of tumor that can be excised safely. I remove as much as possible without risking a gastrointestinal or genitourinary fistula. Removal of ovarian cancer masses helps improve the metabolic and symptomatic status of the patient. It increases the growth rate of the remaining tumor cells and improves the tumor blood supply, which provides a better environment in which the anticancer chemotherapy drugs can work. The success of subsequent chemotherapy, irradiation, or both is inversely proportional to the amount of tumor left in the abdomen after surgery. Therefore aggressive surgery is indicated not

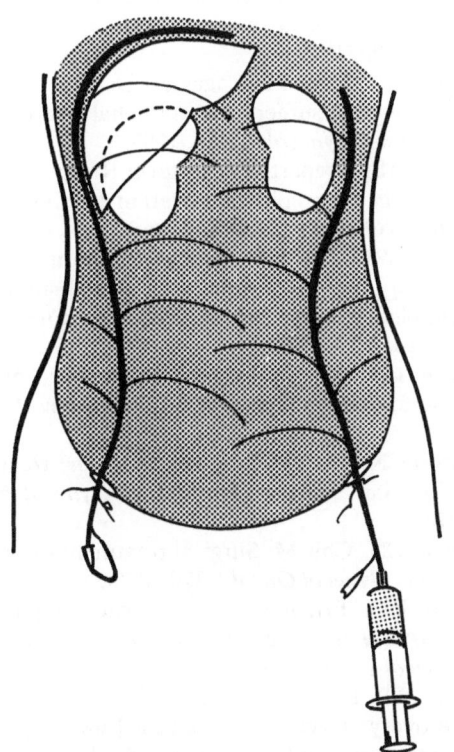

FIGURE 17.9. Cutting multiple holes in the tubes but leaving the ends sealed results in a watering can, or sprinkler, effect when ^{32}P solution is instilled.

so much because it is curative but because it potentiates other forms of treatment. If it is true that the patient is immunized by her own tumor, a point is reached where there is acquired tolerance, or excess antigen may stimulate a great number of antibodies, which may form complexes around the tumor. These blocking factors result in immunologic enhancement that protects the tumor from attack by killer lymphocytes. Therefore the patient's immune response is improved when the volume of tumor has been decreased. Because the tumor is highly immunosuppressive, its removal may convert the patient from being immunoincompetent to being immunocompetent.

Summary

Surgical excision should be approached with a planned, methodical technique. The ideal incision is vertical, extending above the limits of the bulk of the cancer and permitting easy exploration. The abdomen and pelvis should be aspirated before being explored. No attempt should be made to excise the tumor mass until the infundibular ligaments are clamped, cut, suture-ligated, and doubly secured with a free tie. Attacking the tumor before these steps are taken often results in a hemorrhage that curtails any possibility of debulking or removing the cancer. As much tumor should be removed as is possible without inordinate morbidity and mortality and without running a risk of a gastrointestinal or genitourinary fistula.

Bibliography

Bagley CMJ, Young RC, Shine PS, et al: Ovarian carcinoma metastatic to the diaphragm—frequently undiagnosed at laparotomy: a preliminary report. *Am J Obstet Gynecol* 116:397, 1973.

Barber HRK: Surgical aspects of ovarian tumors. In *Selected Topics of Cancer—Current Concepts.* Symposia Specialists, Miami, 1974, p. 161.

Barber HRK: Ovarian cancer: still an enigma. *Dr* 1:17, 1975.

Barber HRK: Surgical management of ovarian cancer. *Curr Ob-Gyn Tech* 1:6, 1975.

Barber HRK, Brunschwig A: Pelvis exenteration

for locally advanced and recurrent ovarian cancer: review of 22 cases. *Surgery* 58:935, 1965.

Brunschwig A: Attempted palliation by radical surgery in pelvic and abdominal carcinomatosis primarily in the ovaries. *Clin Obstet Gynecol* 4:875, 1961.

Brunschwig A: Attempted palliation by radical surgery for pelvic and abdominal carcinomatosis primary in the ovaries. *Cancer* 14:384, 1961.

Buchsbaum HJ, Broady MF, Delgado G, et al: Surgical staging of carcinoma of the ovaries. *Surg Gynecol Obstet* 169:226, 1989.

Cutler SJ, Myers MH, Green SB: Trends and survival rates of patients with cancer. *N Engl J Med* 293:122, 1975.

Day TG Jr, Smith JP: Diagnosis and staging of ovarian carcinoma. *Semin Oncol* 2:217, 1975.

Griffiths CT: Surgical resection of tumor bulk in the primary treatment of ovarian cancer. *Natl Cancer Inst Monogr* 42:101, 1975.

Griffiths CT, Fuller AF: Intensive surgical and chemotherapeutic management of advanced ovarian cancer. *Surg Clin North Am* 68:131, 1978.

Griffiths CT, Parker LM, Fuller AF Jr: Rule of in situ reductive surgical treament in the management of advanced ovarian cancer. *Cancer Treat Rep* 63:235, 1979.

Hacker NF, Berek JS, Lagasse LD, et al: Primary cytoreductive surgery for epithelial ovarian cancer. *Obstet Gynecol* 61:413, 1983.

Helewa ME, Krepart GV, Lotocki R: Staging laparotomy in early epithelial ovarian carcinoma. *Am J Obstet Gynecol* 154:282, 1986.

Hoskins WJ: The influence of cytoreductive surgery on progression-free interval and survival in epithelial ovarian cancer. *Baillieres Clin Obstet Gynecol* 3:59, 1989.

Hudson CN: A radical operation for fixed ovarian tumors. *J Obstet Gynaecol Br Commonw* 75:1155, 1968.

Hudson CN: The place of surgery in the treatment of ovarian cancer. *Clin Obstet Gynecol* 5:700, 1978.

Hudson CN, Chir M: Surgical treatment of ovarian cancer. *Gynecol Oncol* 1:370, 1973.

Knapp RC, Friedman EA: Aortic lymph node metastases in early ovarian cancer. *Am J Obstet Gynecol* 119:1013, 1974.

Parker RT, Parker CH, Wilbanks GD: Cancer of the ovary: survival studies based upon operative therapy, chemotherapy and radiotherapy. *Am J Obstet Gynecol* 108:878, 1970.

Piver MS: Continued controversies in the diagnosis

and treatment of ovarian adenocarcinomas. *J Reprod Med* 22:119, 1979.

Piver MS, Barlow JJ, Lele SB: Incidence of subclinical metastases in stage I and II of ovarian carcinoma. *Obstet Gynecol* 52:100, 1978.

Rosenoff SH, DeVita VT Jr, Hubbard S, et al: Peritoneoscopy in the staging and follow-up of ovarian cancer. *Semin Oncol* 2:223, 1975.

Smith JP: Surgery for ovarian cancer: ovarian cancer. *Adv Biosci* 26:137, 1980.

Symmonds RE: Some surgical aspects of gynecologic cancer. *Cancer* 36:649, 1975.

Tobias JS, Griffiths CT: Management of ovarian carcinoma: current concepts and future prospects. *N Engl J Med* 294:818, 1976.

Way S: Carcinoma of the vulva. In Meigs JV, Sturgis SH (eds): *Progress in Gynecology*. Vol. 3. Grune & Stratton, Orlando, FL, 1957, p. 489.

Wijnen JA, Rosenshein NB: Surgery in ovarian cancer. *Arch Surg* 115:863, 1980.

Young RC, Decker DG, Wharton JT, et al: Staging laparotomy in early ovarian cancer. *JAMA* 250:3072, 1983.

18

Recurrent Cancer of the Ovary: Surgical Treatment

With the increased use of a radical surgical attack on cancer of the cervix during the 1940s, the same approach was attempted when recurrent ovarian cancer was present. There are ten indications for a radical surgical attack on carcinoma of the ovary.

1. The tumor is confined to the pelvis.
2. The tumor is surgically resectable.
3. The patient is young enough and in good enough condition to withstand an extensive surgical procedure.
4. All other forms of therapy have been exhausted, and there is no other modality of treatment left to offer.
5. The duration of symptoms and extent of disease as determined by clinical and biopsy examination indicates that metastasis out of the pelvis is unlikely.
6. Responsible surgeons and their teams must be acquainted with the anatomy and have the technical skill and background to perform the extensive surgery.
7. Thorough knowledge of the natural history of disease is essential.
8. An in-depth knowledge of preoperative and postoperative care is important.
9. An ability to anticipate fluid and electrolyte problems and to correct them in their early stages is necessary.
10. One physician must manage the patient; and although he or she should consult freely, it is that physician's responsibility to give painstaking attention to the most minute details.

Earlier attempts at a radical surgical approach to ovarian cancer were not rewarding. In many instances it was possible to remove the macroscopic disease, but without proper knowledge of chemotherapy and the appropriate drugs cancer usually recurred within a year. In addition, having undergone extensive surgery such as small bowel resection, colectomy, retroperitoneal node dissections, gastrectomy, and removal of large bulky tumors, the patient often experienced fatal metabolic imbalances. Hyperalimentation has changed much of this scenario, and it is now possible to carry these patients in a good nutritional status for long periods. Surgery has come full circle; and with improvement in the use of hyperalimentation and control of the patient through a Swan-Ganz catheter supported by adjuvant chemotherapy, surgeons are once again becoming more aggressive surgically when managing recurrent ovarian cancer.

Cancer of the ovary is characterized by its wide dissemination over peritoneal surfaces of the pelvis, upper abdomen, and omentum and by the frequent involvement of both ovaries, either as spread from the one primarily involved or as bilateral primary growths. The tendency for rapid extension to the upper abdomen, on theoretical grounds, contraindicates radical surgery. Unlike cervical cancer, ovarian cancer is a surface spreader, whereas cancer of the cervix infiltrates structures. Obstruction usually is not caused by an absolute occlusion at one point but by a carcinomatous ileus, which results from malignant cell infiltration of the bowel wall, or mesentery of bowel, preventing peristalsis.

Nonexenterative Radical Surgery

Brunschwig carried out extensive resections, short of pelvic exenteration, on 65 patients. He pointed out that many patients with far-advanced cancer of the ovary—who have often been treated in some fashion or another on one or more occasions—present the clinician with a frustrating problem. Usually such patients have only a short time to live, and immediate relief of symptoms as they evolve is all that is possible. Ironically, many of these patients still appear to be in fair or even good general condition.

Most of the patients exhibited ascites, which in the advanced stage of the disease recurs after previous paracentesis. The large volume of tumor makes it difficult to control the ascites with radioactive substances, external x-ray therapy, or even chemotherapy. If these modalities of treatment do produce a favorable response, it is short-lived in the presence of bulky disease. Debulking the disease usually makes the patient more comfortable, if it can be accomplished without producing inordinate morbidity and mortality. Currently it provides an opportunity to obtain a second response from chemotherapy and from combinations of chemotherapy and immunotherapy.

There were 65 patients in the heterogeneous series reported by Brunschwig. The surgical mortality, defined as death within 30 days of operation, consisted in 7 patients, for an incidence of 11%. Three of the postoperative deaths were patients who of necessity underwent radical upper abdominal excisional procedures involving partial hepatectomy, partial gastrectomy, and partial pancreatectomy. Excluding these three, the mortality rate was 4 among 62 patients, an incidence of 6%.

Among the survivors in this series, three lived 8 to 9 years, and one lived 10 years free of disease; one died of uremia after 5 years, and eight lived for almost a year to 1 year 5 months. Among the patients surviving 8 to 9 years, the patient living 10 years, and the one surviving more than 5 years, the disease, although recur-

rent after previous treatment, had metastasized only locally and was macroscopically entirely resectable. The fact that the involvement was localized, however, was not appreciated until laparotomy had been performed.

Obviously, judgment must be exercised when performing radical excisional surgery in these patients. Patients should not be subjected to operation if they are debilitated or elderly individuals with cancer that has spread beyond the abdomen or if they have advanced disease that is not causing, at the moment, particularly acute and distressing symptoms. Resection is considered only when symptoms (gastrointestinal disturbances) are severe enough to warrant attempted relief at the cost of the discomforts and risks of an operation.

In the absence of emphatic contraindications, laparotomy is indicated in selected patients of the type described because there is always the possibility that the recurrence and metastases are localized and macroscopically resectable. With an increased knowledge of chemotherapy and hyperalimentation, there is new hope for salvaging many of these patients after their tumor is debulked.

Exenterative Surgery for Ovarian Cancer

In some instances the growths and their local extensions appear to be limited to the pelvic structure. When there is peritoneal involvement of the pelvis, pelvic colon, and bladder, or when the cancer has penetrated more deeply into these structures, the question of pelvic exenteration arises as a method of dealing with the situation.

The tendency of such neoplasms toward relatively widespread extension, manifested simultaneously in the pelvis and the upper abdomen, would on theoretical grounds contraindicate these radical procedures. However, because little documentation for the possible palliative effects of incomplete operations on these patients has been recorded, except perhaps for an occasional instance, pelvic exenterations were carried out in a number of cases to ascertain whether they should be more frequently attempted for ovarian cancer, at the moment limited to the pelvis. Twenty-two cases of advanced ovarian cancer—21 previously treated by surgery, irradiation, or both and one fresh case in which the growth macroscopically was confined to the pelvis—were treated by pelvic exenteration.

Fourteen patients were operated on 5 years or more previously, including the single fresh case. Total pelvic exenteration was performed on 13, and one underwent an anterior pelvic exenteration (excision of bladder, vagina, uterus, adnexae, lower ureters, and so on, with preservation of the rectum).

Although the series is small, the 5-year survival rate was 7% among those operated on between September 1947 and the end of 1968. The single long survivor died of uremia without evidence of recurrent cancer 71 months after operation.

During the postoperative course of these patients, there was a high incidence of complications. Of the 11 survivors of the operation, 8 required secondary operations, mostly for intestinal fistulas or intestinal obstruction. All of them had had previous radiation therapy and conservative surgical procedures, which may account for the high incidence of complications.

For 4 of the 11 operative survivors, carcinomatosis was probably the immediate cause of death, the survival period averaging 10 months (7–13 months). Others had cancer present at the time of death, except for the 5-year survivor, who died of uremia without cancer present. Among the remaining seven, the immediate causes of death were intestinal fistula in one, intestinal obstruction in two, uremia in one, hemorrhage in two, and cachexia in one.

Eight patients were operated on during the years 1958 through 1962. Six had total exenterations, and two had anterior pelvic exenterations. One patient is living and clinically well 27 months after operation, but the six others all had carcinoma at the time of death.

The overall surgical mortality, i.e., death within 30 days of operation regardless of cause, was 22.7%. This result contrasts with an overall surgical mortality rate of 15.2% for 576 total and anterior pelvic exenterations done between 1947 and 1961 for cancer of the cervix.

The eventual course of cancer of the ovary is notoriously unpredictable. Patients without treatment may survive many months to several years. In the series reviewed above, the average length of time from the first symptom or previous treatment to pelvic exenteration was 42 months (3.5 years). The extremes were 6 months to 20 years. The average survival after exenteration—excluding the single survivor for 71 months who died of uremia, was brief.

It appears that, in the presence of advanced cancer of the ovary previously treated by conservative surgery, irradiation, or both, the indications for pelvic exenteration may be questioned even though the disease appears confined to the pelvis. The reason for this statement is that usually when the question of this procedure is posed the surgeon is operating in the presence of a recurrent or persistent lesion already treated for some months or years, and the lesion itself is known to have a marked tendency to widespread metastases to the upper abdomen.

The patients dealt with here were all unfavorable candidates for any radical procedure by virtue of the situations presented, and these experiences can hardly serve as a basis for firm conclusions about whether pelvic exenteration is justified for advanced ovarian cancer even when the lesion is apparently limited to the pelvis. Certainly, more experience is necessary before a categoric rejection of the operation. The case of the single long-time survivor (71 months), who eventually died elsewhere of uremia, suggests that some patients, although admittedly few, can be salvaged.

The question may be raised as to why, on the basis of the poor results during 1947 to 1968, further surgical procedures were advised and carried out. The answer is that the symptoms were severe enough to warrant an attempt at relief, and that there is at least a ray of hope, when by clinical history and knowledge of the situation in these patients the alternative was certain, rapid demise. I have yet to witness such patients "dying in peace"—a favorite axiom of the proponents of conservative treatment when faced by patients in advanced stages of cancer. Obviously the patients operated on above were selected. Most of the patients seen with recurrent or advanced widespread cancer of the ovary were not subjected to pelvic exenteration. Patients were operated on only if their neoplasms were macroscopically confined to the pelvis and macroscopically completely excisable.

All patients who underwent pelvic exenteration were selected by nature, as evidenced by the fact that all survived for 1+ to 13 years from the initial therapy to the diagnosis of recurrence. As stated above, those patients were operated on only if their neoplasms were macroscopically confined to the pelvis and macroscopically completely excisable. In general, ovarian cancer does not lend itself to excision by pelvic exenteration because of its spread to the upper abdomen. However, the series of pelvic exenterations did not include any endometrioid tumors. These tumors have less tendency to be bilateral and spread less to the upper abdomen than do other ovarian tumors. In highly selected cases, endometrioid ovarian cancer may be controlled by pelvic exenteration. In summary, it can be stated that the natural history of cancer of the cervix permits radical surgical attack by pelvic exenteration, *whereas ovarian cancers lend themselves to exenteration only if they do not have their usual method of spread and, therefore, violate their natural history*.

Indications for removing the bulk of tumor are as follows.

1. Psychological effect
2. To improve response to X-ray therapy and/ or anticancer drugs
3. To reverse immunosuppression, acquired tolerance, immunologic enhancement, immunoselection, or antigenic modulation

When a patient goes to the operating room with a large abdomen and returns with the same mass, she obviously knows that nothing could be done. Therefore it is important at least to try to reduce the tumor mass.

The *volume of tumor* is important when considering patients for therapy. Radiation therapists believe strongly that nodules larger than 2 cm do not respond in a predictable manner to therapy because the middle of the nodule contains anoxic cells that respond poorly to irradiation. These cells recover and grow. Radiation therapy is not my choice for the treatment of common epithelial ovarian cancer. The anti-

cancer drugs reduce a constant percentage of tumor cells that are in cycle. For example, the same dose kills 99% of 100,000 leukemia cells or 99% of 100 cells, whichever number of leukemia cells is present. Therefore 1,000,000 cells can be reduced to 10,000, and 10,000 reduced to 100, and 100 to 10 or fewer, and then 10 cells to zero. It is obvious why a reduced volume of tumor is important when attempting to achieve a cure.

The *immune response* fails for many reasons. It is important to reverse some of the factors that inhibit a good immune response. The tumor itself is immunosuppressant; therefore removing a bulk of tumor overcomes a great deal of this immunosuppression, which allows the host's own immune response to function more efficiently. *Acquired immunologic tolerance* may occur if a large amount of antigen is released by large tumors, overwhelming the host's immunologic response. After removal of such large tumor masses, the hosts exhibit resistance to the reimplantations of their own tumor cells, suggesting that the intrinsic failure of the immune response was not the cause of the original lack of immune reaction. Rather, the temporary paralysis observed was due to the fact that the system was unable to cope with such a large challenge.

Immunologic enhancement results from enhancing or blocking antibodies present in the serum. It is a humoral response. These antibodies block the antigenic sites on the surface of the tumor and prevent the killer lymphocytes from attacking the tumor. Removing the bulk of the tumor removes a great number of the antibodies that have formed complexes on the surface of the tumor. This argument has been advanced to show that a tumor is destroyed by a cell-mediated mechanism rather than a humoral mechanism.

Immunoselection suggests that cells within a tumor are presumed to be descendants of a single transformed cell. Thus the bulk of the cells have the same antigen. However, through mutation some develop more antigen and attract a greater number of specific antibodies. They are then eliminated while the cells with few antigens continue to grow. The tumor therefore grows relatively slowly at first and often appears to be restrained, but then it progressively acquires more autonomy and greater invasive properties.

Antigen modulation occurs when an antibody is formed and is present, causing the cell to cease synthesizing tumor antigens. It renders ineffective an immunologic reaction against tumor cells. Immunoselection and antigen modulation have not been documented in humans.

Summary

Today's orientation in the management of ovarian cancer is to be aggressive. Radical surgery exclusive of pelvic exenteration has proved to be of value for debulking a volume of disease. When debulking has been accomplished, additional therapy is better able to control the disease. There is only a limited place for pelvic exenteration in the management of ovarian cancer: only when it does not have its usual method of spread and therefore violates its natural history.

The increased use of hyperalimentation and the improved methods of chemotherapy have expanded the indications for an aggressive surgical attack. The immune response of the host fails for many reasons. Because the tumor itself is immunosuppressant, removing it or debulking it allows the host's own immune response to function more efficiently. The tumor produces antigens that stimulate antibody formation. A great volume of tumor may produce an antigen–antibody complex that acts as a blocking agent on the surface of the cell. Removing a volume of tumor decreases the production of antigens and cuts down on the formation of blocking complexes. The killer lymphocytes are then better able to attack the tumor.

Bibliography

Barber HRK: Relative prognostic significance of preoperative and operative findings in pelvic exenteration. *Surg Clin North Am* 49:431, 1969.
Barber HRK, Brunschwig A: Pelvic exenteration for locally advanced and recurrent ovarian cancer. review of 22 cases. *Surgery* 58:935, 1965.
Barber HRK, Graber EA: Surgical aspects of ovarian tumors. In *Selected Topics of Cancer—*

Current Concepts. Symposia Specialists, Miami, 1974, pp. 161–183.
Barber HRK, Kwon T: Current status of the treatment of gynecologic cancer by site—ovary. *Cancer* 38:610, 1976.
Beller U, Beckman EM, Muggia FM, Douglas GW: Surgical treatment for advanced epithelial carcinoma of the ovary. *Surg Gynecol Obstet* 165:279, 1987.
Brunschwig A: Attempted palliation by radical surgery in pelvic and abdominal carcinomatosis primarily in the ovaries. *Cancer* 14:384, 1961.
Griffiths CT: Surgical resection of tumor bulk in the primary treatment of ovarian cancer. *Natl Cancer Inst Monogr* 42:101, 1975.
Griffiths CT: Surgical treatment of advanced disease. In Hudson CN (ed): *Ovarian Cancer*. Oxford University Press, New York, 1985, pp. 213–238.
Griffiths CT, Parker LJ, Fuller AF, Jr: Role of cytoreductive surgical treatment in the management of advanced ovarian cancer. *Cancer Treat Rep* 63:235, 1979.
Hudson CN, Chir M: Surgical treatment of ovarian cancer. *Gynecol Oncol* 1:370, 1973.
Joyeux H, Szawlowski AW, Saint-Aubert B, et al: Aggressive regional surgery for advanced ovarian cancer. *Cancer* 57:142, 1986.
Krebs HB, Goplerud DR: Surgical management of bowel obstruction in advanced ovarian carcinoma. *Obstet Gynecol* 61:327, 1983.
Morris M, Gershenson DM, Wharton JT, et al: Secondary cytoreductive surgery for recurrent epithelial ovarian cancer. *Gynecol Oncol* 34:334, 1989.
Ozols RF, Garvin AJ, Costa J, et al: Advanced ovarian cancer: correlation of histologic grade with response to therapy and survival. *Cancer* 45: 572, 1980.
Piver MS, Barlow JJ, Lele SB, Frank A: Survival after ovarian cancer induced intestinal obstruction. *Gynecol Oncol* 13:44, 1982.
Rubin SC, Hoskins WJ, Benjamin I, Lewis JL Jr: Palliative surgery for intestinal obstruction in advanced ovarian cancer. *Gynecol Oncol* 34:16, 1989.
Rubin SC, Hoskins WJ, Saigo PE, et al: Recurrence following negative second-look laparotomy for ovarian cancer: analysis of risk factors. *Am J Obstet Gynecol* 159:1904, 1988.
Symmonds RE: Some surgical aspects of gynecologic cancer. *Cancer* 36:649, 1975.
Tobias JS, Griffiths CT: Management of ovarian cancer: current concepts and future prospects. *N Engl J Med* 294:818, 1976.

19

Second Look Operation

Early diagnosis of ovarian cancer is a matter of chance rather than scientific discovery. The same frustration confounds any attempt at detecting early recurrence of disease. Currently, laparoscopic examination and laparotomy are the only means available that have a predictable rate of accuracy. Periodic gynecologic examinations have not been helpful. Cul-de-sac aspiration, cytology, and serum enzyme studies have limited application in the initial diagnosis. Tumor markers, such as CA125, CA15-3, CA19-9, NB/70K, LASA-P, carcinoembryonic antigen, α-fetoprotein, human chorionic gonadotropin, acute phase reactive proteins, complement components, and complement inhibitors, if present, can serve to monitor response to treatment. Ultrasonography is employed to evaluate the position and volume of tumor; and if disease is identified with this technique, ultrasonography is employed to monitor therapy. CT scan, MRI, and ultrasonography play a role in identifying cancer in the pelvis and abdomen. They are also useful in monitoring response to treatment.

The second look concept has many interpretations. The one followed in this chapter relates to patients who have had known disease that could not be adequately removed at the time of surgery but in whom the tumor regressed after additional therapy to the point there was no longer any evidence of disease. The other group of patients in whom a second look has been employed consists of those from whom all the disease was removed at the time of the original operation and to whom prophy-

lactic chemotherapy was then given for a period ranging from 6 to 9 months. At this time, in order to judge whether treatment can be stopped in the absence of any palpable disease, an exploratory laparotomy with multiple biopsies is carried out. If disease is palpable or detectable by any means prior to surgery, it is not a second look procedure but a planned type of therapy, hopefully to excise all the tumor or to relieve a complication such as an obstruction, fistula, or abscess.

The second look operation has become an established part of the protocol of many centers for patients with common epithelial or nonepithelial ovarian cancers who have undergone radiation therapy, chemotherapy, or a combination of treatments. *Corynebacterium parvum* and BCG have been used in conjunction with chemotherapy in a limited number of centers. There are no hard data to support the use of either *C. parvum* or BCG when there is a significant volume of tumor present. Their role as agents for immunoprophylaxis remains to be evaluated. When triple or quadruple anticancer chemotherapy is employed and there is no evidence of palpable disease at 6 to 7 months, the patient should undergo exploratory surgery to determine if the disease has been controlled. Using multiple-drug therapy, it has been found that the tumor can be controlled within 6 to 8 months; if it is not, it is because the cells have mutated or become drug-fast, or a cell line remains that is resistant to the therapy. Beyond 6 to 7 months, little is accomplished except to produce immunosuppression. However, using a single alkylating agent which is rarely employed at present, the second look procedure should be delayed for at least 12 to 18 months, depending on the drug that is given. A few centers are doing laparoscopy evaluations at stated intervals to follow the response of treatment in their patients. Evidence of disease is a positive finding, but inability to demonstrate disease does not mean that lesions are not present, and laparotomy is then indicated to evaluate accurately the response to treatment.

The most important question concerning the second look operation is whether it is possible to offer the patient a second chance for cure if disease is present. An attempt is made here to answer this question according to my personal experience and with a review of the literature.

The second look operation was popularized, if not introduced, by Wangensteen, for patients who had cancers arising in the stomach and colon, who had responded to treatment, and who were asymptomatic at the time of the second look operation. About half of these patients were found to have disease present, and only 9% were salvaged by the second look operation. Park, Corscaden, Kottmeier, Rutledge, and Burns and Smith have carried out second look procedures. None of their patients had a dramatic response in the presence of residual or recurrent tumor, despite a change in the therapeutic regimen.

The second look operation gives the surgeon the opportunity to (1) explore the patient and remove all of the residual tumor or reduce the tumor mass and improve the patient's chances with a new treatment regimen; (2) outline the site of the tumor and determine the status of the residual tumor; and (3) devise a plan of therapy for the patient. It is obvious that patients with stage I or II disease in whom all disease has been removed and chemotherapy has been given prophylactically have fewer recurrences than patients with stages III and IV lesions treated therapeutically for residual disease after initial treatment.

It is difficult to interpret the reports in the literature based on the natural history of common epithelial ovarian cancer. The results

from initial therapy for invasive epithelial ovarian cancer range from 15 to 35% 5-year survivals. Therefore 65 to 85% of patients (based on a survival of 15–35%) should present with recurrence after initial therapy. Having treated those patients with a recurrence after a second look operation, the physician faces the question of whether additional treatment has anything to offer.

Tepper et al. reported a series of 17 patients with advanced cancer who had exploratory laparotomy, 3000 rad of radiation therapy, thiotepa, and second look surgery. They reported that 10 of the 17 patients were dead within less than 2 years because of pelvic and abdominal recurrences. Seven survived more than 3 years (41%), four of whom had repeated courses of chemotherapy, irradiation, or both for recurrence. The average survival time of the entire group from the time of diagnosis was 29 months—20 months without a recurrence. For two patients with stage III disease it was 30 months and 23 months, respectively, without a recurrence. Three patients were free of disease at 48, 67, and 77 months, respectively. One had stage IIB disease and two had stage III disease. The respective histologic types of these three patients were papillary serous cystadenocarcinoma, mucinous carcinoma, and granulosa cell carcinoma. The survival of the patients who underwent removal of the tumor was 39 months versus 20 months for those with gross residual tumors.

Wallach et al. performed a second look operation ten times in 240 patients with advanced carcinoma of the ovary treated initially by surgery and postoperative chemotherapy with triethylenethiophosphoramide. After the second look operation, survival ranged from 8 to 100 months. The patient who survived 100 months continued living with a palpable tumor. Therefore eight of ten patients died, and one was living after the second look procedure. Wallach and coworkers reported that the second look operation should be performed in patients with retained ovaries and complete clinical regression of tumor after administration of chemotherapy and in selected patients for whom interval treatment permits surgical clearance of tumor. They concluded that the new drugs may create an expanded role for the second look operation.

Rutledge listed several reasons for reexploration: (1) The patient may have had a sufficient amount of the drug. (2) The tumor may become more localized and possibly resectable for the first time. (3) The benefit from the drug may be exhausted, and it may be time to switch to another drug. (4) The mass may now be suitable for irradiation. (5) It may be suspected that the mass that has served as a guide to the drug action is not cancer, as was originally presumed.

Smith reported that about one in eight of the patients treated at M.D. Anderson Hospital with melphalan have had a second look operation. Among 103 patients who had a second look operation, 65% survived an additional 2 years, and 34% survived 5 years. Twenty-three patients were found to have no cancer by multiple biopsies and cytologic studies, and chemotherapy was stopped. Five of these patients developed recurrent cancer; however, four had received only four cycles of chemotherapy before surgery, and in the fifth patient sampling was probably inadequate at the time of the second look operation. The patient developed distant metastases several months after surgery. Of 103 patients who had a second look operation and were found to have cancer at the time of their surgery, 14 are presently alive 2 to 10 years after surgery without evidence of disease. In 13 of these patients all or almost all of their cancer had been removed at the second look operation, and they had been either continued on chemotherapy or underwent irradiation. Those receiving radiation had a survival rate of only 14% after the second look operation, but 50% of those given chemotherapy survived for 5 years.

Schwartz and Smith reported 186 patients with epithelial tumors of the ovary being managed at the M.D. Anderson Hospital. The patients underwent an exploratory (second look) operation to assess the status of the cancer. Fifty-eight patients were found to have no evidence of disease, and chemotherapy was discontinued. Eight patients with advanced ovarian cancer had no evidence of disease 5 years or more after the negative second look operations and were probably cured by chemotherapy. Seven patients were found to have cancer at second look operations and had a change in management followed by no evidence of disease 5 years or more later. Survival after positive second look operations vary directly with the volume of tumor found at the time of the operation and the amount of tumor left behind at the second look operation.

The survival rate for patients who underwent a second look operation is proportional to the number of cycles of single agent chemotherapy they received before surgery. Among patients who received four or fewer cycles of single agent chemotherapy before the second look operation 2 of 23 (9%) survived 5 years, whereas among those receiving five to nine courses 6 of 19 (32%) survived 5 years, as did 8 of 10 (80%) receiving ten or more courses. All of the patients who received more than 12 cycles of chemotherapy before the second look operation were alive and well. Only patients from whom it was possible to remove all or almost all of the remaining cancer were benefited by a second look operation. Therefore an aggressive approach is indicated at the time of surgery.

It is difficult to answer the initial question about the value of a second look operation. If it is possible to control or reduce the tumor volume so that all or almost all of the remaining cancer can be removed, the procedure has value. However, in most instances this goal is not possible. The greatest contribution of second look operation may be demonstrated if certain drugs (doxorubicin, cis-platinum, and hexamethylmelamine) produce a predictable response after the present first line of drugs fail. Currently, the second look operation serves its greatest purpose in the decision on whether anticancer therapy can be safely stopped. It must be carried out with great caution after radiation therapy or radioactive gold instillation. The complication rate is increased considerably over that reported following treatment with anticancer drugs.

The most important factors correlating with

second look operations are the stage of cancer, the amount of residual tumor left at the initial operation, and the number of courses of chemotherapy administered prior to the second look operation. Survival after second look operations where disease is found varies directly with the volume of tumor remaining at the time of operation and the amount of tumor left behind at the second look operation. Patients who were treated with radiation therapy had a poorer survival rate than those treated with chemotherapy when cancer was found at second look operation.

John McLean Morris reported in an editorial comment in the *Archives of Surgery* (July 1980) that physicians tend to yield to the medical media in the same way that the world yields to news media. When something is published, it becomes a medical fact. A physician may now have to have a sterilized ruler to pare down each metastasis to 1.6 centimeters if one is to cure the patient with ovarian cancer. There has to be an occasional voice from the audience that points out that, although metastatic disease may be missed by the surgeon, diaphragmatic involvement does not occur in stage I carcinoma of the ovary (by staging definition), but only in stage III and IV carcinoma of the ovary. Similarly, removal of aortic nodes is advocated by authors who report no cures when aortic nodes are involved, and irrigation with 10 dl of normal saline solution may, according to some pathologists, give lower yields of tumor cells than in a few milliliters of peritoneal fluid.

Because early tumors do not produce symptoms, ovarian carcinoma has been called the "silent menace." In the international reports on gynecologic cancer published by FIGO in the 20th Volume of the *Annual Report*, 8,273 patients were reported and 4,730 during the years 1979 to 1981 were stages III and IV. Debulking procedures, reexploration, and adjuvant therapy may cause remissions but have failed as yet to produce significant improvement in long term survival figures.

I would like to add to the statement reported by Morris that a registry should be set up to study cases cured by chemotherapy. A structured plan for accepting patients as cured would serve to provide an answer about whether these patients are being cured or their survival is merely prolonged.

It is my belief that a guarded approach should be assumed when reporting on the results from second look operations. It is evident that although no disease is seen occasionally there is unexpected positive cytology on washings or unsuspected nests of tumor cells in some of the random biopsies that are carried out. Piver et al. reported that, on incising the peritoneum in the lumbar gutters, washing the area with saline, and studying the fluid that has been removed a certain number had positive cytology when everything within the peritoneal cavity had been negative. Therefore it is important to reserve judgment about whether these patients have been cured more than 5 years. It would be devastating to find that in those patients reported as cured the operator may have merely reduced the volume to one or a few cells and, in actuality, is reporting on the time it takes to regenerate, from residual microscopic disease, a volume of tumor that is clinically palpable.

Summary

The contribution made by the second look operation has given rise to much controversy. One of the problems has been the lack of a firm definition. The definition chosen for this chapter relates to the apparent regression of disease left at laparotomy but controlled by additional therapy, or to the evaluation of the patient who has no apparent disease after surgery but has been on multiple-agent chemotherapy for 6 to 7 months or has been on a single agent, such as an alkylating agent, for a year to 18 months and is clinically free of disease. With ovarian cancer, the term "second look operation" should be restricted to the surgical exploration of those patients who have completed a course of therapy, without clinical evidence of residual disease, and are being considered for termination of adjuvant chemotherapy. Currently, the most important use of the second look operation is the decision about whether to stop anticancer therapy. Combination anticancer chemotherapy—that includes doxorubicin, platinum (both *cis-* and *para-*), hexamethylmelamine, and cyclophosphamide (Cytoxan)—has proved to be of value as first line treatment. The chemosensitivity testing popularized by Salmon et al. may very well identify a second line of drugs if the combination of the platinums, cyclophosphamide, and hexamethylmelamine fail. Work with the flow cytometer is yielding interesting information on whether the tumor contains more than one or two cell lines, and this information may be valuable when making decisions about treatment. It provides an additional indication for a second look procedure. If disease is palpable or detectable by any means prior to surgery, the operation cannot literally be called a second look procedure. It is a planned procedure carried out to excise known tumor or to relieve a complication and should be called a second operation.

Bibliography

Arhelger SW, Jenson CB, Wangensteen OH: Experience with the "second look" procedure in the management of cancer of the colon and rectum. *Lancet* 77:412, 1957.

Atack DB, Nisker JA, Allen HH, et al: CA125 surveillance and second-look laparotomy in ovarian carcinoma. *Am J Obstet Gynecol* 154:287, 1986.

Block JS, Hacker NF, Lagasse LD, et al: Survival of patients following secondary cytoreductive surgery in ovarian cancer. *Obstet Gynecol* 61:189, 1983.

Copeland LJ, Gershenson DM, Wharton JT, et al: Microscopic disease at second-look laparotomy in advanced ovarian cancer. *Cancer* 55:472, 1985.

Creasman WT, Rutledge F: The prognostic value of peritoneal cytology in gynecologic malignant disease. *Am J Obstet Gynecol* 110:773, 1971.

Feldman GB, Knappl RC: Lymphatic drainage of the peritoneal cavity and its significance in ovarian cancer. *Am J Obstet Gynecol* 119:991, 1974.

Hoskins WJ, Rubin SC, Dulancy E, et al: The influence of secondary cytoreduction at the time of second-look laparotomy on the survival of patients with ovarian carcinoma. *Gynecol Oncol* 34:365, 1989.

Lewis JL Jr, Griffiths T, Morrow CP, et al: Managing ovarian cancer: the second look operation. *Contempt Obstet Gynecol* 12:137, 1978.

Mackman S, Curreri AR, Ansfield FJ: Second look operation for colon carcinoma after fluorouracil therapy. *Arch Surg* 100:527, 1970.

Meyers MA: The spread and localization of acute intraperitoneal effusion. *Radiology* 95:1970.

Morris M, Gershenson DM, Wharton JT, et al: Secondary cytoreductive surgery for recurrent epithelial ovarian cancer. *Gynecol Oncol* 34:334, 1989.

Perez CA, Olson J: Preoperative vs. postoperative irradiation: comparison in experimental animal tumor system. *Am J Roentgenol Radium Ther Nucl Med* 108:396, 1970.

Piver MS, Shashikant BL, Barlow JJ, Gamarra M: Second look laparoscopy prior to proposed secondary look laparotomy. *Obstet Gynecol* 55:571, 1980.

Podratz K C, Malkasian GD, Hilton JF, et al: Second-look laparotomy in ovarian cancer: evaluation of pathologic variables. *Am J Obstet Gynecol* 152:230, 1985.

Rosenoff SH, DeVita VT Jr, Hubbard S, et al: Peritoneoscopy in the staging and follow up of ovarian cancer. *Semin Oncol* 2:223, 1975.

Rubin SC, Lewis JL Jr: Second-look surgery in ovarian carcinoma. *CRC Crit Rev Oncol Hematol* 8:75, 1988.

Rubin SC, Hoskins WJ, Hakes TB, et al: Serum CA125 levels and surgical findings on patients undergoing secondary operations for epithelial ovarian cancer. *Am J Obstet Gynecol* 160:667, 1989.

Rubin SC, Hoskins WJ, Saigo PE, et al: Recurrence following negative second-look laparotomy for ovarian cancer: analysis of risk factors. *Am J Obstet Gynecol* 159:1094, 1988.

Rutledge F, Burns BC: Chemotherapy for advanced ovarian cancer. *Am J Obstet Gynecol* 107:691, 1970.

Salmon SE, Hamburger AW, Soehlen B, et al: Quantitation of differential sensitivity of human-tumor stem cells to anticancer drugs. *N Engl J Med* 298:1321, 1978.

Samuels BI: Usefulness of ultrasound in patients with ovarian cancer. *Semin Oncol* 2:229, 1975.

Schwartz PE, Smith JP: Second-look operations in ovarian cancer. *Am J Obstet Gynecol* 138:1124, 1980.

Smith JP: Chemotherapy in gynecologic cancer. *Clin Obstet Gynecol* 18:109, 1975.

Smith WG, Day TG, Smith JP: Use of laparoscopy to determine the results of chemotherapy for ovarian cancer. *J Reprod Med* 18:257, 1977.

Stanhope CR, Smith JP: Serial determination of marker substances in ovarian cancer. *Gynecol Oncol* 8:284, 1979.

Tepper E, San Filippo LJ, Gray J, Romney S: Second look surgery after radiation therapy for advanced stages of cancer of the ovary. *Am J*

Roentgenol Radium Ther Nucl Med 112:755, 1971.

Wallach RC, Kabakow B, Blinick G: Current status of the second look operation in ovarian carcinoma. *Natl Cancer Inst Monogr* 42:105, 1974.

Wallach RC, Kabakow B, Jerez E, Blinick G: The importance of second look surgical procedures in the staging and treatment of ovarian carcinoma. *Semin Oncol* 2:243, 1975.

20

Role of Radioactive Isotopes in Management of Ovarian Cancer

Study of the atom has evolved from a simple concept to a complex one. There have been many contributions to this subject. Einstein's general theory of relativity and the great theory of quantum mechanics have made it a subject that requires a background in mathematics, physics, and chemistry. The concept of particles, antiparticles, quarks, mesons, and a variety of ongoing basic experiments stimulated by research in theoretical physics have unlocked secrets of the atom and its nucleus. Although all of these concepts are important for an indepth study of the subject, less complex knowledge of nuclear physics is sufficient for clinicians in their work with radioactive isotopes.

A working knowledge of the physics of radioactive isotopes is important for the management of clinical problems. A few definitions and a superficial review of basic principles are presented.

An *isotope* is a chemical element having the same atomic number as another (i.e., the same number of nuclear protons) but with a different atomic mass (i.e., a different number of nuclear neutrons). It is possible for two elements to have isotopes of the same mass number. For instance, all calcium atoms have 20 protons in their nuclei, and all argon atoms have 18 protons. However, some calcium atoms contain 20 neutrons as well, whereas some argon atoms contain 22. The calcium atoms that contain 20 protons and 20 neutrons make up the isotope calcium 40. The argon atoms with 18 protons and 22 neutrons are argon 40. Two atoms that have the same mass number but different atomic numbers are called *isobars*. Calcium 40 and argon 40 are examples of isobars.

A *radionuclide* is an atomic nucleus that decays spontaneously into some other radioactive nuclear species, accompanied by the liberation of energy. The nouns "isotope" and "element" do not always imply distinct species of atom. For example, nuclear isomers are isotopes, but their nuclei differ in terms of energy content. The term "nuclide" has been introduced to specify completely a particular kind of atom on the basis of its nuclear configuration. A nuclide may be defined as a species of atom whose nucleus has a characteristic number of protons, number of neutrons, and energy content. To be a distinct nuclide, an atom must have more than transitory existence; thus nuclear isomers are distinct nuclides, but ordinary excited nuclei that decay promptly to ground state and intermediate products and nuclear reactions are not considered distinct nuclides. If a nuclide happens to be radioactive, it is often designated a radionuclide.

Bremsstrahlung (Brems rays) is a name applied whenever high-speed electrons, regardless of their source, are abruptly slowed down, and their energy is converted to electromagnetic radiation. If the energy is sufficient, the electromagnetic radiation is in the x-ray region. High-energy β-particles, passing close to atomic nuclei, decelerate and give rise to Brems radiation.

All matter is made up of chemical substances that can be divided into two kinds: elements and compounds. An *element* is a distinct kind of matter that cannot be decomposed into two or more simpler kinds of matter. A *compound* is formed when two or more elements combine chemically to produce a more complex type of matter. *Atoms* are the smallest particles of an element that can exist without losing the chemical properties of the element. *Molecules* are the smallest particles of a compound that can exist without losing the chemical properties of the compound.

The atom is an electrical structure with three basic units: proton, neutron, and electron. This concept is adequate for understanding most phenomena in radiologic physics.

The simplest atom is the element hydrogen. It consists of a central nucleus comprising one proton around which one electron moves in a shell or orbit. The proton is a heavy particle carrying a positive charge, and the electron is a much lighter particle with a negative charge of exactly equal magnitude (but of opposite sign) to that of the proton. Therefore almost all of the mass of the atom is in the nucleus, and the positive charge of the nucleus is balanced by the negative charge of the electron to make the atom as a whole electrically neutral (Fig. 20.1).

The next simplest atom is the element helium. Its nucleus comprises two protons and two neutrons, and there are two orbital elec-

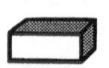

Electron, e$^-$
Mass = $\frac{1}{1845}$
Unit negative
charge

Proton
Mass = 1
Unit positive
charge

Neutron
Mass = 1
No charge

Figure 20.1. Fundamental building blocks of an atomic nucleus. The massive central portion of the atom consists of two major components: positively charged protons and uncharged neutrons. The mass of the protons and that of the neutrons is nearly the same. The number of protons in any atom determines and is designated by the atomic number (Z); the atomic mass (A) is the number of protons and neutrons in the nucleus. The electron has a mass of only 1/1845 of the mass of the proton. It has a negative charge of magnitude equal to that of the proton.

trons moving around the nucleus. A *neutron* is a particle with a mass approximately equal to that of a proton but with no electrical charge. The nucleus of the helium atom therefore has a positive charge of 2 units (because there are two protons) and a mass of approximately 4 units. Also, the two positive charges of the nucleus are balanced by the two negatively charged electrons around the nucleus.

Every element has a mass number and an atomic number. The *atomic number* of an element is the number of protons in the nucleus of an atom of that element; this number is equal to the number of electrons around the nucleus. The *mass number* of an atom is the total number of protons and neutrons in the nucleus. It gives a measure of the mass of the nucleus. Protons and neutrons are known collectively as *nucleons* because they are found in the nucleus. The atomic number is written to the left and above the symbol for the element. For sulfur it is ^{32}S.

The radioactive isotopes now referred to as radionuclides occur as natural or artificial radionuclides. Most radioisotopes remain permanently unchanged. However, some isotopes, especially the heavy ones (which have many more neutrons than protons), are unstable. Their nuclei undergo a process of spontaneous readjustment or transformation with partial disintegration, so they change into isotopes of other elements. During this process they emit ionizing radiation, and this emission of radiation accompanying nuclear transformations is called *radioactivity*.

Naturally occurring radioactivity is found mostly in a few heavy elements, e.g., radium. However, it is now possible to produce artificial radioactive isotopes of all the chemical elements by subjecting them to bombardment by neutrons in the nuclear reactor or atomic furnace where atomic energy is produced. These radiations, whether from natural or artificial radioisotopes, are of three kinds, named after the first three letters of the Greek alphabet: alpha rays (or particles), beta rays (or particles), and gamma rays (electromagnetic energy).

Alpha particles are streams of high-speed helium nuclei (two protons and two neutrons packed tightly together) that have been ejected from radioactive substances.

Beta rays are streams of fast-moving electrons (particles) ejected from radioactive substances with velocities that may be as high as 0.98 of the velocity of light. In soft tissues beta rays can travel distances ranging from small fractions of a millimeter up to about 1 cm, producing ionization in their path.

Gamma rays come from radioactive substances. When they are produced by electrical machines we call them x-rays. They differ fundamentally from alpha and beta radiations in that they are not particles but waves similar to light and radiowaves but with different properties because of their much shorter wavelength.

Where does the beta particle arise? The beta particle is an electron. Because there are no electrons in the nucleus, how can a beta particle be emitted when the nucleus undergoes a process of spontaneous readjustment or transformation? The answer is that the beta particle comes from a neutron in the nucleus. Neutrons change into a proton and an electron, and the electron is then ejected from the nucleus. Emission of this electron or beta particle from the nucleus (beta decay) does not change the mass number (the total number of particles in the nucleus), but it does increase the atomic number by one: $P^{32} \rightarrow {}^{32}S + 1B^0$. To complete the picture, isotopes were found that emitted positively charged electrons or positrons. From where do the positrons come? The answer is that a positron is ejected: ${}^{52}Mn \rightarrow {}^{52}Cr + 1B^0$. Again the atomic mass remains the same, but because the proton is changed to a neutron there is loss of the proton, and the atomic number decreases by one (Fig. 20.2).

Any adjunctive therapy must be directed to the areas involved by ovarian cancer. This type of cancer spreads over the surface of organs and structures rather than infiltrating them early, as do so many other cancers. Ovarian cancer involves the right diaphragm as well as the paraaortic nodes in a high percentage of the patients studied. As much as 80% of the lymphatic drainage of the peritoneum is to the right thoracic trunk by way of the diaphragmatic lymphatics and the retrosternal nodes. On

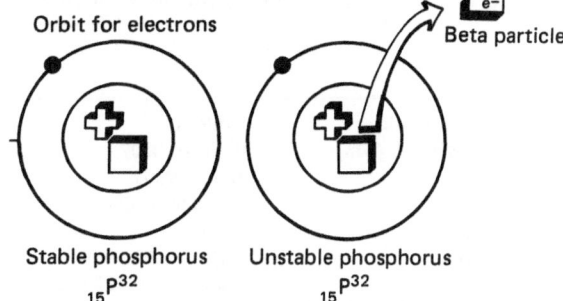

FIGURE 20.2. Beta rays are high-speed electrons that are ejected from the nucleus at speeds approaching the velocity of light rays.

Careful examination about 10 to 15% of stage I ovarian cancers that are encapsulated and unilateral, with no evidence of tumor elsewhere, are found to have metastases to the right diaphragm. Meyers injected radioactive material into the peritoneal cavity of humans and monitored its course. Ascent up the left paracolic gutter was found to be blocked by the left phrenicocolic ligament. Virtually all of the flow was found to progress to the right subhepatic and subphrenic spaces. Radionuclides instilled into the peritoneal cavity covered the serosal surfaces and the omentum, as well as being taken up by retroperitoneal nodes. In 1945 Müller first used radionuclides clinically for management of ovarian cancer. Radioactive zinc (${}^{63}Zn$) was first produced with the cyclotron in 1945 and was used to control malignant effusions. Radioactive gold (${}^{198}Au$) was introduced in 1947. Other isotopes, such as radioactive phosphate (${}^{32}P$) and yttrium (${}^{90}Y$), have been introduced. Currently only two radionuclides, gold and phosphate, are being used. Their characteristics are shown in Table 20.1. It often comes as a surprise that radioactive phosphate is more expensive than radioactive gold. The explanation is that neutrons produced by the fission of uranium 235 can be used to convert natural elements into artificial radioactive isotopes by so-called neutron capture. This method is the preferred way to produce radioactive cobalt 60, gold 198, iridium 192, and many other radioisotopes used in medicine. ${}^{32}P$, which is widely used for radiation therapy, cannot be produced in this simple way be-

TABLE 20.1. Commonly used radionuclides for treatment of ovarian cancer

Characteristic	Gold (^{198}Au)	Chromic phosphate ($Cr^{32}PO_4$)
Physical characteristics	Colloid	Suspension
Particle size MICRA (μm)	0.003–0.0007	0.5–1.5
Emission	Beta—90%	Beta—100%
	Gamma—10%	
Energy (kV)	1700	960
Maximum energy	Beta— 0.97 MeV	Beta—1.7 MeV
	Gamma—0.411 MeV	
Maximum path in tissue (mm)		
	4	4–6
Half-life (days)	2.7	14.3
Dose (mCi)	100–150	10–15
Cost	$64	$250
Side effects	Up to 30, including nausea, vomiting, ileus, temperature elevation, pain at the site of instillation; late dense adhesions and bowel necrosis	Rare
Radiation precautions	Yes, for at least 6.5 days	None

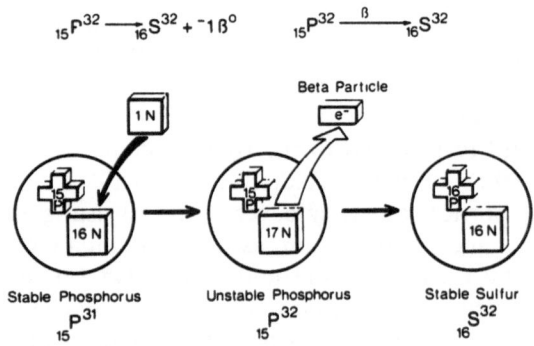

FIGURE 20.3. When stable phosphorus captures a neutron, the resulting nucleus has 17 neutrons, its energy has been raised to a higher level, and it is heavier by the addition of 1 mass unit. The atom is still phosphorus because as yet there has been no change in the number of protons. For this unstable phosphorus atom (phosphorus 32) to return to a stable state, it must eliminate one of its 17 neutrons, which is accomplished by converting one neutron into a proton with the formation of an electron e^-. The electron is ejected from the nucleus as a beta particle.

cause it requires an intermediate step: First, sulfur (^{32}S) is converted by neutron capture to ^{33}S. ^{33}S then decays to ^{32}P, which then must be chemically separated from the sulfur (Fig. 20.3).

Currently, the radionuclides gold and phosphate are most often used. Several important observations have been made following the instillation of these radionuclides.

1. Malignant effusions can be controlled in up to 80% of patients.
2. Little or no control of malignant effusions has been observed in patients with residual bulk disease.
3. Prophylactically, the instillation of radioactive substances has been found to improve survival results, especially with stage I ovarian cancer.
4. In the presence of multiple adhesions, the instillation of radionuclides is followed by a complication rate that offsets the benefit received.
5. In patients who have had external radiation therapy, the instillation of radionuclides increases the complication rate, especially in the gastrointestinal tract.

My experience with radioactive gold has been limited, but I have had considerable experience with radioactive phosphate. The reasons for selecting radiophosphorus was a direct result of the increased complications associated with radioactive gold. The initial complications with radioactive gold were minor and included nausea, vomiting, temperature elevation, and pain. It was the delayed complication rate that was disturbing. The adhesions that followed instillation of radioactive gold were dense. In addition, the serosa of the bowel was thickened and fibrosed, and the intestine often lost its pink color and appeared white. There were some late complications of bowel necrosis and fistula. Among patients treated by radioactive gold who required laparotomy for any reason, the complication rate, particularly of the gastrointestinal tract, was prohibitive. However, radioactive gold is still employed as an adjunctive therapy and is discussed.

Currently, Keetel and Buchsbaum have accumulated the largest experience with radioactive gold as an adjunctive therapy for localized ovarian cancer. In addition to the beta ray, which makes up 90% of the colloid, the gold also gives off a gamma ray. The usual dose of radiogold is 150 mCi instilled into the peritoneal cavity. It has been calculated that the serosa receives 4000 rad, the omentum 6000 rad, and the retroperitoneal nodes and mesenteric lymph nodes 7000 rads (maximum 10,000–30,000 rad). Spilling of activity into the reticuloendothelial system of the liver and spleen accounted for 130 and 250 rad, respectively, and the kidney received 30 rad. Approximately 750 rad of diffuse penetrating gamma radiation has been reported. Keetel found that the ultramicroscopic gold particles are picked up by the peritoneal macrophages and fixed to serosal surfaces. In addition, cells floating in the peritoneal cavity are subjected to a lethal dose of radiation.

The technique used for radioactive gold instillation into the peritoneal cavity was the same as that employed to instill radioactive phosphorus. This technique is described in detail, but first the technique employed by Buchsbaum and Keetel is described as reported by them. The technique is carried out as follows.

1. The patient is asked to void and is then sedated with intramuscular diazepam.
2. The abdomen is prepared with povidine-iodine and draped.
3. The abdominal wall is infiltrated with a local anesthetic, and a long polyethylene catheter is introduced into the peritoneal cavity over a trocar needle. A puncture site is selected that is away from previous scars.
4. After the needle is withdrawn, the catheter is attached to the infusion system. One infusion bottle contains a radiopaque contrast material in normal saline; the other bottle contains normal saline, which is used to flush the gold into the peritoneal cavity. A three-way stopcock controls the flow of liquid.
5. The catheter is fixed to the abdominal wall, and approximately 400 ml of saline with radiopaque medium is introduced into the peritoneal cavity. The distribution of the contrast material is monitored under fluoroscopy. Careful monitoring is necessary to ensure that the catheter tip is in the peritoneal cavity and not in the abdominal wall or the bowel lumen.
6. When contrast material is seen above the liver and in the pelvis, films are obtained.
7. Only after adequate distribution has been documented is the radioactive gold (150 mCi) introduced into the peritoneal cavity. An additional 600 ml of saline is instilled to create a hydroperitoneum.
8. The catheter is then removed, the puncture site sutured, and a collodion dressing applied.
9. In the past, Buchsbaum and Keetel had the patient change positions frequently to aid in the distribution of the isotope. Now they use an electrocircular bed, which allows the patient's position to be changed in a controlled fashion for the first 4 hours.
10. The patient is kept in the supine position, head down, and head up and then in the prone position, head down, head up, for 15 minutes each.
11. After 4 hours she is taken off the bed and housed in a controlled environment for the required 6.5 days.

The radionuclide ^{32}P is instilled after treatment for stage I and II ovarian cancer and for stage III when there is no detectable disease (when disease is limited to the omentum, which is removed, or only small scattered metastases are present). If the patient has had bowel pathology, marked adhesions, is elderly and in poor nutrition, or shows evidence of infection, it is in the best interest of the patient to withhold ^{32}P instillation.

The technique employed for ^{32}P instillation is now described.

1. The only equipment necessary in the operating room is a trocar and a small catheter (a baby-feeding tube), which is threaded through the trocar.
2. Just before the abdomen is closed, the trocar is taken from inside the abdominal incision and brought out in both the right and left lower quadrants. The trocar is passed above the external iliac artery and vein lateral to the psoas muscle to avoid injuring any vessel. Lateral to the epigastric vessels it is pushed through the peritoneum lateral to the rectus muscle and out through the skin. The trocar emerges above the inguinal ligament.
3. The stylet of the trocar is removed, and the small catheter (a baby-feeding tube) is threaded through the trocar and pulled into the abdomen.
4. The trocar is pulled back into the abdominal cavity and removed.
5. Some small extra holes are cut in the catheter, but the tip is left sealed, causing a "watering-can" effect when the ^{32}P is instilled through the tube.
6. The tube is placed high in the abdomen. On the right side it is placed above the liver, and on the left side it is brought high into the abdomen.
7. The skin around the catheter is then stitched in a fashion that resembles the lacing of an old-fashioned ankle-high shoe. The final stitch is left long so it can be tied after the radioactive substance has been instilled and the tube pulled out. This maneuver ensures that there is no leakage of radioactive material from the abdominal cavity.
8. The tubes are slowly withdrawn during the process of the ^{32}P instillation.

During the early part of the project radiopaque material was instilled into the peritoneal cavity to study the distribution. By observing the criteria established (reported above), it was found that the distribution was excellent.

Covington and Hilaris utilized ^{32}P scans for intracavitary distribution studies. Because ^{32}P is a pure beta emitter, the question is raised about its use as a screening agent. Bremsstrahlung x-ray (with energies from 0 to 1.7 MeV) is produced when electrons are slowed down passing by a positively charged nucleus of tissue atoms. Scans are produced by the Bremsstrahlung x-ray. When intracavitary doses (5–20 mCi) of ^{32}P chromic phosphate are used, enough Bremsstrahlung x-ray (about 1% of the total energy) is produced to make good scans, even in large patients. Covington and Hilaris reported that this fact was not appreciated in the past and probably accounts for the lack of use of ^{32}P scans for intracavitary distribution studies. The previous disappointing and poor results using ^{32}P as a scanning agent for detecting tumors were attributable to the small amount of isotope used (usually less than 0.5 mCi); this amount simply did not give off enough Bremsstrahlung x-rays to produce a diagnostic scan. The findings at Lenox Hill Hospital from my own studies agreed with those of Covington and Hilaris. The distribution was generally good when omentectomy was added to hysterectomy and bilateral salpingo-oophorectomy.

It is difficult to compare different series from the literature. However, our results with stage I ovarian cancer were approximately 90% successful when surgery plus ^{32}P comprised the treatment. In other series some form of radiation therapy was used in conjunction with radioisotopes. The combined use of ^{32}P and external x-ray therapy added to our complication rate, and the combination was discontinued. Clark and associates reported a 92.8% and Moore and Langley a 90% 5-year survival in patients treated with radioisotopes for stage I ovarian cancer.

Summary

Since 1955 ^{32}P has been the agent selected when intraperitoneal instillation is chosen for treatment of ovarian cancer and palliation of malignant ascites. Jones et al. developed a chemically inert colloid from ^{32}P in 1944. The advantages that led to the choice of ^{32}P over ^{198}Au were a higher beta energy (and therefore greater tissue penetration), a longer half-life, and absence of gamma radiation. The experience with intraabdominal ^{32}P has demonstrated minimal complications.

The dose of intraperitoneal ^{32}P was estimated from the empirical dose of ^{198}Au, a dose of 10 to 15 mCi of ^{32}P being thought to be equivalent to 100 to 150 mCi of ^{198}Au because of the longer half-life (14.3 days) and more energetic beta particles (0.69 MeV) of ^{32}P. Silver, Blahd, and Van den Brenk et al. have each made statements regarding the dose relations between ^{32}P and ^{198}Au. "The energy delivered by one mCi of chromic phosphate and 1 ml of a solution is about 885,000 rep or more than ten times that of the solution of colloidal gold of the same activity." "In comparison to ^{198}Au, chromic phosphate (^{32}P) has a greater penetration and greater destructive action per disintegration. One microcurie per gram of chromic phosphate ^{32}P will deliver 885 rads in contrast to 1 μCi of gold ^{198}Au, which will deliver 76 rads."

Furthermore, ^{32}P has a longer half-life than ^{198}Au, and its beta radiation is more energetic (and therefore more penetrating). Consideration of these physical properties means that, provided the material is not lost from the cavity, 10 mCi of chromium phosphate delivers approximately the same amount of radiation to the serous wall as 100 mCi of ^{198}Au. While arriving at these conclusions, it was assumed that ^{32}P remains confined to the peritoneal cavity and spreads uniformly over the serous surfaces. Thus the clinical value of a dose of ^{32}P based on these assumptions, and calculated from an initial empiric dose of ^{198}Au, must be viewed with skepticism and concern.

The role of radioactive isotopes in the management of ovarian cancer has not been established. The use of radionuclides for the management of patients with common epithelial ovarian cancer is controversial. Physicians charged with the responsibility of treating patients with ovarian cancer must make their own judgment about whether to include it in their therapy protocol. It is my opinion that it has been beneficial in stage I cancers of the ovary. Although it has been employed for stage II and III cancers where all gross disease has been removed, the survival results are not as dramatic as those reported for stage I. One of the interesting observations made in animals is that although ^{32}P does not seem to accumulate in the nodes in the pelvis or paraaortic area it has been shown to accumulate and destroy nodes in the mediastinum.

The origin of the beta rays and the characteristics of gold 198 and phosphate 32 are discussed. Such discussion is included as a review for those physicians using radionuclides.

Bibliography

Alderman SJ, Dillon TF, Krummerman MS, et al. Postoperative use of radioactive phosphorus in stage I ovarian carcinoma. *Obstet Gynecol* 49:659, 1977.

Aure JC, Hoeg K, Kolstad P: Radioactive colloidal gold in the treatment of ovarian carcinoma. *Acta Radiol [Ther.]* (Stockh) 10:399, 1971.

Bagely CM Jr, Young RC, Schein PS, et al: Ovarian carcinoma metastatic to the diaphragm—frequently undiagnosed at laparotomy: a preliminary report. *Am J Obstet Gynecol* 116:397, 1973.

Blahd WH: *Nuclear Medicine.* McGraw-Hill, New York, 1965.

Buchsbaum HJ, Keetel WC, Lataurette HB: The use of radioisotope as adjunct therapy of localized ovarian cancer. *Semin Oncol* 2:247, 1975.

Clark DGC, Hilaris B, Ochoa M: Treatment of cancer of the ovary. *Clin Obstet Gynecol* 3:150, 1976.

Clark DGC, Hilaris B, Roussis C, et al: The role of radiation therapy (including isotopes) in the treatment of cancer of the ovary (results of 614 patients treated at Memorial Hospital, New York). *Prog Clin Cancer* 5:227, 1973.

Covington E, Hilaris B: ^{32}P scans for intracavitary studies. *Am J Roentgenol Radium Ther Nucl Med* 118:895, 1973.

Decker DG, Webb MJ, Holbrook MA: Radiogold treatment of epithelial cancer of ovary: late results. *Am J Obstet Gynecol* 115:751, 1973.

Feldman GB, Knapp RC: Lymphatic drainage of the peritoneal cavity and its significance in ovarian cancer. *Am J Obstet Gynecol* 119:991, 1974.

Fleay RF: Dosimetry in the use of colloidal isotopes. *Australas Radiol* 15:388, 1971.

Heildelberg JG, Sirota PG, Dewey WC, Rose RG:

Determination of the distribution of P^{32} in phantoms and in patients by detection of bremsstrahlung radiation with a scintiscanner. *AJR* 90: 325, 1963.

Hester LL, White L: Radioactive colloidal chromic phosphate in the treatment of ovarian malignancies. *Am J Obstet Gynecol* 103:911, 1969.

Horowitz DA: Technique of intraperitoneal instillation of radioactive colloids. *Obstet Gynecol* 42:621, 1973.

Jones HB, Wrobei CJ, Lyons WR: A method of distributing beta-radiation to the reticulo-endothelial system and adjacent tissue. *J Clin Invest* 28:783, 1944.

Keetel WC, Fox MR, Longnecker DS, Latourette HB: Prophylactic use of radioactive gold in the treatment of primary ovarian cancer. *Am J Obstet Gynecol* 94:766, 1966.

Meyers MA: The spread and localization of acute intraperitoneal effusions. *Radiology* 95:547, 1970.

Moore DW, Langley JH: Routine use of radiogold following operation for ovarian cancer. *Am J Obstet Gynecol* 98:624, 1967.

Morton ME: Colloidal chromate radiophosphate in high yields for radiotherapy. *Nucleonics* 92:96, 1952.

Müller JH: Curative aim and results of routine intraperitoneal radiocolloid administration in the treatment of ovarian cancer. *Am J Roentgenol Radium Ther Nucl Med* 89:533, 1963.

Priver MS: Radioactive colloids in the treatment of stage Ia ovarian cancer. *Obstet Gynecol* 40:42, 1972.

Reid GW, Watson ER, Chester MS: A note on the distribution of radioactive colloidal gold following intraperitoneal injection. *Br J Radiol* 34:323, 1961.

Rosenshein NB: Radioisotopes in the treatment of ovarian cancer. *Clin Obstet Gynaecol* 10:279, 1983.

Rosenshein NB, Lickner PK, Vogelsang G: Radiocolloids in the treatment of ovarian cancer. *Obstet Gynecol Surv* 34(suppl):708, 1979.

Selman J: *The Basic Physics of Radiation Therapy*. Charles C Thomas, Springfield, IL, 1960.

Silver S: *Radioactive Isotopes in Medicine and Biology*. Lea & Febiger, Philadelphia, 1962.

Van den Brenk HAS, Clarke KH, Holman WP, Winkler C: Studies of the effect of colloidal radioactive chromic phosphate $Cr^{32}PO$, in clinical and experimental malignant effusions. *Br J Cancer* 13:181, 1969.

Veder M, Deland FH, Maruyama Y: Loculation as a contraindication to intracavitary P^{32} chromic phosphate therapy. *J Nucl Med* 17:150, 1976.

21

Role of Chemotherapy in Ovarian Cancer

The pessimism and frustration that exist regarding the treatment of patients with ovarian cancer were well stated by Lewis and Blessing when they observed: "For ovarian cancer seemingly everything works, but practically nothing succeeds." The despair and cynicism reflected in this statement seems justified when reports appear telling of improved therapeutic approaches but statistical mortality rates showing little trend toward improvement at 5 years. Carcinoma of the ovary remains the leading cause of death due to gynecologic cancer, and the results for 1991 were no better than for the previous two decades. New modalities of therapy are helping patients live longer and hopefully more comfortably, but the 5-year-survival rates have not improved.

In contrast to surgery plus irradiation (considered to be the definitive therapy for cancer), chemotherapy—the treatment of cancer with drugs and hormones—can be used effectively for disseminated as well as localized cancer. Chemotherapy has become a reality only since the 1960s. In 1945 nitrogen mustard was found to be effective against lymphomas. Each of the three decades since then has seen important advances in the number of compounds available and in the spectrum of their usefulness. Since that time many drugs have been added to the therapeutic armamentarium. During the 1980s it became clear that, although chemotherapy had long been considered largely a palliative procedure capable of extending but not saving lives, certain kinds of cancer can now be cured by anticancer drug therapy

(chemical treatment). A major goal of current cancer chemotherapy is to achieve cures by prompt, vigorous treatment of such cancers. Combinations of antineoplastic drugs have been used with success, particularly when each drug used acts on the cancer cell in a different way. Progress has been made by using multiple drugs simultaneously as well as in sequence. In patients whose cancers are limited to a bodily region that has an accessible, separate blood supply, the introduction of chemotherapeutic agents into an artery that supplies the cancer tissue has provided substantial benefits.

Certain cancers can be cured by chemotherapy. Chemotherapy now constitutes a major, indispensable therapeutic approach capable of producing cures of particular widespread cancers. Among those cancers responding to chemotherapy are choriocarcinoma, metastatic hydatidiform mole, Burkitt's tumor, acute lymphatic leukemia of children, Hodgkin's disease, embryonal carcinoma of the testis, embryonal carcinoma of the ovary, extraembryonal carcinoma of the ovary, adenocarcinomas of the uterine corpus, and carcinomas in the superficial layers of the skin. Chemotherapy has provided therapeutic benefits but not cures of a number of other types of cancer. Chronic myelocytic leukemia and chronic lymphocytic leukemia, lymphosarcoma, reticulum cell sarcoma, multiple myeloma, polycythemia vera, mycosis fungoides, malignant melanoma, Wilms' tumor, and neuroblastoma are other forms of cancer in which palliation and clinical improvement can be achieved by chemotherapy; and for those patients with disseminated disease, chemotherapy is the preferred means of treatment.

In addition, several types of carcinoma are significantly benefited by anticancer drug therapy. Clinical improvement and significant palliation occur, but long-term freedom from the disease has not been observed in any appreciable fraction of the patients. Carcinomas of the breast, large intestine, stomach, pancreas, prostate, epithelium of the head and neck, thyroid, ovary, and adrenal gland are all subject to palliation in a proportion of the patients when the appropriate anticancer chemotherapeutic drugs are used. The drug regimens differ widely for the cancers mentioned.

With some cancers the effects of the anticancer drugs that have been used so far have been notably unpredictable. Although the tumors may show some response and decrease in size, major clinical benefit has not ordinarily accompanied this regression in patients with carcinomas of the lung, cervix, kidney, or bladder.

Structure of the Cell

Cancer is a disease of the cell. Structures within the cell are visible with the electron microscope. The important structures that have been identified and whose functions have been studied are briefly outlined.

The *nucleus* contains the master chemical deoxyribonucleic acid (DNA) in the chromosomes; the *nucleolus*, found in the nucleus, is considered the storehouse of DNA as well as the transport mechanism for messenger RNA (mRNA). The *cytoplasm* contains the protein-making sites or ribosomes. The *endoplasmic reticulum* is the network to which the ribosomes adhere. *Mitochondria* are the site of energy metabolism and probably produce a limited amount of protein. The *Golgi complex* is thought to play a key role in intracellular synthesis and mobilization of certain proteins and carbohydrate components. The *plasma membrane* is a complex structure through which materials pass in and out of the cell. Plasma membrane is the area of contact between a cell with its neighbors; it permits the passage of ions and molecules, influences the

movement of the cell, and probably plays an important role in controlling growth.

Of all the cell parts that theoretically may become transformed in malignancy, the cell surface is currently the most suspect. Changes in the cell surface control the uptake and release of material from the cell as well as controlling adhesiveness and cohesiveness. These properties may influence invasion and metastasis. It is not surprising that cell surface transplantation antigens are altered in malignancy. Although such tumor-specific antigens are not confined to the surface, it is on the surface of the intact cell that they are most readily detected. The tumor-specific transplantation antigens (TSTA) present on the cell surface are responsible for and sensitive to the immune response in the host, which may result in tumor destruction.

Cell Kinetics or Cell Division

Cellular reproduction (cell division cycle or cell kinetics) is divided into five phases: (1) *growth 1* (G1), which is postmitotic and takes up at least one-half the life cycle of the cell; (2) *synthesis* (S), in which the DNA content is doubled and takes up about 29 to 30% of the life cycle of the cell; (3) *growth 2* (G2), which occurs just before mitosis and takes up about 19 to 20% of the life cycle of the cell; (4) *mitosis* (M), which takes up about 1% of the cell cycle; and (5) *growth 0* (G0), the resting or nondividing phase of the cell. This phase is variable and depends on the type of cancer.

Studies of cell kinetics reveal that certain anticancer drugs have a more predictable effect on different phases of the cell. The alkylating agents attack cells in all phases of the division cycle; antimetabolites attack the cell during the S phase, as does actinomycin D. Vincristine is a mitotic inhibitor and works best during the late G2 phase. Bleomycin has its most significant effect during the G2 phase. The cell is relatively resistant to attack by the anticancer drugs during the resting (G0) phase. Many cells in a tumor population are at one time or another in G0, are at rest, and do not divide until some stimulus triggers the mitotic mechanisms of cell division. Therefore, ac-

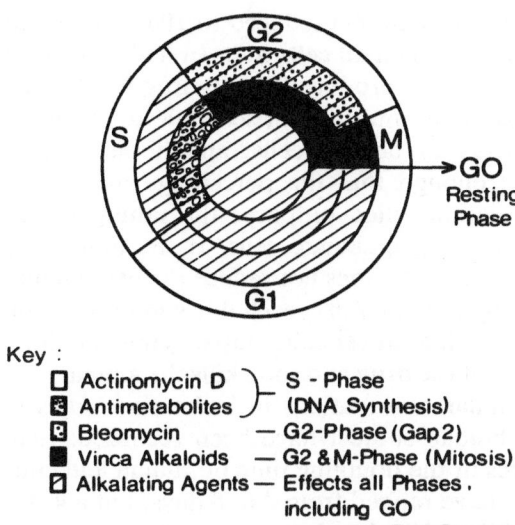

Key :

☐ Actinomycin D ⎤ S - Phase
☒ Antimetabolites ⎦ (DNA Synthesis)
▣ Bleomycin   — G2-Phase (Gap 2)
■ Vinca Alkaloids — G2 & M-Phase (Mitosis)
▨ Alkalating Agents — Effects all Phases ,
                       including GO
                       cross-link DNA Strands

FIGURE 21.1. Cell division phases and the phase of
the cell cycle in which anticancer drugs function.

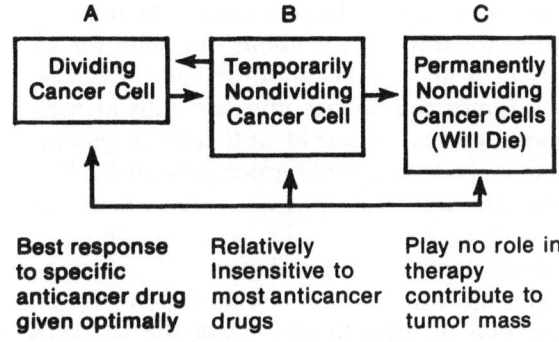

Antineoplastic Chemotherapy Response

FIGURE 21.2. Conceptual model of types of cell
growth in a tumor. It is the basic mechanism of cell
vulnerability to anticancer drug therapy.

cording to the nature of the cytotoxic agent,
cells in the G0 stage are not susceptible to the
drug's action. The reserve compartment of the
hematopoietic system consists of cells during
G0. Most of the drugs now used to treat cancer
have little effect during the G0 phase. Approximately 40 to 80% of the marrow stem cells are
in G0 at any given time. When chemotherapeutic agents cause a decrease in the white
blood cell count, the resting marrow cells temporarily enter the cell cycle and proliferate
rapidly (Fig. 21.1).

Three kinds of cells are theoretically present
in a tumor, as shown in Figure 21.2. The cells
in group A are growing logarithmically and are
sensitive to the best drugs when optimally used
regardless of their mechanisms of action. The
cells in group B have temporarily stopped
dividing and are partially or incompletely insensitive to drugs. They are in G0 or prolonged
G1 and can revert to compartment A. Com-
partments A and B are interchangeable, but
cells in either or both can enter compartment
C. The cells in group C are permanently not
dividing, are not sensitive to drugs, and are no
longer of concern to the chemotherapist. They
are destined ultimately to die. They are of concern to the patient because they contribute to

the tumor mass. Cells in group C never enter
compartment A or B (Fig. 21.2).

One of the principles of modern anticancer
chemotherapy is the use of drugs in relation to
the cell cycle (cell kinetics) in order to ensure
maximum therapeutic response and minimum
toxicity. Currently, no single treatment,
whether with one or several drugs, eliminates
all the tumor cells of a neoplasm. Nevertheless,
the anticancer drugs reduce a constant percentage of tumor cells. This reduction, which is
constant, is in accordance with the first order of
kinetics representing its peculiar rate of reduction. Applying this principle, it is just as easy to
reduce 1,000,000 cancer cells to 10,000 as it is
to reduce 100 cancer cells to 1. Both situations
represent a 99% reduction. The ultimate goal
of cancer chemotherapy is to eradicate the last
cancer cell, which is theoretically possible with
constant chemotherapy. General toxicity,
however, is a limiting factor. Cancer cells may
eventually become resistant to the drugs as a
result of selection from a mixed cell population. This resistance has been shown to result
from the loss of activating enzymes, the induction of synthetic enzymes, or an increase in repair processes. Resistance can be minimized by
the use of suitable drug combinations.

Cancer cell population studies have concluded that each tumor cell divides into two
cells once each *generation time*, that is, the

time for one entire division cycle. The time required for this cycle is about the same for all cells in a given population of cells. Because each tumor cell divides into two cells at each generation time, it is evident that by 10 generations a single cell proliferates into 1000 (10^3) cells. Therefore the growth of many cells following this pattern results in a thousand-fold increase every ten generations.

This growth pattern is referred to as exponential or logarithmic. When the log cells are charted against time, the pattern is a smooth curve. It is possible to gain insight into the effects of drugs on cancerous and normal cells by comparing the growth characteristics of each type. In order to be detected, a tumor must have a volume of at least 1 cc ($1 \times 1 \times 1$ cm) consisting of about 10^9 (one billion) cells. The volume of cells necessary to kill a patient (critical volume) is 1000 cc ($10 \times 10 \times 10$ cm), or about 10^{12} (one trillion) cells. Because these values are 1000-fold (10^3) apart, their separation in time represents ten generations of growth.

Currently, well-prescribed anticancer chemotherapy can reduce the population of lymphocytic leukemia cells from 10^{12} to 10^6 in acute lymphocytic leukemia of childhood. Although the patient is not cured at this point, the disease is in remission. The goal of anticancer chemotherapy is to reduce the last million cells (10^6) to zero. It is accepted that 100% cell kill of leukemic cells is necessary to achieve cure. This assumption is based on work with the mouse leukemic cell. A single leukemia cell implanted into a mouse can multiply and eventually cause the death of the animal. The mouse leukemic cell reproduces in about 12 hours. After an interval of 20 days, one cell can multiply to approximately one billion cells, which is enough to kill the mouse. Because one cell can rapidly become a lethal number of cells, it is probably necessary to kill every leukemia cell to achieve a cure.

Studies have shown that a given dose of drug kills the same percentage of cells, no matter how many are present. For example, the same dose can kill 99% of 100 cells, whichever number of leukemic cells is present in the animal. Therefore 1,000,000 cells can be reduced to

10,000, and 10,000 reduced to 100, and 100 to 10 or less, then 10 cells to 0. In leukemic mice cures can be produced if the drug is administered on an intermittent schedule to allow for recovery of normal cells, and if the dose is large enough that the percentage of the cell population killed outpaces the multiplication of surviving leukemic cells. If the anticancer chemotherapy does not reduce the cell population by at least 75%, each day's multiplication of surviving cancer cells outpaces the inhibiting effect of the drug and soon kills the animal.

Similar observations in leukemia studies in the human subject have been recorded. Estimates of the doubling time of human leukemic cells have ranged from 2 to 8 days, but a 4-day doubling time has been more often assumed. Further calculations indicate that it takes about 160 to 170 days for one cell doubling every 4 days to reach one trillion cells, the number considered lethal for man.

Difference Between Cancer Growth and Normal Tissue Growth

All living things have an inherent capacity to multiply, and they cease multiplication for a variety of reasons. In humans, a cellular brake is required to prevent overgrowth for the benefit of the community of cells. In vitro this mechanism appears to be controlled by an unknown feedback mechanism, probably result-

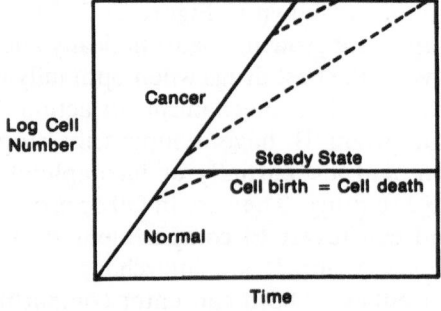

FIGURE 21.3. Lethal number of cells: gompertzian curve. During the early phases of growth, tumor cells grow exponentially; but as the tumor mass increases the time it takes to double its volume increases.

ing from contact phenomena when cells are crowded.

With cancerous growth, cells no longer cease multiplying when they reach a critical mass, and the uncontrolled growth leads to death of the host. During the early phases of growth, tumor cells grow exponentially, but as the tumor mass increases the time it takes a tumor to double its volume increases. This situation is best described as a *gompertzian function*. It is likely that the doubling time is somehow related to crowding and loss of nutrient supply (Fig. 21.3).

Skipper Model or Hypothesis

Survival of animals is related inversely to either the number of cells inoculated or the number remaining after therapy.

1. A single leukemia (or cancer) cell is capable of multiplying and killing the host.
2. A given drug kills a constant fraction (percentage) of cells, not a constant number, regardless of the number of cells present at the onset of therapy.
3. Drug dose and the ability to eradicate cells are related.
4. *Conclusion*: Improved results would occur if therapy is started before the tumor volume is overwhelming.

Commonly Used Criteria for Objective Response and Disease Progression in Solid Tumors

Complete response: complete disappearance of all demonstrable disease

Partial response: at least 50% reduction in the sum of the products of the longest perpendicular diameters of discrete measurable disease, with no demonstrable disease progression elsewhere

No response: no change in the size of any measurable lesion or less than 50% reduction of measurable disease as defined above

Progression: more than 50% increase in the sum of the products of the larger perpendicular diameter of any measurable lesion

The term "cure" indicates that the life expectancy of the treated cancer patient is the same as normal life expectancy, specifically, the same as that of a matched cohort in the general population. When doses are expressed in milligrams per kilogram (mg/kg), the following formula can be used to convert roughly to milligrams per square meter (mg/m^2): mg/kg $\times$ 40 = mg/m^2. Depending on the drug, there may be an upper limit to the single dose given to patients weighing more than 70 kg.

Response Criteria: Measurability of Disease

The following categories regarding response criteria are recognized.

1. *Measurable, dimensional*: The malignant disease is measurable (metric system) in two dimensions by a ruler or calipers; surface area is determined by multiplying the longest diameter by the greatest perpendicular diameter (i.e., metastatic pulmonary nodules, lymph nodes, and subcutaneous masses). Institutions performing life-size liver scans may use clearly defined biopsy-proved malignant hepatic nodules measuring more than 5 cm in diameter as measurable disease.
2. *Measurable, unidimensional*: The malignant disease is measurable (metric system) in one dimension by ruler or calipers (i.e., mediastinal adenopathy, malignant hepatomegaly, or abdominal masses). Malignant hepatomegaly may be measured if the liver descends 5 cm below the costal margin by adding the measurements below the costal margins in the midclavicular line and the tip of the xiphoid. Measurements below the costal margin should be made in the midclavicular lines during quiet respiration.
3. *Nonmeasurable, evaluable*: The malignant disease is evident on clinical (physical or radiographic) examination, but it is not measurable by ruler or calipers (i.e., pelvic and abdominal masses, lymphangiotic or confluent multinodular lung metastases, skin metastases). When applicable, photographs (including identification, date, and scale) should be taken before and during therapy to document response (i.e., skin and subcutaneous metastases, inflammatory

breast cancer, intraoral lesions, recurrent rectal cancer). Chemical values and pathologic markers should be measured during therapy but are not used to evaluate response.

Determination of Overall Response

Progression at any site indicates disease progression, despite objective responses at other sites. If the organ's site responses are greater than known change designations, the overall response is partial. If there is no change of the evaluable disease, it does not detract from the complete or partial response at measurable sites, but the patient's overall response is still only partial.

Duration of Response

The period of complete response should last from the date the complete response was first noted to the date progressive disease was first noted. For those who achieve only partial response, only the period of overall response lasts from the first day of treatment to the date of first observation of progressive disease.

Date of First Recurrence

The date of first recurrence should be based on the onset of a sign. The date of first detection of a palpable lesion is acceptable only when the diagnosis of tumor involvement is subsequently established. The diagnosis of recurrent disease by roentgenography or scanning should be dated from the first positive record, even if determined in retrospect. Time to recurrence or death is measured from the first day of therapy. These data should be recorded by those responsible for the care of the patient. The dates of first recurrence, relapse, metastases, and death should be confirmed by an independent reviewer whenever possible. Data based on suspicion alone should be reviewed to establish their accuracy.

Diagnosis of Recurrence

One or more of the following must be positive for a diagnosis of recurrent disease to be acceptable: histology or cytology; progression

of lesion originally considered suspicious only; response of lesion to specific therapy; autopsy.

Chemosensitivity Testing

Chemosensitivity testing is carried out in patients with malignancies in order to improve therapy by means of individual (selective) cytotoxic chemotherapy. A bioassay technique offers the promise of facilitating drug selection for cancer chemotherapy. This technique may be described as a quantitation of differential sensitivity of human tumor stem cells to anticancer drugs. When evaluating the technique the evaluator should expect no more than is achievable with studies of sensitivity of bacteria and antibiotics. The current definition of sensitivity in most reports is an operational one. However, it has been shown that there is a fairly high correlation between in vivo and in vitro sensitivity responses.

Various test methods and evaluation procedures have been developed for the purpose of chemosensitivity testing. A distinction can be made among long-term culture methods (i.e., more than 30 hours), short-term culture methods (i.e., less than 30 hours), and those that require less than 3 hours. The in vitro and in vivo correlations attained so far provide promise for an additional method of predicting response to a given anticancer drug.

In the 1978 report of Salmon et al., drug sensitivity testing was noted to take 2 to 3 weeks. The authors reported that the assay may be helpful for identifying drugs that might otherwise not be considered for therapeutic trial. With new testing, the answer can be obtained in a much shorter time. Salmon and colleagues reported that in many assays a "plateau" phenomenon occurred in which increasing lethality was not observed above a relatively low dosage level. For cycle-nonspecific drugs, such as the alkylating agents, the plateau is thought to reflect the fraction of drug-resistant cells present in the sample. Because many of their patients were clinically resistant to alkylating agents, this explanation seemed reasonable. For drugs active only on proliferating stem cells (i.e., vinblastine and methotrexate), the plateau effects may be due to the presence of a proportion of tumor stem cells that were not cycling during the period of in vitro drug exposure. This possibility will undoubtedly be clarified with extended drug incubation.

Salmon et al. reported that logistics and time constraints of this assay may present major problems. Thus far they have focused attention on the study of accessible cancers that can be readily converted to single cell suspensions containing a sufficient number of viable tumor stem cells. The number of drugs and the variations in duration of drug exposure are limited to some extent by the amount of tumor available and relatively low cloning efficiency. Although the cloning efficiency of human tumor cells is low, it is comparable to that observed in normal human bone marrow granulocytic and erythroid progenitors in vitro. It is important to emphasize that the responsible physician must work with a single cell suspension containing a sufficient number of viable tumor stem cells.

Currently, clinicians rely on their experience or choose well-proved therapy regimens of the recently reported prospective randomized therapy studies. However, test systems are being developed and are available for predictive tests. The methodology for sensitivity testing for cancer chemotherapy includes in vitro and in vivo methods and models. The in vitro methods (long term and short term) include monolayer cultures, organ cultures, free-floating slices cultures, single cell suspension, and fragment cultures. The in vivo models include cultivation in animals (fusion chambers) and heterotransplantation (immunologically deprived animals, nude mice, or rats).

Evaluating test samples requires experience. To be able to detect effects of cytotoxic substances on tissues or cells, the following possibilities are available: (1) morphologic evaluation; (2) cell count; (3) enzyme assays; (4) tracer incorporation studies, such as autoradiography; and (5) radioactive biochemical methods. It must be pointed out at this time that clinical problems cannot be simulated exactly with animal transplantation tumors.

A further limiting factor for all pretherapeutic tests is the unknown reaction of the organism to a given chemotherapy. It may include the vascularity of the tumor, the amount of necrosis, the type of cell present, and the patient's own metabolic status. The success of a chemotherapeutic agent depends mainly on the effects of the drug used on the tumor cells and on the host cell as well. The action of cytotoxic drugs on hematopoiesis is mostly the limiting factor when establishing dose levels of drugs. Some suggest determination of the therapeutic index. The chemosensitivity of tumor cells is determined at the same time as the reaction of bone marrow cells to cytostatic agents in the same patient. It can be concluded that if the cells of the bone marrow react more strongly than tumor cells the side effects are going to be greater than the benefits of therapy, which offers a prognostic value for a pretherapeutic test. However, when comparing the rate of uptake of label by tumor systems and the bone marrow systems, it may well be that it is the relative rate of division of the two cell systems that is being tested, not the drug resistance of the tumor.

The disadvantage for all methods remains the heterogeneity of cell populations in human tumors, so it is not known if the pretherapeutic investigations are taking place in cells that are representative of the respective tumor. There are methods that give a predominance of stem cells. Therefore the goal of further efforts must be to develop better methods of preparation, adequate cell preparation, and identification methodology to obtain as many representative and viable tumor cells as possible.

Certain criteria are necessary for routine clinical use. A predictable test should be (1) available in a short time, (2) simple, (3) well producible, and (4) as inexpensive as possible. The results can now be available after 8 to 10 hours. However, with monolayer and organ cultures a few days are required for evaluation; with tumor colony assays it is 2 to 3 weeks; and with the in vivo test models it is several months. Evaluation by means of autoradiography likewise requires several days. Rapid advances are being made in the field of chemosensitivity assays, which promise a method for facilitating drug selection for a given tumor. However, it must be emphasized that the clinician should expect no more from this procedure than is achievable with studies of sensitivity of bacteria and antibiotics. Optimally, drugs that are active in vitro may also be active in vivo, and a maximum cytotoxic concentration can be predicted.

Flow Cytometry

Flow cytometry has quickly moved from the laboratory to being a clinical tool. It is beginning to play a significant role in the study of DNA content in cells. The question now asked is: Will the expanded use of flow cytometry in oncology render clonogenic assays obsolete?

By plotting a frequency distribution of fluorescence intensity, the relative DNA content of cells can be displayed, and the relative number of cells in each phase of the cell cycle can be determined. DNA analysis can help determine the best time to administer chemotherapy. By staining bone marrow cells with a DNA stain, the percent of abnormal cells in S phase can be monitored. An appropriate schedule can be determined to administer the S phase-specific drug, maximizing the kill of only abnormal S phase cells.

To verify the long-term success of treatment, DNA analysis can monitor effects of chemotherapy by determining the relative number of cells in a tumor population at regular intervals. Aneuploid cell populations in each phase of the cell cycle can be identified. These cells, containing an abnormal amount of DNA, appear as separate populations on a DNA histogram, which provides verification of the tumor populations present.

Flow cytometry also has the ability to measure the DNA content of individual chromosomes and sort them for further study. This method provides a quick, relatively easy, accurate method for performing "flow karyotyping." Numerous studies have been reported on its use as a research and clinical method to monitor the treatment of ovarian carcinoma.

DNA Histogram

The flow cytometer efficiently and accurately analyzes a large number of cells from tissue samples and generates a frequency histogram that provides the following information.

The DNA Index (DI) provides a measure of DNA content of the cell. A normal diploid cell has a index of 1.0 and a tetraploid cell has a index of 2.0. Abnormal DNA content (aneuploidy) is frequently associated with tumors and correlates with poor prognosis. These tumors are usually poorly differentiated and steroid-receptor negative.

The percentage of cells in S-phase in the tumor indicates the number of cells actively synthesizing DNA. It measures the proportion of cells in the proliferative phase of the cell cycle (S, G_2, and M phases). It is often referred to as the S-phase fraction or cell cycle distribution (CCD). A high S-phase fraction indicates a poorly differentiated and aneuploid tumor likely to be ER-negative and PR-negative. A value is high if percentage of S is >10.0

Cycling index (CI) measures the rate of cellular proliferation and thus tumor activity. CI distinguishes G_0 (resting cells) from S, G_2, M, and G_1 phases of the cell cycle. It may be reported as Cell Proliferative Index (CPI). Recurrence is significantly more frequent with more active tumors having high proliferative rate, regardless of stage.

Aggressive tumors have a higher proportion of mitotically active cells. Cells with lower proliferative activity are associated with a more favorable prognosis. KI-67 is a cell proliferation market used to determine tumors that are mitotically active. When elevated, studies suggest that it is an indicator of poor patient prognosis.

The cycling index (CI) or Synthesis index (SI) is abnormal when the high S-phase cycling cells is >6.0%.

Multidrug Resistance in Cancer Patients

An ancient pump protein that flushes toxins out of cells may be to blame if cancer therapy fails. The question that is asked repeatedly is why chemotherapy eventually fails when at first it appeared to be so successful. Why are some cancers curable by chemotherapy alone, whereas others are unaffected by drugs and are apparently incurable? These questions are not new. Indeed, the resistance of parasites and infectious-disease organisms to antibiotics is as old as chemotherapy itself. German chemist Paul Ehrlich, the "father of chemotherapy," had envisioned magic bullet drugs that would cure many of the diseases that plague mankind, but after decades of experience with antimicrobial drugs he stated that drug resistance had followed the development of new drugs like a faithful shadow.

Cancer chemotherapy has its roots in antimicrobial chemotherapy that had been under development since the turn of the century, and therefore clinical resistance to anticancer chemotherapeutic drugs was not entirely unexpected. Work prior to World War II showed that tumors transplanted into mice were capable of developing pervasive resistance to experimental drugs. Since then experimental tumors resistant to every class of anticancer drugs have been isolated. All organisms, including cells within the cancer patient's tumor, seem to have the capacity to become resistant to drugs that would otherwise kill them.

The multiple-drug resistance concept had two theories proposed to explain it. One theory proposed that a permeability barrier prevents drug entry into the cells. The other suggested that an efflux pump, a mechanism that actively pumps drugs out of the cell once they get inside, is at work in the resistant cell. The latter model was based on observations of the kinetics of drug flow into and out of B cells. It was found that when a resistant cell was temporarily poisoned with cyanide to inhibit energy production the cell behaved like a drug-sensitive one: It could not keep out the drug. When the cyanide was washed out and normal metabolism restored, the cell could once again exclude the drug. Furthermore, the cell was then able to pump out the drug that had accumulated while it was poisoned. An instant energy-dependent drug-efflux pump seemed to be the simplest explanation.

It was shown that P-glycoprotein resides in the cell membrane, and it may act to pump toxins out of the cell. The protein chain appears to snake back and forth 12 times across the lipid by a layer of the membrane, forming a 12-sided pore. The part of the protein outside the cell bears sugar chains; two large, nearly identical domains protrude into the cell. They include regions that bind the cellular energy carrying compound ATP, which probably produces the energy that drives the efflux.

Multidrug resistance enables a cell to withstand the effects of toxic molecules that vary in size, structure, and site of action in the cell. A common anticancer drug acts in the nucleus of drug-sensitive cells, interfering with the cell transcription of DNA and its synthesis during cell division. When resistance develops, it could be either a passive barrier or an active pump in the cell membrane that explains the simultaneous resistance to a variety of anticancer agents. The monoclonal antibody research tool for the detection of P-glycoprotein, a determinant of multidrug resistance, has been isolated and was found to be amplified in many cases of multiple drug resistance. P-glycoprotein has been found to confer drug resistance by serving as a pump actively removing drugs from the cell. Drug resistance may be partially blocked by calcium channel blockers, such as verapamil, which binds to P-glycoproteins. P-glycoprotein is present in numerous cell lines selected from multidrug resistance in vitro. During clinical investigations, P-glycoprotein has been found in: (1) ovarian cancer ascites cells; (2) acute nonlymphoblastic leukemia; (3) breast cancer; and (4) colon cancer. Research is currently being conducted to determine if P-glycoprotein serves as a prognostic indicator for response to chemotherapy. To date it is of interest as an early warning of developing resistance, allowing the oncologist to redirect therapy.

The principal groups of anticancer drugs used in practice are outlined in the following sections.

Antimetabolites: Folic Acid Antagonists

A. Chemistry
   1. Derivatives of folic acid
   2. Component parts of the folic acid molecule
      a. Plexidine nucleus
      b. *p*-Aminobenzoic acid
      c. Glutamic acid
   3. Folinic acid is the formyl-containing

Formation

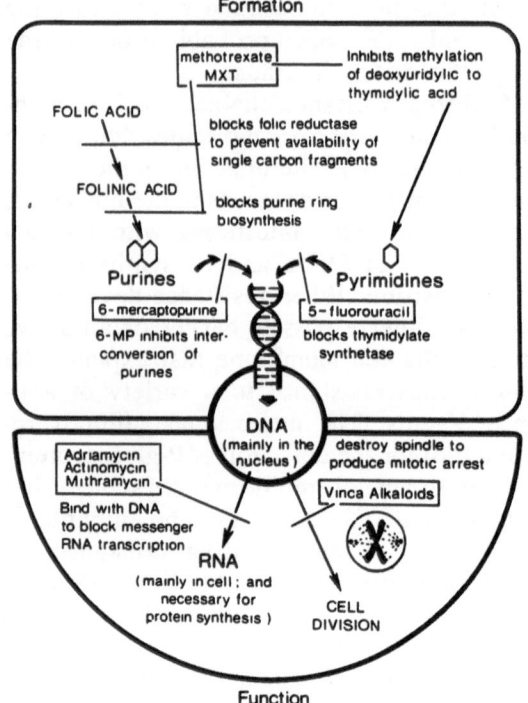

FIGURE 21.4. Mechanism of action of anticancer drugs at the cellular level.

analogue of reduced folic acid. It is called synthetic citrovorum factor of leucovorin.

B. Mechanism of action
1. Blocks folic acid reductase to prevent availability of single carbon fragment; which blocks purine ring biosynthesis (Fig. 21.4).
2. By a lesser action it inhibits methylation of deoxyuridylic acid to thymidylic acid, blocking pyrimidine synthesis.

C. Toxicity
1. Mouth lesions
2. Ulceration of the gastrointestinal tract
3. Bone marrow depression
4. Susceptibility to infection
5. Alopecia
6. Hyperpigmentation
7. Teratogenic properties

D. Method of administration and dosage
4-Amino-N^{10}-methyl-pteroylglutamic

acid, amethopterin, methotrexate: 2.5–5.0 mg/day PO or 5–25 mg/day IV or IM for 5 days

E. Uses
1. Choriocarcinoma
2. Cancer of the ovary
3. Cancer of the breast
4. Cancer of the cervix (in combination with other anticancer drugs)

Purine Antimetabolites

A. Chemistry
6-Mercaptopurine
B. Mechanism of action
1. Blocks purine ring biosynthesis
2. Inhibits interconversion of purines
C. Toxicity
1. Leukopenia
2. Thrombocytopenia
3. Stomatitis
4. Nausea and vomiting
D. Method of Administration
Usual dose: 2.0–2.5 mg/kg/day PO or 500 mg/m^2/day IV for 5 days every 10–14 days
E. Uses
1. Acute lymphatic leukemia
2. Choriocarcinoma (occasionally)

Pyrimidine Antimetabolite: fluorouracil (5-FU)

A. Mechanism of action
1. Blocks thymidylate synthetase
2. Inhibits methylation of deoxyuridylic to thymidylic acid, blocking pyrimidine synthesis
B. Toxicity
1. Myelosuppression
2. Stomatitis
3. Gastrointestinal ulceration
4. Nausea and vomiting
5. Alopecia
6. Cerebellar ataxia
C. Method of administration
1. 12 mg/kg/day × 3
2. Smaller dose, 1–2 times weekly for maintenance

Glutamine Antagonists: azaserine (0-Diazoacetyl-1-serine); DON (6-Diazo-5-oxo-1-norleucine)

A. Chemistry
  1. Diazo compounds, closely related in structure to glutamine
  2. Derived from both filtrates of *Streptomyces*
B. Mechanism of action
  1. Interference of the donation of an amino group by glutamine to various biochemical needs in the body, thereby blocking the conversion of formyl glycineamide ribonucleotide (FGAR) to formyl glycineamidine ribonucleotide (FGAM)
  2. A step in purine biosynthesis in which glutamine acts as an amine donor under the influence of an amidotransferase
C. Toxicity
  1. Mouth lesions
  2. Gastrointestinal tract disturbances
  3. Leukopenia
  4. Thrombocytopenia
  5. Liver damage
D. Methods of administration and dosage
  1. Azaserine: 5–10 mg/kg/day IV; ×10 or more
  2. DON: IV 0.2 mg/kg/day
E. Uses
  1. Choriocarcinoma (rarely now)
  2. Childhood acute leukemia

Polyfunctional Alkylating Agents

A. Chemistry

$$H_3CN \begin{array}{c} CH_2CH_2Cl \\ \diagup \\ \diagdown \\ CH_2CH_2Cl \end{array} \longrightarrow CH_3N \begin{array}{c} CH_2 \\ \diagup \quad \diagdown \\ R^1 \quad CH_2 \end{array} \begin{array}{c} CH_2 \\ \diagdown \\ CH_2 \end{array}$$

B. Mechanism of action
  1. Important sites of action appear to be on the nucleic acids, probably within the nucleus, as suggested by the following observations.
    a. They are mutagenic.
    b. They are carcinogenic.
    c. They preferentially deactivate DNA-containing viruses.
    d. They inactivate the pneumococcal and *Hemophilus influenzae* transforming principles.
  2. Alkylation (insertion of an alkyl group) may interfere with synthesis of cross-linking in a number of places. Prevents H bonding between chains of DNA.
  3. A monofunctional compound produces nuclear energy by a sheet mass effect; has only one active alkyl group.
  4. Polyfunctional agents are 50 to 100 times more active than the monofunctional group.
    a. They are cross-linking agents.
    b. Reactive atoms bridge two chromosomal strands or react at two points on a chromosome.
C. Toxicity
  1. Delayed death: 3 to 7 days after exposure to LD_{50} dose
  2. Decrease in antibody production
  3. Increased susceptibility to infection
  4. Diarrhea
  5. Ulceration of the gastrointestinal tract
  6. Hemorrhagic cystitis
  7. Involution in size of lymph nodes, thymus, and spleen
  8. Progressive fall in the leukocytes and platelets in the peripheral blood
  9. Decrease in spermatogenesis
  10. Teratogenic effect
D. Methods of administration and dosage
  1. Mechlorethamine HCl (H_2NCH_1, Mustargen): 0.4 mg/kg IV single or divided doses
  2. Chlorambucil (Leukeran): 0.1–0.2 mg/kg/day PO (6–12 mg/day)
  3. Melphalan (Alkeran; L-phenylalanine mustard (L-PAM); L-sarcolysin): 0.2 mg/kg/day PO × 5; 2–4 mg/day maintenance
  4. Cyclophosphamide (Endoxan, Cytoxan): 200 mg/day IV for 5 days; 50 mg/bid PO
  5. Triethylenethiophosphoramide (TSPA, thiotepa): 0.2 mg/kg IV × 5 days
  6. 1,4-Dimethanesulfonyloxybutane

(Busulfan, Myleran): 2–6 mg/day PO, 150–250 mg/course
7. Nitrosourea alkylating agents [1,3-(2 chloroethyl)-1-nitrosourea (BCNU): 100 mg/m² IV every 6 weeks
E. Uses
 1. Carcinoma of the ovary
 2. Hodgkin's disease
 3. Lymphomas
 4. Burkitt's tumor
 5. Multiple myeloma
 6. Cancer of the breast
 7. Neuroblastoma
 8. Carcinoid
 9. Leukemias

Antibiotics

A. Mechanism of action
Form a complex with DNA involving selective binding at the guaninecystosine segments, with a specific block in the DNA-dependent RNA synthesis (inhibits formation of mRNA).
B. Toxicity
 1. Damage to bone marrow and intestinal epithelium
 2. Nausea and vomiting
 3. Diarrhea
 4. Skin eruption
C. Methods of administration and dosage
 1. Actinomycin D (dactinomycin; Cosmegen): 0.01 mg/kg/day IV × 5 days or 0.04 mg/kg/week
 2. Daunomycin: 0.8–1.0 mg/kg/day IV × 3–6 days; total dose never to exceed 25 mg/kg
 3. Mitomycin C (Mutamycin): 0.06 mg/kg IV × 2 weekly if blood counts permit
 4. Doxorubicin (Adriamycin): 50–75 mg/m² IV in single or divided doses every 2 weeks
 5. Mithramycin: 25 μg/kg IV every other day × 3–4 days
D. Uses
 1. Lymphomas
 2. Leukemias
 3. Solid tumors
 4. Embryonal tumors
 5. Trophoblastic disease

6. Carcinoid
7. Lower calcium level (mithramycin)

Doxorubicin Hydrochloride (Adriamycin)

A. Mechanism of action
Intercalation between base pairs of DNA, which inhibits DNA-dependent RNA synthesis
B. Methods of administration
 1. 0–75 mg/m² IV single dose every 3 weeks
 2. 30 mg/m², IV single dose, days 1–3 inclusive every 4 weeks
 3. Administered through running intravenous infusion. [If any of the drug leaks out of the vein, the tissue must be infiltrated immediately with an ample amount of sodium bicarbonate.]
 4. Avoid giving to patients with significant heart disease; reduce dosage in patients with impaired hepatic function.
C. Toxicity
 1. Gastrointestinal
  a. Nausea and vomiting—usually mild to moderate
  b. Diarrhea
  c. Stomatitis
 2. Hematologic (major)—dose-limiting toxicity
  a. Leukopenia occurs 10-14 days after administration. The counts return to normal approximately 21 days from the date of administration.
  b. Thrombocytopenia and anemia follow a similar pattern but are less common.
 3. Cardiac
  a. Electrocardiographic changes (e.g., sinus tachycardia, ST segment depression, voltage reduction, and arrhythmias) are indications to stop or defer treatment.
  b. Congestive cardiac failure secondary to a diffuse cardiomyopathy indicates that treatment be discontinued.
 4. Dermatologic
  a. Alopecia develops 3 to 4 weeks after

the initial dose. Hair usual regrows completely within 2 to 5 months after cessation of therapy.
   b. Local irritant if injected subcutaneously.
   5. Red urine (not hematuria)
D. Uses
   1. Ovarian cancer
   2. Sarcomas in the pelvis

Mitotic Inhibitors: Vinka Alkaloids

A. Chemistry
   1. Dimeric indole-dihydroindole alkaloids
   2. Periwinkle plant
B. Mechanism of action
   Arrest of mitosis in metaphase by destruction of spindles
C. Toxicity
   1. Nausea and vomiting
   2. Diarrhea
   3. Leukopenia
   4. Neurotoxic paresthesias
   5. Palsies
   6. Peripheral neuritis
   7. Alopecia
   8. Ileus
D. Methods of administration and dosage
   1. Vinblastine (Velban): 0.10–0.15 mg/kg/week IV
   2. Vincristine (Oncovin): 0.030–0.075 mg/kg/week IV
E. Uses
   1. Choriocarcinoma
   2. Lymphoma
   3. Leukemia
   4. Hodgkin's disease

Enzymes: L-Asparaginase

Normal cells can synthesize their own supply of asparagine. It appears that asparagine-dependent cells lack an enzyme, asparagine synthetase, which in normal cells converts aspartic acid to asparagine. Certain types of leukemia (e.g., acute lymphoblastic) have an asparagine dependence, which provides an explanation for the effect of L-asparaginase. The tumor activity of L-asparaginase is also found with transplanted rat tumors and primary dog lymphosarcoma. The final indications for using the enzyme in the treatment of malignancy remain to be determined.

A. Method of administration and dosage
   50–200 IU/kg/day IV or 200-1000 IU/kg IV 3–7 days each week for 28 days
B. Uses
   Acute lymphoblastic leukemia

Nonalkylating Agent Therapy: Hexamethylmelamine (HMM, HXM)

A. Synonyms: none
B. Administration
   1. 12 mg/kg/day PO for 21 days with a 4-week rest period or a low-dose regimen of 8 mg/kg/day PO for periods up to 90 consecutive days.
   2. The total daily dosage should be divided into four parts and given 1.5 to 2.0 hours after each meal and at bedtime. This regimen may avoid some of the gastrointestinal side effects commonly seen.
C. Toxicity
   1. Gastrointestinal
   2. Myelosuppression
   3. Neurologic
   4. Alopecia—rare
   5. Skin—infrequent
D. Mechanism of Action
   Hexamethylmelamine is still an investigational drug and has been in clinical trial for more than 10 years. Although hexamethylmelamine structurally resembles triethylenemelamine, a known alkylating agent, it is thought not to act as an alkylating agent at present. Its activity is more like that of antimetabolites, as it inhibits the incorporation of thymidine and uridine into DNA and RNA. Prolonged exposure of cells to hexamethylmelamine also inhibits protein synthesis. It is cell-cycle-specific for the S phase.
E. Uses
   1. Bronchiogenic carcinoma
   2. Ovarian cancer

cis-Diamminedichloride Platinum

Chapter 22 presents cis-platinum in detail.

A. Synonym: CPDD
B. Administration
   1. 80 mg/m² IV every 3 weeks
   2. 15–20 mg/m² IV for 5 days, repeated every 3 weeks
   3. 50 mg/m² IV as a single dose each week
   4. 60–75 mg/m² every 3 weeks
   5. Most commonly used in combination with other anticancer drugs
C. Toxicity
   1. Gastrointestinal
   2. Hematologic
   3. Renal insufficiency
   4. High frequency other toxicity
D. Mechanism of action
   It is one of the many new platinum compounds being investigated for antitumor activity. Upon loss of a chlorine atom, the drug binds to DNA, high molecular weight RNA, and transfer RNA. The resulting inhibition of DNA synthesis persists for several days after administration of the drug. It is a cell-cycle-nonspecific agent.
E. Uses
   1. Bladder carcinoma
   2. Ovarian carcinoma
   3. Testicular carcinoma

Carboplatinum (CarboP); (cis-Diammine 1,1-cyclobutane Dicarboxylate Platinum II)

Carboplatinum for injection is a significant stride toward improving outpatient chemotherapy. As a cis-platinum analogue, carboplatin provides efficacy and numerous clinical benefits for the patient. It has the classic antitumor activity noted for the platinum compounds but with a more tolerable toxicity profile. Compared with cis-platinum, carboplatin is

1. Significantly less nephrotoxic and neurotoxic
2. Easier to administer in the physician's office or in the outpatient setting
3. Significantly less emetogenic
4. More convenient for patients and staff
5. Significantly less ototoxic

A. Mechanisms of action
   Carboplatin produces predominantly interstrand DNA cross-links rather than DNA-protein cross-links. This effect is apparently cell-cycle-non-specific. The aquation of carboplatin, which is thought to produce the active species, occurs at a slower rate than in the case of cis-platinum. Despite this difference, it appears that both carboplatin and cisplatin induce equal numbers of drug DNA cross-links, causing equivalent lesions in biologic effects. The difference in potency for carboplatin and cisplatin appear to be directly related to the difference in aquation rates.
B. Toxicity
   1. Myelosuppression is dose-related and reversible.
   2. Thrombocytopenia and leukopenia/neutropenia are dose-limiting toxicities. The nadir usually occurs at about day 21 in patients receiving single-agent therapy.
   3. Anemia, frequently observed, is cumulative with increased doses of carboplatin.
   4. Nausea and vomiting are generally of mild to moderate severity and may be dose-related. Vomiting usually begins 6 to 12 hours after carboplatin is administered and may continue for 24 hours.
   5. Anorexia may occur.
   6. Taste alterations may occur.
   7. Renal and electrolyte changes have not been significant, although renal tubular damage resulting in a reversible increase in serum creatinine has occurred on occasion.
   8. Prior aminoglycoside therapy can potentiate renal toxicity associated with carboplatin therapy.
   9. Hypersensitivity to carboplatin has been reported in 2% of patients.
   10. Peripheral neuropathy rarely occurs.
   11. Mild, reversible elevations of liver

function tests have been reported in up to 24% of patients receiving carboplatin.

12. A variety of other adverse effects occur, such as alopecia, constipation, diarrhea, mucositis, taste alterations, tinnitus, and visual disturbances.

C. Methods of administration and dosage
Carboplatin for injection as a single agent has been shown to be effective at a dosage of 360 mg/m² (IV) on day 1 every 4 weeks.

D. Uses
Carboplatin was initially marketed for palliative treatment of patients with ovarian cancer that has recurred after prior chemotherapy, including patients who have been previously treated with *cis*-platinum. However, it is now being used as a first line drug either alone or in combination with other chemotherapeutic agents.

Ifosfamide (Ifex)

A. Mechanism of Action
Ifosfamide has been shown to require metabolic activation by microsomal liver enzymes to produce biologically active metabolites. Activation occurs by hydroxylation at the ring carbon atom 4 to form stable, intermediate 4-hydroxy-ifosfamide. This metabolite rapidly degrades to the stable urinary metabolite 4-ketoifosfamide. Opening of the ring results in formation of the stable urinary metabolite 4-carboxyifosfamide. These urinary metabolites have not been found to be cytotoxic. *N,N*-bis(2-chloroethyl)-phosphoric acid diamide (ifosphoramide) and acrolein are also found. Enzymatic oxidation of the chloroethyl side chains during subsequent dealkylinization produces the major urinary metabolite dechloroethyl ifosfamide and dechloroethyl cyclophosphamide. The alkylated metabolites of ifosfamide have been shown to interact with DNBA.

In vitro incubation of DNA with activated ifosfamide has produced phosphot-riesters. Treatment of the intact cell nuclei may also result in formation of DNA-DNA cross-links. DNA repair most likely occurs in G1 and G2 phase cells.

B. Contraindications
Continued use of ifosfamide is contraindicated in patients with severe depressed bone marrow function and in patients who have demonstrated a previous hypersensitivity to it.

C. Laboratory tests
1. During treatment, the patient's hematologic profile (particularly neutrophils and platelets) should be monitored regularly to determine the degree of hematopoietic suppression.

2. Urine should be examined regularly for red blood cells, which may presage hemorrhagic cystitis.

D. Toxicity
1. Urinary system: Urotoxic side effects, especially hemorrhagic cystitis, may occur.

2. Hematopoietic system: When ifosfamide is given in combination with other chemotherapeutic agents, severe myelosuppression is frequently observed.

3. Central nervous system: Neurologic manifestations consisting in somnolence, confusion, hallucinations, and sometimes coma have been reported.

Mesna (Mesnex)

Mesna is used as a detoxifying agent to inhibit the hemorrhagic cystitis induced by ifosfamide. The active ingredient is a synthetic sulfhydryl compound: sodium 2-mercaptoethanesulfonate with the molecular formula $C_2H_5NaO_3S_2$ and molecular weight 164.18. In the kidney, the mesna disulfide is reduced to the free thiol compound, mesna, which reacts chemically with urotoxic ifosfamide metabolites, resulting in their detoxification.

Warning

Mesna has been developed as an agent to prevent ifosfamide-induced hemorrhagic cystitis.

It does not prevent or alleviate any of the other adverse reactions or toxicities associated with ifosfamide therapy, nor does it prevent hemorrhagic cystitis in all patients. Mesna is usually given combined with ifosfamide therapy.

Ifosfamide may be used in combination with other certain approved antineoplastic agents. It is indicated for third-line chemotherapy of germ cell testicular tumors. However, it is now being explored for use in some of the gynecologic cancers.

Etoposide (VP-16 Vepesid)

Etoposide (VP-16) is a semisynthetic derivative of podophyllotoxin, which is used for treatment of certain neoplastic diseases.

A. Mechanism of action
   Etoposide has been shown to cause metaplasia and to arrest and check fibroblasts. Its main effect, however, appears during the G2 phase of the cell cycle in mammalian cells. Two dose-dependent responses are seen. At high concentrations (10.0 μg/ml or more), lysis of cells entering mitosis is observed. At low concentrations (0.3–10.0μg/ml) cells are inhibited from entering prophase. It does not interfere with the microtubular assembly. The predominant macromolecular effects of etoposide appear to block DNA synthesis.
B. Toxicity
   1. Hematologic
   2. Gastrointestinal
   3. Hypotension
   4. Allergic reaction
   5. Alopecia
   6. Infrequently reported: aftertaste, rash, fever, pigmentation, abdominal pain, constipation, dysphasia, transient cortical blindness, possibly radiation recall dermatitis
C. Method of administration
   Injection, oral capsules
D. Uses
   1. Refractory testicular tumors
   2. Small cell lung cancer
   3. Ovarian cancer
   4. Gestational trophoblastic disease

VIP (Vepesid, Ifosfamide, Platinol)

The combination Vepesid/ifosfamide/platinol (VIP) is currently being explored as second- and third-line therapy for ovarian malignancies. It offers the potential for long-term remission and cure. When used as a salvage therapy for refractory testicular tumor, the VIP regimen "can induce long-term remission and a cure in a cohort of poor prognosis (patients) otherwise incurable." Studies have shown the effectiveness of this combination when administered over a fractionated dosage schedule along with the intermittent dosage of the uroprotective agent mesna injection.

Intraperitoneal Chemotherapy

Treatment of ovarian carcinoma that persists after aggressive surgery and chemotherapy is rarely successful. Abdominal irradiation may benefit those with minimal disease, but there is usually a high morbidity rate.

The rationale for utilizing intraperitoneal chemotherapy to treat ovarian cancer is based on the following facts. (1) The anticancer agents have direct contact with tumor cells. (2) Cytotoxic agents with low lipid solubility and a high molecular weight clear the peritoneal area slowly compared to clearance of the systemic circulation; this situation results in low systemic clearance in the circulation while achieving high levels in the peritoneal cavity. (3) The low systemic clearance allows use of higher doses of drugs than could be safely given systemically. (4) Drugs that are metabolized in the liver to nontoxic substances have a pharmacologic advantage.

Because the use of intraperitoneal chemotherapy depends on diffusion of the drug inwardly from the peritoneally exposed surface of the tumor, it has been generally assumed to be most successful in patients with minimal disease. The ideal drug for intraperitoneal use would have the following properties.

1. Large peritoneal/plasma concentration gradient
2. Steep dose-response relation over the concentration range to be used
3. No local peritoneal toxicity

Cisplatin has been delivered safely in a dose of up to 270 mg/m^2 with simultaneous intravenous sodium thiosulfate. Thiosulfate was selected as a neutralizing agent on the basis of its ability to protect against cis-platinum-induced renal toxicity in the murine model. It is thought to react covalently with cis-platinum, the resulting complex not being toxic or possessing antitumor activity.

Not only has a pharmacokinetic advantage for peritoneal cavity drug exposure been demonstrated, but the systemic delivery of active cis-platinum is increased twofold (at an intraperitoneal dose of 270 mg/m^2) over that observed with an intravenous dose of 100 mg/m^2. Major toxicities of intraperitoneal chemotherapy include abdominal pain (chemical serositis) and infection.

Cisplatin is the only known effective intraperitoneal chemotherapeutic agent used for second-line chemotherapy. It appears to be effective, however, only for small residual cancer (1cm or less).

Traditionally, the treatment for ovarian cancer has been surgery followed by x-ray therapy. Chemotherapy was reserved for the far-advanced and recurrent ovarian cancers. The results from this treatment have been poor, despite the fact that a more aggressive surgical program has been carried out and that supervoltage has been introduced with innovative plans for administering the radiation. Ovarian cancer is a surface spreader and is found over the kidneys and liver in stage III. Because it is necessary to shield the liver and kidneys with lead to prevent radiation hepatitis and nephritis, these patients are selected for therapeutic failure when radiation therapy is applied to the whole abdomen. Metastatic cancer has been found between the liver and diaphragm in about 10 to 12% of what was initially thought to be stage I ovarian cancer. It is obvious that x-ray therapy would be of little help for these patients. As a consequence of the inability to control ovarian cancer in most instances with surgery and radiotherapy alone, chemotherapy is being increasingly employed for the management of this cancer.

Whether chemotherapy has increased the overall survival is difficult to estimate, but it has made life more comfortable for a great number of these unfortunate patients. Each medical center has its own criteria, but in general patients with metastases and ascites have been chosen for chemotherapy. Chemotherapy given in a well-controlled manner does not produce as much morbidity as radiation therapy delivered to the upper abdomen. Following a response, and in the absence of palpable disease, a second look may be undertaken to determine whether the patient is a candidate for (1) excision of any remaining cancer or (2) continued chemotherapy.

Laparoscopic examination has been employed to evaluate and monitor the response of the tumor to therapy. The presence of tumor confirmed by biopsy appears to have more significance than negative findings after laparoscopic examination. Negative findings at laparoscopy should be followed by an exploratory laparotomy.

Until 1979 single-agent chemotherapy of the alkylating group had proved most valuable for treating common epithelial ovarian cancer. After the 1978 report of Young et al. there was a shift to combination chemotherapy. Prior to this time, the combination chemotherapy that had been employed had not produced as good a result as those reported by Young except for the treatment of germ cell and gonadal stromal tumors. It may well be that the combination of anticancer drugs may eventually be alternated or perhaps different drug combinations rotated on a monthly basis. It is not common practice today but may some day prove valuable for controlling the different cell lines that are present in any given ovarian carcinoma.

Combination chemotherapy is always given using an intermittent protocol. There is evidence that the combination chemotherapy is most effective in patients with limited amounts of residual disease. Age, stage, and histologic type of tumor have historically been used for evaluating response to treatment, but these factors are probably less important than the extent of residual disease after operation and the histologic grade. Future prospective clinical trials will have to include such stratification factors to ensure comparability of groups so an informed judgment can be made concerning the management of these patients.

Because Bruce has shown that when chemotherapeutic agents lower the white blood count the resting marrow stem cells temporarily enter the cell cycle and proliferate rapidly, it follows that spacing of chemotherapeutic agents, as in the intermittent regimen, should give the best results. However, a study of several investigations using either the continuous or intermittent regimen produced essentially the same results. The combination of chemotherapy and radiation therapy has not proved any more successful than when each is given alone, and in fact there is increased morbidity.

Hexamethylmelamine is a derivative of the alkylating agent triethylenemelamine but probably does not act primarily as an alkylating agent. The drug, given in a dosage of 6 to 8 mg/kg/day PO in divided doses, causes occasional nausea and vomiting but appears to be associated with fewer bone marrow depression complications than other alkylating agents. The principal toxicity is peripheral neuropathy, which usually prevents the drug from being given for more than 8 to 9 months. Smith and coworkers have reported that it is effective in an occasional patient who does not respond to melphalan or Actinomycin D (Act), 5-fluorouracil (Fu), cyclophosphamide (Cy) regimens.

Cis-dichlorodiammineplatinum (II) (*cis*-platinum II diamminedichloride) has proved to be the keystone drug for treatment of common epithelial ovarian cancer. *Cis*-platinum was first introduced as a possible anticancer drug by Rosenberg and colleagues in 1965, and it has since been shown to have antineoplastic activity in many in vitro and in vivo animal systems. As a single agent its response rate in previously treated patients is not impressive; but when combined with doxorubicin, ifosfamide, or etoposide it holds promise as an additional modality of therapy for recurrent and advanced ovarian cancer. The toxicity noted has been typical of that found with heavy metals and includes elevated blood urea nitrogen levels, tinnitus, anemia, nausea, vomiting, and myelosuppression.

Cis-platinum has many biologic properties similar to those of alkylating agents in terms of its effect on DNA synthesis and its cross-linking of DNA (see Chapter 22).

Doxorubicin (Adriamycin) is an antitumor antibiotic. Subject of a great deal of research and clinical evaluation, studies have shown that it is active as a single agent in previously untreated patients and in those in whom alkylating agent therapy fails. It has its greatest effect as one of the components of a combination regimen. Doxorubicin has produced alopecia, gastrointestinal toxicity, and stomatitis. The prevention of doxorubicin-induced hair loss with scalp hypothermia has produced only indifferent results in my hands. Several ongoing trials comparing the drug alone and in combination with an alkylating agent or *cis*-platinum have been carried out and favor the combination. Currently the most commonly selected chemotherapy combination is platinum plus cyclophosphoramide.

Combination Chemotherapy for Ovarian Cancer

One of the most widely accepted hypotheses in cancer research is that the initial event leading to malignancy is a change in a single cell. Following this change there may be a series of events within succeeding generations of cells, culminating in many malignant cells, which may develop into a mass as a solid tumor or may be at once widespread throughout the body, as in the leukemias.

A major problem of cancer chemotherapy has been the development of resistance to the action of a specific drug to which a cancer was initially susceptible. Resistance is apparently caused by the development of mutant or genetically altered cells that are no longer subject to damage by the drug. However, such cells may be responsive to a different drug.

Many of the advances in the treatment of the leukemias and lymphomas have been associated with schedules consisting of two or more drugs given concomitantly or sequentially. Agents that produce toxicity in different organs are said to have independent toxicity. They can be combined frequently at full doses to produce increased damage to the tumor but little or no increased toxicity to the patient. Methotrexate and 6-mercaptopurine, both antimetabolites and both producers of damage to the bone marrow and gastrointestinal tract, would be expected to have additive toxic effects. Data show, however, that when 60 to 70% of the normal doses of the two drugs are combined, the combined toxicity is no greater than the toxicity of either drug alone.

DeVita and Schein have reported that there are important reasons to consider combination anticancer therapy for ovarian carcinoma. Ideally the combination includes drugs with proved antitumor activity against epithelial ovarian tumors that have an acceptable toxicity. The drugs should have different mechanisms of action. Several studies are under way to test the designated combinations and to compare them directly with a parallel group treated by a single alkylating agent. This approach should answer the question of whether combination therapy is superior to alkylating agents used alone. Preliminary studies have reported improved survival with combination chemotherapy.

Intraaortic Infusion

The credit for introducing intraarterial infusion into clinical medicine belongs to Klopp and coworkers, who reported the use of nitrogen mustard injected directly into the artery supplying a tumor site. The technique used at Lenox Hill Hospital employs a catheter passed by way of the femoral artery and threaded into the aorta to any desired level or by way of the brachial artery into the aorta. The latter method is preferred because it allows the patient more mobility. Multiple anticancer drugs are pumped into the aorta with an infusion pump. The drugs are given sequentially in anticipation of blocking tumor cells at different phases of the cell cycle. The drug schedule is as follows.

1. Cyclophosphamide (Cytoxan) 200–400 mg to run for 24 hours, repeated for a second 24 hours.
2. Actinomycin D 1 mg to run for 8 hours.
3. Vincristine 1 mg to run for 6 hours.
4. Doxorubicin (Adriamycin) 50 mg to run for 24 hours.
5. No anticancer drug then for 48 hours.
6. Entire cycle of drug therapy is then repeated. Multiple cycles are given in anticipation of controlling the cancer.

The use of intraaortic infusion is being presented for its historical value. However, in the future anticancer drugs may be available that will act better if given by the intraaortic method.

Progestational agents have been employed for the management of endometrioid ovarian carcinoma. If this type of therapy is used, it should be given in pharmaceutical doses and not physiologic doses, that is, medroxyprogesterone acetate (Depo-Provera) 400 mg IM each day for 10 days, then once a week for 1 month, then once a month for a long time. Megestrol acetate (Megace), 40 mg 4 times a day by mouth, is given daily. In the presence of an elevated follicle-stimulating hormone (FSH) or luteinizing hormone (LH) titer, Depo-Provera has a more predictable action on the suppression of gonadotropins than does Megace by mouth. The progestogens may be used concurrently with any of the anticancer drugs.

Taxol

Taxol is any of a genus (*Taxus*) of evergreen shrubs and trees of the yew family, having red, cup-like, waxy cones containing a single seed, broad flattened leaves that are needles, and fine-grained elastic wood.

In 1977 Taxol was chosen for development as an antineoplastic agent because of its unique mechanism of action and good cytotoxic activity against the intraperitoneally implanted B16 melanoma and the human MX-1 mammary tumor xenograft. Taxol inhibits normal cellular replication in vitro by promoting microtubule assembly and stabilizing tubulin polymers against depolymerization. Clinical trials began in 1983.

Taxol functions as a mitotic spindle poison and is a potent inhibitor of cell replication in vitro. After exposure to Taxol, there was an increase in the mitotic index of P388 cells and inhibition of human HeLa and mouse fibroblast cells during the G2 and M phases of the cell cycle. Although this inhibition is thought to be secondary to Taxol-induced disruption of mitotic spindle formation, the drug acts in a manner unique from that of other known mitotic inhibitors. Unlike other plant-derived toxins, such as colchicine and podophyllotoxin, which inhibit microtubule assembly, Taxol promoted the assembly of calf brain microtubules in vitro and stabilized them against depolymerization by either low temperatures (4° C) or calcium chloride (4 mM), conditions that normally cause rapid disaggregation of microtubules.

Microtubules are cellular structures that play an essential role in mitosis and another function such as cell migration. The microtubular cytoskeleton is thought to play a role in determining the polarity of migrating cells. Experiments suggest that migrating cells must be able to both polymerize and depolymerize their cytoplastic microtubules in order to migrate. Thus the inhibition of HeLa BALB/c fibroblast cell replication in the presence of low concentrations of Taxol may be secondary to the cells' inability to depolymerize the cytoplasmic microtubules. This observation may help explain the mechanism of action of Taxol and partially account for its observed antitumor activity.

The toxic effects of Taxol in all species investigated were most evident in tissues with high cell turnover, such as hematopoietic, lymphatic, gastrointestinal, and reproductive systems. Throat-related lesions were dose-dependent and reversible with the exception of mandibular lymph node inflammation (rats) and tonsillitis (dogs), which were secondary to Taxol-induced immunosuppression. Effects on other tissues were relatively minor, with no histologic confirmation of toxicity suggested by clinical signs.

A major obstacle in the development of Taxol is limited drug supply. Taxol is derived from a lengthy fermentation of bark obtained from the western yew, *Taxus brevifolia*; a method of synthesis has not been developed. Therefore there are a limited number of clinical trials. If drug supply is sufficient and the ongoing phase 2 trials in ovarian caner confirm the activity reported during the initial trial, a phase 3 trial may be undertaken at this disease site. If drug supply is sufficient, limited phase 2 trials will be performed, particularly for those disease sites in which activity was observed during phase 1 or for those that occur frequently.

Currently the Division of Cancer Treatment (National Cancer Institute) plans to keep the Investigation of New Drug (IND) protocol for Taxol open to support clinical studies, the number of which will be limited by drug availability. Taxol, which has shown activity against ovarian and breast cancers but which can be obtained only in limited supplies, may be available on a compassionate basis. One kilogram of taxol has been set aside for compassionate use in 1991 through 1992.

Summary

Unfortunately, progress in the management of ovarian cancer has been painfully slow. It is a tragedy that more than 100,000 women have succumbed to this disease during the 1980s. Ovarian cancer is now the leading cause of death from gynecologic cancer. These women literally vomit themselves to death. They are often ravishingly hungry, but one bit of food or a drink causes them to vomit. At this point the art of medicine must take over from the science of medicine. Unlike the terminal stage of many other cancers, during which the patient gradually becomes comatose, the ovarian cancer patient is usually alert right up to the time of death. The best therapy for each stage of the disease is not known.

The impressive responses of some patients to a single alkylating agent has suggested an expanded role for chemotherapy. There is an urgent need to explore the potential of multiple-drug therapy as new anticancer drugs prove to have activity against ovarian cancer. It is important to compare standard alkylating agents with new, active agents as well as combination chemotherapy regimens. The newer chemotherapeutic agents must be systematically investigated in patients who have failed existing standard methods of treatment in order to identify new agents of promise for the management of this disease. Subsequent clinical trials should compare newer therapies to optimal existing treatment within each stage. Such studies will define the role of chemotherapy in the management of ovarian cancer and will enable patients to enjoy the benefits of continually improving forms of therapy.

Chemotherapy now constitutes a major, indispensable therapeutic approach that is capable of producing cures of particular kinds of widespread cancer. It has produced some spectacular results in ovarian cancer patients. In contrast to surgery and radiation therapy, chemotherapy—the treatment of cancer with drugs and hormones—can be used effectively for disseminated as well as localized cancer. Chemotherapy has become an accepted modality of treatment only since the 1960s. Each of the decades since its introduction has seen the addition of new drugs with a wide spectrum of usefulness. Originally chemotherapy was used only for palliation, but now it is the primary treatment for several malignancies. A major goal of current cancer chemotherapy is to achieve cures by prompt, vigorous treatment of those cancers that have responded to anticancer drugs.

It remains for the gynecologist and chemotherapist to explore the best method and regimen to control ovarian cancer as well as the role of these agents in prophylaxis as well as therapy. Combinations of chemotherapeutic agents have been used with substantial success for certain cancers, particularly if each of the drugs used acts on the cancer cell in a different way. Major improvements in the treatment of certain cancers have been achieved by using several of the active drugs simultaneously, as well as by using different drugs in sequence. This approach must be thoroughly explored by systemically investigating these regimens in the various families of ovarian cancer.

Chemotherapy occasionally produces a cure among a broad spectrum of cancers, including ovarian cancer. The cancers that can be cured by chemotherapy are not always those that grow most rapidly. Moreover, not all are from the same primitive embryonic tissue; many organ classes are represented. Furthermore, curative chemotherapy is not usually the product of a single drug or a single technique of drug use. Rather, many drugs are involved, sometimes in combination with each other, sometimes with surgery or irradiation. Ovarian cancer was previously treated with a single alkylating drug; and if that failed, the second- and then third-line drugs were added. Currently, programs have been established to study systematically and in detail the value of multiple-drug therapy for the initial chemotherapeutic regimen. The high degree of specificity between a particular tumor and a particular drug or drug combination implies that no universal chemotherapeutic cure can be anticipated. The complexity of special drugs and regimens for special tumors can also be construed to mean that a drug that fails in treatment of one kind of cancer may exhibit major activity against another. Until a laboratory test such as chemosensitivity testing or flow cytometry is established to identify the best anticancer drug or combination of drugs for a given tumor, treatment will continue to depend on empiric factors as well as on past and present clinical experience.

The sensitivity of cancer cells to drug action depends on a variety of possible factors. Many of these factors are not known, and there are few tests to guide the clinician in selecting and administering anticancer drugs. The anticancer drug must reach the cancer cell surface in the right concentration, enter the cell, remain active or become active through enzymes present in the cell, reach a critical target site, and combine with it. It is ideal if the anticancer drug combines with the critical target site at a time when chemical processes on which the cell depends for its viability or reproduction are in progress. It is important to eliminate the bypass pathways in the cell that would negate the effect of the anticancer drug. The chain is no stronger than its individual links, and failure of the whole chain can result from the failure of any one step. Thus any anticancer drug given via the wrong regimen to a mass of cancer cells that is biologically not susceptible to its action at that time is a failure of judgment regarding the use of chemotherapy. Such an error introduces a degree of toxicity without therapeutic help. Better drug design and better understanding of the biologic characteristics of each cancer type, and indeed of each cancer, can advance the effectiveness of chemotherapy. Unfortunately, studies on the treatment of ovarian cancer only recently have been directed toward these goals.

It is obvious that much work remains to be done before the use of chemotherapy for ovarian cancer reaches the stage it has for choriocarcinoma, the leukemias, and many embryonal tumors. Many studies now under way, however, should provide guidelines for the chemotherapeutic treatment of ovarian cancer that will give a predictable chance for cure in an increased number of patients.

The response of treatment and progress of the patient can be evaluated using the Karnofsky Performance Status scale, as follows.

100 Normal; no complaints; no evidence of disease
90 Able to carry on normal activity; minor signs or symptoms of disease
80 Normal activity with effort; some sign or symptoms of disease
70 Cares for self, unable to carry on normal activity or do active work
60 Requires occasional assistance but is able to care for most personal needs
50 Requires considerable assistance and frequent medical care
40 Disabled; requires special care and assistance
30 Severely disabled; hospitalization is indicated, although death not imminent
20 Very sick; hospitalization necessary; active support treatment is necessary
10 Moribund; fatal process progressing rapidly
0 Dead

Performance status, according to the Union International Cancer Control (UICC)/Eastern Cooperative Oncology Group (ECOG) scale is as follows.

0 Ability to carry out all normal activity without restriction
1 Restricted in physically strenuous activity but ambulatory and able to do light work
2 Ambulatory and capable of all self-care but unable to carry out any work; "up and about" more than 50% of waking hours
3 Capable of only limited self-care; confined to bed or chair more than 50% of waking hours
4 Completely disabled; cannot carry on any self-care; totally confined to bed or chair

Bibliography

Bagley CM, Young RC, Canellos GP, et al: Treatment of ovarian carcinoma: possibilities for progress. *N Engl J Med* 287:856, 1972.

Barber HRK: Editorial Comment. In Barber HRK, Graber EA (eds): *Surgical Disease in Pregnancy.* Saunders, Philadelphia, 1974, p. 718.

Barber HRK: *Manual of Gynecologic Oncology.* Lippincott, Philadelphia, 1980.

Bruce WR: A model system for examining the action of anticancer agents at the cellular level in vivo. *Natl Cancer Inst Monogr* 24:249, 1967.

Bruce WR, Meeker BE, Valenote FA: Comparison of the sensitivity of normal hematopoietic and transplanted lymphoma colony-forming cells to chemotherapeutic agents administered in vivo. *J Natl Cancer Inst* 37:233, 1966.

Brulé G, Eckhardt SJ, Hall TC, Winkler A: *Drug Therapy of Cancer.* World Health Organization, Geneva, 1973.

Carter SK, Bakowski MT, Hellmann K: *Chemotherapy of Cancer.* John Wiley & Sons, New York, 1977.

Connors TA, Roberts JJ (eds): Platinum coordination complexes in cancer chemotherapy. In *Recent Results in Cancer Research.* Vol. 48. Springer-Verlag, Berlin, 1974.

Dean JC, Salmon SE, Griffith KS: Prevention of doxorubicin-induced hair loss with scalp hypothermia. *N Engl J Med* 301:1427, 1979.

DeVita VT, Schein PS: The use of drugs in combination for the treatment of cancer. *N Engl J Med* 288:998, 1973.

Ehrlich CE, Einhorn L, Williams SD, Morgan J: Chemotherapy for stage II–IV epithelial ovarian cancer with *cis*-dichlorodiammine platinum II, Adriamycin, and cyclophosphamide: a preliminary report. *Can Treat Rep* 63:281, 1979.

Gove ME, Fryatt I, Wiltshaw E, et al: Treatment of relapsed carcinoma of the ovary with cisplatin or carboplatin following initial treatment with these compounds. *Gynecol Oncol* 36:207, 1990.

Hryniuk WM, Bertino JR: Rationale for selection of chemotherapeutic agents. *Adv Intern Med* 15:267, 1969.

Kaufmann M: Clinical applications of in vitro chemosensitivity testing: ovarian cancer. *Adv Biosci* 26:189, 1980.

Klopp CT: Fractionated intraarterial cancer chemotherapy with methylbisamine hydrochloride, preliminary report. *Ann Surg* 132:811, 1950.

Lewis B, Young R: Adjuvant and first line chemotherapy for ovarian cancer: ovarian cancer *Adv Biosci* 26:165, 1980.

Lewis GC, Blessing J: Ovarian cancer: use of multiple modality programs involving surgery, radiation therapy and chemotherapy. *Cancer* 40:588, 1977.

Manetta A, MacNeill C, Lyter JA, et al: Hexamethylmelamine as a single second live agent in ovarian cancer. *Gynecol Oncol* 36:93, 1990.

Parker RT, Parker CH, Wilbanks GD: Cancer of the ovary: survival studies based upon operative therapy, chemotherapy, and radiotherapy. *Am J Obstet Gynecol* 108:878, 1970.

Pratt WB, Ruddon RW: *The Anticancer Drugs.* Oxford University Press, New York, 1979.

Rosenberg B, Van Camp L, Kregas T: Inhibition of cell division in *Escherichia coli* by electrolysis products from a platinum electrode. *Nature* 205:698, 1965.

Rowkinsky EK, Donehower RC, Jones RJ, et al: Microtubule changes and cytotoxicity in leukemic cell lines treated with Taxol. *Cancer Res* 48:4093, 1988.

Salmon SE, Hamburger AW, Soehnlen B, et al: Quantitation of differential sensitivity of human-tumor stem cells to anticancer drugs. *N Engl J Med* 298:1321, 1978.

Silver RT, Lauper RD, Jarowski CI: *A Synopsis of Cancer Chemotherapy.* Yorke Medical Group, New York, 1977.

Skipper HE, Schabel FM, Wilcox WS: Experimental evaluation of potential anticancer agents. XIII. On the criteria and kinetics associated with curability of experimental leukemia. *Cancer Chemother Rep* 35:1, 1964.

Smith JP: Chemotherapy in advanced ovarian cancer. *Natl Cancer Inst Monogr* 42:141, 1975.

Smith JP, Rutledge F, Wharton JT: Chemotherapy of ovarian cancer: new approaches to treatment. *Cancer* 30:1565, 1972.

Taxol Clinical Brochure, the Division of Cancer Treatment. National Cancer Institute, Bethesda, 1983.

Thigpen TL, LaGasse L, Bundy B: Phase II trial of *cis*-platinum in treatment of advanced ovarian adenocarcinoma. *Proc Am Assoc Cancer Res* 20:84, 1979.

Van Eden EB, Falkson G, Van Dyk JJ, et al: 5-Fluorouracil, imidazole-4-carboxamide, vincristine and BCNu given concomitantly in the treatment of solid tumors in man. *Cancer Chemother Rep* 56(I):691, 1972.

Wallace HJ, Higby DJ: Phase I evaluation of *cis*-platinum II diammine chloride (PDD) and a combination of PDD plus Adriamycin. In *Recent Results in Cancer Research.* Vol. 48. Springer-Verlag, Berlin, 1974, p. 167.

Watkins E Jr, Sullivan RD: Cancer chemotherapy by prolonged arterial infusion. *Surg Gynecol Obstet* 118:3, 1964.

Webb NJ, Malkasian GD, Jorgensen EO: Factors influencing ovarian cancer survival after chemotherapy. *Obstet Gynecol* 44:564, 1974.

Wiltshaw E, Kroner T: Phase II study of *cis*-dichloro-diammineplatinum (II) in advanced adenocarcinoma of the ovary. *Cancer Treat Rep* 60:55, 1976.

Young RC: Chemotherapy of ovarian cancer: past and present. *Semin Oncol* 2:267, 1975.

Young RC, Chabner BA, Hubbard ST, et al: Advanced ovarian adenocarcinoma: a perspective clinical trial of melphalan (L-PAM) versus combination chemotherapy. *N Engl J Med* 299:1261, 1978.

Young RC: Ovarian carcinoma: an optimistic epilogue. *Can Treat Rep* 63:333, 1979.

Young RC, Hubbard SP, DeVita VT: The chemotherapy of ovarian cancer. *Cancer Treat Rep* 1:99, 1974.

22

Platinum Drugs

Diamminedichloroplatinum (DDP) was first synthesized in 1845 and was known as Peyrone's chloride. However, it was not until 1965 when Rosenberg showed the inhibition of cell division in *Escherichia coli* by electrolysis products from a platinum electrode that interest in *cis*-platinum was restimulated.

Cis-Diamminedichloroplatinum (II)

Cis-diamminedichloroplatinum (II) is one of a number of platinum coordination complexes with antitumor activity. The potential of this compound as an antitumor agent was recognized through an observation made by Rosenberg et al. that a certain group, VIII B transition metal compounds, inhibit bacterial division. They had shown that during studies to investigate the effect of an electromagnetic field on the division of *Escherichia coli* the cells were made to lengthen and form a filamentous appearance, and cell division was inhibited. It became clear that cell division was being inhibited not by the electromagnetic field but by an electrolysis product of the platinum electrode. Additional studies showed that a platinum compound was more effective than several other group VIII B transition metal compounds in inhibiting cell division in cultures of gram-negative bacilli. It was shown that it was a *cis* compound that caused filamentous growth, whereas the *trans* isomer had no effect. In 1970 Rosenberg and his colleagues tested the antitumor activity of several platinum compounds and demonstrated that DDP was effective against sarcoma 180 and L1210 leukemia in mice. The efficacy of the platinum compounds has since been confirmed in animals as well as in humans. These compounds represent an entirely new class of anticancer drugs. Additional tests on animal tumor cell systems showed potent antitumor activity for at least two *cis* compounds. One of them, *cis*-[PtCl$_2$ (NH$_3$)$_2$], now known as *cis*-platinum, was chosen for further testing, and clinical trials were started in 1971.

When the results using *cis*-platinum for testicular teratomas and ovarian adenocarcinomas were reported it was obvious that the agent had a definite therapeutic usefulness. Great fear, however, was expressed regarding the nephrotoxicity. Such problems can now be overcome, at least in the short term, if the patients receive adequate hydration in association with the drug, with or without mannitol to induce diuresis.

Description

Cis-platinum (*cis*-diamminedichloroplatinum) is a heavy metal complex containing a central atom of platinum surrounded by two chloride atoms and two ammonia molecules in the *cis* position (Fig. 22.1). It is a white, lyophilized powder with the molecular formula PtCl$_2$H$_6$N$_2$ and a molecular weight of 300.1. It is soluble in water or saline at 1 mg/ml and in dimethylformamide at 24 mg/ml. It has a melting point of 207°C.

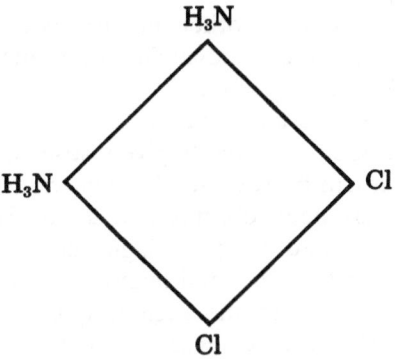

FIGURE 22.1. Molecular structure of *cis*-platinum.

Action

Cis-platinum has biochemical properties similar to those of bifunctional alkylating agents, producing interstrand and intrastrand cross-linkings in DNA. It is apparently cell-cycle-nonspecific. After a single intravenous dose, *cis*-platinum concentrates in liver, kidneys, and the large and small intestines in animals and humans. *Cis*-platinum apparently has poor penetration in the central nervous system.

Rosenberg thought that platinum compounds disrupted antigenic masking on animal tumor cells, exposing what he thought might be new antigens at the cell surface that generate a host immune reaction. He noted the appearance of densely stained patches associated with the tumor cell membranes but not with normal cell membranes, and he identified them as possibly masking antigens containing DNA. Most nucleic acids and nuclear proteins are weaker antigens and may escape host immune surveillance. Rosenberg originally concluded that *cis*-platinum worked through an immune mechanism.

Plasma levels of radioactivity decay in a biphasic manner after an intravenous bolus dose of radioactive *cis*-platinum to patients. The initial plasma half-life is 25 to 49 minutes, and the postdistribution plasma half-life is 58 to 73 hours. During the postdistribution phase, more than 90% of the radioactivity in the blood is protein-bound. *Cis*-platinum is excreted primarily in the urine. However, urinary excretion is incomplete, with only 27 to 43% of the radioactivity being excreted within the first 5 days after administration in humans. There are insufficient data to determine if biliary or intestinal excretion occurs. Abdominal scans show high levels of radioactivity in the kidney, liver, and intestine. Little drug is excreted in the feces. Scans of the head show little radioactivity in the brain area, an observation that suggests poor penetration into the cerebrospinal fluid. In the animal distribution study, rather high levels of DDP were found in the ovary, a localization that may contribute to the efficacy of the drug against ovarian carcinoma.

Pharmacology and Use

Cis-platinum is routinely administered by intravenous infusion. It is supplied as a lyophilized powder containing sodium chloride, mannitol, and hydrochloric acid for pH adjustment. It is reconstituted by adding 10 ml of sterile water for injection USP to the vial, which results in a concentration of 1 g/ml. The solution is stable at room temperature for at least 8 hours; but if this preparation is diluted into a solution with a low concentration of chloride, the drug is converted, probably to the aquo form. Further conversion to the biologically inactive neutral hydroxy ligands also occurs slowly in such solutions, but it has not been demonstrated to occur to a significant extent under clinical conditions of administration. After administration, the high chloride concentration of the plasma and extracellular fluids favors the persistence of unaltered DDP, which, as a neutral species, can cross cell membranes. The relatively low chloride concentration of the intracellular milieu favors the formation of the reactive mono- and di-aquated species. Upon loss of a chloride atom, the drug binds to DNA, high molecular weight RNA, and transfer RNA. The resulting inhibition of DNA synthesis persists several days following administration of the drug. It is a cell-cycle, nonspecific agent.

Dosage and Administration

Dilute half of the total dose to be given in about 150 ml of sodium chloride injection USP and infuse over 1 hour. Repeat with the remaining dose fraction over the next hour. The reconstructed drug product is stable for 8 hours at room temperature, protected from light. It should not be refrigerated. Prior to using this drug, the patient must be properly hydrated with 5% dextrose in water USP and 0.45% sodium chloride USP with appropriate potassium supplements. Hydration must result in urine output of at least 100 ml/hr for 4 consecutive hours before drug administration. Then a loading dose of 12.5 g of mannitol is given intravenously followed by an infusion of 0.5 g/hr to maintain urine output at a minimum of 100 ml/hr for 2 hours of administration of *cis*-diamminedichloroplatinum (II) and for 6 hours thereafter. Some investigators substitute furosemide for mannitol infusions. This regimen can be safely administered to outpatients.

Contraindications

Cis-platinum is contraindicated in patients with preexisting renal impairment and should not be employed in myelosuppressed patients or in those with hearing impairment. It is also contraindicated in patients with a history of allergic reactions to *cis*-platinum or other platinum-containing compounds.

Adverse Reactions and Toxicity

Nausea and vomiting are side effects that are nearly universal, often severe and protracted. They start at 1 hour, can last up to 12 hours (average 4–6 hours), and may persist up to a week in an especially sensitive patient.

The major dose-limiting effect is nephrotoxicity. Clearly dose-related, this nephrotoxicity is manifested by elevations in blood urea nitrogen (BUN) and creatinine levels, and a decrease in creatinine clearance. It has been reported that with doses above 3 mg/kg the incidence of irreversible elevations of the serum creatinine level is higher than 50%. Lower dose levels and the use of adequate hydration and mannitol-induced diuresis usually prevent significant renal toxicity. Pathologic changes in the kidney consist in focal, acute necrosis primarily affecting the distal convoluted tubules and collecting ducts, dilation of the convoluted tubules, and formation of casts. It is possible

that therapy with other nephrotoxic drugs, such as gentamicin and cephalothin, augments the nephrotoxicity of DDP.

Tinnitus is usually the earliest sign of ototoxicity. Seen in patients given doses over 80 mg/m², it can be reversed in most cases. Ototoxicity has been observed in up to 31% of patients treated with a single dose of *cis*-platinum (50 mg/m²) and manifests as tinnitus or hearing loss in the high frequency range (4000–8000 Hz). Decreased ability to hear normal conversational tones occurs occasionally. The ototoxicity effects may be more severe in children receiving *cis*-platinum. Hearing loss may be unilateral or bilateral and tends to become more frequent and severe with repeated doses. It is not clear at this time whether *cis*-platinum-induced ototoxicity is reversible. Careful audiometric monitoring should be performed prior to initiation of therapy and to subsequent doses of *cis*-platinum. Although this protocol is ideal, it is not always practical.

Myelosuppression

There is little hematologic toxicity at doses of 1 mg/kg. However, at doses of 3 mg/kg there is definite myelosuppression, with the nadir seen after 7 to 10 days. This bone marrow toxicity is reversible. Recovery is usually seen by 20 days. Myelosuppression occurs in 25 to 30% of patients treated with *cis*-platinum. Leukopenia and thrombocytopenia are more pronounced at doses higher than 50 mg/m². Anemia (a hemoglobin decrease of more than 2 g/dl) occurs at approximately the same frequency and with the same timing as leukopenia and thrombocytopenia.

Hyperuricemia

Hyperuricemia has been reported to occur at approximately the same frequency as the increases in BUN and serum creatinine. It is more pronounced after doses higher than 50 mg/m², and peak levels of uric acid generally occur 3 to 5 days after the dose. Allopurinol therapy for hyperuricemia effectively reduces uric acid levels.

Neurotoxicity

Peripheral neuropathy is generally less common than ototoxicity, although one study showed an incidence of up to 33%. Loss of taste and seizures have also been reported. Neuropathies resulting from *cis*-platinum therapy may occur after prolonged therapy (4–7 months); however, neurologic symptoms have been reported to occur after a single dose. *Cis*-platinum therapy should be discontinued when symptoms are first observed. Preliminary evidence suggests that peripheral neuropathy is irreversible in some patients.

Anaphylaxis

There have been several reports of patients experiencing anaphylactic reactions to DDP. Such reactions consist in facial edema, wheezing, tachycardia, and hypertension within a few minutes of drug administration. These reactions may be controlled by intravenous epinephrine, corticosteroids, or antihistamines. Other toxicities reported to occur infrequently are cardiac abnormalities, anorexia, and elevated serum glutamic oxaloacetic transaminase.

Hypomagnesemia

One retrospective study showed a significant number of patients with tetany or muscle cramps who required hospitalization. This effect is not clearly dose-related. A postulated mechanism is a defect in the renal tubular conservation of magnesium.

Carboplatin (CarboP)

Carboplatin for injection is a significant stride toward improving outpatient chemotherapy. As a *cis*-platinum analogue, carboplatin provides efficiency and numerous clinical benefits for patients. It also provides a classic antitumor activity noted for platinum compounds with a more tolerable toxicity profile. Compared with *cis*-platinum, carboplatin is:

1. Significantly less nephrotoxic and neurotoxic

2. Easier to administer in the office or in the outpatient setting
3. Significantly less emetogenic
4. More convenient for patients and staff
5. Significantly less ototoxic

Carboplatin for injection is a cytotoxic complex structurally related to *cis*-platinum. It has been developed in an effort to retain or improve on the therapeutic activity of *cis*-platinum while reducing or eliminating the dose-limiting adverse effects, i.e., nephrotoxicity, neurotoxicity, nausea, and vomiting (commonly associated with *cis*-platinum). However, carboplatin reacts with nucleophilic sites on DNA, causing predominantly intrastrand and interstrand cross-links rather than DNA–protein cross-links. These cross links are similar to those formed with *cis*-platinum but are formed later.

Approximately 70% of the administered dose was excreted as carboplatin in the urine within 24 hours. The urinary excretion of carboplatin is rapid, with most being excreted within 12 to 16 hours. It was not found to be bound to plasma proteins, and no significant quantities of free, ultrafilterable, platinum-containing species other than carboplatin were present in the plasma. However, the platinum from carboplatin degradation species was irreversibly bound to plasma proteins (approximately 30%) and was eliminated with a minimum half-life of 5 days.

Carboplatin is a platinum coordination compound that is used as a cancer chemotherapeutic agent. The clinical name for carboplatin is platinum diammine[1,1-cyclobutane dicarboxylate(2-)-0,0′], also called SP-4-2.

Oncopharmacology

Carboplatin, like *cis*-platinum, produces predominantly interstrand DNA cross-links rather than DNA–protein cross-links. The effect is apparently cell-cycle nonspecific. The aquation rate of carboplatin, which is thought to produce the active species, occurs at a slower rate than in the case of *cis*-platinum and accounts for the differences in potencies for carboplatin and cisplatin. Despite this difference, it appears that both carboplatin and *cis*-platinum induce equal numbers of drug–DNA cross-links, causing equivalent lesions and biologic effects. The difference in potency for carboplatin and *cis*-platinum appears to be directly related to the difference in aquation rates.

Indications

Originally, carboplatin was indicated for the palliative treatment of patients with ovarian carcinoma recurrent after chemotherapy, including patients who have been previously treated with *cis*-platinum. However, now it is used as a first line of therapy either alone or with other anticancer drugs.

Contraindications

Carboplatin is contraindicated in patients with a history of severe allergic reactions to *cis*-platinum or other platinum-containing compounds or mannitol. Carboplatin should not be employed in patients with severe bone marrow depression or significant bleeding.

Adverse Reactions

Adverse reactions include the following.

1. *Hematologic toxicity*. Bone marrow suppression is the dose-limiting toxicity of carboplatin.

2. *Thrombocytopenia*. Platelet counts below $50,000/mm^3$ occur in 24% of the patients treated. The nadir occurs at about day 21 in patients receiving single-agent therapy. By day 28, 90% of the patients have platelet counts above $100,000/mm^3$, 74% have neutrophil counts above $2000/mm^3$, and 67% have leukocyte counts above $4000/mm^3$. Anemia is frequently observed and is cumulative with increased doses of carboplatin.

3. *Myelosuppression*. It may be more pronounced in patients who have had previous treatment with *cis*-platinum or radiation therapy, or when carboplatin is combined with other myelosuppressive agents. The risk for severe myelosuppression may also be increased with increasing age, renal impairment, poor performance status, or extensive prior chemotherapy.

4. *Gastrointestinal reactions*. Nausea and vomiting are generally mild to moderate in severity and may be dose-related. Vomiting usually begins 6 to 12 hours after carboplatin is administered and may continue for 24 hours. Nausea alone may occur. Anorexia, which usually resolves within 24 hours, has been reported.

The gastrointestinal symptoms may be more pronounced in patients who had prior *cis*-platinum or other emetogenic therapy such as radiation therapy. Other gastrointestinal symptoms that have been reported are diarrhea and constipation.

5. *Taste alterations*. These changes are experienced by the patient as either a decrease in taste acuity (hypogeusia) or an unusual/unpleasant taste sensation (dysgeusia).

6. *Renal and electrolyte changes*. Clinically significant nephrotoxicity, however, despite the fact that carboplatin has usually been administered without high-volume fluid hydration or forced diuresis have not been reported. Renal tubular damage resulting in a reversible increase in serum creatinine has occurred on occasion. Prior aminoglycoside therapy can potentiate renal toxicity associated with carboplatin therapy.

Before initial therapy is undertaken, BUN, serum creatinine, and creatinine clearance values should be evaluated to establish baseline renal function. BUN and serum creatinine tests should be repeated before each course of carboplatin. No prehydration or diuresis is necessary before treatment with carboplatin.

Patients who have reduced renal function before treatment with carboplatin are at greater risk for severe hematopoietic toxicity. Reduced dosage is indicated if creatinine clearance is less than 60 ml/min.

7. *Hypersensitivity to carboplatin*. Reported in 2% of patients, these reactions usually occur as a rash, urticaria, erythema, pruritus, bronchospasm, and hypotension. These reactions can be successfully managed with epinephrine, corticosteroids, and antihistamines.

8. *Peripheral neuropathy* (rarely). Its incidence is increased in patients over 65 years of age and in those previously treated with *cis*-platinum.

9. *Ototoxicity*. This problem has been reported in only 1% of patients receiving standard doses of carboplatin for injection. Patients who have received prior therapy with *cis*-platinum or who have had a previous hearing loss should have baseline audiometry testing before receiving carboplatin. Testing should be repeated if a hearing loss is noted by the patient. The patient should be questioned before each course of therapy regarding changes in hearing.

10. *Liver function abnormalities*. Mild, reversible elevations of liver function tests have been reported in up to 24% of patients receiving carboplatin. High doses of carboplatin—more than four times the recommended dose—have resulted in severe abnormalities. Liver function tests should be evaluated before initial therapy with carboplatin and before each subsequent course.

11. *Miscellaneous effects*. Other reported adverse effects include alopecia, constipation, diarrhea, mucositis, taste alterations, tinnitus, and visual disturbances.

Dosage

Carboplatin for injection as single-agent therapy has been shown to be effective in patients with ovarian carcinoma, primary or recurrent, at a dosage of 360 mg/m^2 IV on day 1 every 4 weeks. Patients with impaired kidney function with creatinine clearance values below 60 ml/min are at increased risk for severe myelosuppression. It is therefore recommended that for patients with impaired baseline kidney function the first carboplatin dosage should be reduced by 50%. Subsequent dosage adjustments (decreases or increases) should take into account the patient's tolerance and the degree of myelosuppression observed.

Carboplatin is usually administered by an infusion lasting 15 minutes or longer. There is no need for pretreatment or posttreatment hydration or forced diuresis.

New analogues of cisplatin are being identified and evaluated. An exciting new platinum compound currently being evaluated is ormaplatin (formerly tetraplatin), another second generation platinum analogues developed in an attempt to reduce toxicity. Like carboplatin, it has less nephro- and neurotoxicity. Ormaplatin has been found to be more potent than cisplatin when tested against various human ovarian cancer cell lines. This drug has been shown to have activity in cell lines that have been made resistant to cisplatin. Unlike other platinum compounds, ormaplatin was not crossresistant with cisplatin and carboplatin in vitro.

Summary

It is accepted that *cis*-platinum has been added to the armamentarium of the chemotherapist. *Cis*-platinum is effective as a single agent, but when administered in combination with other drugs it seems to increase the complete remission rate as well as the partial remission rate. Currently, the drug is under intensive investigation by a number of groups around the world, and an evaluation of the accumulated material identifies the exact role that *cis*-platinum has to play, particularly in the treatment of common epithelial ovarian cancer.

To give meaning to these studies, it is important to have a careful histologic evaluation with grading of the tumor and meticulous clinical staging. It is also important to record accurately the severe side effects and the cost of therapy. All of these factors can be measured against the complete and partial response rates.

Cis-platinum is emerging as one of the most effective drugs for the management of common epithelial ovarian cancer. It is undergoing extensive trials as a single agent as well as one of the drugs in combination therapy. Wiltshaw and Kroner have reported that *cis*-platinum has shown significant activity in ovarian cancer, with a response rate of 26%.

Bibliography

Bruckner HW, Cohen CJ, Wallach RC, et al: Treatment of advanced ovarian cancer with cis-dichlorodiammine-platinum (II): poor risk patients with intensive prior therapy. *Cancer Treat Rep* 62:555, 1978.

Ehrlich CE, Einhorn L, Williams SD, Morgan J: Chemotherapy for stage III–IV epithelial ovarian cancer with cis-dichloro-diammine-platinum (II),

Adriamycin and cyclophosphamide: a preliminary report. *Cancer Treat Rep* 63:281, 1979.

Hollinshead A, Stewart T: Specific active immunotherapy and specific active immunoprophylaxis in lung cancer. Reprinted from Moore M (ed): *Basis for Cancer Therapy 2, Advances in Medical Oncology Research and Education.* Pergamon Press, New York, 1979.

Hoskins WJ: The influence of cytoreductive surgery on progressive-free interval and survival in epithelial ovarian cancer. *Bailliends Clin Obstet Gynaecol* 3:59, 1989.

Howell SB, Zimm S, Markman M, et al: Long-term survival of advanced refractory ovarian carcinoma patients with small-volume disease treated with intraperitoneal chemotherapy. *J Clin Oncol* 5: 1607, 1987.

Leh FKV, Woo W: Platinum complexes: a new class of antineoplastic agents. *J Pharm Sci* 65:315, 1976.

Markman M: Intraperitoneal cisplatinum chemotherapy in the management of ovarian carcinoma. *Semin Oncol* 16(4; suppl 6):79, 1989.

Markman M, Hakes T, Reichman B, et al: Intraperitoneal cisplatin and cytarabine in the treatment of refractory or recurrent ovarian carcinoma. *J Clin Oncol* 9:204, 1991.

McClay EF, Howell SB: A review: intraperitoneal cisplatin in the management of patients with ovarian cancer. *Gynecol Oncol* 36:1, 1990.

McDermott DF, Jaffee EA, Coleman M, Pasmantier MW: The effect of surgical debulking on the response of patients with ovarian carcinoma to chemotherapy. *Am J Clin Oncol* 11:520, 1988.

Newman CE, Ford CHJ, Jordan JA (eds): *Ovarian Cancer: Proceedings of the International Symposium on Ovarian Cancer, 1979, Birmingham, Alabama.* Pergamon Press, Oxford, 1980.

Ozols RF: Editorial: intraperitoneal therapy in ovarian cancer: time's up. *J Clin Oncol* 9:197, 1991.

Pratt WB, Ruddon RW: *The Anticancer Drugs.* Oxford University Press, New York, 1979.

Rosenberg B: Possible mechanisms for the antitumor activity of platinum coordination complexes. *Cancer Chemother Rep* 59:589, 1975.

Rosenberg B, Renshaw E, van Camp L, et al: Platinum-induced filamentous growth in *Escherichia coli. J Bacteriol* 93:716, 1967.

Rosenberg B, van Camp L, Grimley EB, Tomson AJ: The inhibition of growth and cell division in *Escherichia coli* by different ionic species of platinum (IV) complex. *J Biol Chem* 242:1347, 1967.

Rosenberg B, van Camp L, Krigas T: Inhibition of cell division in *Escherichia coli* by electrolysis products from a platinum electrode. *Nature* 205: 698, 1965.

Rosenberg B, van Camp L, Trosko JE, Mansour VH: Platinum compounds: a new class of potent antitumor agents. *Nature* 222:385, 1969.

Rozen C, Weig M, von Hoff DD, et al: Cis-diammine-dichloro-platinum (II): a new anticancer drug. *Ann Intern Med* 86:803, 1977.

Tomson AJ: The interaction of platinum compounds with biological molecules. *Recent Results Cancer Res* 48:38, 1974.

Wiltshaw E: A review of clinical experience with cis-diammine-dichloro-platinum (II). *Biochemistry* 60:925, 1976.

Wiltshaw E: Cis-platinum in adenocarcinoma of the ovary, a critical review. *Adv Biosci* 26:179, 1980.

Wiltshaw E, Kroner T: Phase 2 study of cis-dichloro-diammine-platinum (II) (NSC-119875) and advanced adenocarcinoma of the ovary. *Cancer Treat Rep* 60:55, 1976.

23

Role of Radiation Therapy in Management of Ovarian Cancer

Controversy has developed over the role of external x-ray therapy for the management of patients with common epithelial ovarian cancer. Although it is accepted that external x-ray therapy has a place in the treatment of the gonadal stromal tumors and germ cell tumors exclusive of the extraembryonal tumors, its role in the therapy of the common epithelial ovarian cancers has diminished in prominence. There are several reasons: (1) A study carried out at the M.D. Anderson Hospital compared melphalan (Alkeran) to radiation therapy as postoperative therapy. The radiation therapy was associated with more serious toxicity and a greater economic cost to the patient but did not improve the surgical rate; therefore chemotherapy was selected as the treatment of choice. (2) The response of the common epithelial ovarian cancer and its type of superficial spread over the liver and diaphragm interfered with optimal treatment. (3) There have been few reports of radiation therapy studies showing improved results with this modality, and some have emphasized toxicity. Orthovoltage, kilovoltage, and now megavoltage have not shown any increase in the 5-year survival. (4) There has been an increasing number of reports of studies on single chemotherapeutic agents or combinations of drugs showing high response rates. (5) The addition of *cis*-platinum to a multiple-drug regimen has produced an increased survival rate in most series.

Protocol for the management of ovarian carcinoma at Lenox Hill Hospital has phased out external therapy as the second-line therapeutic modality for the common epithelial ovarian carcinoma. Radiation therapy is now reserved for selected stage IV patients in whom the disease involves supraclavicular and inguinal nodes; it has been helpful when there is localized disease against the pelvic wall. When disease on the pelvic wall can be outlined with metallic clips, it is possible to deliver a high dose of radiation to this area without damaging an excessive amount of normal tissue. It is obvious that it must be combined with systemic chemotherapy to achieve maximum effect. It is not given for stage I, II, or III carcinoma for reasons stated in other chapters of this book. However, it must be reemphasized and restated that external x-ray therapy has a place in the management of gonadal stromal tumors and germ cell tumors exclusive of the extraembryonal tumors. These tumors not only appear to be radiosensitive, their natural history and method of spread provides a better clinical setting for the administration of external x-ray therapy.

Because external irradiation is frequently for the management of ovarian carcinoma, the use of irradiation and the most frequently employed methods of giving the therapy are discussed.

Ovarian cancer is not a single entity but encompasses a group of diseases with different biologic behaviors, all spreading diffusely over the surface of organs throughout the abdominal cavity. It may also spread to the retroperitoneal lymph nodes, particularly along the paraaortic chain. Even with early disease, when the tumor has been limited to one ovary and has been completely removed, there is the possibility of contamination of the peritoneal cavity. It is therefore accepted by many physicians that irradiation of the entire abdomen is the logical therapy for ovarian carcinomas.

Technique for External X-Ray Therapy

Kottmeier's technique is to administer the therapy through two large anterior and two corresponding posterior fields while protecting the kidneys and liver. His protocol has progressed from the conventional x-ray therapy (200–400 kV) aimed at the large fields as described above (with the occasional addition of later fields), to the use of supervoltage. Kottmeier's results do not indicate that supervoltage radiation improves results, but from a physical point of view it has several advantages. The wide-field technique attempts to deliver a total dose of 2000 rad over 6 weeks, and no more than 3000 rad can be delivered in 5 to 6 weeks to such a large volume of the abdomen. A daily dose of 200 rad to the lower abdomen is well tolerated, but it is inadvisable to exceed 100 rad per day to the upper abdomen.

Delclos and colleagues reported on another technique using three or four fields. It is a modification of the static field method. The treatment, which is given with megavoltage, is not better tolerated than the static-field method because the tissue volume irradiated at any one time is the same. Although a higher dose is given to the central volume, which may be desirable in selected situations in which a higher dose is warranted around the paraaortic area, it can be better accomplished using a megavoltage unit at an 18- to 25-MeV level, with a field within a field, or with an additional boost after completion of whole abdominal irradiation. There is an increased incidence of gastrointestinal complications with this method of treatment.

Often treatment must be interrupted because of nausea, diarrhea, malaise, temperature elevation, fatigue, loss of appetite, and a considerable drop in the blood count. It is un-

likely that this dose will be lethal in any significant number of tumors, except the pure dysgerminoma.

The other technique popularized by Delclos is the moving strip technique for treating the whole abdomen from the pelvic floor to the diaphragm over the course of 30 to 40 days. The technique was introduced in Manchester, England, in 1957. It can be used with any supervoltage unit by proper correction of depth dose and penumbra effect, provided the beam is wide enough to cover the abdomen from side to side.

This technique treats a volume of tissue eight times by the beam and four times by the penumbra (12 days total). The whole treatment time, to cover the area from the pelvic floor to the diaphragm, extends from 30 to 40 days. A tumor dose of 2500 to 2700 rad, measured at the midline of the patient along a sagittal plane, can be delivered safely. The dose delivered to the tumor has a much greater biologic efficiency because it is given in a much shorter time than with the static-field technique. Because only a fragment of the abdominal cavity and surrounding tissues is irradiated at any one time, tolerance is also better. The dose given by this technique is equivalent to about 3200 to 3400 rad given in 3.5 weeks by the static-field technique. After irradiation of the whole abdomen, Delclos et al. added 2000 rad in 2 weeks to the pelvis (15 × 15 cm fields) by means of a 25-MeV photon beam (from a betatron or linear accelerator).

The volume of tissue described by Delclos et al. is divided into a series of contiguous segments, and the field is moved from one end of the volume to the other. Lines 2.5 cm apart are marked on the front and back of the patient. On the first day a single strip is treated from the front, and on the second day an identical opposite field is irradiated from the back. Thereafter one 2.5 cm wide strip is added daily until four strips have been irradiated front and back. Next the 10 cm strip is moved 2.5 cm up every day by alternating front and back until the last strip is reached. The field is then reduced by one strip of 2.5 cm daily. During the last 2 days, a single 2.5 cm strip is irradiated. The kidneys are shielded from the posterior beam by two half-value layers (HVLs) of lead placed on a satellite platform (which reduces the dose to the kidneys to about 50% of the tumor dose). The right side of the liver (three strips) is shielded both front and back with one HVL of lead. To compensate for the lower dose at both ends of the irradiated volume, the treatment is started one strip below the lower margin of the pelvic field (placed at midpubis) and completed one strip above the diaphragm, which should be localized by fluoroscopy. As reported above, the pelvis then receives an additional 2000 rad.

The patients tolerated the moving-strip technique better than they did the static field method. There was little weight loss during treatment despite the high incidence of nausea and diarrhea. The hemoglobin and hematocrit remained fairly constant, but the lymphocytes and platelets dropped by 60% of the original value during the first 2 weeks and then started to return toward normal after therapy was completed. The diarrhea tended to appear by the second week of treatment and then decreased, whereas the nausea was more marked during the fifth week at the time of the most intense treatment to the upper abdomen.

The Princess Margaret Hospital in Ontario, Canada, employs a moving-strip technique. However, there is a difference in their technique from the moving strip technique reported by others. To irradiate the whole abdomen, the irradiation field has been extended superiorly to cover the diaphragm. At the Princess Margaret Hospital, routine radiologic verification of the superior border invariably demonstrated the domes of the diaphragm to be above the xiphisternum. It is uncommon in this hospital's experience for a field less than 40 cm in length to cover the peritoneal cavity adequately from the floor of the pelvis to the domes of the diaphragm. In early publications from the M.D. Anderson Hospital, diagrams suggest that the xiphoid process was used to define the superior border. At the Princess Margaret Hospital, in randomized studies utilizing a cobalt 60 moving strip technique, only 1 of 78 (1.5%) patients developed serious bowel complications during the median period at risk of 62 months. The prescribed midplane abdominal dose was 2250

rad in ten fractions (plus a pelvic boost) compared to 2800 rads and 3300 rads in eight fractions reported by others. The physical cost of the lower dose treatment is small, and the benefit is large. Based on a failure analysis, it was concluded is that it is the effectiveness of abdominal irradiation in controlling occult upper abdominal disease that has resulted in the improvement. The current status of treatment for patients with ovarian cancer at the Princess Margaret Hospital considers irradiation to be the postoperative treatment of choice for patients with poorly differentiated stage I and all those with stage II and III cancer who have no gross residual disease or only a small amount of pelvic residual disease. When the disease is more extensive, the group obtains few cures with irradiation, and they prefer to use chemotherapy as the initial approach. It is estimated that only about 55% of patients fall into the favorable group, and the remainder are considered in the unfavorable group.

The common epithelial ovarian carcinomas arise from the germinal epithelium. This histogenetic origin might imply a high degree of radiosensitivity. However, experience has shown that in general these tumors have limited radiosensitivity. Among the germ cell tumors, the dysgerminoma has a highly radiosensitive response; and among the gonadal stromal tumors (granulosa cell), the response in general is excellent but does not equal that of the dysgerminoma. The other germ cell tumors (embryonal teratomas) and the extra-embryonal tumors (endodermal-sinus tumors and choriocarcinoma ovarian tumors) are relatively radioresistant. Thus for the common epithelial ovarian tumors, radiation therapy is severely handicapped by frequent widespread anatomic distribution of tumors of limited radiovulnerability.

Consequently, for those physicians who use radiation therapy in patients whose ovarian cancer is grossly limited to the pelvis, it seems preferable to irradiate this restricted tumor and tissue volume to a potentially cancericidal dose. This approach is chosen in preference to treating the entire peritoneal cavity to a lower and likely ineffective dose limited by patient tolerance. However, it has been shown that the

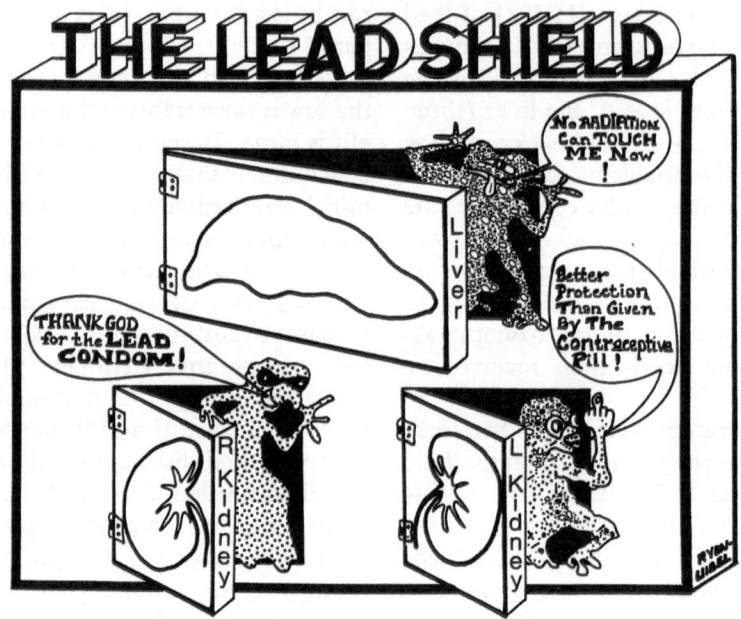

FIGURE 23.1. Cancer cell being protected by a lead shield and thereby avoiding a cancericidal dose during abdominal radiation therapy.

failures among this group occur with disease in the upper abdomen. In addition, the number of patients who fall strictly within the stage II group makes up a small number in any series. It is becoming increasingly clear that it is not logical just to irradiate the pelvis when common epithelial ovarian cancer is being treated.

The patient does not tolerate radiation therapy of the entire peritoneal cavity to cancericidal dosage. Therapy is initially limited by the nausea, vomiting, diarrhea, weight loss, fatigue, lack of appetite, and drop in the blood count. These complications are reversible, but the most serious problem is nonreversible damage to the kidneys and liver by doses required to control cancer (Fig. 23.1).

Currently, a moving-strip technique has been employed to irradiate the entire peritoneal cavity. This technique has been proposed in an attempt to improve the dose-time relation, but such improvement is achieved at the expense of delivering a homogeneous dose of radiation to anatomic structures and the tumor, which results from the daily variation in position. Hot spot damage to the intestines may result.

Experience indicates that radiation should have its optimal application for patients with stage II ovarian cancer. The results in stage I do not show any advantage to the addition of external x-ray therapy. The radioactive isotopes play a significant role in increasing the 5-year survival rate in stage I common epithelial ovarian cancers. Use of external radiation therapy in patients with stage III disease is compromised by the need to reduce the dosage to large tissue volumes. Local irradiation for palliative purposes occasionally is useful in patients with stage III and IV disease.

Because laparotomy is necessary for the diagnosis of tumors in situations in which radiation therapy is likely to be useful, irradiation has followed definitive surgery. Therefore preoperative irradiation, frequently preferred for other clinical problems, has not been adequately evaluated. The work reported on the poor response rate to radiation therapy when tumor masses are larger than 2 cm precludes the use of preoperative x-ray therapy except in highly selected cases.

In the past in some institutions, the uterus was not removed so it could be used as a container for radium. Because the radiation level decreases by the inverse square law, little is delivered to the area surrounding the uterus. Now, however, available external radiation therapy allows adequate dose distribution throughout the pelvis. Therefore the uterus, which is frequently involved by ovarian cancer, should be removed at the time of initial definitive therapy.

External radiation therapy is supplied by machines producing x-rays, gamma rays, or electrons. In addition, machines producing protons, neutrons, and mesons are under intense investigation. X-ray machines range from very low to very high voltages (10,000 volts = 10 KeV to 70,000,000 volts = 70 MeV). In general, the higher the voltage, the greater is the penetration of the x-rays. X-ray therapy with voltage over 1 MeV, called supervoltage therapy, is used for deep-seated cancers. The principal advantage of supervoltage machines compared with ordinary 250 KeV machines is the greater penetration and less severe skin reaction.

Protons, helium ions, and free ions are heavily charged particles. The particles pass through matter and travel at nearly a straight line and come to a stop after passing through a certain depth of absorbent, depending on their initial energy. The rate of energy loss increases sharply near the end of the range. There the dose reaches a peak known as the *Bragg peak*. The dose falls off rapidly beyond the Bragg peak. Neutrons interact with tissue and release actively ionizing, heavily charged particles. Most of the dose is contributed by recoiling protons from hydrogen and tissue. Current research with neutron therapy has promise but has not added significantly to the survival of those treated for gynecologic cancer. Ionizing radiation cuts through chromosomes much like a Gigli saw. Unless something is introduced to block the two ends of the chromosome from joining, the ends join often with no loss of function. On the other hand, the particle radiation is large and tears gaping holes in the chromosomes, often damaging them beyond repair.

The negative pi mesons, or *pions*, are negatively charged particles with the mass 273 times

that of an electron. Pions can be produced in any nuclear interaction if the energy of the primary particle is sufficient to create the rest mass of a pion. Radiotherapy employing pions with energies between approximately 70 and 440 MeV is of interest, as these particles have ranges in tissue of approximately 6 and 15 cm, respectively. Pions travel through tissue in a manner similar to that of any other heavily charged particle and stop after traveling a given range, which depends on the initial energy.

As the pion goes through tissue, it transfers little of its energy, and it gives rise to a sharply defined maximum near the end of the range (Bragg peak). It delivers more dose at depth than at the entrance and practically no dose beyond the calculated depth to be treated. Obviously, then, it should not be as destructive to normal tissue as conventional radiotherapy, which has been demonstrated—a strong plus for pion therapy. Complications following conventional radiotherapy are feared by both patient and physician. It may now be possible to put these fears to rest. With available methods of delivering radiation therapy, there is no way of giving a tumoricidal dose to organs deep in the abdomen (i.e., the pancreas) and spare the spinal cord. With the meson beam, the therapist is able to match the shape of the tumor by controlling the energy level, which results in a considerable reduction in the incidence of transverse myelitis.

A unique characteristic of the pions is that they are captured by the nuclei of the medium when they come to rest because of the negative charge on the meson. These nuclei then disintegrate into short range and heavily ionizing fragments, thus constituting so-called star production and providing a way to monitor the dose of pions delivered at a particular level. During the cascade, characteristic x-rays are evident. They are called *pi mesic x-rays* and are used to monitor the amount of radiation delivered. This method delivers maximum radiation to the cancer while sparing adjacent normal tissue.

The pion beam offers the attractive possibility to the radiotherapist of localizing radiation to the tumor. It can be directed to a region where the absorbed dose is high and the radiation has a high degree of biologic effectiveness and low dependence on oxygen. At the same time, the normal tissues in the path of the incident ray are exposed to lower doses of radiation than is the tumor, and the radiation involved is also of lower biologic effectiveness.

During radiation therapy one of the important physical parameters is the sharpness of the beam, usually referred to as the *penumbra*. With the sharp beam, the normal tissue adjacent to the outer edge of the beam is not damaged. The pions qualify for achieving this goal. Prior to the introduction to particle therapy, the limiting factor of therapy was damage to normal tissue. Now another obstacle to delivering a cancericidal dose has been overcome. This point has been reviewed because, if current work continues to be as productive as the initial experiments, a new modality for therapy for ovarian cancer may be added to the armamentarium of the clinician.

The most common teletherapy machine is the cobalt 60 unit. Practically every department of radiation therapy now has a cobalt machine. These units produce a fairly homogeneous (clean) beam of 1 MeV and 1.3-MeV gamma rays.

Radiation therapy makes use of the ionizing radiations —x-rays and electrons produced by manmade machines and gamma rays, which emanate from naturally or artificially radioactive elements—to destroy cells by injuring their capacity to divide. The "law" for Bergonie and Tribondeau, formulated in 1906, stated that x-rays are more effective on cells that have a greater reproductive activity; the effectiveness is greater among cells that have a larger dividing future and those whose morphology and function are last fixed. The radiosensitivity of cells and tissues is proportional to their reproductive capacity and inversely proportional to their degree of differentiation. Because the central attribute of cancer cells is their sustained, uncontrolled, lawless proliferation, injury to this property is precisely what is desired. Although some rapidly dividing normal cells are also killed during the radiotherapeutic eradication of a cancer, the large reservoir of similar normal cells outside the irradiated field is readily able, in most instances, to replenish the supply and to repair the irradiated tissues. Thus in favorable cases the cancer gradually disappears completely during treatment, the acute radiation reaction in the normal tissues then slowly subsides, and a year or more later the patient may present no external evidence whatever of having been treated.

Oxygen and Radiosensitivity

It has long been known that cells are nearly threefold more radiosensitive in the presence of oxygen than in its absence. Many cancers outgrow their blood supply, and the presence of necrotic foci within them strongly suggests that cancer cells that have come to be more than 150 to 200 μm from the nearest capillary are severely hypoxic or anoxic. Oxygen concentration diminishes as the distance from the capillary increases. Cells near the necrotic center may actually be anoxic. Oxygen concentration falls to zero at 150 μm from capillaries, and cells even more distant are anoxic. Such anoxia may underlie the observation that the zone of living cells is rather constant in width. Diffusion of oxygen across the zone and its eventual exhaustion may determine how many cells can live as the tumor mass increases. The source of oxygen and nutrients may be pushed too far away from cells at the center, and many of the cells may die. Such hypoxic or anoxic cells would be radioresistant compared to normally oxygenated ones adjacent to the stroma. It may well be that, in the usual course of events, they get damaged and become part of the necrotic center of the tumor, but because they are hypoxic they may survive a normal course of radiotherapy.

The radiation therapists have reported that a tumor mass of 2 cm or more has a large residue of hypoxic cells after x-ray therapy. These hypoxic cells may not die and in fact may begin to divide and give rise to a recurrence of the tumor. This possibility has caused therapists to reevaluate their positions and has resulted in their reluctance, if not refusal, to treat such patients. Thus it is suggested that the recurrent growth of many cancers after an initially good radiotherapeutic response may be due to the

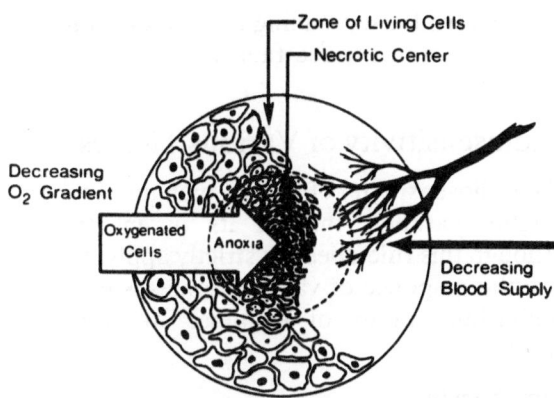

FIGURE 23.2. Tumors have ectopic regions. The mass of cells grows outward from its interior. Oxygen concentration diminishes as the distance from the capillaries increases. Cells near the necrotic center may actually be anoxic. Such hypoxic or necrotic cells would be radioresistant compared to normally oxygenated ones near the periphery.

survival of microscopic foci of such hypoxic, radioresistant tumor cells that, after shrinkage of the tumor, are once again brought into proximity with blood vessels, can obtain oxygen and nutrients, and thereupon resume active proliferation (Fig. 23.2). To eliminate all of the cells in the necrotic center, it would take three times the dose that it takes to kill cells in a well-oxygenated environment. It is not possible to deliver this level of radiation therapy because of fear of damaging the intestine.

Radiobiology

Radiobiology is the study of the action of ionizing radiation on living things. It is now established that the killing of cells by ionizing radiation, in vivo and in clonal cell culture, is an exponential function of dose, beyond an initial low-dose range in which the survival curve exhibits a "shoulder." When the same total dose is split into two fractions separated in time by an increasing interval, survival increases for the first 2 to 4 hours, decreases during the next 3 to 4 hours, and finally increases again with concomitant restoration of the shoulder to the survival curve. It is thus apparent that the shoulder represents a recov-

ery process, which is operative at low doses but becomes overwhelmed as the dose increases. Split dose recovery is diminished by low temperature, by certain chemical agents (e.g., actinomycin D), and at least in some cells by hypoxia, suggesting that it is an energy-consuming enzymatic process. However, neither the identity of the molecular lesion nor the mechanism of its repair is known at this time.

The goal of radiotherapy must be to sterilize essentially all of the clonogenic cells of the tumor while avoiding damage to normal tissues beyond their capability to repair. The rationale for a treatment regimen cannot be based on the expectation that tumor cells are more sensitive than normal cells, as there is no evidence that this is the case. Indeed, there is every indication that at least a proportion of tumor cells are more resistant than normal cells because they are hypoxic. The differential effect of a treatment regimen on tumor cells compared to normal cells must therefore exploit the difference in kinetics between the two cell populations concerned.

The body of experimental data accumulated during recent years has shed a good deal of light on what has come to be called the four R's of radiobiology: (1) repair of sublethal damage; (2) redistribution of cells within the cell cycle; (3) repopulation, that is, division and regrowth of cells following a treatment; and (4) reoxygenation, the term used for the process by which the proportion of hypoxic cells in a tumor tends to return to its original value after disturbance caused by a dose of radiation.

DNA Breaks

The linear energy transfer (LET) is a measure of the average rate of energy loss along the track of an ionizing particle. It is the energy released (usually in kiloelectron volts) per micrometer of medium (tissue) along the track of any ionizing particle. LET is not a static or constant value; it is different even for the same particle over different portions of the track because, although charge on a particle is a constant factor, the velocity continually changes (decreases) all along the particle track. Each interaction (excitation or ionization) involves a loss of energy from the particle and a concomitant deceleration. As a result, LET gradually increases along a particle track and increases dramatically just before the particle comes to rest. This peak in the rate of energy dissipation is called the *Bragg peak*. Particles with different degrees of charge produce different tracks. Highly charged particles interact frequently; consequently they have a high LET, and the ionization along their tracks is dense. Particles with lesser degrees of charge are sparsely ionizing, and they have a lower LET.

The radiobiologic effects on cells may be due to molecular, enzyme, or nuclear damage. The principal macromolecular target in the cell is its nucleus, particularly the DNA. The nuclear damage includes inhibition of cell division, chromosome mutation, and nuclear damage. In bacteria it has been shown that ionizing radiation produces both single- and double-strand breaks in DNA, and several lines of evidence suggest that the double-strand breaks account for most of the lethal events. X-rays can go through a chromosome like a Gigli saw; and if conditions are right, the two portions of the chromosome join as they were before and no damage results. However, potentiators such as the halogenated, thymidine analogues (5-bromodeoxyuridine), if given during x-ray therapy, may be incorporated into DNA in place of thymidine and inhibit cell growth. Other potentiators, such as hydroxyurea, bind to DNA and may thus interfere or compete with the binding of a repair enzyme to a site of injury. Certain nuclear particles, notably protons, neutrons, and negative pi mesons (pions), have attracted attention as substitutes for x-rays and electrons because they are much less dependent on oxygen and, in the case of pions, have unique properties that would make possible a much more precise and selective localization of the beam energy to the volume occupied by the cancer. Unlike x-rays, which cut through a chromosome like a Gigli saw, the particles such as protons, neutrons, and pions are large particles; and when they pass through a chromosome a large piece of the chromo-some is torn loose, making it more difficult for that chromosome to reestablish itself.

Radiosensitivity of Various Tissues

The radiosensitivity of a given malignant tumor roughly parallels that of its parent tissue, although this rule does not strictly apply; therefore the response of various tissues is listed in diminishing order of response to radiation therapy.

Lymphocytes
Erythroblasts, myelocytes
Myeloblasts
Epithelial cells
    Basal cells of testis
    Basal cells of ovary
    Basal cells of skin
    Basal cells of secretory glands
    Pulmonary alveolar cells and bile ducts
Endothelial cells
Connective tissue cell
Renal tubular cells
Bone cells
Nerve cells
Brain cells
Muscle cells

Summary

In my protocol for common epithelial ovarian cancer, external x-ray therapy has been reserved for selected patients with stage IV carcinoma of the ovary in whom the disease involves supraclavicular or inguinal nodes (or both). Radiation therapy is not given for stages I, II, or III. Some medical centers routinely apply radiation therapy to all stage II ovarian cancer patients—those with disease against the pelvic side wall.

The natural history of germ cell and gonadal stromal ovarian cancers permits a more rational external x-ray therapy program. Indeed, both groups (except for the embryonal and extraembryonal germ cell cancers) respond well to x-ray therapy. The dysgerminoma spreads to paraaortic nodes, and a limited part of the abdomen can then be irradiated with cancericidal doses. The gonadal stroma are characterized by local spread, late recurrence, and recurrence within the pelvic cavity, which provides the opportunity to treat the patient successfully with external x-ray therapy.

Currently, external x-ray therapy is being reevaluated as a modality of therapy for management of common epithelial ovarian cancer. Princess Margaret Hospital in Toronto, Canada, has been treating patients with a moving-strip technique that covers a field of 40 cm. The position of the diaphragm is identified by x-ray studies so the area can be adequately irradiated. In summary, the Princess Margaret Hospital group considers radiation to be the postoperative treatment of choice for patients with poorly differentiated stage I cancer and all stage II and III cancer patients who have no gross residual disease in the upper abdomen or only a small amount of pelvic residual tumor. When the disease is more extensive, these physicians have obtained few cures with irradiation and so prefer to use chemotherapy as the initial approach. (Approximately 55% of their patients are eligible for treatment with chemotherapy.)

The case against external x-ray therapy includes the observation that the common epithelial ovarian cancer is a surface spreader, moving over the liver and diaphragm as well as along the bowel. Damage to the bowel limits the effectiveness of a cancericidal dose to the entire pelvis. Radiation therapists also state that it is difficult to cure lesions that are 2 cm or larger, and every gynecologist knows that with most stage III and IV tumors a volume greater than 2 cm is left at the time of the initial surgery. Epithelial cells, especially those of the common epithelial ovarian tumors, are considered only relatively radiosensitive. Woodruff has advanced the concept that the ovary and the entire peritoneal cavity comprise a mesothelial structure, and whatever stimulates the ovary to produce a tumor is also stimulating other areas. It is his observation that many stage III cancers do not represent metastatic lesions but multiple primaries. This situation changes the interpretation of the disease, and instead of being a "localized" disease it moves into a more unfavorable category that should be treated as a systemic disease. A 1979 editorial in the *British Medical Journal* did not even mention radiotherapy as a treatment method for ovarian cancer.

There are several studies using combined-modality therapy, including chemotherapy and radiotherapy. Both of these treatment methods are active against ovarian cancer; yet a way of combining the two to obtain an additive effect on survival has been elusive. The simultaneous use of large-field irradiation and chemotherapy is limited by myelosuppression, although the possibility of low-dose systemic *cis*-platinum or intraperitoneal administration of chemotherapy during a course of whole abdominal irradiation has been described as an innovative approach. Fuks and coworkers were the first to attempt improving survival in patients with large residual disease by systematically employing a combined modality approach in sequence: primary surgery→ combination chemotherapy→ secondary cytoreductive surgery→ abdominopelvic radiotherapy. The preliminary work on this approach showed promise, but more time is needed to evaluate it.

A much larger study was begun in Italy in 1980 using a sequential combined modality approach. Stage III and IV cancers were stratified by residuum and then randomized between *cis*-platinum, cyclophosphamide/*cis*-platinum, and cyclophosphamide (Cytoxan)/doxorubicin (Adriamycin)/*cis*-platinum (CAP). After six cycles, laparotomy was performed; and depending on the findings, patients were given consolidation treatment with nothing, radiophosphorus, moving-strip abdominopelvic radiotherapy, or CAP. The percentage of residual tumor is greater than 30%. However promising these two series have been, they have not received widespread support in the United States. The morbidity rate has increased, and therefore gynecologists are less inclined to use it.

An attempt has been made in this chapter to review briefly the types of radiation therapy and radiobiology that may help the clinician manage patients with ovarian cancer.

Bibliography

Bagley CM, Young RC, Shine PS, et al: Ovarian carcinoma metastatic to the diaphragm—frequently undiagnosed at laparotomy. *Am J Obstet Gynecol* 116:397, 1973.

Bleehen NM: Prospects from radiobiology. In Halman KE (ed): *Recent Advances in Cancer and Radiotherapeutics: Clinical Oncology*. Williams & Wilkins, Baltimore, 1972.

Buschke F, Parker RG: *Radiation Therapy in Cancer Management*. Grune & Stratton, Orlando, FL, 1972, p. 276.

Bush RS, Allt WEC, Beal A, et al: Treatment of epithelial carcinoma of the ovary: operation, irradiation and chemotherapy. *Am J Obstet Gynecol* 127:692, 1977.

Bush RS, Dembo AJ: Current status of treatment for patients with ovarian cancer: ovarian cancer. *Adv Biosci* 26:115, 1980.

Dalrymple GV, Gaulden ME, Kollmorgen GM, Vogel HH, Jr: *Medical Radiation Biology*. Saunders, Philadelphia, 1973.

Delclos L, Braun EJ, Herrera JR, et al: Whole abdominal irradiation by cobalt 60 moving strip technique. *Radiology* 81:632, 1969.

Delclos L, Fletcher GH: Postoperative irradiation for ovarian carcinoma with the cobalt-60 moving strip technique. *Clin Obstet Gynecol* 12:993, 1969.

Delclos L, Murphy M: Evaluation of tolerance during treatment, late tolerance, and better evaluation of clinical effectiveness of the cobalt 60 moving strip technique. *Am J Roentgenol Radium Ther Nucl Med* 96:75, 1966.

Delclos L, Smith JP: Ovarian cancer, with special regard to types of radiotherapy. *Natl Cancer Inst Monogr* 42:129, 1975.

Dembo AJ: Radiotherapeutic management of ovarian cancer. *Semin Oncol* 11:238, 1984.

Dembo AJ: The role of radiotherapy in ovarian cancer. *Bull Cancer (Paris)* 69:275, 1982.

Dembo AJ, Bush RS, Beale FA, et al: A randomized clinical trial of moving strip versus open field whole abdominal irradiation in patients with invasive epithelial cancer of the ovary. *Int J Radiat Oncol Biol Phys* 9(suppl):97, 1983.

Editorial. cancer of the ovary. *Br Med J* 3:687, 1979.

Fazehas JT, Maier JG: Irradiation of ovarian carcinoma: a prospective comparison of the open field and moving strip techniques. *Am J Roentgenol Radium Ther Nucl Med* 120:118, 1974.

Fletcher GH: Clinical dose-response curve of subclinical aggregates of epithelial cells and its practical application in the management of human cancers. In Friedman, M. (ed): *Biological and Clinical Basis of Radiosensitivity*. Charles C Thomas, Springfield, IL, 1974, pp. 485–501.

Fuks Z: External radiotherapy of ovarian cancer: standard approaches and new frontiers. *Semin Oncol* 2:253, 1975.

Fuks Z, Rizel S, Anteby SO, et al: The multimodal approach to the treatment of stage III ovarian carcinoma. *Int J Radiat Oncol Biol Phys* 8:903, 1982.

Hall EJ: *Radiobiology for the Radiologist*. Harper & Row, New York, 1973.

Heintz BL, Fuks Z, Timpson RL, et al: Results of postoperative megavoltage radiotherapy of malignant surface epithelial tumors of the ovary. *Radiology* 114:695, 1975.

Kjellgren O, Jonsson L: Bone marrow depression in the pelvis after megavoltage irradiation for ovarian carcinoma. *Obstet Gynecol* 105:849, 1969.

Kottmeier HL: Radiotherapy in the treatment of ovarian carcinoma. *Clin Obstet Gynecol* 4:865, 1961.

Martinez A, Schray MF, Howes AE, et al: Postoperative radiation therapy for epithelial ovarian cancer: the curative role based on 24-year experience. *J Clin Oncol* 3:901, 1985.

Myers MA: The spread and localization of acute intraperitoneal effusions. *Radiology* 95:547, 1970.

Parmley TN, Woodruff JD: The ovarian mesothelioma. *Am J Obstet Gynecol* 120:234, 1974.

Perez CA, Bradfield JS: Radiation therapy in the treatment of carcinoma of the ovary. *Cancer* 29:1027, 1972.

Pizzarello DJ, Witcofski RL: *Basic Radiation Biology*. Lea & Febiger, Philadelphia, 1972.

Rosenhoff R, Young R, Bagley C, et al: Peritoneoscopy: a valuable tool for initial staging and "second look" in ovarian cancer. *Proc Am Assoc Cancer Res* 15:171, 1974.

Wharton JT, Delclos L, Gallagher S, et al: Radiation hepatitis induced by abdominal irradiation with cobalt 60 moving strip technique. *Am J Roentgenol Radium Ther Nucl Med* 117:73, 1973.

Woodruff JD: The pathogenesis of ovarian neoplasm. *Johns Hopkins Med J* 144:117, 1979.

24

Autoimmune and Immunodeficiency Diseases

Ovarian cancer often resembles an autoimmune disorder. These patients may be difficult to cross-match, and it has been observed that they have an antibody that interferes with cross-matching. Such an antibody, which may occur in patients who have not been transfused, reacts against normal tissue but does not recognize the ovarian cancer antigen. It can be suppressed after cortisone treatment. For 2 to 3 days following this therapy it is possible to cross-match the patient. In addition, the use of anticancer drug treatment gives the patient a sense of well-being long before there is any effect on tumor volume. These observations are suggestive but not conclusive that an autoimmune disorder results from the ovarian cancer.

Autoimmune Disorder and Autoimmune Disease

Autoimmunity is the reaction of the immune system against the body's own tissue. The autoantigens–autoantibodies refer to antigen–antibody systems where antibodies are formed to self-molecules. Autoreactive cells are lymphocytes with receptors for autoantigens. These cells can potentially produce an autoimmune response but do not necessarily do so.

Burnet proposed the theory to explain the way the body is normally tolerant to its own tissue by saying that autoreactive cells were effectively forbidden and so were clonally deleted during embryologic development. It is now known that autoreactive B cells are present, but they are not normally active.

It is accepted that self-tolerance is maintained at the level of the T cell; self-reactive T cells are clonally aborted or functionally deleted. It has been proposed that with autoimmune disease autoreactive B cells become activated by a mechanism that bypasses the tolerant T cells. For example, a cross-reactive exogenous antigen binding to a T cell could produce help for an autoreactive B cell. Alternatively, polyclonal stimulators such as the Epstein-Barr virus or lipopolysaccharide could stimulate the B cell directly.

The control of some autoreactive cells is considered to depend on T suppressors. If there is a failure of the T suppressors or if autoantigens become associated with 1a molecules and preferentially stimulate autoreactive T cells, autoimmunity may result. Autoimmune diseases occur when autoimmune reactions result in pathologic tissue damage. In general, they are either organ-specific or organ-nonspecific.

Organ-specific autoimmune diseases are primarily directed toward particular tissues, for example, autoantibodies to thyroid and Hashimoto's thyroiditis or to pancreatic islet cells in autoimmune diabetes. Different types of organ-specific autoimmunity tend to occur together in particular individuals and their relatives.

Organ-nonspecific autoimmune diseases have antibodies to autoantigens with a wide tissue distribution, such as anti-DNA and systemic lupus erythematosus. These conditions often produce type III immune complex-mediated hypersensitivity reaction.

Advanced and recurrent cancer of the ovary may display clinical features similar to those found in an autoimmune response. For this reason a brief discussion on autoimmune disorders is included here, and a correlation of the findings regarding advanced and recurrent ovarian cancer is discussed.

Clinical and experimental observations show that individuals can sometimes respond immunologically to certain of their own antigens (self-antigens). These important exceptions to the principle of self-tolerance help analyze its fundamental mechanisms, and they are frequently associated with disease. It is often not clear, however, whether these anomalous responses cause, or are the result of, disease. Hence it is necessary to emphasize the distinction between an *autoimmune response*, in which an individual makes antibodies or becomes allergic to a self-antigen, and an *autoimmune disease*, which is a pathologic condition arising from an autoimmune response. Autoimmune reactions can be both antibody-mediated and cell-mediated. Autoimmunity reflects a loss of immunologic tolerance to tissue and cellular antigens. Immunologic tolerance is the result of an active physiologic process and is not simply the lack of an immune response. Before the pathogenetic processes that lead to autoimmunity are discussed, it is important to review the roles of B cells and T cells (suppressor and helper) and the mechanisms involved.

Immunodeficiency

Immunodeficiency is often identified by the increased frequency of infection in patients. Impaired immunity is a consequence of many pathogenic infections, but primary immunodeficiency is inherited and may affect any part of the immune system, including complement components, granulocytes, macrophages, and lymphocytes.

There are a variety of immunodeficiencies and abnormalities, including X-linked agammaglobulinemia (Bruton's disease), variable hypogammaglobulinemia, DiGeorge syndrome, severe combined immunodeficiency (SCID), acquired immunodeficiency syndrome (AIDS), thymoma, myeloma, Bence Jones protein disorder, and heavy chain disease.

Background

Experiments, clinical observations, and studies of experiments of nature (Bruton's agammaglobulinemia, DiGeorge syndrome, Swiss agammaglobulinemia) have led to the concept of two cell systems of immunity: T (thymus-derived) lymphocytes, which are concerned with cell-mediated immunity, and B (probably bone marrow-derived) lymphocytes. These two cell lines represent independent lines of differentiation but have a common precursor stem cell.

Pluripotent stem cells originate in the yolk sac and migrate to the fetal liver and then to the bone marrow. These stem cells differentiate into the cells of all the major hematopoietic elements. Lymphocytes, the primary cells involved in all immunologic reactions, are classified in two subpopulations according to their origin and functions. T lymphocytes derive their immunologic maturity from the thymus and are responsible for cell-mediated immunity; B lymphocytes mature in an unknown site, probably in the bone marrow, and are responsible for antibody-mediated immunity. A number of receptors and antigens have been identified on the surface of human lymphocytes, and these surface markers serve to evaluate lymphoid cell populations in a variety of human diseases.

Lymphoid stem cells can function as prethymic cells and are processed in the thymus under the influence of thymosin or thymopoietin to differentiate into T cells. T lymphocytes represent 80% of the circulating peripheral blood lymphocytes and are responsible for protection against certain infective agents such as fungi, intracellular facultative bacteria and most of the viruses, rejection of tissue transplants, and delayed-type hypersensitivity. The effector functions are performed by the pharmacologically and biochemically active chemical mediators, the lymphokines, which are produced by the T cells when they are exposed to specific antigens or nonspecific mitogens. These lymphokines (transfer factor, lymphocyte transforming activity, migration inhibition factor, and lymphotoxin) probably have both specific and nonspecific functions. The immunocompetent T lymphocyte produces sensitized T-lymphocyte subpopulations. These sensitized T lymphocytes release a helper factor that enables immunocompetent B cells to respond to antigens that they are otherwise unable to recognize.

The sensitized subpopulation of lymphocytes may produce suppressor T cells, which regulate the B-cell response to some antigens. Accumulated data indicate that the interaction of certain antigens with the thymocytes during tolerance induction results in a turning off of B cells, so they no longer cooperate with T cells to produce antibodies. Suppression by T cells can be mediated by both specific and nonspecific means. It has not been determined if there are two distinct subpopulations of lymphocytes for helper and suppressor functions. The same T-cell population under different circumstances may function as either helper or suppressor T cells. It may be that specialized populations of T lymphocytes send "on and off" signals to effector cells.

Lymphoid stem cells are processed by an alternate pathway that is poorly understood in man but that has been extensively studied in birds and in the bursa of Fabricius. The precursor cells under the influence of a hormone-like substance (bursin) are processed in the liver and later in the bone marrow to differentiate into B lymphocytes. In response to antigenic stimulation, the immunocompetent B cells differentiate into plasma cells, which produce antibody. These immunocompetent B cells may be stimulated by a helper factor from a sensitized T-lymphocyte population to produce a K cell. The K cell can act in the presence of an antibody to destroy a cell; it does not need complement to complete this action. B lymphocytes are responsible for protection against bacteria.

In addition to the T cells (helper T cells, suppressor T cells, and tolerant T cells) and B cells (variant K cells) there is a third immunologic component consisting of natural killer (NK) cells. The NK cells were discovered when it was observed that animals have some natural resistance to tumors that is not mediated by B or T cells. The process is different from immunity acquired by various exposures. It can be enhanced or suppressed, but not greatly; immunization, then, is rather ineffectual in terms of stimulating NK cell immunity. It is stimulated by viral infections, possibly through production of interferon. The NK cells are probably a type of lymphocyte, but at present scientists are not certain of that.

Burnet's Clonal Selection Theory

Burnet's clonal selection theory has become the central dogma of immunology. The immune system is capable of responding to a wide variety of naturally occurring and synthetic immunogens. This diversity of recognition and response is provided by the sum of different specificities of the entire lymphocyte mass. Burnet proposed that during prenatal development pluripotent lymphocyte precursors differentiate in the absence of immunogens into a diverse array of individually unique lymphocyte clones. All of the cells within the clone bear identical immunogen receptors. These events occur while the immune system is still immature. According to Burnet, lymphocytes acquire their specificity prior to the immunogen encounter. The capacity in the immune system to recognize and respond to a diverse variety of immunogens is provided by thousands of lymphocyte clones, each with a single, unique specificity. Once the immune system has matured, around the time of birth, an individual possesses a full complement of cells with which to recognize immunogens.

Experimentation has confirmed that Burnet's clonal selection theory supports the following concepts: (1) a lymphocyte acquires its specificity prior to immunogen encounter; (2) a lymphocyte's specificity is restricted; (3) lymphocyte activation occurs at the cell surface; and (4) an immunogen selectively expands clones of reactive cells. One would expect that the proportion of an individual's unimmunized lymphocytes that are capable of reacting with any single purified immunogen is small. Up to this time, it is possible to account for four characteristics of the immune response: Immunity is (1) acquired; (2) remembered; (3) specific; and (4) transferred with antibodies or with lymphocytes. Normal individuals do not mount immune responses against their own cells and molecules. Any theory of immunologic responsiveness must accommodate the fact that under normal circumstances the immunologic system is able to distinguish self from nonself.

Self Versus Nonself

Burnet proposed that while lymphocyte precursors are proliferating and acquiring diverse specificity during fetal development, lymphocytes of all specificities appear, including cells capable of recognizing cell antigens. During this time of emerging antigen-recognizing cells, relevant (self), antigens coexist without mutual adverse effect. At some defined developmental stage—approximately the third intrauterine month in humans—cells confronted by relevant (self) antigens are deleted; the remaining antigen-reactive cells, which are theoretically capable of recognizing only nonself-antigens, persist. Thus under normal circumstances, immunologically mature individuals do not react against self-antigens because self-reactive cells have been deleted. Beyond this developmental stage, encounters between nonself-antigens and appropriate antigen-recognizing cells lead to immunity. With Burnet's mechanism for self-tolerance (unresponsiveness toward self), lymphocytes that have specificity for self-antigens are called forbidden clones and do not participate in adult immunity. Thus self-antigens are not immunogenic because of the deletion of potentially reactive cells.

An autoimmune disease can generally be defined as one in which an autoantibody or a sensitized lymphocyte reacts with host tissue. This definition does not mean that the autoantibody or lymphocyte plays a causative role in the disease. Autoimmunity may arise whenever there exists a state of immunologic imbalance in which B-cell activity is excessive and suppressor T-cell activity is diminished. This imbalance occurs as a consequence of

viruses, drugs, genetic factors, environmental factors, carcinogens, or cancer itself. A central mechanism in this concept involves a disturbance of the delicate balance between suppressor and helper activity of the regulatory T cells. Either an excess of helper T-cell activity or a deficiency of suppressor T-cell activity could lead to the development of autoimmunity. The mechanisms by which such a balance may be upset are complex but may involve many factors, including viral factors and the abnormal product ion of thymic hormones. It is the imbalance between B-cell production and suppressor T cells that is important in autoimmune diseases. The impaired immunoregulation is then expressed by the production of an increased number of B cells.

Similarities can be seen between autoimmune disease in humans and the disease in the New Zealand black mouse, particularly in reference to genetic susceptibility, immunodeficiency, and thymic injury. Genetic susceptibility to autoimmunity is reflected by the high incidence of autoimmune phenomena in families of patients with immunologic deficiencies and in families of patients with systemic lupus erythematosus. Inherited immunodeficiency syndromes are associated with a high incidence of autoimmunity as well as increased risks of infection and malignancy.

It has repeatedly been reported that there is a connection between immune disorders and malignant transformation of lymphoid tissue. This connection is illustrated by the high incidence of reticulum cell sarcoma in association with certain autoimmune disorders, such as Sjögren syndrome, and the association of Coombs-positive hemolytic anemia with reticulum cell sarcoma, chronic lymphocytic leukemia, and malignant lymphomas.

Finally, viruses are associated with autoimmune syndromes in humans. Although viruses have not been reported as a causative agent of malignancy in humans, there is indirect and suggestive evidence that a virus or viruses may play an etiologic role in Burkitt's lymphoma and possibly in myelogenous leukemia. Work in progress with the enzyme reverse transcriptase may provide more information. Not only has it been established that a virus can cause a malignancy such as Marek's disease in chickens (a lymphomatosis), but a vaccine has been produced that immunizes chickens against the disease.

Cancer of the ovary is usually advanced when first diagnosed, with 60 to 80% of the cases in stages III and IV. It has been well established that cancer is markedly immuno-suppressive. In animal models and humans it has been shown that a growing cancer is accompanied by a high titer of suppressor serum. The serum blocks the cancer so the T lymphocytes are unable to attack the cancer cells. This response is seen in vivo but does not occur in vitro unless suppressor serum is added to the culture. The action involves the humoral mechanism and is the result of a cell-free anti-body being secreted by the B cell or plasma cell. The hypothetical question raised is whether advanced cancer of the ovary is ever an autoimmune disease. To my knowledge, there is no documentation that there is an ex-cess of helper T-cell activity or a deficiency of suppressor T-cell activity in patients with can-cer of the ovary.

In an ovarian cancer project at Lenox Hill Hospital, an autologous antibody was isolated by eluting it from the surface of the tumor cell, and an antigen was identified but has not yet been purified. While working on this project, the research team observed that these patients were difficult to cross-match and that they pos-sessed an antibody that interfered with their typing and cross-matching. The research asso-ciate, Brent Dorsett, then identified an anti-body that reacted with normal tissue but did not recognize the ovarian cancer antigen. Con-versely, the ovarian cancer antibody identified the ovarian carcinoma but did not recognize normal tissue. After treatment with cortisone for 2 to 3 days, it was possible to suppress the antibody that was interfering with the cross-match, and successful cross-match was accom-plished.

This observation suggests but does not prove that an autoimmune disease is present in pa-tients with advanced and recurrent ovarian cancer. Moreover, the use of anticancer drugs often gives these patients a sense of well-being long before there is any effect on tumor volume. These factors raise the question of the possibility of an autoimmune disorder or dis-ease in these patients. Researchers in the Blood Bank Center at Lenox Hill Hospital, however, were unable to confirm this observa-tion.

Immune Complexes

Type III hypersensitivity results from deposi-tion of immune complexes in blood vessel walls and tissues. Complexes can activate platelets and basophils in humans via Fc receptors to release vasoactive amines, which cause endo-thelial cell retraction and increased vascular permeability leading to complex deposition. Complexes also activate complement, releasing C3a and C5a. Both C3a and C5a activate baso-phils, and C5a increases vascular permeability and is chemotactic for polymorphonuclear neutrophils (PMNs) as well. PMNs, which fail in the attempt to phagocytize the depositive complexes, release their granules to the ex-terior, causing local tissue damage. Complexes tend to deposit at sites of high pressure, filtra-tion, or turbulence, such as in the kidney or at the bifurcation of the arteries.

Immune complex clearance is normally effected by cells of the reticuloendothelial sys-tem. The factors that affect clearance include (1) the size of the complexes; (2) the class affinity of the antibody; (3) the valence of the antigen; and (4) the amount of the complexes. The fourth factor explains why immune com-plex disease occurs in the presence of infec-tions that release large amounts of antigen and in autoimmune disease where there is a ready supply of autoantigen.

Immune complex diseases result when exces-sive immune complex deposition occurs in par-ticular organs. Serum sickness is a type III reaction that occurs in individuals given injec-tions of foreign serum. Antibodies are made to the serum antigens, and there is massive im-mune complex formation, producing nephritis and arteritis. The Arthus reaction is a skin reaction manifesting as an area of redness and swelling that is maximum 5 to 6 hours after in-tradermal injection of antigen. It is caused by IhG binding to the injected antigen, triggering inflammation by type III mechanisms.

With increasing frequency, reports indicate that a wide variety of chronically debilitating diseases are thought to be caused by circulating soluble immune complexes, including the collagen diseases, that is, vascular diseases, rheumatoid arthritis, glomerular nephritis, and possibly chronic inflammatory bowel disease. The antigen–antibody complexes are deposited in the blood vessels of affected organs and initiate damage by activation of the complement system, eliciting an inflammatory response. Intensive research using plasmapheresis as a modality of therapy for immune complex disease state is in progress.

The identification and interest in circulating soluble immune complexes has resulted from the introduction of methods that have been developed for detecting these circulating immune complexes, and their presence has been confirmed in a variety of diseases. However, mere detection does not mean that they cause the disease state. Work is now under way to identify what is cause and what is effect. It has been reported that elevated levels of immune complexes are found during pregnancy and that the levels fall after delivery. This phenomenon suggests that certain types of immune complex modulate the immune response in an advantageous manner, possibly preventing material rejection of mosaic foreign antigens—the fetus. Facilitation or enhancement of malignant tumor growth may also be due to certain types of immune complex.

Immune complexes are being identified with increasing frequency in the field of cancer. Indirect evidence of several tests suggests that immunologic processes accompany many malignancies. Work in progress indicates that immunologic reactions often occur in patients with cancer, an observation confirmed by frequent demonstrations of antigen–antibody complexes in the plasma of patients and by evidence that the complement system has been activated. The presence of such immune complexes has been demonstrated by a number of tests, including C1q-deviation test and competition with aggregated gamma globulin receptors on cells of the Raji lymphoblastic cell line. It is conceivable that work now in progress with plasmapheresis will provide a method for removing harmful immune complexes and perhaps even some of the blocking antibodies that reduce the effectiveness of definitive treatment for malignancy.

Hybridomas

When a foreign substance enters the body of a vertebrate animal or is injected into it, antibodies are produced. The antibody response to a typical antigen is highly heterogeneous. It represents a mixture of many antibody molecules of variant charge, size, and such biologic properties as the ability to fix complement and to agglutinate or precipitate antigen. This heterogeneity is reflected in the diffuse nature of the immunoglobulin band, and such antisera are compared to the homogeneous albumin peak observed on serum electrophoresis. Furthermore, the relative amounts of the different, specific antibody types that constitute such antisera vary considerably among animals and even vary from one bleeding to the next in a single animal.

Antibody-secreting normal cells cannot be maintained in a culture medium. However, cells that secrete antibodies can be made immortal by fusing them with tumor cells and cloning the hybrid. Each clone is a long-term source of substantial quantities of a single, highly specific antibody. In 1975 Kohler and Millstein learned how to fuse mouse myeloma cells with lymphocytes from the spleen of mice immunized with a particular antigen. The resulting hybridmyeloma, or *hybridoma*, cells expressed both the lymphocyte property of specific antibody production and the immortal character of the myeloma cells. Such hybrid cells can be manipulated by the techniques applicable to animal cells in permanent culture.

Individual hybrid cells can be cloned, and each clone produces large amounts of identical antibody to a single antigenic determinant. The individual clones can be maintained indefinitely, and at any given time samples can be grown in culture or injected into animals for the large-scale production of monoclonal antibody. Highly specific monoclonal antibodies produced by this general method have proved to be a remarkably versatile tool in many areas of biologic research and clinical medicine. It is now possible to generate monoclonal antibodies against many antigens. Through hybridoma technology, these immunologic reagents can be made available in large quantity and can be regenerated indefinitely. Such tailor-made, homogeneous antibodies are likely not only to improve the reliability—and reduce the cost—of immunoassays but should also permit the development of new diagnostic procedures and therapeutic modalities for human diseases. It is anticipated that the ability to produce monoclonal antibodies through hybridoma technology may supply a method for making an early diagnosis of ovarian cancer. It is conceivable that these antibodies may be used as immunotherapy at some time and perhaps as an initial step will be used as immunoprophylaxis in patients identified as being at high risk for the development of ovarian cancer.

Summary

Autoimmunity is both a major immunologic phenomenon in clinical medicine and an important immunobiologic clue to the workings of the immune system. It may arise whenever there is a state of immunologic imbalance in which B-cell activity is diminished. This imbalance occurs as a consequence of genetic, viral, and environmental mechanisms acting singly or in combination. A central mechanism has also been postulated and involves an imbalance between suppressor and helper T cells. Either an excess of helper T-cell activity or a deficiency of suppressor T-cell activity could lead to the development of autoimmunity. If the B cell is overstimulated or underregulated, autoimmunity may result. If the imbalance of regulatory signals results in excessive B cell proliferation, malignant lymphomas may develop as they do in some New Zealand mice.

Aging, the response to bacterial and viral infections, and specific immunologic diseases may give rise to a condition similar to autoimmunity. Individuals may respond immunologically to certain of their own antigens (self-antigens). These important exceptions to the principle of self-tolerance help to analyze its fundamental mechanisms and are frequently associated with disease. It is important to emphasize the distinction between an *auto-immune response*, in which an individual makes antibodies or becomes allergic to a self-antigen, and an *autoimmune disease*, which is a pathologic condition arising from an autoimmune response. Autoimmune reactions can be both antibody-mediated and cell-mediated. Autoimmunity reflects a loss of immunologic tolerance to tissue and cellular antigens. Immunologic tolerance is the result of an active physiologic process and is not simply the lack of an immune response.

When treating patients with ovarian cancer, I have observed that it was often difficult to cross-match their blood before transfusions. At first it was thought that previous transfusions had stimulated antibodies to the platelets and leukocytes of the original donors. However, it was noted that some had antibodies present but had not been transfused before. Antibody was identified that did not recognize the cancer antigen but that reacted to the normal tissue of the host. Treatment with a corticosteroid suppressed the antibody and permitted a compatible cross-match of blood. At this time the antibody has not been studied in more detail. The research team in the Blood Bank Department were not able to confirm this observation, which suggests but does not prove that an autoimmune disorder or disease may accompany advanced or recurrent ovarian cancer.

Hybridomas are cells produced by the physical fusion of two different cells. Polyethylene glycol and Sendai virus are often used to effect the fusion. A hybridoma cell and its progeny contain some chromosomes from each fusion partner, although some others are usually lost. Immune responses in antibody populations may be described according to the number of responding cells as monoclonal, oligoclonal, or polyclonal according to whether the response is due to one, a few, or many clones.

Monoclonal antibodies are homologous antibodies produced by a single clone. They are usually made from hybridomas, which are prepared by fusing immunized mouse or rat spleen cells with a nonsecretor myeloma using polyethylene glycol. The fusion mixture is plated out in HAT medium (hypoxanthine/aminopterin/thymidine). Aminopterin blocks a metabolic pathway that can be bypassed if hypoxanthine and thymidine are present, but the myeloma cells lack this bypass and consequently die in HAT medium. Spleen cells also die naturally in culture after 1 to 2 weeks, but fused cells survive because they have the immortality of the myeloma and the metabolic bypass of the spleen cells.

The decade of the 1990s will undoubtedly produce significant advances in both the diagnosis and management of ovarian cancer. Work with the immune complexes and the new hybridoma technology should produce significant advances in diagnosis and treatment for ovarian cancer.

Bibliography

Allison AC: Unresponsiveness to self-antigens. *Lancet* 2:1401, 1971.

Allison AC, Denman AM, Barnes RD: Cooperating and controlling function of thymus-derived lymphocytes in relation to autoimmunity. *Lancet* 2:135, 1971.

Altman A, Cohen IR, Feldman M: Normal T cell receptors for alloantigens. *Cell Immunol* 7:134, 1973.

Barber HRK: *Immunobiology for the Clinician*. John Wiley & Sons, New York, 1977.

Barber HRK: The immune complex in diagnosis. *Diagn Gynecol Obstet* 2 (1):3, 1980.

Barber HRK: Introduction to immunology. *Mt Sinai J Med* 47:427, 1980.

Barnes EW, Irvine WJ: Clinical syndromes associated with thymic disorders. *Proc R Soc Med* 66:151, 1973.

Belohradsky BH: Meeting report of the second international workshop on primary immunodeficiency diseases in man. *Clin Immunol Immunopathol* 2:281, 1974.

Bretscher P: A model for generalized autoimmunity. *Cell Immunol* 6:1, 1973.

Burnet FN: *The Clonal Selection Theory of Acquired Immunity*. Cambridge University Press, Cambridge, 1959.

Burnet FN: *Cellular Immunology*. Cambridge University Press, Cambridge, 1970.

Christian CL, Phillips PE: Viruses and autoimmunity. *Am J Med* 54:611, 1973.

Cooper MD: Meeting report of the second international workshop on primary immunodeficiency diseases in man. *Clin Immunol Immunopathol* 2:416, 1974.

Fudenberg HH, Stites DP, Caldwell JR, Wells JV: *Basic and Clinical Immunology*. Lange Medical Publications, Los Altos, CA, 1976.

Gershon RK: T cell control of antibody production In Cooper MD, Warner NL (eds): *Contemporary Topics in Immunology*. Vol. 3. Plenum, New York, 1974.

Glasser DL, Silvers WK: Genetic determinants of immunological responsiveness. *Adv Immunol* 18.1, 1972.

Harris JE, Sirkovics JG: *The Immunology of Malignant Disease*. Mosby, St. Louis, 1970.

Hemet R, McKern T (eds): *Monoclonal Antibodies*. Plenum Press, New York, 1980.

Kohler G, Millstein C: Continuous cultures of fused cells secreting antibody of predefined specificity. *Nature* 256:495, 1975.

Levy JA: Autoimmunity and neoplasia: the possible role of C-type viruses. *Am J Clin Pathol* 62:258, 1974.

Marx JL: Slow viruses: role in persistent disease. *Science* 181:1351, 1973.

McDevitt HO, Bodner WF: Histocompatibility antigens, immune responsiveness and susceptibility to disease. *Am J Med* 52:1, 1972.

Millstein C: Monoclonal antibodies. *Sci Am* 243(4):66, 1980.

Paterson PY: Multiple sclerosis: an immunologic reassessment. *J Chronic Dis* 26:119, 1973.

Rowley DA: Specific suppression of immune responses. *Science* 181:1133, 1973.

Siegel MM, Good RA (eds): *Tolerance, Autoimmunity and Aging*. Charles C Thomas, Springfield, IL, 1972.

Steinberg AD, Baron S, Talal N: The pathogenesis of autoimmunity in New Zealand mice: induction of antinucleic acid antibodies by polymosinic polycytidylic acid. *Proc Natl Acad Sci USA* 63:1102, 1969.

Stutman O: Lymphocyte subpopulations in NZB mice: deficit of thymus dependent lymphocytes. *J Immunol* 109:602, 1972.

Thomas L: Experimental mycoplasma infections as models of rheumatoid arthritis. *Fed Proc* 32:143, 173.

Wybran JL, Levin AS, Spitler LE, Tudenberg HH: Rosette-forming cells, immunological deficiency diseases and transfer factor. *N Engl J Med* 288:710, 1973.

Yaltan DE, Roberts SB, Scharff MD: Hybridomas and monoclonal antibodies. *Lab Management* 19(1):19, 1981.

25

Tumor Markers in Ovarian Cancer

All vertebrates have a defense system that protects them from disease-causing microorganisms. Its deliberate exploitation has conquered many infectious diseases and has long been a major achievement of medical science in terms of preventing suffering and saving lives.

The progressive and inexorable nature of cancer has led many physicians and laymen alike to believe that humans are incapable of defending themselves against it. There was a time, however, when many infectious diseases that are now easily eradicated or cured seemed almost as relentless in their course as does cancer today. Attempts to fight cancer immunologically go back to the early days of immunology.

A primary goal of cancer research is to define differences between normal and neoplastic cells that can be used as a point of attack in tumor diagnosis, prophylaxis, and therapy. Even if no qualitative differences exist, quantitative differences may be large enough to serve the same purpose.

Early in the twentieth century it was hoped that dissimilarities between normal and neoplastic cells could be demonstrated by immunologic methods, and that vaccination against cancer could be demonstrated. However, work with outbred animals showed that the rejection of tumor by previously immunized animals was, in a great number of instances, attributable to sensitization to the normal alloantigens (HL-A) that were present in the animal in which the tumor originated (and therefore in the tumor) but not in the recipients.

Recognition of this response to the normal alloantigens rather than to a specific tumor antigen set back the field of tumor immunology. An accepted view followed that tumor-specific antigens could not possibly exist because they would confer a selective disadvantage on the cells that carried them and lead to their immediate elimination by immunologic mechanisms. The fact that neoplasms often metastasize to the lymph nodes was viewed as an additional indication that an immunologic defense against cancer could hardly play a role.

When inbred strains of mice were developed in quantity, the pieces of the puzzle began to fall into place. It was now possible to analyze the conditions that either allowed transplants of normal and neoplastic tissues to grow in their hosts or led to their rejection.

The modern scientific study of the relation of immunity to cancer was undertaken by Gross during the 1940s and later by Prehn and Main during the 1950s with extensive work on experimental transplantable tumors and the phenomena causing a rejection of grafted normal and cancerous tissue in inbred animals. For the first time there was firm evidence that a tumor-associated antigen was present on the surface of a tumor cell. The background for the identification of tumor markers is reviewed here.

Immunology is a relatively new medical discipline. However, the concept of immunity is an ancient one and is properly termed the study of resistance to infection. As a scientific discipline, immunology encompasses immunity dealing with the adaptive response to infective agents; immunochemistry, concerned with the chemical nature of antigens and antibodies; and immunobiology, which deals with the activity of the cells of the immune system and their relation to each other and their environment. As a biologic science, immunology includes developmental biology, genetics, biochemistry, microbiology, anatomy, and medicine. These basic concepts are fundamental for understanding the principles and practices of modern medicine. Currently, the term "immunity" has taken on an expanded role; it is now defined as the property whereby the lymphoreticular system makes a memorized response to an antigenic stimulus. It may result in a state of positive reaction known as *sensitization* or in one of negative reaction known variously as immunologic tolerance, acquired tolerance (former term: "immunologic paralysis"), or immunosuppression. It is a complex state arising from the properties of the individual, community, race, and species; but the most striking thing about it is the specific nature of its protection in individuals after recovery from infection.

Histocompatibility Complex

Ongoing work in the histocompatible antigens has made significant contributions to the understanding of disease states. Population genetic studies in man have revealed extraordinary high association between certain HL-A genotypes and human disease. For example, virtually every patient with ankylosing spondylitis expresses HL-A-B27 antigen on their cells. Although the meaning of these associations at the cellular and molecular level is unclear, the relation of the major histocompatibility complex to disease susceptibility in man will undoubtedly have increasing importance as more is learned.

The chromosomal region that encodes for the glycoproteins that function as strong histocompatibility antigens includes other genetic loci as well. In mice, genes exist that determine whether the animal makes little or a great deal of antibody in response to certain antigens. Genes that appear to govern the level of immune responsiveness to antigens in this manner are called IR genes. Analysis of segregate populations of mice reveals that some IR genes are closely linked to genes in coding for major histocompatibility antigens, giving rise to the concept of a major histocompatibility complex (MHC). Thus some genes within the MHC encode for histocompatibility antigens, others are involved in determining the amount of antibody produced in response to certain antigens. A large number of IR genes have been identified within the MHC of the mouse, each governing immune responsiveness to a different antigen. Although the gene product of any particular IR gene is not known, the activity of each gene is expressed through T lymphocytes. Thus it appears that the T lymphocytes help B lymphocytes to promote antibody production through the action of IR genes.

Certain viruses are known to cause cancer in the mouse. It has been found that the susceptibility to viruses that cause cancer (*oncogenic viruses*) is determined by genes within the MHC. The MHC therefore includes several kinds of gene: those that encode for histocompatibility antigens important in allograft immunity; those that govern the amount of antibody produced in response to antigenic challenge, termed IR genes; and genes governing susceptibility to oncogenic viruses. Histocompatibility antigens encoded for by genes within the MHC are not in and of themselves responsible for susceptibility to disease. However, the tight association between the MHC antigenic phenotype in certain diseases suggests that the genes governing disease susceptibility are tightly linked to genes governing the histocompatibility antigens. Exploration of this field of histocompatibility antigen research is providing an exciting period in understanding genetic engineering.

Modern Era

The future of modern immunology was born when Jenner discovered that inoculation with cowpox crusts protected man against smallpox. The next advancement in immunology was made through the contributions of Louis Pasteur. Roux and Yersin then demonstrated the existence of an exotoxin elaborated by the diphtheria bacillus. The existence of tumor-specific antigens was suspected by the medical scientists of that era. In 1895 Héricourt and Richet attempted passive immunization with antisera produced in animals injected with human tumors. The results were highly unpredictable. In 1906 Bashford claimed that prior inoculations of tumor and whole blood in mice prevented the growth of transplants of a mammary adenocarcinoma. He noted that established transplants of spontaneous cancers were not affected. Seven decades later and millions of dollars spent on research have not resolved the problem. However, the advances made since the 1960s arouse hopes of cure with certain cancers and promise the opportunity for early diagnosis in others, all within the foreseeable future.

Cancer-specific antigens were first identified in a little-quoted study by Gross in 1943. He described the failure of mice to accept transplants of a specific cancer after they had been immunized with material from the same cancer growing on syngeneic mice. The rebirth of tumor immunology as an active field of research may be said to have occurred in 1957 when Prehn discovered that mice immunized against syngeneic methylcholanthrene-induced fibrosarcomas by inoculation of living sarcoma tissue followed by surgical removal of the growing tumor were resistant to subsequent grafts of the same tumor. In addition, immunization with normal tissue did not confer resistance to the tumor grafts. The mice that had become resistant to the tumors still accepted skin grafts from the primary hosts of these tumors. Different methylcholanthrene-induced sarcomas were found to have individually distinct antigens; mice that were immunized against one tumor still accepted the grafts of other tumors.

Tumor-specific transplantation antigens (TSTAs) have been demonstrated not only in chemically induced tumors but also in tumors induced by viruses. A great number of tumor-associated antigens have been identified. Although the syngeneic donor-host relationship seldom pertains in humans, other experimental methods have clearly shown that many human tumors have tumor-associated antigens: colonic cancers (Gold and Freedman, 1965); ovarian cancers (Levi et al., 1969; Ioachim et al., 1973; Knauf and Auerbach, 1974); bronchial cancers (Yashi et al., 1968); mammary cancers (Edynak et al., 1971); urothelial carcinomas (Bubenik et al., 1970); neuroblastoma (Hellström et al., 1968); melanoma (Morton et al., 1968; Jehn et al., 1970); lymphomas (Smith et al., 1967; Buffé et al., 1970; Order et al., 1971); leukemia (Harris et al., 1971); and sarcomas (Morton et al., 1968; Wood and Morton, 1971). The 125th monoclonal antibody screened was designated OC125 and its antigenic determinant was called CA125.

The progressive nature of cancer has led many physicians and laymen to believe that humans are incapable of defending themselves against cancer. Until closely inbred mice were available for studies, the results of tumor transplants were unpredictable and difficult to explain. However, when genetically pure strains of animals became available for study, experiments on tumor immunity using the techniques employed in the earlier studies showed clearly that previous success was related to the presence in the tumor of genetically incompatible transplantation antigens of the original host, and that tumor regression, when it occurred, was consequent to homograft rejection rather than to immunity to tumor-specific antigens.

With this tool available, extensive work on experimental transplantable tumors and the phenomenon causing the rejection of grafted normal and cancerous tissue in animals was carried out. A major conceptual advance was established when it was demonstrated that cancers do arouse a specific immune response in the organism within which they appear. Antigenic differences represent the first known qualitative distinctions between cancer cells and their normal counterparts. These qualitative differences between normal and cancer cells had escaped other methods of investigation but were revealed by immunologic techniques. Such techniques took advantage of the extraordinary power of discrimination of the immune defense mechanism itself. Cancer immunology appears to be on the threshold of an era in which it will be possible to establish an early diagnosis. It was these advances that prompted us to undertake a multidisciplinary approach to the problem of ovarian cancer and to make early diagnosis through an immunologic method, the keystone of the project.

Cancer of the ovary is the leading cause of death from gynecologic cancer. The constant challenge presented by ovarian cancer is that 13,000 women die from ovarian cancer each year, and the 5-year results were no better in 1992 than they were during the previous two decades. It is a sobering statistic to realize that more than 100,000 women at the height of their social and economic productivity die from ovarian cancer. Because early diagnosis is a matter of chance rather than scientific discovery, it follows that it is not possible to treat ovarian cancer with any predictable degree of certainty for cure. In the present state of our knowledge, early diagnosis is the key to successful treatment.

The definition of an ovarian tumor is difficult because of the diversity of histogenetic types of neoplasms originating in the ovary. It is considered a family of diseases, rather than a single, distinct entity. The ovary is complex in terms of its embryology, histology, steroidogenesis, and potential for malignancy. It is made up of germ cells, gonadal stromal cells, and mesenchymal tissue, each with its own potential to form tumors. The ovary is unique not only because it gives rise to a variety of cancers, but also because it is itself a favorite site for metastases from other organs.

This chapter summarizes work on tumor markers concerning the immunology of cancer. The application of immunologic methods to the study of human tumors has made significant progress. It has been demonstrated that there is immunity to autologous tumors manifested by both tumor and cellular reactions. A number of tumor-associated antigens have been discovered, and they are discussed in this chapter.

Immunologic Means of Cancer Detection

In the cancer cells of animals or, more specifically, on the cell membrane of these cancer cells, there are antigens (associated with DNA and RNA viruses) that are shared by all cancer cells produced by a particular virus. These antigens are referred to as *common antigens*. Cancer cells produced by chemical carcinogens also have antigens on their cell membranes, but they are different in each tumor produced by the carcinogen and are referred to as *unique antigens*. This rigid separation of antigens has been challenged, and now it is thought that both can be present with one or the other playing the major role.

Antigens have also been found in human cancers. Burkitt's tumor has antigens that have been identified, and the same antigen is associated with infectious mononucleosis. A common as well as a unique antigen has been found in melanomas. The finding of a common antigen in melanomas suggests a possible viral origin for this cancer. An antigen that appears to be a common antigen has also been identified in epithelial ovarian cancers.

Fetal Antigens

A new type of antigen, called *fetal antigen*, has been identified in association with human cancers. These antigens are released from the cancer cells and can be detected in the bloodstream. They are found in the fetus, most often during the first two trimesters, and disappear before birth. They reappear later in cancerous cells. Apparently during the first two trimesters a gene is functioning that is repressed during the third trimester or at birth. It is derepressed during carcinogenesis.

The two most commonly studied fetal antigens are the carcinoembryonic (CEA) and the α-fetoprotein antigens (AFP). Other fetal antigens are leukemia-associated antigen (LAA), fetal sulfoglycoprotein antigen (FSA), and placental alkaline phosphatase. All of these antigens offer promise as useful agents in the development of diagnostic tests.

Of great interest has been the discovery of one particular group of materials: the embryonic-specific fetal antigens. It has been shown that they are associated with human and animal tumors and that they can be released into the body fluids. These antigens have been found in diverse tumors of the mouse, rat, and hamster, where they occurred spontaneously or were induced by physical, viral, and chemical agents. It has been proposed that they represent a universal oncologic phenomenon termed *retrogenetic expression*.

Tumor-associated macromolecules fall into two groups. The first group comprises those macromolecules that reside within or on tumor cells; they have not yet been shown to be released, and they may be detected because of their influence on the host's cellular and humoral systems. That is, they are present in tumors and body fluids without known metabolic effects (CEA, LAA, FSA, and polypeptides) and in tumors and body fluids with metabolic effects (placental alkaline phosphatase, placental-type hormones, and related products). The other group consists of those macromolecules that are not present in or on tumor cells but are released from the tumor cells into the body fluids. The ectopic production of hormones, their subunits, and related materials and fetal-associated macromolecules are the principal examples.

Carcinoembryonic Antigen

The carcinoembryonic antigen (CEA) was first described by Gold and Freedman in 1965. The heterologous (produced in another species) antibodies to CEA were produced by injecting saline extracts of colon cancer into rabbits. Adenocarcinoma of the human colon does not extend more than 6 or 7 cm beyond the tumor. Because the resection always includes some of the surrounding normal tissue, it was possible to obtain both normal and tumor tissue from the same person. Therefore it was possible subsequently to absorb the rabbit antiserum with the corresponding normal bowel obtained during resection of the primary tumor mass, permitting the researchers to circumvent the problem of distinguishing tumor-specific from individual-specific antibodies in the final antiserum preparations.

Initially, an antigen common to all adenocarcinomas of the bowel was demonstrated by a variety of immunologic techniques. Subsequently, a similar antigen was found in the embryonic gut and was called CEA. The antigen was identified during the first two trimesters but was absent at birth. It was suggested that the gene producing CEA during early embryonic life had been repressed. Later in adult life, when CEA was found in association with adenocarcinoma of the gut, it was thought that the repressed gene had been derepressed. The stimulus for the derepression may have been a virus, a carcinogen, failure of the immunologic surveillance mechanism, age, or some unknown factor.

It has been reported that CEA is found in association with a variety of tumors, both entodermal and nonentodermal. Because the serum from patients with both entodermally and nonentodermally derived carcinomas had elevated levels of CEA, an antigenic site common to several tumors was hypothesized to exist on CEA.

The CEA has been characterized as a glycoprotein with a molecular weight of 200,000. Studies raise doubts that CEA is a homogeneous material. It appears that its activity is similar to that of blood group A substance. Chemical analysis reveals a repeating unit of N-acetylglucosamine, which seems to be partly responsible for the antigenicity of CEA. The correlation between blood groups and malignancies is currently receiving a great deal of attention.

Radioimmunoassay Tests

There are several modifications of radioimmunoassays being used. Todd uses a so-called triple-isotope/double-antibody assay. The Hansen method uses a zirconyl phosphate gel (Z-gel), whereas the Gold test uses ammonium sulfate to precipitate the antibody-bound CEA. In general, antigens combine with their appropriate antibody to form an antigen–

antibody complex. With the Roche method, which uses the radioimmunoassay, the unknown sample is first added to the antibody and incubated, after which the radioactive-labeled antigen is added and incubated. The reaction of antigen with antibody is essentially irreversible. The test can be summarized in this manner: Basically a radioimmunoassay utilizes a standard antigen that has been tagged with an isotope and an antibody that is going to react with it. Anything that interferes with that reaction is measured in terms of the amount of isotope that does not precipitate. This value is then translated to represent (and is called) CEA (or whatever is being tested).

Conclusion on CEA

The normal value for CEA is 2.5 ng/ml. It is now accepted that the CEA assay is not a screening method for cancer of the colon. However, it does provide a means of monitoring the results of therapy. If the CEA level is elevated before surgery, and within 2 to 18 days after complete resection of a colonic tumor it falls to a baseline level, any rise can be interpreted as suggestive of cancer reactivation. CEA is not specific for the diagnosis of cancer, and the amount present has significance in making a diagnosis. It is possible to divide CEA values into three groups: below 2.5 ng/ml is normal; 12.5 to 40.0 ng/ml is intermediate; and above 40 ng/ml is high. Patients with benign disease, malignant tumors, or inflammatory and regenerative disorders may fall into the normal or intermediate groups, whereas levels in excess of 40 ng/ml are practically diagnostic of malignancy. The CEA level is elevated in up to 40% of women with stage I ovarian cancers and in a relatively higher percentage of those with stage II, III, or IV disease.

α-Fetoprotein

Serum α-fetoprotein (AFP) assays have currently gained an important place in the diagnosis and differential diagnosis of hepatocellular and testicular tumors. The observation that the AFP level may be elevated before the detection of tumors by other means has important implications. In addition, successful therapy is associated with a decline in AFP to normal, and it rises again when the tumor recurs.

α-Fetoprotein is known to be a product of the human fetal liver, gastrointestinal tract, and yolk sac. It has been shown that the endodermal sinus tumor, which is of vitelline origin, invariably gives a positive test for AFP. Because the outcome of disease does not appear to depend on the level of AFP, there is a suggestion that a homeostatic control exists for AFP production in the tumor cells. This situation, however, does not seem to be true for teratocarcinoma. The test's greatest value lies in the study of hepatomas of the liver, endodermal sinus tumors of the ovaries, and teratocarcinomas of the ovary. In addition to AFP, there are α_2H-fetoprotein (α_2 HF), βS-fetoprotein, and (gamma) γ-fetoprotein (γFP).

A specific protein of embryonal and fetal serum in mammals, AFP is an α-globulin. It is the dominant serum protein during embryonic development and during early life. The normal AFP level in fetal blood is 4 to 5 mg/liter, but during development the concentration gradually falls. During adult life the titer ranges from 2 to 15 ng/ml. AFP is a well-characterized protein with a molecular weight of about 70,000 daltons, and it comprises a single polypeptide chain. Its physiochemical properties are close to those of serum albumin.

α-Fetoprotein acts as an albumin substitute early. It also binds estrogen and may suppress lymphocyte activity. AFP synthesis starts at the same time as embryonic hematopoiesis. AFP is synthesized in the yolk sac, where the first blood islets are formed and which is the principal source of AFP in the embryo. During this time fetal hepatocytes are responsible for AFP synthesis. As the process of liver hematopoiesis begins to fade and hepatocytes progressively differentiate, AFP synthesis ceases or, to be more precise, falls to between one hundred-thousandth and one millionth of its maximal value. It can be concluded that AFP is one of the most distinct and well-defined biologic markers of certain tumors. Its presence in adult serum is evidence of hepatocellular carcinoma or teratocarcinoma of the ovary and testis. AFP can be used as a specific diagnostic indication of these tumors; and because there is usually a specific correlation between AFP dynamics in the patient's blood or tumor progression or regression, it can be used to monitor the effectiveness of treatment.

It is a specific tumor marker for the endodermal sinus tumor of the ovary, embryonal carcinoma of the ovary, and ovarian teratomas, which may be present in either of these tumors. It is not elevated in epithelial ovarian carcinomas. Elevated also in most patients with endodermal sinus tumor of the ovary, it decreases with response to therapy and increases with recurrence, making it an almost perfect tumor marker for endodermal sinus tumors.

CA 125

The murine monoclonal antibody OC 125 reacts with antigen CA 125, present in most nonmucinous epithelial ovarian carcinomas. The 125th monoclonal antibody screened was designated OC 125, and its antigenic determinant was called CA 125. An assay has been developed by Bast and Knapp to detect CA 125 in the serum. With this assay, originally only 1% of 888 apparently healthy persons and 6% of 143 patients with nonmalignant disease had serum CA 125 values above 35 U/ml. It was found that rising or falling levels of CA 125 correlated with progression or regression of disease in at least 93% of the cases originally reported. It became obvious that the determination of CA 125 levels was an important aid for monitoring response to treatment in patients with epithelial ovarian cancer.

Mucinous and borderline tumors as well as germ cell tumors of the ovary do not have consistently elevated CA 125 levels, which represents a serious limitation of the assay.

Although CA 125 is useful for diagnosing ovarian cancer, it can also be elevated in patients with (1) gynecologic cancers that arise from coelomic epithelium derivatives (fallopian tubes, endometrium, endocervix); (2) pancreatic, breast, colon, or lung cancer; (3) endometriosis; (4) pancreatitis; (5) pelvic inflammatory disease; (6) peritonitis; (7) renal failure; (8) liver cirrhosis; and (9) hepatocellular carcinoma with ascites.

Although a rise or a fall in the CA 125 level is suggestive of progression or regression of the disease, approximately 15% of patients with falling CA 125 levels have exhibited progression of their ovarian cancer.

If the CA 125 level falls to normal within 3 months of chemotherapy usually the second look laparotomy is negative, whereas if it has not fallen within the normal range by 3 months usually persistent disease is found. The day-to-day variation of the assay is approximately 10 to 15%, and a doubling or halving of the antigen level is considered significant.

The reasons for the consistent elevations of serum CA 125 levels in patients with benign conditions, as well as certain metastatic gynecologic and nongynecologic cancers, have not been fully elucidated. It may be explained by a "leak" in the tumor-vascular interface, as has been proposed, rather than by irritation of the coelomic epithelium.

There are a variety of CA antigens: CA 15-3, CA 19-9, and one that is not associated (NB/70K). CA 19-9 was originally detected in a colorectal carcinoma cell line. CA 19-9 determinant is a sialylated Lewis blood group A determinant expressed on a mucin-like glycoprotein of more than 500,000 daltons. CA 19-9 is found in sections of approximately 40% of ovarian cancer but has been detected in serum of only 20% of ovarian cancer patients, which greatly limits its value in clinical practice.

The combined use of serum assays for markers CA 15-3 and CA 125 has been found to increase significantly the specificity of the tests for identifying women with ovarian cancer. However, used by itself it has limited value in following patients with ovarian cancer. It has proved to have some value for evaluating patients with metastatic bone carcinoma secondary to breast cancer.

An ovarian carcinoma antigen (OCA) has been studied. Although OCA shares determinants with CEA, no correlation has been found between OCA and CEA levels in serum specimens. OCA is elevated in sera from approximately 75% of patients with stage I through stage IV disease. Similar levels of OCA were found in sera of 10% of apparently healthy individuals. Although initial attempts to use OCA for monitoring ovarian carcinoma were disappointing, a 70,000 dalton moiety, NB/70K, has been isolated from OCA that is immunochemically distinct from CEA. A radioimmunoassay has been developed to detect NB/70K in serum. Both the level of NB/70K and the frequency of values of more than 11 KU/ml correlated with the increasing stage and residual tumor burden but not with tumor histologic type or grade.

Fetal Sulfoglycoprotein Antigen

Fetal sulfoglycoprotein antigen (FSA) occurs in gastric juice in the fetus and in 96% of patients with gastric carcinoma. Certain immunologic studies indicate that FSA and CEA share common antigenic determinants. FSA production has also been reported to precede the development of overt carcinoma. The difficulty of interpreting this fact is that the incidence of FSA-positive patients with peptic ulceration far exceeds their known incidence of malignant change (approximately 2%). The successful removal of gastric cancer need not be followed by a decline of FSA levels in gastric juice.

α_2H-Fetoprotein is detected in the fetal liver and serum up to the end of the second postnatal month. It is elevated in adults with various tumors, including hepatoma, cholangiocarcinoma, and lymphoma. After the third postnatal month, elevated levels are uncommon in children with noncancerous conditions.

βS-Fetoprotein is elevated in the serum of patients with hepatocarcinoma, cholangiocarcinoma, gastric carcinoma, leukemia, and lymphoma. It is present in the serum until the seventh postnatal month.

Leukemia-associated antigen (LAA) is derived from the tumor cell membrane and is not found in the sera of normal persons or of patients with hepatomas. Unfortunately, serum LAA need not decline during remission.

There are two types of AFP: AFP-1 and AFP-2. The AFP-1 type does not occur in the serum of healthy persons, pregnant women, or patients with nonneoplastic disease, but it may be found in the fetus as well as in the serum of a few patients with tumors. The AFP-2 type has been found not only in breast carcinomas themselves but also in normal breast tissue.

Lipid-Associated Sialic Acid in Plasma

Levels of lipid-associated sialic acid (LSA) reflect the release of cell membrane glycolipids. The LSA level has been noted to be elevated in a variety of nongynecologic malignancies and may be correlated with stage of disease, tumor burden, and recurrence of cancer. Preliminary data suggested that LSA in plasma (LSA-P) is elevated in 62% of ovarian cancer patients with clinical evidence of disease and in 53% of cervical cancer patients with clinical evidence of disease.

Currently there are reports indicating that the tumor-associated antigen CA 125 and the nonspecific tumor marker measured by LSA-P combined appear to offer more effective surveillance of patients known to have ovarian cancer than single markers alone. However, more observations are needed before these two markers can be proved to identify the presence of occult disease.

Tissue Polypeptide Antigen

Tissue polypeptide antigen (TPA) has been shown to be a component of the endoplasmic reticulum and plasma membrane. It is a polypeptide with specific antigenic properties that have been identified in a variety of species. It is a tumor-associated antigen that occurs in human placenta, human cancer tumors, and body fluids of cancer patients. TPA is present in the membrane structures of human cancer cells and can be detected there by its effects of cytotoxic antibodies or the localization of fluorescent, monospecific anti-TPA antibodies.

Released from growing and multiplying human cancer cells in vitro, TPA can be specifically demonstrated by the culture medium hemagglutination inhibition technique. Because TPA is produced by propagating tumor cells, it could be expected to appear also in placenta and fetuses, and indeed it does, particularly in the placenta. High levels of TPA were found in all of the individual placentas.

Further studies of TPA have disclosed that the antigenic specificity of the TPA molecule is not limited to the human species; it is present in a wide variety of animal species, ranging from apes through hoof-bearing animals and rodents to certain fish.

It has the ability to inhibit stimulation of lymphocytes by phytohemagglutinin in cell culture and to stimulate the uptake of radioactive thymidine in cultures of peripheral blood lymphocytes from immunized horses. It has also been found in patients with inflammatory changes of other origin. Studies have revealed close agreement between TPA level and the clinical course of patients with metastases from mammary carcinoma. It has proved to be a good method for monitoring the progress of the patient during therapy. In most cases TPA was reduced to normal levels before remissions were evident from the clinical parameters studied. Therefore the test is considered to be worthwhile for governing the treatment of critically ill patients. Useless drugs can be discarded and replaced by more potent or more specific drug therapy before there is evidence of further progress of cancer, detected by roentgenography or scintigraphy.

Enzymes

Numerous enzymes are being studied in ovarian tumors and identified as markers, including glycosyltransferases and glycosidases. Other miscellaneous tumor markers under study include pregnancy-associated macroglobulin (PAM, PZP) and fibrin-fibrinogen degradation products. Acute-phase reactant proteins are under intensive study. The levels of acute-phase reactant proteins, complement components, and inhibitors have been measured in sera of patients with stage IV ovarian carcinoma. Markedly elevated α_1-acid glycoprotein, α_1-antitrypsin, and haptoglobin levels, as well as levels of C3, C4, C3PA, and the inactivator of C3 (C3 bINA) have been reported in a controlled series. Laparotomy and tumor extirpation produced a temporary decrease of the

level of all but α-proteins. Chemotherapy brought about a decrease in the serum level of acute-phase reactant proteins, complement components, and C3 bINA, with a concomitant rise in total protein level. Measuring acute-phase reactants and complement inhibitors may be an additional tool for evaluating the efficiency of chemotherapy in patients with advanced cancer of the ovary.

Hollinshead identified tumor-associated antigens, as well as nucleoprotein, which are inhibitory antigens on the surface of the cell membrane. Rosenberg thought that the platinum complexes disrupted antigenic masking on animal tumor cells, exposing what he thought might be tumor antigens at the cell surface that generate a host immune reaction. He noted the appearance of densely stained patches associated only with the tumor cell membranes, not with normal cell membranes, and identified them as possibly masking antigens containing DNA. Most nucleic acids and nucleoproteins are weak antigens and may escape host immune surveillance. Hollinshead was able to isolate the tumor-associated antigen and its masking substance, which she identified as a nucleoprotein (DNA) inhibitory antigen (IA) in clusters or patches on the cancer cell plasma membrane. This observation has opened up an entirely new field and offers hope that an ovarian cancer vaccine is possible.

Hormones (Ectopic Hormone Production and Malignancies Susceptible to Hormone Influences)

The ectopic hormone syndromes represent an important aspect of oncology. Inappropriate hormone production can also serve as an index of tumor activity, as the hormone levels decline with successful therapy.

There are certain similarities between hormones and neoplasia. The immunologic defenses are decreased among the very young and the very old. It is in these same age groups that we find decreased production of hormones. In addition, tumor antigens are most often found on the cell membranes, and antigens in this position are considered to be the most important for producing antibodies specific for mounting a defense against that particular cancer. The similarity between hormone synthesis and tumor antigen has a similar pattern of action. The specificity of the hormonal response depends on the existence of unique receptors in the cell membrane. The peak incidence of tumors occurs at a time when there is maximum hormone imbalance, i.e., during puberty and the prepubertal months, as well as during the perimenopausal and early menopausal years.

Attempts to explain why nonendocrine tumors should produce ectopic hormones has given rise to much discussion. It is generally if not totally accepted that if humans start from one cell that cell must carry all the potential genetic and phenotypes of the body. The next question raised is why some genes function and others are repressed. Only time and additional studies can give us these answers. One theory that has aroused much interest is the so-called depressor-deletion hypothesis proposed by Gellhorn. This theory proposes that as a tumor becomes progressively less well differentiated it loses the depressor that modifies the biosynthetic mechanisms present in the multipotential or embryonic cell. Another theory suggests that embryonic cells at a very early stage of development migrate into the mucosa of the alimentary tract and may give rise to endocrine glands. The scattered neuroendocrine cells have the potential to develop into a variety of hormone-producing tumors.

There are also other hypotheses concerning the origin of the nonendocrine neoplasms that produce hormones, i.e., the derepression of existing genes and the random production of "new" material. In the genetic hypothesis it should be restated that all cells of an organism may contain the same DNA information and therefore are capable of synthesizing an unlimited number of proteins. As cellular differentiation progresses, the cell is limited to the production of a limited number of proteins and enzymes. As neoplasia develops, the gene is derepressed, and its capability to synthesize a particular protein or hormone may be restored. The hormone should be similar to the original hormone. This situation has been reported in erythremia, hypercalcemia, and Cushing syndrome. The aberrant protein synthesis hypothesis suggests that with the development of neoplasia abnormal cells develop that would synthesize new or altered DNA. In most instances it would be anticipated that the hormones produced by the neoplasms would be different from the natural hormones. This hypothesis is confirmed in patients with neoplasms that cause hypoglycemia or hyperthyroidism. In these cases the hormone produced by the neoplasm is immunologically different from the natural hormone.

Paraendocrine Tumor Activity

There are several humoral syndromes associated with neoplasia: hyperadrenocorticism, hypercalcemia, hypoglycemia, erythremia, hyperthyroidism, precocious puberty, inappropriate secretion of antidiuretic hormones, atypical carcinoid syndrome, and ectopic human chorionic gonadotropin secretion. The latter syndrome is discussed in detail.

Ectopic Human Chorionic Gonadotropin Secretion

Human chorionic gonadotropin (hCG) and human luteinizing hormone (hLH) are glycoproteins with similar biologic activity. Both hormones are composed of an α-subunit and a β-subunit. The β-subunit confers immunologic and biologic specificity. The placenta secretes hCG, which is found normally during pregnancy. hLH is secreted by the pituitary and is found in the peripheral blood of both males and females after puberty. Because hCG is found normally only during pregnancy, its detection under any other circumstance implies that an hCG-secreting tumor is present. Until recently most antisera to hCG could not discriminate between hCG and hLH. The development of an antiserum specific for the β-subunit has now been described and documented.

It has been shown that approximately 40% of all tumors, including those in men, secrete hCG, and the incidence climbs to 90% among embryonal ovarian tumors and testicular tumors. This finding confirms reports that differentiated somatic cells do carry information for all the potential cell phenotypes of the body, and it has been demonstrated by nuclear transplantation into an enucleated egg; this egg with a transplanted nucleus can support the development of a fertile adult.

Precocious sexual maturity has followed the production of a gonadotropin-like material elaborated by a tumor. In these tumors there were no teratoid or trophoblastic elements that could have produced the gonadotropin. One is left with the conclusion that it represents cellular dedifferentiation and derepression of a gene.

A radioimmunoassay has been developed that selectively measures hCG in serum or plasma samples containing both hCG and hLH. Using that assay system, a large number of serum or plasma samples from patients with documented tumors have been assayed for the presence of immunoreactive hCG. Adenocarcinoma of the stomach, ovary, pancreas, and hepatoma are the tumors most commonly associated with ectopic hCG secretion, and the incidence of ectopic hCG secretion ranged between 17 and 40% in those selected tumor types. Significantly, 30% of epithelial ovarian cancers and up to 90% of the embryonal ovarian carcinomas are associated with measurable amounts of this hormone.

Heterogeneity has been observed among the hormonal peptides secreted by tumors. hCG is composed of two dissimilar, noncovalently linked subunits. In a variety of tumor tissue extracts, samples of serum or urine contained not only hCG but either or both subunits of hCG. Rare tumors have had only free α-subunits or free β-subunits present.

Lymphocyte function in vitro is altered by hCG. High concentrations of hCG inhibit the response of lymphocytes to phytohemagglutinin. The trophoblasts have antigens on their surfaces that have a negative charge, as do the lymphocytes. The fact that like charges repel each other may explain why the pregnancy (allograft) is not rejected. In addition, the antigens of the trophoblast stimulate an antibody response, and these antibodies have been shown to function as blocking or enhancing antibodies in many instances. Because it has been shown that many tumors produce hCG, the blocking antibodies formed may protect the tumor from the killer lymphocytes. Whether hCG, encountered during normal pregnancy or in patients with tumors ectopically secreting it, exerts any physiologic effect on the immune system in humans is unknown. If hCG were to exert a significant immunosuppressive effect, one might expect to see a significant difference in the clinical course of patients with tumors that ectopically secrete hCG compared to patients with comparable tumors not ectopically secreting hCG. Such studies have not yet been undertaken.

Ferritin

A purified antigen identified as ferritin by electrophoretic, chemical, and immunologic criteria has been studied by Marcus. It has been found in breast cancer, and researchers at Lenox Hill Hospital reported that both normal ovary and the common epithelial tumors contained ferritin as well. However, there was no reaction between the purified ferritin and the antisera raised in the rabbit or the antibody extracted from ascitic fluid. It was concluded after additional studies that the common epithelial ovarian cancer antigen was not ferritin.

Regan Alkaline Phosphatase Isoenzyme

The Regan isoenzyme is heat stable, and at least one component of the enzyme has a molecular weight around 200,000 daltons. The alkaline phosphatase enzymes are known to occur in serum and are derived from the liver, bones, lung, intestinal tract, and placenta. The placental alkaline phosphatase enzyme does not occur in fetal tissues, blood, or serum but does occur in maternal serum during the third trimester of pregnancy. It is never found in the serum of normal male subjects. The enzyme, first detected in a patient named Regan who had lung cancer, has been found in association with a variety of cancers. When alkaline phosphatase is present it is a useful method for monitoring tumor progression or regression. It can be detected in malignant serosal exudates. In any patient with an elevated serum alkaline phosphatase level found by routine methods, reexamination should be carried out to determine if the placental alkaline phosphatase is responsible for the maternal elevation. If it is, the patient should be carefully evaluated to detect or eliminate the possibility of a latent neoplasm.

Stolbach et al. found the isoenzyme in the serum of 30 to 40% of patients with cancer of the ovary and in 50 to 70% of malignant effusions from the abdomen in patients with carcinoma of the ovary.

Human Placental Lactogen

Human placental lactogen has been reported to be elevated in as many as 76% of patients with common epithelial ovarian tumors, but it is considered more specific for germ cell ovarian tumors containing ectopic trophoblastic tissue.

Biomarker Profiles

Cancer Antigen 125

An immunoradiometric assay using a monoclonal antibody (OC 125) has 88% sensitivity for detecting nonmucinous epithelial ovarian carcinoma and 60% sensitivity for detecting uterine cancer.

NB/70K (Dianon Marker; DM/70K)

A radioimmunoassay can detect human ovarian tumor-associated antigen NB/70K using monoclonal antibody NB12123. A sensitivity of 70% is found for ovarian carcinoma. Elevated levels have been associated with other gynecologic malignancies as well as with carcinoma of the lung and breast.

Lipid-Associated Sialic Acid

Lipid-associated sialic acid (LASA) is a biomarker useful in a wide range of malignancies that reflect an alteration in the surface membranes of malignant cells. The LASA-P (LASA in plasma) test measures total gangliosides and glycoproteins by the biochemical extraction and partition method of Katopodis. Sensitivities range between 77% and 97% de-

pending on the cell origin of the neoplasm. Studies have shown improved predictive value when the LASA-P test is combined with other biomarkers in biomarker profiles.

Carcinoembryonic Antigen

An enzyme immunoassay with CEA uses a monoclonal antibody against glycoprotein produced by immature or malignant cells originating in the gut. Elevated values are associated with carcinomas of the rectum, colon, lung, and breast.

Carbohydrate Antigen 19-9

An immunoradiometric assay using a monoclonal antibody against sialylated Lewis antigen (blood group substance) is useful for pancreatic, gastric, hepatic, recurrent colorectal carcinoma, and ovarian cancer. This antigen, CA 19-9, is also termed gastrointestinal cancer-associated antigen (GICA). Patients who are $Le_a^- b^-$ test negative with this assay.

Immunosuppressive Acidic Protein

A radioimmunodiffusion assay measures a type of α_1-acid glycoprotein. This immunosuppressive acidic protein (IAP) suppresses phytohemagglutination-induced lymphocyte blast formation and the next lymphocyte reaction in vitro. Sensitivities of 84% or higher are found for adenocarcinoma of the lung, pancreas, and ovary, as well as for leukemia and lymphoma.

Human Chorionic Gonadotropin, β-Subunit

An enzyme immunoassay measures the β-hCG ordinarily produced by the placenta and used as an indicator of pregnancy. β-hCG is also produced by tumors of germ-cell origin, such as testicular and ovarian cancers, as well as some lung cancers.

Tissue Polypeptide Antigen

An immunoradiometric assay for molecules derived from the cytoskeleton of epithelial cells, tissue polypeptide antigen (TPA) is useful for the management of many cancers.

Comment

The CA 125, CEA, hCG, and LASA-P tests have been approved by the U.S. food and Drug Administration. The others are for investigational use only, but probably some will be released within a short period of time for routine diagnostic purposes.

Ovarian Cancer Vaccine from Tumor-Associated Antigens

The subject of ovarian cancer antigen is covered in Chapter 27. However, a short description is included here with the tumor markers.

Heterologous antisera produced against pools of ovarian carcinoma tissue have reacted consistently and specifically with the tissues of origin in immunodiffusion and immunofluorescence tests. The highly absorbed sera showed no reaction with normal ovarian tissues, normal human serum components, and various other neoplasms. These investigations have suggested the presence of a specific antigenic component in carcinomas of the ovary. The antigen did not cross-react with the carcinoembryonic antigen (CEA) and was not revealed in fetal tissues. Present attempts to purify and fully characterize this antigen are aimed toward its possible use in a much needed diagnostic test for the early detection of carcinoma of the ovary.

It has been demonstrated that effusions obtained from patients with ovarian cancer contain sizable amounts of free and complexed immunoglobulins. Salt precipitation procedures have recovered antibodies that, after purification and concentration displayed a high degree of specificity against ovarian cancer cells. It is hoped that autologous antibodies recovered from peritoneal effusions can be utilized in sensitive radioimmunoassays, which are greatly needed for the early detection of ovarian cancer, the leading cause of death due to gynecologic neoplasia.

The ovarian cancer project has progressed rapidly using urea to split the complexes and to identify the more potent antibodies using a nephelometer. The work with immune complexes has provided insights into some of the chemistry related to ovarian cancer as well as its production and clinical picture. Work with the hybridomas has been started, and it is shown that this work will result in the development of monoclonal antibodies that can be used for early diagnosis and possibly even immunotherapy and immunoprophylaxis.

A mouse monoclonal antibody (MoAb) produced with affinity-isolated OCAA (Ovarian Cystadenocarcinoma Associated Antigen) has been designated FEN-1, and preliminary immunohistologic observation demonstrates reactivity against endometrioid and serous ovarian carcinomas. It does not react against mucinous tumors, nor does it cross-react with gastrointestinal neoplasms. There was no reactivity seen against fetal tissue, placenta, or normal tissue except goblet cells of normal colonic mucosa. MoAb FEN-1 did not react against lymphoid neoplasms, sarcoma, melanoma, or inflammatory or mesothelial cells. The antibody reacted with 80% of the endometrioid ovarian carcinomas tested on fixed tissue.

Currently there are projects under way to provide a genetically engineered vaccine. More work is required to evaluate the role a vaccine may play in ovarian cancer management

Summary

At present it is possible to measure a significant number of tumor markers in the serum of ovarian cancer patients. The development of such tumor markers is essential for early diagnosis. However, with the exception of α-fetoprotein and human chorionic gonadotropin, most lacked sensitivity as well as specificity.

In general, the tumor markers have been categorized as: (1) carcinoplacental antigens; (2) fetal antigens; (3) tumor-associated antigens; and (4) miscellaneous tumor markers. Detection of tumor-associated antigens in serum is possible because these substances are released in the circulation (1) during the time of cell death or lysis, (2) by abnormal permeability of the cell membrane, and (3) by normal divestment of the cell membrane into the circulation.

The presence of tumor-associated markers (macromolecules) in association with human tumor is now well established and accepted.

They occur either on the surface of the cell membrane or within the cell. The tumor markers (antigens) may be released into the body fluid. Many are also known to be present in fetal tissues, and some possess biologic activity.

To be clinically useful, tumor antigens must meet the following criteria.

1. The antigen must pass from the tumor into the body fluids at an early point in the life of the tumor.
2. The antigen must aid in the differential diagnosis.
   a. The tumor markers must be found only with tumors.
   b. Ideally, the antigen is site-specific or tumor-site-specific.
3. The titer or amount of tumor marker or antigen should decline with successful therapy.
4. The titer should rise early when recurrence develops.
5. It must be readily measurable by routine laboratory methods.

Tumor markers are being identified at an increasingly rapid rate. Confusion results if the same marker is assigned different names. Obviously, the ideal plan to coordinate the work of various investigators would include a registry with liberal exchange of material and a committee to identify the marker with an acceptable name.

None of the currently recognized tumor-associated markers that occur in body fluids are specific for malignant tumors; quantitative rather than qualitative differences exist among inflammatory disease and benign and malignant CA 125 tumors. Despite this fact, CA 125, CEA, AFP, and hCG have been accepted for their clinical application and value. They aid in tumor diagnosis and monitoring the effects of therapy.

A number of tumor markers frequently are seen in elevated titers in association with particular tumors. Measurement of each marker, hormone, and their products can make available a group of tests that, studied collectively, may supply help in detection, differential diagnosis, and prognostic assessment. Immunological Parameters Laboratories developed the capacity to quantify each of the known means by which humans immunologically resist infections, intoxications, and cancer. By outlining the immunologic parameters or spectra, it may be possible to observe functional heterogeneity between tumors of identical morphology or between cells of the same tumor. Such a finding could have behavioristic, histogenetic, and etiologic significance.

Ectopic production and secretion of hormones by a wide variety of tumors were initially recognized by signs and symptoms of excess circulating biologically active hormones. The development of more sensitive techniques has made it evident that not all tumors secrete biologically active hormones. Some of the forms of polypeptide hormones may not be active biologically even though present in high concentrations, whereas others secrete small amounts that cannot be detected clinically. Modern technology has made it possible to test for the ectopic production and secretion of hormones produced by a wide variety of tumors. Several new syndromes have been identified, and it is easier to identify those previously described. Every hormone known to be normally secreted by endocrine organs or the placenta has been documented to be secreted ectopically by a great number of tumors. Several of these hormones may be used as biochemical markers of malignancy for both screening and monitoring patients with documented or suspected tumors.

There are certain striking similarities between hormones and neoplasia.

1. Immunologic defenses are decreased among the very young and the very old.
2. Hormone production is low among the very young and the very old.
3. Tumor antigens are most often on the cell membrane.
4. Hormone action starts on the cell membrane.
5. Human chorionic gonadotropin may represent a surface antigen.
6. The peak incidence of many tumors, especially of the urogenital tract, occurs during the prepubertal or pubertal years.
7. The peak incidence of many tumors (breast,

uterus, and ovary) occurs during the peri- and postmenopausal years, at the time of marked hormone changes.

8. When the feedback mechanism in the endocrine system fails, there is overstimulation from the pituitary hormones, causing a disease state. A similar situation presents when the helper T cells overstimulate the B cells and are not inhibited by the suppressor T cells. This situation leads to the production of autoantibodies and an autoimmune state. If the stimulation is severe enough, a malignancy in the form of a lymphoma has been produced in the New Zealand mouse.

Endocrine-active substances that are of interest to the gynecologist and that are produced by aberrant hormone activity by tumors include gonadotropins, lactogens, thyrotropins, and adrenocorticotropins, as well as calcium-mobilizing and erythropoietic substances.

Bibliography

Abelev GI: Alpha fetoprotein in oncogenesis and its association with malignant tumors. *Adv Cancer Res* 14:295, 1971.

Alexander P: Fetal "antigens" in cancer. *Nature* 235:137, 1972.

Alpert ME, Uriel J, DeNechaud B: Alpha feto globulin in the diagnosis of human hepatoma. *N Engl J Med* 278:964, 1966.

Baldwin RW: Tumor specific antigens associated with chemically induced tumors. *Rev Eur Etud Clin Biol* 25:593, 1970.

Baldwin RW, Erubleton MJ: Demonstrations by colony inhibition methods of cellular and humoral immune reactions to tumor-specific antigens associated with aminoazo-dye-induced rat hepatomas. *Int J Cancer* 7:17, 1971.

Barber HRK: *Immunobiology for the Clinician.* John Wiley & Sons, New York, 1977.

Barber HRK, Dorsett BH: The immune system in gynecologic malignancy. *Mt Sinai J Med* 47:539, 1980.

Barber HRK, Dorsett BH: Immunologic aspects of gynecologic cancers. *Cancer* 48:472, 1981.

Barber HRK, Kwon T: Hormones and cancer (ectopic hormone production and malignancies susceptible to hormone influences). *J St Barnabas Med Center* 22, 1975.

Barlow JJ, Bhattacharya M: Tumor markers in ovarian cancer: tumor-associated antigens. *Semin Oncol* 2:203, 1975.

Bast RC JR, Klug TI St John E, Jennson E, Niloff JM, Lazarus H, Berkowitz RS, Leavitt T, Griffiths CT, Parlav L, Zurakwski VR Jr, Knapp RC: A radioimmunoassay using monoclonal antibody to monitor the course of epithelial ovarian cancer. *N England J Med* 309(15):883, 1983.

Benham FJ, Povey S, Harris H: Placental-like alkaline phosphatase in malignant and benign ovarian tumors. *Clin Chim Acta* 86:201, 1978.

Bhattacharya M, Barlow JL: Tumor markers for ovarian cancer. *Int Adv Surg Oncol* 2:155, 1979.

Bragshaw KD, Wass M, Searle F: Ovarian cancer serum markers: ovarian cancer. *Adv Biosci* 26:57, 1980.

Braunstein GD, Vaitukaitis JL, Carbone PP, et al: Ectopic production of human gonadotropin by neoplasms. *Ann Intern Med* 78:39, 1973.

Bubenik J, Perlmann P, Helmstein K, Moberger G: Immune response to urinary bladder tumors in man. *Int J Cancer* 5:39, 1970.

Buffé, D, Rimbault C, Lemerle J, et al: Presence d'une ferro-proteine d'origin: tissulaire, Lα₂H dans le serum des enfants porteurs de tumeurs. *Int J Cancer* 5:85, 1970.

Coligan JE, Eagan ML, Todd CW: Detection of carcinoembryonic antigen by radioimmune assay. *Natl Cancer Inst Monogr* 35:427, 1972.

Dorsett BH, Ioachim HL, Stolbach L, et al: Isolation of tumor-specific antibodies from effusions of ovarian carcinomas. *Int J Cancer* 16:779, 1975.

Edynak EM, Hirshant Y, Old LJ, Trempe GL: Antigens of human breast cancer. *Proc Am Assoc Cancer Res* 12:75, 1971.

Fishman W, Raam S, Stolbach LL: Markers for ovarian cancer: Regan isoenzyme and other glycoproteins. *Semin Oncol* 2:211, 1975.

Freedman SO: Carcinoembryonic antigen: current clinical applications. *J Allergy Clin Immunol* 50:348, 1972.

Gall SA, Walling J, Pearl J: Demonstration of tumor-associated antigens in human gynecologic malignancies. *Am J Obstet Gynecol* 115:387, 1973.

Gellhorn A: The unifying thread. *Cancer Res* 23:961, 1963.

Giancotti FR, Dorsett BH, Qian H, et al: Ovarian cancer-associated antibodies recovered from ascites: their use for the isolation of ovarian cancer-associated antigen to produce monoclonal antibodies. *Gynecol Oncol* 37:24, 1990.

Giancotti FR, Dorsett BH, Weaver SC, et al: Description and characterization of an endometrioid ovarian cancer cell line. *Gynecol Oncol* 35:330, 1989.

Gold P: Antigenic reversion in human cancer. *Annu Rev Med* 22:85, 1971.

Gold P, Freedman SO: Demonstration of tumor-specific antigens in human colonic carcinomata by immunologic tolerance and absorption techniques. *J Exp Med* 121:439, 1965.

Gross L: Intradermal immunization of C3H mice against a sarcoma that originated in animals of the same line. *Cancer Res* 3:326, 1943.

Haber E: *Radioimmunoassay: Principles and Practical Applications*. Little, Brown, Boston, 1974.

Harris R, Viza D, Todd R, et al: Detection of human leukaemia associated antigens in leukaemic serum and normal embryos. *Nature* 233:556, 1971.

Hellström I, Hellstrom KE, Pierce GE, Bill AH: Demonstration of cell-bound and tumoral immunity against neuroblastoma cells. *Proc Natl Acad Sci USA* 60:1231, 1968.

Hollinshead A.: Active specific immunotherapy. In: Anderson MD (ed). Immunotherapy of Human Cancer. New York, Raven Press, 1978.

Hollinshead A, Stewart T: Specific active immunotherapy and specific active immunoprophylaxis in lung cancer. In Moore M (ed): *Advances in Medical Oncology Research and Education. Vol. 6. Basis for Cancer Therapy II*. Pergamon Press, Oxford, 1979.

Ioachim HL, Dorsett BH, Sabbath M, et al: Antigenic and morphologic properties of ovarian carcinoma. *Gynecol Oncol* 1:130, 1973.

Jehn UW, Nathanson L, Schwartz RS, Skumen M: In vitro lymphocyte stimulation by a soluble antigen from malignant melanoma. *N Engl J Med* 283:329, 1970.

Knauf S, Auerbach GI: Ovarian tumor specific antigens. *Am J Obstet Gynecol* 119:966, 1974.

Laurence DJR, Munro N: Fetal antigens and their role in diagnosis and clinical management of human neoplasms: a review. *Br J Cancer* 26:335, 1972.

Levi MM, Keller S, Mandl J: Antigenicity of a papillary serous cystadenocarcinoma tissue homogenate and its fractions. *Am J Obstet Gynecol* 105:856, 1969.

LeGerfo P, Krupey J, Hansen HJ: Demonstration of an antigen common to several varieties of neoplasia. *N Engl J Med* 283:138, 1971.

Margariti PA, Benedetti-Panici P, Villani L, et al:

Tumor markers in the ovarian carcinoma. *Eur J Gynecol Oncol* 1:77, 1980.

Mitchison NA: Immunologic approaches to cancer. *Transplant Proc* 2:92, 1970.

Morton DL, Malmgren RA, Holmes EC, Ketcham AS: Demonstration of antibodies against human malignant melanoma by immunofluorescence. *Surgery* 64:233, 1968.

Order SE, Porter M, Hellman S: Hodgkin's disease: evidence of a tumor associated antigen. *N Engl J Med* 285:471, 1971.

Prehn RT, Main Im M: Immunity to methylcholanthrene-induced sarcomas. *J Natl Cancer Inst* 18:769, 1957.

Rosenberg B: Possible mechanism for the antitumor activity of platinum coordination complexes. *Cancer Chemother Rep* 59:589, 1975.

Shuster J: Immunologic diagnosis of human cancers. *Am J Clin Pathol* 62:243, 1974.

Smith JB: Alpha fetoprotein: occurrence in certain malignant diseases and review of clinical applications. *Med Clin North Am* 54:797, 1970.

Smith RT, Klein G, Klein E: Studies of the membrane phenomenon in cultured and biopsy cell lines from the Burkitt lymphoma. In Dausset J, Hamberger J, Mathé G (eds): *Advances in Transplantation*. Williams & Wilkins, Baltimore, 1967, p. 483.

Stolbach LL, Krant MJ, Fishman WH: Ectopic production of an alkaline phosphatase isoenzyme in patients with cancer. *N Engl J Med* 281:757, 1969.

Stone M, Bagshawe KD, Kardana A, et al: β-Human chorionic gonadotropin and carcinoembryonic antigen in the management of ovarian cancer. *Br J Obstet Gynaecol* 84:375, 1977.

Tee DEH, Wang M, Watkins J: Antigenic properties of human tumors: tumor-specific antigens. *Eur J Cancer* 1:315, 1965.

Vaitukaitis JL: Peptide hormones as tumor markers. *Cancer* 37:567, 1976.

Van Nagell JR, Meeker WR, Parker JC Jr, Harralson JD: Carcinoembryonic antigen in patients with gynecologic malignancy. *Cancer* 35:1372, 1975.

Wood WC, Morton DL: Host immune response in common cell-surface antigen in human sarcomas. *N Engl J Med* 284:569, 1971.

Yashi A, Matsumura Y, Carpenter CM, Hyde L: Immunochemical studies on human lung cancer antigens soluble in 50% saturated ammonium sulfate. *J Natl Cancer Inst* 40:663, 1968.

26

Sex Steroid Receptors

Sex steroid hormone receptors provide the means by which estrogen and progesterone influence their target tissues. Receptor assays have proved clinically useful for the management of breast cancer. Their application to study of the ovary is currently undergoing intensive investigation.

Intracellular receptors for estrogen and progesterone in the hormone-specific target tissues are being examined with increasing frequency. Some human ovarian malignancies respond favorably to hormone therapy. To obtain more information about the endocrine properties of these malignancies Jähne and coworkers measured estrogen and progestin receptors in 21 malignant ovarian tumors and compared the findings with those from 29 benign tumors and 28 tumor-like ovarian lesions. There were marked differences in steroid receptor distributions among the three groups. Only 38% of the malignant tumors simultaneously contained measurable amounts of both receptors, whereas the corresponding figure was 76% for benign tumors. Malignant tumors were receptor-negative more often than were the benign lesions (29% and 7%, respectively.

Mechanisms available at this time to change hormone receptor responses are essentially limited to the following alternatives: (1) levels of receptors in target tissue; (2) hormone quality and quantity; (3) interference by other steroids; and (4) temporal effect of the complex in the nucleus. The measurement of how readily the receptor complex separates from the hormone and if it can provide reusable receptors remains to be explained.

It is obvious that the role of hormone receptors in the management of ovarian tumors is proving to be clinically useful. To have a better understanding of the role of hormone receptors in ovarian tumors, a general review of estrogen and progesterone receptors is presented.

The endometrium, ovary, and breast comprise the upper genital tract. These organs have a great deal in common; for example, many of their responses are hormone-associated. When cancer arises in these organs, there is great epidemiologic similarity. The endometrium, ovary, and breast have been shown to have estrogen and progesterone receptors. Most of the work on the receptors has been done on the breast and endometrium, but the ovary is currently receiving a great deal of attention. This chapter covers general background material on work that has been reported on the endometrium, ovary, and breast.

A new era in cancer endocrinology started with the discovery that breast cancer cells retain the ability to incorporate and retain estrogens, both in vitro and in vivo. The road of discovery has been uphill, held back at first by the use of outmoded methodology; but it has now progressed to the use of more sophisticated techniques, and much information is now available to us. For those interested in this problem, it is important to be familiar with the background of the hormone-dependent and hormone-independent tumors. The concept of utilizing the available data on hormone receptors in clinical oncology would eliminate much of the guesswork of spotting the high-risk patient, allow more logical selection of patients whose therapy should be monitored, and provide a method for selecting and controlling management of recurrent endometrial cancer.

Cells that depend on hormones for optimal growth and function contain specific steroid-binding proteins, so-called hormone receptors. The work of Jansen et al. on the selective binding of estradiol by rat uterus opened up this field of research. The interaction of the hormone with target cells takes place by a two-step mechanism. Perhaps there are as yet an undetermined number of steps. A discussion of the discoveries that have been reported follows.

Receptor Research

During the early 1970s Jensen and coworkers demonstrated that estrogen would bind to an intracellular (cytoplasmic) molecule, designated the *receptor*. This binding initiates a chain of events leading to an effect on cell growth. Following this discovery, a great deal of information began to accumulate. It has been shown, for instance, that the cell membrane is freely permeable to the steroid molecule, which then binds to the cytoplasmic receptor to form a steroid–receptor complex. This complex is directed by an enzyme-dependent step that translocates to the nucleus, where it interacts with the chromatin to result in the transcription of specific mRNA segments, which in the cytoplasm interact with tRNA and rRNA to cause new protein to be produced, a process designated *translation*. This new protein is the end-product of steroid hormone reaction. If this step does not occur, the steroid is unable to exert an effect on the cell. It has been shown that, although a receptor must be present for the steroid to affect the cell's growth, its mere presence does not necessarily signify that the cell will respond to the hormone, as many steps are necessary for the hormone to exert an effect. It is accepted that the absence of a receptor indicates that there is little chance of the cell responding to the hormone.

The major clinical value of steroid hormone receptors is for patients with breast cancer. Patients whose tumors were found to contain estrogen receptor (ERs) had about a 60% chance of responding to endocrine therapy, which included ablative therapy such as oophorectomy (performed in the premenopausal woman) or adrenalectomy, as well as additive therapy with estrogens. Later it was shown that antiestrogen therapy such as tamoxifen produced a similar response. It was also reported that patients whose tumors were ER-negative were found to have only about a 5% response rate to endocrine therapy.

There are exceptions to this rule, and it has been shown that a small number of patients with ER-negative tumors do respond to hormonal therapy. Other studies have shown that these exceptions may be due to false-negative assays, which in turn may be due to several factors: ERs are heat-sensitive, and unless the tissue is carefully handled a false-negative assay may result. False-negative assays may result for the following reasons, among others.

1. Tumors are heterogeneous, and the sample assayed may not be representative of the rest of the tumor. This argument supports sampling several sections of the tumor.
2. Receptor assays measure cytoplasmic binding, and the ER may be stored in the nucleus. Projects are under way to study the ERs in the nucleus.
3. Receptor assays are competitive binding assays; the receptor may already be occupied by another molecule with high binding affinity, thereby preventing the radiolabeled ligand from binding to the receptor.

There are also false-positive assays. Although the use of ER analysis improves the response rate to endocrine therapy for patients with breast cancer from 30% in unselected cases to about 60% in patients who are ER-positive, many patients still fail to respond. There are many possible reasons for these apparent false-positive assays.

1. There may be defects in translocation, transcription, translation, or another step in the biochemical pathway that results in new protein synthesis being altered.

2. The protein produced may not be relevant to the cell's growth even when a complete pathway is present.
3. The tumor heterogeneity may mean that most of the tumors are not representative of the portion assayed.
4. The binding observed may not be true receptor binding but merely binding to another molecule in the cell cytoplasm with no subsequent biochemical pathway to follow. Thus not all binding is true receptor binding.

Cellular Mechanisms of Hormone Action

At the cellular level, hormones increase the activity of certain enzymes selectively, thereby predictably modifying cellular function. Although the polypeptide hormones and the steroid hormones initiate their action after they have made contact with the cell membrane, there are differences in their overall action in bringing about the end result.

Cyclic AMP

Most of the polypeptide hormones affect cellular metabolism through the adenyl cyclase system. Simply, the circulating hormones bind rapidly and reversibly to a hormone-specific receptor on the surface of the cell membrane. This binding results in activation of the enzyme adenyl cyclase which in turn converts adeno-sine triphosphate (ATP) to cyclic 3',5'-adenosine monophosphate (AMP) (Fig. 26.1). Phosphodiesterase rapidly converts cyclic AMP to inactive AMP. Before its inactivation, cyclic AMP activates an enzyme, adenyl cyclase, which modifies cellular function. The hormone dissociates from its receptor site as the hormone concentration outside the cell falls. The specific hormone as "first messenger" and cyclic AMP as a "second messenger," as just outlined, may be similar for such hormones as insulin and the growth hormone, which have not been shown to activate adenyl cyclase but may work through an as yet undetermined second messenger.

Steroid Hormone Action

The ability of tissue to bind hormones is secondary to specific hormone receptors located within or on the surface of cells. These receptors apparently interact with a given hormone by combining with it, thereby initiating biochemical events characteristic of the function of that particular hormone. Among the naturally occurring estrogens, estradiol (the most potent) has a higher affinity for the receptor than does estrone or estriol. The synthetic steroid mestranol does not bind to ERs and is known to require demethylation to ethinyl estradiol to become active. Ethinyl estradiol binds with an affinity similar to that of estradiol. Thus mestranol is best considered a "prohormone." Diethylstilbestrol, though not a steroid, binds avidly to ERs and is an active estrogen. Other nonsteroidal compounds, such as tamoxifen, bind with the ERs, translocate to the nucleus, and bind to chromatin; but they do not influence gene transcription in an "estrogenic" fashion. By occupying receptors and nuclear receptor sites, these compounds make the cell refractory to estrogen stimulation and thus are designated *antiestrogens* or *estrogen antagonists*.

The steroid hormone enters the cell, presumably by passive diffusion, and combines with a specific receptor protein. This reaction is labeled *uptake*. The steroid hormone–receptor complex is next activated so it can enter the nucleus. Entrance of the activated complex into the nucleus is labeled *translocation*. Once

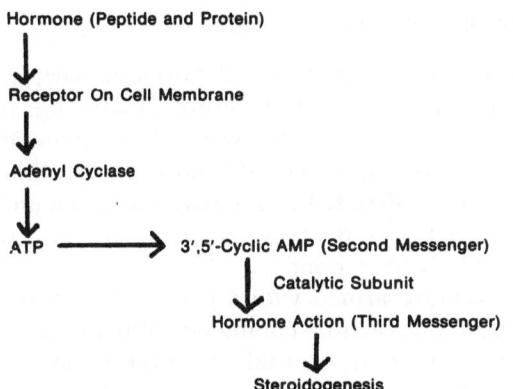

FIGURE 26.1. AMP as a second messenger for hormone action.

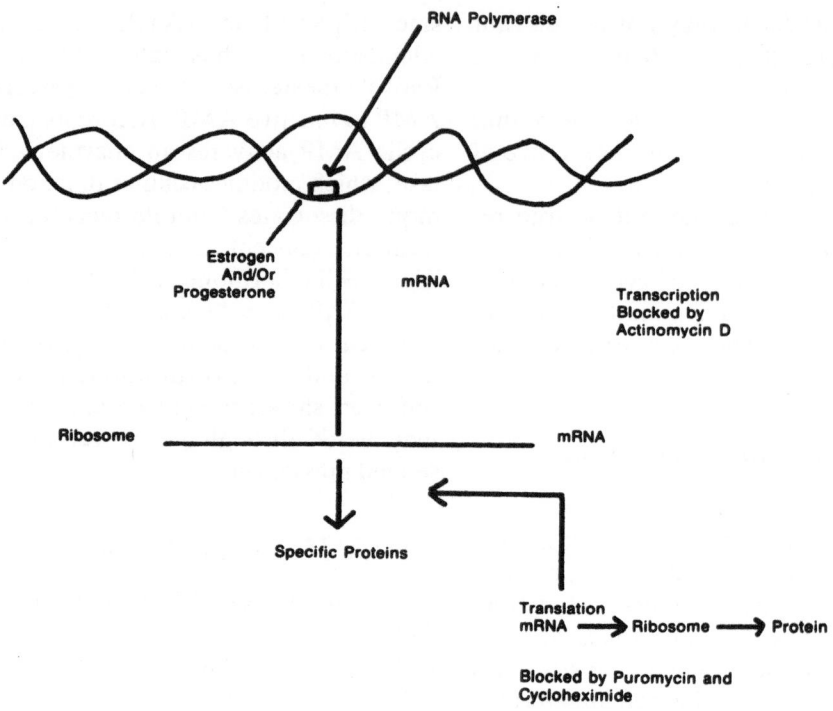

FIGURE 26.2. Estrogen and progesterone modifying nuclear gene expression.

inside the nucleus, the steroid hormone–receptor complex associates with nuclear chromatin, an event labeled *retention*. The interaction of steroid hormones with nuclear chromatins stimulates RNA synthesis, which in turn leads to the synthesis of certain cell proteins (Fig. 26.2). To expand the mechanism of action of estrogens in more detail, it has been shown that estrogens, whether administered pharmacologically or secreted by endocrine-active tissue, are carried bound to a plasma transport protein. Estrogens are able to enter the cytoplasm of all cells regardless of whether they are target tissues. However, in the cytoplasm of target tissues are found specific protein molecules that we term *receptors*. These proteins can bind biologically active estrogens with great affinity and great specificity. Following this initial binding step, the steroid–receptor complex undergoes temperature-dependent activation. This activation allows the steroid–receptor complex to enter the nucleus of the cell and bind to the chromatin, the location of the genetic information of the cell.

Once bound to the chromatin, the interaction of the steroid–receptor complex with the genetic information of the cell leads to an elaboration of new species of RNA. These RNA molecules then pass into the cytoplasm of the cell, where they then can be usefully translated on polysomes to program amino acids into new proteins that lead to the induced effects of the steroid hormone (Fig. 26.3).

Usefulness of the Assay

Clearly the aim of work with hormone receptor mechanisms is directed toward identifying, in advance, those patients who will respond to hormone therapy. With this information, therapy can be avoided in nonresponsive patients and can be used earlier in patients who are most likely to respond.

Therefore armed with a general knowledge of hormone action combined with increased awareness that steroid hormones do act through a receptor mechanism, it seemed reasonable to examine human breast cancer for

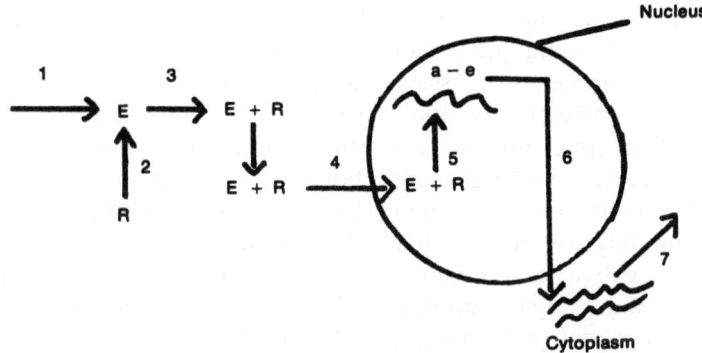

FIGURE 26.3. Steps in the formation of enzymes after the estrogen has entered the cell. (1) Free estrogen enters cell by passive diffusion; (2) uptake; (3) activation; (4) translocation; (5) association with nuclear protein and its labeled retention: (a) chromosomes untwist, (b) nucleotides are accepted, (c) RNA polymerase catalyzes, (d) mRNA is formed, (e) mRNA is released; (6) production of RNA messenger; (7) protein synthesis, enzymes, and cellular response characteristic of the hormone.

the presence of ERs. The first two groups to explore this question were Terenius in Europe and Jansen in the United States. It was their basic assumption that, because steroid hormones interact with target tissues through a receptor mechanism and because cytoplasmic receptors are necessary for steroid responsiveness, it might in fact be possible to predict, by examining the tumors for hormone receptors, which patients would respond to hormonal therapy. If the receptor were present, the tumor would be more likely to respond to hormonal manipulation; if the receptor were absent, the tumor would be independent of hormonal manipulations that one might institute in the management of these patients. Strong evidence has been provided that the risk of early recurrence is two to three times higher in ER-poor tumors than in ER-rich tumors. This increased risk is apparently independent of the status of lymph nodes. It is obvious that once it was established for breast tissue the method would be then adapted to studying most of the hormone-associated tumors.

Assays for Receptors

The assay for hormone receptors in breast cancer patients usually calls for a minimum of 500 mg of tumor tissue. Moreover, the tumor must be available within 15 minutes after removal from the breast by biopsy. It is better to perform the assay on a biopsy specimen than on a mastectomy specimen. The lengthy surgical procedure required for the mastectomy may injure the tissue, and there is unavoidable delay while processing the specimen. It is important to trim off the normal tissue and to be certain that the specimen is truly neoplastic.

By a variety of assay techniques, it has been possible to demonstrate steroid hormone receptors for estrogen in many human breast cancer samples. Essentially, these receptors appear in every way to be similar to those in nonmalignant tissue. They are protein, are free-floating in the cytoplasm of the cell, have limited binding capacity, have high binding affinity, and have great specificity for steroid molecules; they are able to translocate the steroid bound to them into the nucleus. The fact that they are present in normal tissue as well as in tumor tissue seems to contradict the statement of their usefulness for identifying tumors that will respond to hormone manipulation. Although there is a large difference in the anticipated assay test and its prediction for response to hormone manipulation, the finding of positive or negative ERs does provide guidelines for establishing treatment.

It is important to remember that when

assaying cancer samples for steroid receptors through any of the several techniques, and speaking about a positive or negative assay, one must have a specific correlate in mind. That is, "positive" and "negative" are qualitative measures of how much receptor is present in the tumor. A statement that a certain amount of receptor binding versus another amount is positive or negative is completely arbitrary. Unless there is some way of knowing with what the number correlates (e.g., clinical responsiveness), the number is meaningless. Therefore a competitive binding assay is utilized. Tritium-labeled estradiol is incubated with particle-free extract of the tumor. The particle-free extract is known as the *cytosol*. If the tumor extract contains ERs, they will bind with labeled hormone, and the resulting labeled receptors can be quantified. The results are reported in femtomoles per milligram of cytosol protein. A femtomole is 10^{-15} mol (*femten*: fifteen; Danish). It is critical to recall that such studies are done on crude samples that are mixtures of cell populations. Although binding sites are reported as numbers (usually in terms of femtomoles) of binding per gram of tissue or milligram of cytoplasmic protein, they are misleadingly accurate-sounding numbers, because one is talking about binding in terms of milligrams or grams of tissue in general, not specifically cancer tissue. Cancer specimens are almost invariably mixtures of unknown proportions of cancer cells and stroma.

The important question regards the data that demonstrate ERs in approximately 60 to 65% of fresh human breast cancer samples from primary tumors. These data have been presented at numerous meetings sponsored by the National Cancer Institute Breast Cancer Task Force. However, there are still questions that must be answered. In general, "positive" usually means something close to the limit of detectability of whatever assay method was used by a given investigator. Usually if any number of sites could be detected, the assay was called positive for ERs. This receptor protein satisfied all the criteria outlined previously, that is, its ability to distinguish between different steroids of varying estrogen potential and its ability under artificial assay conditions to translocate estrogen to the nuclei of cells.

The question most important to clinicians was whether the presence or absence of the ER protein was associated with hormone responsiveness. In general, there is an almost complete correlation between lack of response to hormone manipulation and lack of receptor. It has been reported that fewer than 10% of those whose tumors lack ERs respond to hormone therapy, whether ablative or additive. The logical question is to ask why even these 10% respond if they lack receptor, but as yet there is no clear definition of what constitutes positive or negative. It is this particular area that requires more investigation before reliable statements can be made.

It is important to address this question. It may be that the receptor in the sample is present in such small quantities that it is below the limit of the present detectability of the assay. Tumor cells themselves may contain sufficient receptor. Another consideration is that the tissue analyzed is not always homogeneous but is, rather, heterogeneous; it is difficult at this time to determine accurately the amount of homogeneous tissue present.

Twice as many patients whose tumors are known to contain hormone receptors have objective clinical regressions following hormonal therapy as those whose therapies are prescribed in an arbitrary manner. The question, however, of why there is not a 100% response has again not been answered.

Because receptors have wide application in all areas of tumor study, it is important to know the general uses of this measurement and the mechanism by which the patients whose tumors contain ERs fail to respond to hormonal therapy. The next question is whether the cost benefit ratio justifies the overall management of patients with cancer.

Using the breast as a model, it has been observed that the size of the tumor at the time of operation is known to be a poor indicator of prognosis. Moreover, ERs are independent of tumor size. It has also been observed that increasing histologic grade of the tumor is a poor indicator of prognosis, and the presence or absence of ERs is not definitely correlated with the prognosis.

The presence or absence of positive axillary lymph nodes is well known to be the most significant clinical prognosticator of tumor recurrence. Axillary involvement with tumors is not associated with the presence or absence of ERs. It is increasingly obvious that with our present technology it is important that clinical acumen be used when interpreting the results of the receptor assays.

The patients whose tumors contain ERs but fail to respond to hormone therapy present one of the greatest challenges in the field of oncology. It has been observed that there are several biologic steps that take place on the way to the cell producing its final protein or enzyme. It is obvious that at any one of these steps there may be a derangement that interferes with the function of the cell. In addition, there must be tumors that rapidly metabolize steroids to some inactive form. Last but not least is the fact that the tumor receptor assay may be correct but the hormonal therapy is inadequate. It may represent the fact that the tumor is dependent on other steroid hormones, such as androgens, so if one removes estrogen, endogenous androgen stimulation may be sufficient to keep the tumor growing.

It has been shown that estrogen treatment stimulates not only tissue growth but also the appearance of progesterone receptors. This point has proved to be an advance in the combination of estrogen and progesterone receptors that has added to our knowledge of tumor responsiveness and has increasingly correlated with clinical response. In initial studies it has been shown that most tumors that lack ERs also lack progesterone receptors (PRs), which is what had been anticipated. It is interesting to note that among tumors that contain ERs only about two-thirds had PRs. This figure represent the proportion of ER-positive tumors that respond to estrogen therapy. It is now accepted that a correlation of the ERs and PRs give a more important and accurate prognostic value than do the ERs alone.

Endometrial Carcinoma

Researchers and clinicians have observed that there are many biologic similarities between endometrial and breast carcinoma. Each of these neoplasms is susceptible to stimulation by estrogen at physiologic concentrations, and in some cases both are responsive to therapy with pharmacologic doses of steroids and antiestrogen therapy. It is becoming increasingly obvious that the description of the mechanism of interaction of steroid hormones with mammary tissue is similar to that found in the endometrium.

Receptor studies in endometrial tissue have proved that there are receptors for estradiol and progesterone. In addition, it has been demonstrated that the concentration of these receptors varied throughout the menstrual cycle. It has been observed that during the premenstrual cycle estradiol is secreted by the developing follicles and the concentration of estradiol receptors in proliferative endometrium is high. The luteal phase develops following ovulation; it is maintained by corpus luteum and is accompanied by the onset of significant ovarian secretion of progesterone. The estradiol secretion, which was high during the proliferative phase, begins to diminish markedly at this point. Measurements of the estradiol receptors reveal that there is a decrease of receptors not only in the cytosol but also in the nucleus. Conversely, there are a few progesterone receptors during the early proliferative phase, but they increase to a maximum at the time of ovulation. Because estradiol secretion is maximum at this point, it is thought that the PRs increase as a result of estrogen stimulation. Additional studies have shown that receptors are present in both the glandular and stromal cells of the human endometrium.

The next logical step is to use the findings of the receptor measurements in the normal endometrium and to apply them to hyperplastic tissue, such as adenomatous hyperplastic, through the various stages to the invasive stage of cancer. Researchers have reported that hyperplastic endometrial tissue from postmenopausal women has estradiol receptor concentrations comparable to those found during the proliferative phase of the endometrium. As one might predict, specimens of well-differentiated endometrial adenocarcinoma from postmenopausal women show a large variability in estradiol receptor content. The average values are higher than those seen in normal secretory endometrium but lower than those of proliferative tissue. The same variability and puzzling findings have been reported in the endometrium as had been reported in breast tissue.

Concentrations of PR have been reported to decline with the loss of differentiation in endometrial carcinoma. The use of this observation may explain some of the unpredictable results that arise during the treatment of endometrial carcinoma. Martin and Hähnel reported that the tissues from 30 cases of endometrial carcinoma and 44 cases of cervical cancer were examined for ER activity. Twenty of the endometrial and nine of the cervical tumors contained ER levels above 4 fmol/mg of protein. The proportion of ER-positive tumors was significantly greater in adenocarcinoma of the cervix than in squamous carcinoma of the cervix. Tissue from three mixed mesodermal tumors of the uterus, two carcinomas of the vagina, a carcinoma in situ of the cervix, and a carcinoma in situ of the endometrium were ER-negative. One ovarian carcinoma and a single case of uterine sarcoma were ER-positive. This point has interesting implications in terms of the relation to hormone therapy.

Clinical experience has shown that endometrial carcinoma is significantly more frequent in women with an abnormal endocrine constellation, for example, as associated with polycystic ovarian syndrome, severe obesity, liver disease, and a variety of ovarian tumors. It has also been shown that neoplastic proliferation of the tumor can often be reduced by high doses of progestin. These observations have raised the question if some alteration of human uterine estrogen or progesterone receptor system could be involved in the genesis of endometrial cancer. Because of the therapeutic effects, it may be expected that tumor cells containing PRs will regress after appropriate progestin therapy, whereas cells that have lost their complex endocrine regulatory unit will not.

Epidemiologic studies support this concept: Patients whose uteri are exposed over long periods to estrogen in the absence of progesterone are at high risk for the development of endometrial hyperplasia and carcinoma. This situation is found, for instance, in postmeno-

pausal women and in patients with estrogen-secreting ovarian tumors. There has been a debate in the literature relative to the increased risk of cancer of the endometrium in women who take estrogen after the menopause.

It has been documented that the source of estrogen in postmenopausal women is not the ovaries but, indirectly, the adrenal gland. The secretion of large amounts of androstenedione by the adrenal has been confirmed, and it is known that it is converted extraglandularly to estrone estradiol and other estrogens. Postmenopausal patients with endometrial carcinoma have been shown to have either increased secretion of androstenedione or increased conversion of androstenedione to estrone. Obese postmenopausal women are at high risk of developing endometrial cancer and can convert androgens at a significantly higher rate.

A great deal of work has been done on the association between carcinoma of the endometrium and hormone stimulation. Paradoxically, carcinoma of the endometrium occurs at a time when the hormone titer is decreasing. There may be explanations for this phenomenon, namely, low doses of estrogen may serve to stimulate hormone secretion, whereas normal or high titers may act as a feedback mechanism and serve as controls or regulators of hormone secretion.

A brief review of the estriol/estradiol-estrone ratio may serve to clarify the problem. Estriol has been considered a noncarcinogenic estrogen, whereas estradiol and estrone have been cast in the role of being carcinogenic. It is concluded that estriol acts as an antagonist of the carcinogenic activity of estradiol-estrone. Oriental women, who have a low incidence of cancer of the endometrium, breast, and ovary (which are hormone-dependent organs) compared to caucasian women, have a high estriol titer between the ages of 15 and 19 years. However, as each group moves toward age 40, the difference decreases until it is negligible. Because there is little difference at the time the incidence of carcinoma in these three organs begins to increase, it must be concluded that estriol serves to protect the immature cell. This situation may be similar to the group of cases reported in which the immature cells were damaged and 14 to 20 years later a malignancy in the form of müllerian-type clear-cell adenocarcinoma of the vagina appeared. The role of stilbestrol is difficult to evaluate, as the estrogens are growth stimulants but not cell transformers.

Estrogen receptors were determined in cytosol by Hähnel and his research team. They also measured the DNA content of the tissues and the protein content of the cytosols. The plasma concentrations of estradiol, estrone, testosterone, sex hormone-binding globulin, and follicle-stimulating hormone (FSH) were examined at the same time. Hähnel et al. found that there was no evidence that low receptor concentration in the tissues was associated with high blood levels of estradiol or estrone, or vice versa. It was observed that the average DNA content in ER-positive endometrial carcinomas was higher than that in ER-negative carcinomas. The characterization and measurement of hormone receptors in the tissues has opened up a new field, but it is only the beginning. More intensive investigative efforts directed toward elucidation of the interrelation between the plasma hormone fractions and their concentrations in tissue, between free and receptor-bound hormones in the tissue, and finally between the hormone–receptor complexes of the cytoplasm and their nuclear counterparts are at present some of the most promising approaches to a better understanding of the hormone sensitivity of cancer.

Hausknecht and Gusberg measured the urinary metabolites of estradiol in normal postmenopausal women and postmenopausal women with endometrial carcinoma. They found no statistical difference in excretion of the classic estrogen or in the estriol quotient. Aleem et al., studying plasma estrogen in patients with endometrial hyperplasia, challenged this concept. It has been suggested that there is an increased peripheral conversion (two to three times normal) of estrogen precursors (i.e., androstenedione) in postmenopausal women who produce an excess amount of estrone, which in turn may produce endometrial hyperplasia in older women. Gusberg showed that there is a higher estrone/estradiol ratio in the blood of postmenopausal women

with endometrial cancer. He found also that postmenopausal women with endometrial cancer excrete less total estriol glucuronide compared to estrone glucuronide than normal postmenopausal women and suggested that the protective effectiveness of estriol had been lost. Gusberg also reported a significantly higher conversion rate of Δ4-androstenedione to estrone in postmenopausal women with endometrial cancer. Rubin et al., measuring circulating estrone and estradiol concentrations, showed the mean ratio once again to be significantly higher in women with cancer. Gusberg reported that it appears that the postmenopausal prehormone is androstenedione and the notable postmenopausal estrogen is estrone. Additional studies reported another point that cannot be adequately explained: 90% of patients with endometrial carcinoma have ovarian stromal hyperplasia.

Nordqvist investigated the influence of steroid hormones in human endometrial carcinoma and organ culture heterotransplants. Progesterone impaired the success of organ cultures, and estrogen given simultaneously was found to potentiate these cytostatic and cytolytic effects. In culture, the endometrial carcinomas showed a marked dose-dependent sensitivity to progesterone, which reduced the mean DNA synthesis to 46% and the RNA synthesis to 39% of control values. Among the series of endometrial carcinomas treated with high-dose progesterone, about 75% showed decreased survival in organ cultures and significantly reduced RNA synthesis in vitro and in vivo.

Luteinizing hormone secretion in patients with endometrial carcinoma is seven times greater than in the normal population. It can be reduced to normal limits with the administration of 17α-hydroxyprogesterone acetate. This change (i.e., the LH elevation) cannot be demonstrated in women with ovarian or breast carcinoma.

The use of oral contraceptive pills containing estrogen and progesterone has been said to offer protection against carcinoma of the endometrium, although there are women who have developed endometrial cancer while on sequential contraceptives. Perhaps this medication does not give the protection that the combined medication for 21 days does, especially now that a minimal dose of estrogen is given.

The mechanism of action of the progesterones has not been elucidated. It is not known whether they have a suppressant effect, if there is a change in sex steroid components or sex steroid support of the tumor, or if there is direct action on the neoplastic cell itself. It has been noted that if the vaginal smear shows that the continuous estrogen effect has been suppressed by progesterone there is usually uninterrupted tumor progression. It also has been postulated that progestins seem to work better if there has been no prior irradiation. Kistner made the point that, if there is remission with one agent but it is followed by eventual failure, switching to another progestin may produce a further remission.

A reasonable goal of studies on endometrial carcinoma is, at this moment, to establish a relation between PR concentrations, therapeutic effectiveness of progesterone, and responsiveness of the neoplastic tissue. It should be evaluated morphologically or by biochemical measures, such as induction of estradiol-17β-dehydrogenase in vitro or in vivo.

Pollow et al. reported that the results of the progesterone binding studies done on 30 endometrial carcinomas demonstrated that there is a strong correlation between the number of PRs contained in a tumor specimen and the degree of differentiation of this tumor. The concentration of progesterone binding sites in undifferentiated tumors was low, whereas well-differentiated tumors contained a relatively high concentration of these sites. For estradiol receptors, the contrary was the case. Similar results for progesterone binding in human endometrial carcinoma were reported by Richardson et al. These findings may explain why in undifferentiated carcinomas treatment with progestins achieve little, whereas in well-differentiated tumors long remissions have been achieved even in patients with metastases.

For the whole range of steroid receptor concentrations in the different types of endometrial carcinoma, the following might be con-

sidered: First, the total PR concentration is an integrated value for the whole tumor. Because each tumor is a mixture of various cell types, the receptor concentration varies inversely with the proportion of connective tissue and directly with that of specific neoplastic cells. Second, it is possible that the receptor concentration in a given cell reflects its degree of differentiation. Finally, it is possible that a given endometrial carcinoma contains a mixture of cells, some of which have normal PR levels and other that have no receptors.

Interest in both ERs and PRs in normal human endometrium and endometrial cancer has taken a giant step forward. Breast cancer has been more widely studied for various reasons: (1) Jensen first described the estrogen receptor in breast cancer; and (2) there are approximately 38,000 new cases of endometrial cancer a year and more than 100,000 breast cancers reported annually. From these figures alone it is obvious that there is a greater pool of tissue to study among patients with breast cancer than among those with endometrial carcinoma.

Similar lines of study for endometrial carcinoma have been established using breast cancer as the model. Antiestrogens have been employed for the treatment of endometrial carcinoma following success administering antiestrogens to patients with breast cancer who are ER-positive. Antiestrogens, when administered pharmacologically, are transported in the plasma and readily enter all cells, regardless of whether they are in target tissues; and once again, as with estrogens, these molecules combine with the ERs. However, their action is more than simply to prevent the binding of radioactive estrogen to the receptor. It is clear from a variety of experiments that antiestrogens can bind to the receptor and activate it, and that antiestrogen bound to the ER can then translocate to the nucleus and bind to chromatin sites. At this time, little is known about what occurs at this level. However, in terms of two criteria—nuclear occupancy time and salt extractability—we do know that these complexes have biologic behavior that is different from normal ER complex behavior, and we presume that an important additional activity of these antiestrogenic compounds involves this nuclear interaction. Thus antiestrogens can exert their effect by two mechanisms. First, they can compete with the biologically active estrogens for the receptor protein and thus prevent their binding; and second, these antiestrogen compounds combine to the receptor themselves. The resulting antiestrogen–ER complexes can then translocate to the nucleus, where they can alter the transcriptive processes of the cell in a manner that leads to tumor regression.

Receptors in Ovarian Cancer

The ovary is unique in that it not only is the source of estrogen and progesterone but is itself a target organ for both these hormones. Punnonen et al. have reported that there are high-affinity cytoplasmic ERs in the endometrium, myometrium, and ovary of climacteric women. However, the ER levels of the ovary were low in all the cases studied. Pasqualini and Nguyen reported specific binding sites for progesterone and for the synthetic progestin in the cytosol and nuclear fractions of the fetal uterus of the guinea pig. Similar specific binding sites were found in the fetal ovaries and at the end of gestation reached comparatively high concentrations. Therefore it is evident that there are ERs and PRs in normal ovaries.

Reports show that common epithelial ovarian cancer occasionally responds well to hormonal therapy. It is estimated that about one-fourth of these tumors show a partial response when the patient presents with an inoperable situation. Although work is just being reported on receptors in ovarian cancer, it indicates that receptors are found in some ovarian cancers. Holt et al. reported that 50% contain a significant number of ERs and 16% contain a significant number of PRs. No association was found between receptor titers and histologic types, differentiation, or stage of the tumors. In this series, 8 of 16 women with primary ovarian adenocarcinomas had ERs or PR-like components (or both); among those with metastases who were tested, one-third retained estrogen binding. Hoffman and Siiteri have performed ER and PR assays on 32 primary ovarian epithelial tumors. Two-thirds of the tumors were ER-rich and one-fourth were PR-rich. Six clear-cell and mucinous carcinomas were receptor-poor. Among the remaining 26 endometrioid and seropapillary carcinomas, endometrioid carcinomas were more frequently rich in ERs and PRs. ER titers tended to be higher in less-differentiated lesions from older women, and PR titers were higher in well-differentiated tumors from premenopausal women.

Estrogen binding occurred in specimens from women with no histories of exposure to exogenous estrogen. Because tamoxifen and nafoxidine could inhibit estradiol binding, it is likely that antiestrogens will prove beneficial against some ovarian cancers.

Although the ovaries produce sex-steroid hormones, their projection is regulated by the pituitary. Reports have indicated that ovarian epithelial malignancies may contain all classes of steroid hormone receptor, but in relatively low concentrations. No large series has been investigated, and there is only minimal information available concerning the endocrine responsiveness to ovarian cancer. It has been shown that some patients respond to endocrine therapy.

Ovarian cancer that has been grown in long-term tissue cultures has proved to contain both ERs and PRs and may become a model for studying the actions of steroid hormones in ovarian cancer. The presence of steroid hormones may allow selection of candidates to participate in the formal trial of endocrine therapy to enable correlation of receptor data with response to therapy.

Work in Progress on Receptors

It has been reported that receptors can be manipulated and will become more sensitive to steroid hormone manipulation. It has been shown that induction of receptors may become possible within malignant cells in vivo, which may result in a conversion of a hormone-resistant tumor to one that is hormone-sensitive.

Projects in progress are investigating the coupling of cytotoxic agents to steroid hormones, and the administration of this endocrine-chemotherapy molecule to patients whose tumors contain the appropriate steroid hormone receptor. This method has the potential of delivering large quantities of a cytotoxic drug directly to the tumor. It also has the potential of imaging with radioactive isotopes. The project is in its infancy, and the early data have been somewhat disappointing, but other approaches are being undertaken and hopefully will be more successful.

Alterations in the Receptor Systems During Aging

The ovary has membrane receptors that are fairly specific for gonadotropins and that provide a stimulus for intracellular steroid pathways. The end result is that there is secretion of estrogen (as estradiol primarily) and other intermediate steroids, including progesterone. It has been confirmed that estrogens and progesterones act at appropriate target organs and require their own intracellular receptors for response.

Estrogen has been described as initially decreasing between the ages of 26 and 29; however, more evident effects are seen during the perimenopausal (36–45) and menopausal (45–55) years. At the time of the perimenopausal period, estrogens decrease in terms of production and serum levels. Estrogen has ubiquitous activity through body cells, and the primary method for expression is through the presence of intracellular ERs. Presuming that receptor protein decreases with aging, this biochemical pathway could further reduce the activity of the steroids in the cells. Studies have shown that not all the cells of the body age equally, and the receptor systems may be responsible for this differential. Focal centers of aging may occur within the body and may be causally related to these receptor systems.

A considerable amount of work on receptor aging has been done in rodents and has shown diminished ER protein in the endometrium. Indirect evidence of reduced ER protein in the breasts of menopausal women has been reported. Data reported in the literature suggest that there is a loss of estrogen and progester-

one that may reduce cell metabolism in various tissues of the body. A great deal of work is in progress that shows receptors are fundamental to end-organ expression of hormones. Tissues dependent on estrogen or its effects have an increase in the rate of senescence during the perimenopause and menopause. Because the incidence of cancer increases with age, valuable information about transformation of cells to a malignant process will undoubtedly result by determining the full extent of these intracellular receptors.

Receptors

Estrogen Receptors

The ER test measures receptor expression and reports the tumor as ER-positive or ER-negative. ER-negative tumors are aggressive and rarely respond to endocrine therapy. ER status is a strong, independent predictor of recurrence and survival. ER-negative is defined as less than 10 fmol ER/mg cytosol protein.

Progesterone Receptor

Progesterone receptor expression is reported as positive or negative. Reports indicate that the presence of PRs has greater predictive value than that of ERs and is better correlated with the outcome of endocrine therapy. A PR-positive report may indicate false-negative ER results. PR-negative is defined as less than 10 fmol PR/mg cytosol protein.

Epidermal Growth Factor Receptor

The epidermal growth factor receptor (EGFR) assay is investigational. EGFR-negative tumors carry a prognosis similar to that for ER-positive disease, even in ER-negative tumors. Ninety-five percent of EGFR-positive tumors are ER-negative. EGFR-negative status may thus define a subgroup of ER-negative patients with better survival. EGFR negative is defined as less than 5 fmol/mg of protein.

HER-2/Neu Oncoprotein

An assay for the protein product of the HER-2-neu oncogene has been developed. Amplification of this gene is significantly greater in patients with early relapse and poor survival. With node-positive diseases the test may predict outcome better than either the ER or PR assay.

Sex-Hormone-Binding Globulin

Plasma protein binds estradiol, making less estradiol available for diffusion into cells. Tamoxifen increases sex-hormone-binding globulin (SHBG).

Comment

The assays for EGFR and the HER-2/neu oncoprotein (H2n) are investigational but may be soon approved for diagnostic purposes. At present, they may not be used for diagnostic or prognostic purposes.

Summary

The ovary has membrane receptors that are fairly specific for gonadotropins and provide a stimulus for intracellular steroid pathways. The end result is that there is secretion of estrogen, primarily as estradiol, and other intermediate steroids including progesterone. It has been confirmed that estrogens and progesterones act at approximate target organs and require their own intracellular receptors for response.

Steroid hormones circulate in extremely low concentrations. To respond with specific and effective actions, target cells require the presence of intracellular receptor protein.

Steroid hormones are rapidly transported across the cell membrane by simple diffusion. The factors responsible for this transfer are unknown, but the concentration of free (i.e., unbound) hormone in the bloodstream is an important determination of this action. Once within a target cell, the hormone is quickly bound by a protein receptor, a large protein that may or may not consist of subunits.

The function of the receptor is to transmit the hormone's message to the chromatin material. After binding to the hormone, the receptor undergoes transformation, also called activation, a conformational change that allows initiation of RNA transcription.

The specific hormone message is then transmitted by means of protein synthesis in the ribosomes, brought about by specific RNA. The principal action of steroid hormones is the regulation of intracellular protein synthesis by means of the receptor mechanism.

Tissue responsiveness to hormone is determined not only by the presence of a specific receptor but also by the intracellular concentration of that receptor. Responsiveness may be modified by effecting receptor concentration. Estrogen increases target tissue responsiveness to itself and to progesterone by increasing the concentration of its own receptor and that of the intracellular progesterone receptor.

Biologic activity is maintained only while the receptor is joined with the hormone. Therefore the dissociation rate of the hormone–receptor complex is a factor in the biologic response. A hormone effect is also influenced by the half-life of the nuclear chromatin bound complex. Estrogen increases the concentration of its own receptor in a process called receptor replenishment. Substances that interfere with replenishment of the estrogen receptor, with time, decrease receptor concentration and therefore exert an antiestrogen effect. Progesterone, clomiphene, and testosterone limit tissue response to estrogen by blocking the replenishment of cytoplasmic estrogen receptors.

Increasing intraovarian androgens may suppress receptors for estrogen and play a regulatory role in ensuring that only one follicle reaches the point of ovulation.

At the time of the perimenopausal period both the production and serum levels of estrogens decrease. Estrogen has ubiquitous activity throughout body cells, and the primary method for expression is the presence of intracellular estrogen receptors. Presuming that receptor protein decreases with aging, this biochemical pathway could further reduce the activity of the steroids in the cell. Studies have shown that not all the cells of the body age equally, and receptor systems may be responsible for this differential. Focal centers of aging may occur within the body and may be causally related to these receptor systems.

A considerable amount of work on receptor aging done in rodents has shown a diminished estrogen receptor protein in the endometrium. Indirect evidence of reduced estrogen receptor protein in the breasts of menopausal women has also been reported. The date reported in the literature suggests that there is a loss of estrogen and progesterone, which may reduce cell metabolism in various tissues of the body. Work is in progress that shows receptors are fundamental to end-organ expression of hormones. Tissues dependent on estrogen or its effect have an increased rate of senescence during the perimenopause and menopause. Because the incidence of cancer increases with age, valuable information on cells that participate in the malignant process will undoubtedly result by determining the full extent of these intracellular receptors.

Bibliography

Aleem FA, Moukhtar MA, Hung HC, Romney SL: Plasma estrogen in patients with endometrial hyperplasia and carcinoma. *Cancer* 38:2101, 1976.

Baranczuk RJ: A new tool in the fight to control advanced breast cancer. *Diagn Med* 26:1, 1978.

Barber HRK; Kwon TH: The endometrium. In Nealon Jr RF (ed): *Management of the Patient with Cancer*. 2nd Ed. Saunders, Philadelphia, 1976.

Clark JH, Park EJ, Anderson JN: Nafoxidine, mode of action on estrogen receptor systems. *Nature* 251:446, 1974.

Dao TL: Chemotherapy for women with breast cancer. *Female Patient* 3(11):61, 1978.

Dapunt O, Daxenbichler G, Margerter HJ, et al: The role of steroid receptors for hormonal therapy of mammary and genital carcinomata. *Eur J Gynecol Oncol* 1:37, 1980.

Eskin BA (ed.): *The Menopause Comprehensive Management*. Masson, New York, 1980.

Farley AL, O'Brien TE, Moyer D, Taylor CR: The detection of estrogen receptors in gynecologic tumors using immunoperoxidase and the dextran-coated charcoal assay. *Cancer* 49:2153, 1982.

Galli M, DeGiovanni C, Nicoletti G, et al: The occurrence of multiple steroid hormone receptors in disease-free and neoplastic human ovary. *Cancer* 47:1297, 1981.

Geisinger KR, Kute TE, Pettenati MJ, et al: Characterization of a human ovarian carcinoma cell with estrogen and progesterone receptors. *Cancer* 63:280, 1989.

Gusberg SB: The dysfunctional and the neoplas-

tic: clinical investigation in the service of patient care in endometrial cancer. *Am J Obstet Gynecol* 116:175, 1973.

Hähnel R, Martin JD, Masters AM, et al: Estrogen receptors and blood hormone levels in endometrial carcinoma. *Gynecol Oncol* 8:209, 1979.

Hausknecht RV, Gusberg SB: Estrogen metabolism in patients at high risk for endometrial carcinoma. *Am J Obstet Gynecol* 105:1161, 1969.

Hoffman PG, Siiteri PK: Sex steroid receptors in gynecologic cancer. *Obstet Gynecol* 55:648, 1980.

Holt JA, Caputo TA, Kelly KM, et al: Estrogen and progestin binding in cytosols of ovarian adenocarcinoma. *Obstet Gynecol* 53:50, 1979.

Hoover R, Gray LA Sr, Fraumeni JF Jr: Stilbestrol (diethylstilbestrol) and the risk of ovarian cancer. *Lancet* 2:533, 1977.

Hubay CA, Arafah B, Gordon NH, et al: Hormone receptors: an update and application. *Surg Clin North Am* 64:1155, 1984.

Jähne O, Kauppila A, Syrjälä P, Vihko R: Comparison of cytosol estrogen and progestin receptors status in malignant and benign tumors and tumor like lesions of the human ovary. *Int J Cancer* 25:175, 1980.

Jansen EV, Suzuki T, DeSombre ER: A two-step mechanism for the interaction of estradiol with rat uterus. *Proc Natl Acad Sci USA* 59:632, 1968.

Kistner RW: Treatment of carcinoma in situ of the endometrium. *Clin Obstet Gynecol* 5:1166, 1962.

Knat DR: Estrogen and endometrial carcinoma. *Obstet Gynecol Surv* 32:267, 1977.

Martin JD, Hänel R: Oestrogen receptor studies in carcinoma of the endometrium, carcinoma of the uterine cervix and other gynecological malignancies. *Aust NZ J Obstet Gynaecol* 18:55, 1978.

McGuire WL, Clark GM: The prognostic role of progesterone receptors in human breast cancer. *Semin Oncol* 10(suppl 4):2, 1983.

McGuire WL, Raymond JP, Banheu EE: Progesterone receptors: introduction and overview. In McGuire WL, et al (eds): *Progesterone Receptors in Normal and Neoplastic Tissues*. Raven Press, New York, 1977, p. 1.

Mortel R, Levy C, Wolff JP, et al: Female sex steroid receptors in postmenopausal endometrial carcinoma and biochemical response to an antiestrogen. *Cancer Res* 4:1140, 1981.

Myers AN, Moore GE, Major FJ: Advanced ovarian carcinoma: response to antiestrogen therapy. *Cancer* 48:2368, 1981.

Nelson JF, Holinka CF, Finch CE: Loss of cytoplasmic estradiol binding capacity during aging in uteri of 57/6 mice. *Proc Endocrinol Soc* 58:349, 1976.

Nordqvist S: Hormonal responsiveness of human endometrial carcinoma studied in vitro and vivo. Student-litteratur, Lund, Sweden, 1969.

Nordqvist S: Survival and hormonal responsiveness of endometrial carcinoma in organ culture. *Acta Obstet Gynecol Scand* 49:275, 1970.

Nordqvist S: Endometrial cancer: fact and theories. *Pathol Annu* 8:282, 1973.

Pasqualini JR, Nguyen EL: Progesterone receptors in the fetal uterus and ovary of the guinea pig: evolution during fetal development and induction and stimulation in estradiol primed animals. *Endocrinology* 106:1160, 1980.

Pollow K, Schmidt-Gollwitzer M, Nevinny-Stacket J: Progesterone receptors in normal and neoplastic tissue. McGuire WL, Raymond JP, Baulieu ET (eds). New York, Raven Press, 1977.

Punnonen R, Kouvonen I, Lövgren T, Rauramo L: Uterine and ovarian estrogen receptor levels climacteric women. *Acta Obstet Gynecol Scand* 58:389, 1979.

Rao BR, Meyer JS: Estrogen and progestin receptors in normal and cancer tissue. In McGuire WL et al (eds): *Progesterone Receptors in Normal and Neoplastic Tissues*. Raven Press, New York, 1977.

Richardson GS, McLaughlin DT, Scully RE: Progesterone specific binding by cytosols of human endometria. *J Steroid Biochem* 5:329, 1974.

Roth GS: Altered biochemical responsiveness and hormone receptor changes during aging. In Behnke J, Finch G, Morneut G (eds): *The Biology of Aging*. Plenum Press, New York, 1978, p. 291.

Roth GS: Hormone receptor changes during adulthood and senescence: significance for aging research. *Fed Proc* 38:1910, 1979.

Rubin BL, Gusberg S, Butterly J, et al: Screening test for estrogen dependence of endometrial carcinoma. *Am J Obstet Gynecol* 114:660, 1972.

Schindler AE, Ebert A, Friedrich E: Conversion of androstenedione to estrone by human fat tissue. *J Clin Endocrinol Metab* 35:627, 1972.

Schriber JR, Erickson GF: Progesterone receptor in the rat ovary: further characterization and localization in the granulosa cell. *Steroids* 34:459, 1979.

Schriber JR, Hsueh AJW: Progesterone receptor in rat ovary. *Endocrinology* 105:915, 1979.

Sherman AJ, Woolf RB: An endocrine basis for endometrial carcinoma. *Am J Obstet Gynecol* 77:233, 1959.

Shimar K, Kitayama S, Nikano R: Gonadotropin binding sites in human ovarian follicles and corporea lutea during the menstrual cycle. *Obstet Gynecol* 69:800, 1987.

Taylor RW, Bush MG: The use of estradiol uptake and binding sites studies in endometrial and ovarian carcinoma. *Postgrad Med J* 49:77, 1973.

Terenius L: Oestrogen binding in the mouse uterus. *Acta Endocrinol (Copenh)* 57:669, 1968.

Terenius L, Johansson H, Rimsten A, Thorem L: Malignant and benign mammary disease: estrogen binding in relation to clinical data. *Cancer* 33: 1364, 1974.

27

Biologic Response Modification

Biologic response modifiers (BRM) are compounds that modify an immune response, usually enhancing it. They include immuno-potentiating bacterial products, chemicals such as polynucleotides, physiologically active molecules such as thymic hormones and interferon, and the true adjuvants, which are administered with the antigen. A number of these substances have been used in an attempt to potentiate immune reactions in cancer patients and those who suffer from immunodeficiency.

The term biotechnology encompasses many activities that have in common the fact that they all harness the fundamental abilities of living organisms. One of the most impressive achievements of science has been the explosion of knowledge about the chemical composition of organisms and the way these chemicals interact to create the phenomenon scientists recognize as life. Organisms are sometimes compared to chemical factories. The strength of this analogy lies in its emphasis on the chemical nature of life—the fact that growth, development, and reproduction depend on chemical reactions. However, the analogy does obscure some of the most fundamental characteristics of organisms, many of which are directly relevant to biotechnology.

With genetic engineering there is a reweaving of the threads of life. The possibility of transferring genes from one organism to another is an alluring prospect, as genetic engineering can reduce the cost and increase the supply of an enormous range of materials now used in medicine, agriculture, and industry.

Furthermore, there are many substances that occur naturally in only small quantities, which might well prove invaluable if they were available in sufficient quantities for their potential to be examined.

A major attraction of employing microbes as the factories for producing these materials is that scientists and technologists have a great deal of experience in growing such organisms inexpensively and efficiently on a large scale. Growers and bakers have been doing it for a millennia, and the modern pharmaceutical industry has developed a level of sophistication that will underpin many of the biotechnologic industries.

The basic principles of genetic engineering were developed only during the 1980s, and since then there has been astounding progress that has provided us with a set of tools of remarkable power and sophistication. In outline, genetic engineering involves inserting new genetic information into an organism—usually a bacterium—to endow it with novel capabilities. It does not follow a single fixed set of procedures. The choice of method depends on the gene to be transferred and the type of organism that is to receive the new genetic information. The choice even depends to some extent on personal preferences of the scientists involved.

The biotechnologic applications of genetic engineering consist in four main stages: (1) obtaining the gene that codes for the product the microbial factory is to manufacture; (2) inserting the gene into the microbes; (3) inducing the microbes to start synthesizing the foreign product; and (4) collecting that product.

Biologicals and Biologic Response Modifiers

The body's inherent biochemical capacity for killing cancer cells plus the new genetic technology gives biologic response modification, or *biomodulation*. Biologic response modification is the new wave in cancer treatment and is generating excitement among scientists, patients, the public—even on Wall Street, with the latest glamour stocks being those of the biotechnology firms. This field is expanding to include infectious diseases and a variety of hereditary disorders.

The use of biologicals and biologic response modifiers for the treatment of cancer is of recent origin. Biologicals may be defined as any product of a mammalian organism, and biologic response modifiers are those agents and approaches that alter biologic responses during the host–tumor interaction. The field encompasses traditional immunotherapy as well as molecular biology, recombinant genetics, and hybridoma technology, all of which produce highly purified biologic substances with anticancer activity. The recognition of growth, differentiation, and maturation factors, as well as the possibility of making antagonists or competitive inhibitors to factors that support neoplastic growth, infectious diseases, and hereditary disorders provides an additional biologic approach in this area.

Genetic Engineering

Genetic engineering has brought about a revolution in the field of biology. It will continue to be the front and center of research. Genes will be implanted into bacteria, resulting in the production of any desired protein or enzyme in large quantities. Medicine has already reaped many rewards from recombinant techniques that manufacture proteins in quantities by moving human genes into microorganisms. These genes can program the production of commercial quantities of human insulin, human growth factor, interferon, and genetically

engineered vaccines. It is possible that by the turn of the century cancers of the reproductive tract will be controlled by this technology. DNA probes and recombinant DNA experiments will change obstetrics and gynecology in all of its aspects as it is known today. Gene therapy is medicine's next frontier. It is now possible to isolate a single gene from the organism's total DNA and to introduce recombinant DNA to a bacterial cell to produce an altered organism.

Recombinant DNA technology, commonly referred to as genetic engineering, has provided science with the tools for the biosynthesis and subsequent mass production of a significant number of biologicals. It should revolutionize the treatment of cancer by the next century.

The process involves incorporation (recombination) of a segment of a DNA molecule containing a desired gene into a vector, usually a plasmid, which in turn is inserted into a host organism, usually *Escherichia coli*, although other bacteria, yeast, fungi, and sex and mammalian cells have been used. *E. coli* is cloned, and the organism producing the desired protein or polypeptide is selected. This clone is mass-produced by fermentation techniques, and the protein molecule is harvested and purified. The resultant product is a highly purified protein solution generally with more than 95% purity and a highly specific activity, containing the greatest possible amount of biologic activity per milligram of protein.

By genetic engineering, it is possible to produce in fairly large quantities α-, β-, and γ-interferon. At this point in time interferon has been approved for use only with hairy-cell leukemia. However, the potential for it to be used for a variety of other conditions is being investigated. It has shown promise in treating condyloma acuminatum, which has reached epidemic proportions.

Interleukins

Interleukins are a group of antigen nonspecific factors involved in lymphocyte activation and differentiation. There are three main groups: interleukin-1 (IL-1), which is a lymphocyte-activating factor; interleukin-2 (IL-2), which is a T cell growth factor; and interleukin-3 (IL-3), which is one of the colony-stimulating factors. The interleukins are produced by cell lines of several lineages that induce proliferation of lymphocytes.

Interleukin-1 is produced by macrophages and other antigen-producing cells. It acts on T cells to induce IL-2 receptors. In IL-2 the T-cell growth factor is produced by activated T cells. It is necessary for long-term proliferation of T cells and can act on previously stimulated B cells.

Adoptive immunotherapy describes the transfer of lymphocytes from a normal or immunized donor into a cancer patient to create activated killer (LAK) cells. In one variation, the lymphocytes removed from a patient are exposed to IL-2 in the laboratory. The cells are then transferred back into the same patient. Highly publicized IL-2 trials conducted at the National Cancer Institute are an example of this type of adoptive immunotherapy. Bone marrow transplantation also falls into this category because bone marrow contains a variety of mature immune cells and their forerunners.

Thymic Hormone

Thymic hormones, produced by the thymus, are factors that play a role in differentiation during development of T lymphocytes within the thymus and in their maintenance at the periphery. Some of these factors have been isolated from the thymic epithelium, and they tend to decline with age concomitantly with thymic atrophy. Five thymic hormones and factors have been isolated: thymosin (factor 5), thymopoietin-1 (and thymopoietin-2), thymic hormone factor, thymostimulin (TP-1), and thymulin.

Restorative immunotherapy is a direct or indirect restoration of immunologic function in a patient whose immune system is weakened. It is often used in conjunction with attempts to boost immunity above normal in such patients. An example is the use of thymic hormones, which convert T-lymphocyte precursors into functional T lymphocytes. Specific thymic hor-

mones generate production of helper and suppressor T lymphocytes, which act against tumor cells. Restorative biomodulators include cyclophosphamide, prostaglandin antagonist, and monoclonal antibodies directed against suppressor T cells. Cyclophosphamide (Cytoxan), a chemotherapeutic agent in use for years, is being used experimentally in low doses as a biomodulator to kill suppressor cells.

Tumor Necrosis Factor

The tumor necrosis factor (TNF) is produced by macrophages and is cytotoxic for some tumor cells and some karyocytes. The necrosis is induced by lipopolysaccharide (LPS) stimulation and exhibits direct cytotoxic activity in vitro. Clinical trials with these molecules are in progress now that preparations of good pharmaceutical quality are available.

Lymphokines, a group of protein substances produced by white blood cells, play a role in the body's immune system. Lymphotoxin, IL-2, interferon, and migration inhibition factor (macrophage migration inhibition factor) are just a few of the many lymphokines that are being studied. TNF is a substance known as a lymphokine of the body's natural immune system. There is evidence that it causes the same side effects in patients as do most lymphokines (e.g., chills, fever, headache, mild nausea, and weakness).

The story of the discovery of TNF began with William B. Coley, a surgeon at Memorial Hospital in New York City from 1892 to 1931. During the late nineteenth century he and a few other physicians had some success in treating cancer by infecting the patient with live bacteria. There were, however, serious problems with this approach; and infection could not be induced in some patients. Moreover, during the preantibiotic era, the difficulty of controlling the infections that did result was cause for concern. Coley therefore developed a vaccine of killed bacteria, which came to be known as Coley's toxins. These toxins reproduced many of the symptoms of bacterial infection, such as fever and chills, but they could be administered without fear of producing an actual infection. Tumors in some patients treated with the toxins diminished or disappeared, but as was the case with infection by live bacteria the results were inconsistent. Coley's decision to treat cancer patients with microbes made good sense; when his toxins were successful, they almost certainly induced macrophages in the human body to produce TNF and other factors that in combination exerted anticancer effects. His work was ignored for some time because there was no understanding of how the toxins worked, which itself was delayed until inflammation and immunity were understood. The critical molecules involved in these processes have now been identified and isolated. In retrospect, patients who did not respond were those who were unable to produce TNF or other cytokines, which activate the inflammatory and immune processes that are destructive to cancer. Now that TNF and many of the other factors elicited during the course of an infection have been identified, work is under way to see if there may not be a more effective version of Coley's toxin.

Tumor necrosis factor, which is an immunomodulator, has the ability, at least in the laboratory, to kill tumor cells while sparing normal cells. An α-TNF has been identified, and a substance formerly known as lymphotoxin has been renamed β-TNF. TNF seems to have some regulatory function in the body and may play a role against infections in support of interferon.

Macrophage Activating Factor

Macrophage activating factor (MAF) increases the microbicidal and cytotoxic capacity of macrophages; it is now known to be partly due to interferon-gamma (IFN-γ). Activated macrophages have the capacity to kill tumor cells nonspecifically but selectively. They recognize transformed (malignant) cells as foreign and are selectively cytotoxic to those cells but not to nonmalignant cells. MAF is a lymphokine; it has not been synthesized or genetically engineered. Some studies have confirmed that IFN-τ is an MAF, but there are MAF activities demonstrable even after removal of the interferon.

Granulocyte Macrophage Colony-Stimulating Factor

Unlike the other lymphokines that affect cells known as lymphocytes, the granulocyte macrophage colony-stimulating factor (CSF) stimulates cells called macrophages. The word macrophage literally means "big eater." Macrophages are scavenger cells that remove dead cellular debris, which they digest and remove.

Macrophages also have powerful killing effects against certain foreign organisms in tumor cells. Granulocyte macrophage CSF stimulates macrophages and causes them to proliferate and release their killer substances. The granulocyte macrophage CSFs may be to the killer macrophage what IL-2 is to the killer lymphocyte.

Growth and Transforming Factors

Current work indicates that the control and regulation of cellular growth and differentiation is under the control of a variety of proteins known as growth factors. Epidermal growth factor (EGF) stimulates the growth of epithelial tissues in vivo and in vitro. It has not been well characterized, but it seems to be similar to the murine growth factor, which has been well studied.

Transforming growth factors (TGFs) are secreted by transformed cells and have the capacity to transform normal cells and reduce anchorage-independent growth in semisolid media. They are related to the EGF. Secretions of these factors has been associated with the presence of oncogenes. A TGF has been identified in the urine of patients with disseminated cancer. Further understanding of this substance may add another biologic approach to treatment.

Interferons

Interferons (IFN) are a group of molecules that limit the spread of viral infection. There are three types: IFN-α and IFN-β, produced by leukocytes and lymphocytes, and IFN-γ, produced by activated T cells. Interferons from activated or virally infected cells bind to receptors in nearby cells, inducing these cells to make antiviral proteins. IFN-γ also modulates immune responses and enhances natural killer (NK) cell activity. An increasing number of sexually transmitted diseases are of the viral type, and it is obvious that much attention is being given to the use of interferons for combating these diseases, particularly condyloma acuminatum.

Interferons are polypeptides and are the first group of lymphokines/cytokines to have been identified. They are also the first anticancer agents to have been genetically engineered. IFN-α and IFN-β production is induced within 4 to 6 hours after viral stimulation, primarily by leukocytes and fibroblasts, respectively, whereas IFN-τ is produced by lymphocytes 2 to 3 days after antigenic stimulation. They all have a variety of functions, including inhibition of viral replication, modulation of various immune functions, and inhibition of cellular proliferation.

They have all been produced by genetic engineering. In addition to their antiviral activity, which is the definitive basis for interferon's biologic activity, the interferons are immunomodulatory and have the capacity to stimulate intracellular enzyme systems, with a resultant profound effect on protein synthesis. They also prolong and inhibit cell division, inducing an antiproliferative effect.

The question is often raised about the rumors that interferon cures the common cold. It has been shown that if you spray interferon in the nose it can prevent growth of the common cold virus and stops the virus's infestation quickly. However, interferon seems to cause a secondary reaction in the nose much like the symptoms of the cold itself—a decided disadvantage. The studies just cited were done with IFN-α. It is possible that IFN-β does not have those side effects, but this question must be explored.

There is a hope that interferon can be used to treat a variety of virus diseases, such as shingles, vocal cord papillomatosis, kidney cancer, and perhaps melanoma. Chronic hepatitis affects about 400 million people, mostly in tropical areas. There are a number of studies indicating that these people may be helped by interferon treatment, which eliminates the chronic virus state and retrovirus, after which liver function becomes normal.

Interferon deserves a special place in current research programs. It was one of the major factors that helped spawn the genetic engineering industry. Future treatment strategies undoubtedly will involve interferon in combination with some of the drugs that are being produced by genetic engineering. It may well be the one drug in the orchestration of different substances that nature intends for us to use to fight cancer.

Monoclonal Antibodies

Monoclonal antibodies are homogenous antibodies produced by a single clone. A *clone* is a group of cells derived from a single original cell; the cells are therefore genetically identical. A *line* is a group of cells grown under defined conditions from an initially heterogeneous population. Only occasionally is such a line monoclonal. "Monoclonal," "oligoclonal," and "polyclonal" refer to whether the line is from one, a few, or many clones, respectively.

Hybridomas are cells induced by the physical fusion of two different cells. Polyethylene glycol and Sendai virus are often used to effect the fusion. A hybridoma cell and its progeny contain some chromosomes from each fusion partner, although some others are usually lost. Immune responses and antibody populations may be described according to the number of corresponding cells as monoclonal, oligoclonal, or polyclonal.

Monoclonal antibodies are usually made from hybridomas that are prepared by fusing immunized mouse or rat spleen cells with a nonsecretor myeloma using polyethylene glycol or a virus such as Sendai. Although normal cells are mortal, tumor cells may be immortal. For that reason, Kohler and Milstein selected mouse myeloma cells to fuse with lymphocytes from the spleen of mice immunized with a particular antigen. The resulting hybrid-myeloma or "hybridoma" cells—expressed the lymphocytes' property of specific antibody production and the immortal character of the myeloma cells. Individual hybrid cells can be cloned, and each clone produces large amounts of identical antibody to a single antigenic determinant. The individual clones can be maintained indefinitely. This form of genetic engineering immortalizes immunity.

The fusion mixture between an immunized spleen cell and a myeloma cell is plated out in HAT medium (hypoxanthine/aminopterin/thymidine). Aminopterin blocks a metabolic pathway, which can be bypassed if hypoxanthine and thymidine are present; but the myeloma cells lack the bypass and consequently die in HAT medium. Spleen cells also die naturally in culture after 1 to 2 weeks, but a few cells survive, as they have the immortality of the myeloma and the metabolic bypass of the spleen cells. Some of the fused cells secrete antibody, and the supernatants are tested in a specific assay. Wells that contain the desired antibody are used to clone the antibody. Cloning by limiting dilution is a process in which a cell population is diluted successfully and set up in culture so there are wells containing only one cell. The progeny of this cell are continued as a clone. Cloning is done by culturing cell populations in soft agar, which prevents the cells from moving. Colonies that develop around a single clone are removed by micromanipulation in culture.

Through recombinant DNA techniques, bacteria, yeast, and other organisms can become factories for the production of human protein such as interferon, insulin, human growth hormone, and a variety of vaccines. This point is significant because natural collection of these proteins is a costly, time-consuming, frustrating process.

Most current antineoplastic drugs are poorly selected poisons that attack fast-growing cells. Monoclonal antibodies (MABs) are more specific and can be coupled with drug, toxin, radionuclei, or liposome carrying one of the above. Monoclonals coupled to other anticancer agents are showing promise against a few cancers.

Currently there are studies under way using Ricin, which is one of the ribosomal inhibiting proteins under investigation as an MAB conjugate partner. Ricin A-chain has toxic potency of one molecule per cell. It deactivates the 60 S ribosomal subunits and blocks protein biosynthesis, killing the cancer cell. Ricin B-chain mediates cell binding.

Tumor cell antigens and antibody receptors move between the cell interior and coated pits on the cell surface. Once bound, receptor and immunotoxin are taken in by the cell. Receptors and ligands accumulate in endosome sacs inside the tumor cells. pH changes separate the antibody from the receptor, which goes back to the cell surface. The immunotoxin is stored in a lysosome. The therapeutic problem is how to get the toxin out of seclusion in the lysosome. Much work is being done to solve this problem, and progress is slow but steady.

It is clear that we are entering a new era of cancer treatment. Historically, all efforts have been focused on eradication of cancer by cytotoxic modalities. Extirpation by surgery, sterilization by radiotherapy, and eradication of the last cell by chemotherapy have been major approaches to cancer treatment to this point. With the advent of biologicals and biologic response modifiers, several other approaches are now possible. In addition to manipulating the immune system in a manner favorable to the patient, one can use specific clues from the immunologic system to formulate specific pharmaceuticals that may be of use in cancer treatment.

Molecular biology and recombinant technology have made available highly selective biologic molecules that can be manufactured as highly purified pharmaceuticals. These new pharmaceuticals are likely to be of significant value for the treatment of cancer. They are currently being used in the fight against ovarian cancer. These approaches represent a strategically different way of developing therapeutics, and biotherapy is now a fourth modality of cancer treatment.

Future of Biologic Response Modifiers

No one has actually been cured by biologic response modifiers. However, widespread disease is not often cured by any means. Medical ethics dictates that new treatments be tested on advanced cases when established treatments offer no hope. Thus the most difficult cases are used to test these substances. The future of biologic response modifiers rests on the answer to a crucial and fundamental question: What causes the body to perceive harmful tumor antigen as self? Once the body has decided that the tumor antigen is part of itself, any attempt to destroy that balance can have only limited success. Initially, the body recognizes a tumor antigen as harmful. Its ability then changes, and the body accepts the tumor antigen as self. Thus suppressive cells are produced that inhibit the immune system's attempt to attack the tumor cells. Drugs can be used to reduce this suppression, but the effects are short term. If physicians can understand why the body sees the tumor antigen as part of itself, it would be possible to use biomodulation to intervene at a critical point. Until scientists understand what is involved in the determinants of self, they cannot reach their potential for treating patients by modulating the immune system.

My sequential treatment plan is as follows.

1. Restore immunity to normal by treating the patient with a thymic hormone or low-dose cyclophosphamide (cytoxan).
2. Give a vaccine to stimulate the patient's own cells.
3. Activate the patient's immune cells to a greater degree with IL-2.
4. Monoclonal antibodies can be used to target killer cells and to act effectively as carriers for killer molecules (toxins, drugs, or radioactive isotopes).

The use of MABs as carriers is receiving a great deal of attention. Most current antineoplastic drugs are poorly selected poisons that attack fast-growing cells. MABs are more specific and can be coupled with drug, toxin, radionuclei, or liposomes carrying one of the above. MABs coupled with other anticancer agents are showing promise against breast cancer, lung cancer, and malignant melanoma. Clinical trials with conjugated MABs are under way.

Ricin is one of the ribosomal inhibiting proteins that is under investigation as a monoclonal conjugate partner. It is described above.

Summary

Biomodulation was introduced during the late 1960s with the development of bacille Calmette Guérin (BCG), an organism similar to the tuberculosis bacillus, which was found to activate the immune responses in animals with leukemia. BCG cured some animals and led to prolonged survival of others. During the early 1970s it was used experimentally on humans, mostly leukemia cases, with limited success. However, it did give rise to studies that led to genetic engineering.

Biologic response modification is the combination of the body's inherent biochemical capacity to kill cancer cells joined with the new genetic technology. Having put them together, biologic response modification (biomodulation) has been achieved. A major classification of biologic response modifiers is as follows.

Immunomodulating agents
Interferons and interferon inducers
Thymosins
Lymphokines and cytokines
Interleukins
Tumor necrosis factor
Macrophage activating factor
Lymphotoxins
Growth and transforming factors, antigens
Effector cells
Monoclonal antibodies
Miscellaneous approaches
Genetic engineering with recombinant DNA
   or gene splicing

Recombinant DNA technology, commonly referred to as genetic engineering, has provided scientists with a tool for the biosynthesis and subsequent mass production of a significant number of biologicals. The process involves the incorporation (recombination) of a segment of DNA molecule containing a desired gene into a vector, usually a plasmid, which in turn is inserted into *Escherichia coli*, although other bacteria, yeast, insects, and mammalian cells have been used. *E. coli* is cloned, and the organism producing the desired protein or polypeptide is selected. This clone is mass-produced by fermentation techniques, and the protein molecule is harvested and purified. The resultant product is a highly purified protein solution generally with more than 95% purity and a high specific activity.

Over the next few years, DNA technology will be used in tandem with classic procedures in advanced microbiology laboratories. There is enormous potential for these techniques, and there are no doubts about the exciting future they promise pathologists, microbiologists, and all clinical laboratories. The results of these new techniques will provide clinicians with precise diagnostic and prognostic tools and therapy.

Bibliography

Barber HRK: Biological response modification. *Infec Dis Lett Obstet Gynecol* 10(1):7, 1988.

Barber HRK: Present status of tumor immunology in clinical gynecology. *Am J Reprod Immunol* 20(4):140, 1989.

Carter PW: Monoclonal antibodies and the biological approach to cancer. *J Biol Response Modifiers* 4:325, 1985.

Cherfas J: *Man-made Life*. Oxford, Basil Blackwell, 1982.

Garnet MC, Embleton MJ, Jacobs E, Baldwin RW: Preparation and properties of drug carrier antibody and conjugate showing selective antibody directed cytotoxicity in vitro. *Int J Cancer* 31:661, 1983.

Jackson DA, Stich MS (eds): *Recombinant DNA Debate*. Prentice-Hall, Englewood Cliffs, NJ, 1979.

Kennet G, McKearn T (eds): *Monoclonal Antibodies*. Plenum Press, New York, 1980.

Kohler G, Milstein C: Continuous culture of few cells secreting antibody of predefined specificity. *Nature* 256:495, 1975.

Lenard WJ, Depter JM, Kanehisa N, et al: Structure of the human interleukin-2 receptor gene. *Science* 230:633, 1985.

McAuliffe S, McAuliffe K: *Life for Sale*. Coward, McCann & Goeghejan, New York, 1981.

Moertel CG: On lymphokines, cytokines and breakthrough. *JAMA* 256:341, 1986.

Wiseman A (ed): *Principles of Biotechnology*. Surrey: University Press, 1983.

28

Immunotherapy and Immunopotentiation

The modern era of tumor immunotherapy started with William B. Coley, a surgeon at Memorial Hospital in New York at the end of the last century. As stated in Chapter 27, Coley had successfully treated sarcomas using live bacteria. The treatment produced a marked febrile course resulting in some spectacular results, but unfortunately the results were inconsistent and unpredictable. He next turned to using vaccines prepared from killed bacteria and again had some success, but the therapy proved to be nonspecific. Interest waxed and waned, but advances in molecular biology and understanding of the mechanism of drugs and multiple lesions on the cell has currently resulted in a revival of interest in this field.

Definition

The immune response is regulated by lymphocytes through positive and negative controls as well as feedback from soluble factors including antigen, antibody, lymphokines and interleukins. Antibody regulates its own control of synthesis in several ways. The following actions are important: (1) binding to antigen, thereby preventing the antigen from activating lymphocytes; (2) binding to Fc receptors on B (and possibly T gamma) cells (in the presence of antigen it causes cross-linking of the antigen receptors and Fc receptors, which is inhibitory to the cell); and (3) antibody–antigen complement produce complexes which localize in germinal centers where they stimulate B and T cells and induce memory.

Immune regulation falls into three classes.

1. *Antigen-specific interactions* are confined to cells that bind a particular antigen. These interactions are mediated either by antigen-specific factors or by direct cell-cell contact across an antigen bridge. The interaction is usually major histocompatibility complex (MHC)-restricted.
2. *Idiotype-specific interactions* are confined to cells and antibodies that express particular idiotypes on their antigen receptors; they are not usually MHC-restricted. Both antigen-specific and idiotype-specific interaction have a carrier that interacts with a B cell, producing the idiotype antibody to the hapten phosphorylcholine.
3. *Nonspecific interactions* affect lymphocytes regardless of their idiotype or antigen specificity. In practice, the structural organization of the lymphoid system dictates that the effects of the nonspecific signals are localized.

Immunotherapy is the treatment of disease by active or passive immunization. The most basic concept of tumor immunology is that there are certain characteristic antigens in or on tumor cells that distinguish them from normal host cells. These antigens are capable of eliciting humoral and cell-mediated immune responses. The manipulation of these responses to achieve tumor rejection is of considerable clinical interest.

Basic Principles of Tumor Immunity

Helper/suppressor factors released by T cells either enhance or suppress the release of other lymphocytes. They are often antigen-specific. In some systems they act by binding to antigen-presenting cells and thus modify the responses of lymphocytes with which they come in contact. The classic helper factors released by T_h cells act on macrophages or B cells; it is thought to be MHC class II restricted. Suppressor factor is released by T_s cells and acts primarily on T cells.

Immunity is the property whereby the lymphoreticular system makes a memorized response to an antigenic stimulus. It may result in a state of positive reaction known as sensitization or in one of the negative reactions (diminished or absent) known variously as immunologic tolerance, immunologic paralysis, or immunosuppression. It is not strictly correct therefore to use immunization as a synonym for sensitization or stimulation.

Despite these immunologic defenses, however, tumors develop in and kill animal and human hosts. A variety of mechanisms have been postulated to explain this phenomenon. The most efficient cures involve the potentiation of normal biophysical or biochemical processes or the countering of abnormal processes that lead to or accompany disease. Cancer presents few examples of this ideal at present, but studies of host resistance are an early step in this direction.

Many factors, such as intercellular communication, metabolic peculiarity, biochemical selection, and hormonal requirements, may be involved in host resistance. The immune activities of the lymphoreticular system have received the greatest attention and are the main topic of this chapter.

It is important to differentiate between *immunoprophylaxis*, which is the administration of an immunostimulator or an immuno-potentiator when all gross disease has been removed, and *immunotherapy*, which is given to control or eradicate macroscopic disease. The goal of immunotherapy is to eliminate the last cancer cell. It is hopefully achieved by manipulating the host immune response to tumor-specific antigens, thereby providing a systemic modality that, alone or in combination with conventional therapies, can kill the malignant cells.

The first-order kinetic cell kill by anticancer drugs (fixed percentage killed rather than fixed number killed per effective dose) is that, with a small tumor burden total cell kill can be achieved with a reasonable number of repetitive doses. A large tumor cell burden leaves residual cells that would eventually develop resistance and start to grow again.

The critical differences now existing between immunotherapy and chemotherapy are as follows

1. Immunotherapy is postulated to kill tumor cells by zero-order kinetics (fixed number).
2. Immunotherapy is therefore considered able to control only small cell numbers.
3. Regression of advanced disease cannot be used as a predictor for adjuvant choice.
4. The correlation of test results, which indicate immune response enhancement, to tumor cell control has still not been established.
5. The efficiency of immunomodulation with regard to specific diseases also remains to be established.

The commonly used criteria for objective response and disease progression in solid tumors are as follows.

Complete remission: complete disappearance of all demonstrable disease

Partial response: more than a 50% reduction in the sum of the products of the largest perpendicular diameters of discrete, measurable disease with no demonstrable disease progression elsewhere

No response: no change in the size of any measurable lesion or less than 50% reduction of measurable disease as defined above

Progression: more than 50% increase in the sum of the products of the largest perpendicular diameter of any measurable lesion

To make progress with immunotherapy, it is important to have a method that accurately measures the volume of tumor, such as that used to measure human chorionic gonadotropin (hCG) titers during the treatment of choriocarcinoma.

Rationale for an Immunologic Approach to Cancer Therapy

For more than 100 years the disappearance of cancer after severe infection has been reported. Coley during the 1890s noted the disappearance of cancer following a severe streptococcal infection (erysipelas). He therefore began to treat cancer patients with a variety of live bacterial cells and later with killed bacteria cells. Despite some promising results, though, he found no consistent therapeutic benefit. Interest in the use of toxins as immunopotentiators has waxed and waned since the beginning of the century.

Clinically, a frequent observation is that patients with empyema following pneumonectomy for cancer do better than those who have an uncomplicated postoperative course. It has also been reported that the simultaneous injection of a specific bacterium and an antigen increases the immune response to that antigen. The tubercle bacillus (bacille Calmette Guérin; BCG) was found to be one of the most effective bacterial adjuvants for immunostimulation. Complete Freund's adjuvant is a water-in-oil emulsion adjuvant in which killed, dried tubercle bacilli are suspended in the oil base. This adjuvant is especially effective for stimulating cell-mediated immunity; and in some animals, such as the guinea pig, it potentiates production of certain immunoglobulin classes.

It is recognized that the growth rates of various types of cancer are markelly different. Furthermore, and perhaps of greater interest, growth rates of specific histologic types vary considerably in different patients. Rarely, certain types of cancer undergo either temporary or permanent spontaneous regression. The world's literature has been surveyed and demonstrates the phenomenon of spontaneous regression.

A review of the literature shows that clinical and laboratory observations suggest the presence of host immunity factor in patients with malignant disease. These features include the following.

1. Spontaneous regression of tumor
2. Prolonged survival after incomplete removal of tumor
3. Sudden appearance of widespread metastases many years after apparently successful treatment of the primary lesion
4. Regression and metastases after treatment of the primary tumor
5. Histologic evidence of increased histiocytic, lymphocytic, and plasmacytic activity in the area of some tumors and regional lymph nodes
6. Evidence suggesting enhancement of tumor growth by adrenocorticosteroids and certain carcinostatic drugs
7. Low incidence of successful autografts of tumor tissue in cancer patients

This evidence indicates that host mechanisms are operative in human malignant disease, and such responses may have an immunologic basis.

Immune Defense System

The most effective cures of diseases that our philosophy can conceive involve the potentiation of normal, biophysical, or biochemical processes, or the countering of abnormal processes that lead to or accompany disease. Cancer presents few examples of this ideal at present, but studies of what has become known as host resistance are clearly an early step in this apparently logical direction. There are multitudinous factors (e.g., intercellular communication, metabolic peculiarity, biochemical selection, and hormonal requirement) that may be involved in host resistance. The immune activities of the lymphoreticular system have received the greatest attention and are the main topic of this discussion.

The immunology of human cancer has excited interest for a number of years. There is a body of circumstantial clinical and pathologic evidence that there may be a host response in human ovarian cancer. Scientific data suggest the presence of tumor-associated antigens and antibodies with some antitumor activity. Currently, characterization of the antigen is incomplete. Because an antigen is anything that reacts with the antibody whose formation it stimulated, it can be stated that a tumor-associated antigen is present in ovarian cancer. However, the antigen has failed to be immunogenic in the sense that, when purified, it fails to stimulate production of a specific antibody in animals. Evidence exists that there is blocking activity in the serum of patients with progressive disease and that these factors disappear when the patient is responding to treatment.

Pursuit of an immune response in human malignancy has challenged scientists but has continued to escape specific identification. There is great difficulty when transposing data from animal models to the human. In addition, there seems to be a difference between experimentally induced tumors and those arising spontaneously. Spontaneous tumors were long considered to lack tumor-specific transplantation antigens. It was impossible, for example, to immunize mice against spontaneous sarcomas by the techniques successfully employed to immunize them against methycholanthrene-induced tumors. Similarly, immunization with heavily irradiated cells of spontaneously occurring mammary carcinomas in the mouse did not induce resistance to these tumors. The latter finding has since been attributed to specific immunologic tolerance to the mammary tumor antigen that develops in newborn mice after exposure to the virus in their mother's milk. Tumor-specific transplantation antigens of mammary tumors have been readily demonstrated by immunizing mice that had been raised free of the virus. Thus mammary tumor cells indeed have foreign antigens, even if they are not immunogenic under certain conditions. During the 1990s, immune complex studies and work with the hybridomas should provide answers to many of the problems that have prevented progress in the diagnosis and management of ovarian caner.

Immunotherapy for ovarian cancer has not yet emerged from the experimental stage. However, there are indications that it may prolong the disease-free interval and possibly make easier the induction of second remissions. At present, its most important role is in the management of patients with minimal residual disease. Terry has reported that although there are good reasons to explore the possible effectiveness of BCG, *Corynebacterium parvum*, levamisole, interferon, and a host of other agents, the lack of information about tumor antigens and the patients' potential response to these antigens makes it likely from the outset that empiric efforts to stimulate immune responses would have a low probability of success. Further attempts at general stimulation or activation of the immune system with bacterial or chemical agents will probably not be fruitful until there is more information about cancer cells. Additional trials incorporating changes in dose, route of administration, treatment schedule, or any of the other countless treatment variables that clinical investigators can introduce are not likely to produce results of any importance.

The antigens on the surface of cancer cells are generally weak, and although they do arouse a specific response in the host the response is also weak. If the tumor cell has the ability to stimulate a specific immune response, why does the cancer continue to grow in the presence of a mechanism designed to control its growth? The explanation may be that the rate of growth exceeds the capacity of the immune response. However, studies in animals have disclosed more specific reasons for failure of the immune response to prevent the start and growth of cancer. These reasons are discussed in the next section.

Failure of the Immune Response

Immunosuppression

Many factors contribute to immunosuppression, including aging, the neoplastic process itself, anticancer drug therapy, radiation therapy, genetic defects, neonatal thymectomy, and, to a lesser extent, antibiotics, anesthetics, analgesics, and hypnotics. In reality, it is difficult to separate the contributions of drugs and disease in bringing about immunosuppression. One of the most potent factors to bring about a state of immunosuppression is the cancer itself; and as it progresses, the degree of immunosuppression increases. If there is to be any attempt to use immunotherapy, the disease must first be debulked.

Immunologic Tolerance

In a broad sense, immunologic tolerance may represent a specific form of immunosuppression. It is usually associated with exposure to an antigen during embryonic or early neonatal life, before the immune system has matured. It may, however, occur later in life. The tolerance theory for the progress of cancer is offered as an explanation for the theory that cancer arises from a single cell clone. Work on choriocarcinoma has suggested this mechanism. When it occurs, the host is not immunologically tolerant in general but tolerant only for that specific tumor antigen.

Acquired Tolerance (Immune Paralysis)

The currently preferred term is *acquired tolerance*. It is induced by injecting very small or very large doses of antigen. The tolerance persists for as long as that antigen remains in the body. In clinical practice it has been suggested that acquired tolerance (immune paralysis) occurs in the host with large tumors. After removal of such a large tumor mass, the host exhibits resistance to the reimplantation of her own tumor cells. This fact suggests that the intrinsic failure of the immune response was not the cause of the original lack of immune reaction. Rather, the temporary paralysis resulted from the system's inability to cope with too great a challenge.

Immunologic Enhancement (Blocking Antibodies)

The phenomenon of immunologic enhancement was discovered during the course of transplantation experiments. It was anticipated that animals transplanted with grafts of foreign cancer cells, then given injections of antiserum against cancerous cells, would rapidly reject the grafts. However, it was found that not only were the cancer cells tolerated, but rejection was delayed. The antibody produced and then injected was an enhancing or blocking antibody, in contrast to a cytotoxic antibody. These antibodies may have coated the tumor by forming an antigen–antibody complex at the surface membrane. This complex covering the surface would then prevent the killer lymphocytes from attacking the tumor.

Immunoselection

Cancer develops from a clone of cells. Some of these cells mutate and form more antigen than others. The cells then attract more antibodies and are eliminated from the cell population, leaving the cells with weaker antigens as survivors. The colony of cells with weak antigens grows slowly and may sneak through the immunologic defenses of its host. When the host is finally sensitized, it may be too late to mount an effective attack against an already established, fast-growing tumor.

Antigen Modulation

As soon as antibody is formed, cancer cells of certain animal leukemias cease synthesizing antigens. As a result, the immunologic defense becomes ineffective. (This response has not been documented in humans.)

It is a tribute to the minds of scientists that they observed that cancer occasionally regressed after an infection. BCG, an antituberculosis vaccine introduced in 1921, is presently under controlled observation in the field of immunotherapy. The disappearance of cancer after severe infection has been reported for more than 100 years. During the early 1900s Coley noted the disappearance of cancer after a severe streptococcal infection. He therefore began to treat cancer patients with a variety of bacterial toxins; despite a few promising results, however, he reported no consistent therapeutic benefit. Interest in the use of toxins as immunopotentiators waxed and waned until the present time. Clinically, it was repeatedly observed that those patients with empyema following pneumonectomy for lung cancer did better than those who had an uncomplicated postoperative course. In addition, it has been reported that the simultaneous injection of certain bacteria with an antigen increased the immune response to the antigen. Tubercle bacilli were found to be among the most effective bacterial adjuvants for immunostimulation. Complete Freund's adjuvant is a water-in-oil emulsion adjuvant in which killed, dried tubercle bacilli are suspended in the oil phase. This adjuvant is especially effective for stimulating cell-mediated immunity; and in some animals (e.g., the guinea pig), it potentiates production of certain immunoglobulin classes.

Immunotherapy and Immunopotentiation of Cancer

For orientation purposes the immunotherapy of cancer can be outlined as follows.

I. Active immunization against cancer
    A. Active immunization *against oncogenic virus*
    B. Active immunization *against cancer cells*
        1. Autochthonous or autologous cells
        2. Allogeneic cells
        3. Attenuated cells
        4. Soluble tumor antigens
    C. Modification of antigenicity
II. Passive immunization against cancer
    A. Passive immunization
    B. Adoptive immunization
        1. Allogeneic lymphocyte transfer
        2. Transfer factor
        3. Immune RNA
        4. Autologous lymphocyte stimulated in vitro with a mitogen: phytohemagglutinin (PHA)
        5. Bone marrow transplant
        6. Thymosin
III. Nonspecific and miscellaneous immunization
    A. Coley's toxin
    B. BCG (bacille Calmette Guérin)
    C. Vaccinia, pertussis vaccine, poly-IC
    D. MER (methanol extraction residue of BCG)
    E. Maruyama vaccine
    F. *Cornybacterium parvum*

    G. Levamisole
    H. DNCB (dinitrochlorobenzene)
    I. Chalones
    J. Interferon and interferon inducers
    K. Deblocking factor
    L. Neuraminidase, *Vibro cholerae* (VCN)
    M. Concanavalin A (con A)
    N. Viruses
    O. Müllerian inhibiting substance (MIS)

Active Immunization

Active Immunization Against Oncogenic Viruses

In general, immunization implies a method of protection rather than an active form of treatment. Traditionally, an antigen has been given to stimulate an immune response to that antigen. This process is called *active immunity*.

Oncogenic viruses may be antigenic, provoking an immune response against their own capsid antigens and providing a means of preimmunization against the agent itself. The results of animal studies show that immunization with an oncogenic virus provides complete protection against tumor development. If immunization is carried out shortly after infection with the virus, it is still preventive; but when performed after the tumor appears, it is usually ineffective.

Vaccination against Marek's lymphomatosis has provided poultry growers with protection for their fowl against the development of malignancy, despite the fact that the virus is still present and continues to grow. It is interesting that the virus that causes lymphomatosis is a DNA virus related to the Epstein-Barr (EB) virus, which in turn is associated with Burkitt's lymphoma. EB virus is also related to a virus found in association with nasopharyngeal cancer and infectious mononucleosis.

At this time, no virus has been proved to cause human cancer. Work in progress with the enzyme reverse transcriptase may help to discover a viral etiology for cancer. Despite the lack of hard data to support this hypothesis, successful vaccination against Marek's lymphomatosis raised hope that a similar active immunization may one day be achieved for controlling cancer in humans.

Active Immunization Against Cancer Cells

Active specific immunotherapy uses autologous or allogeneic tumor cells as presumptive antigen. Immunization may be in the form of whole tumor cells or subcellular fractions, such as membranes or extracts. A variety of antigenic stimuli have been employed to produce active immunization against cancer cells. This phase of research has lagged behind active immunization against oncogenic viruses.

Autologous or autochthonous (derived from the subject herself) and allogeneic (same species, different genetic pattern) cells have been used in an attempt to arouse active immunization against cancer cells. This type of immunization is based on the assumption that related tumors have common antigens.

Otherwise, the patient's own tumor would be required for use in an attempt at this type of immunization. The use of autologous cells assumes that although the in situ tumor apparently stimulates all of the immunologic response of which the patient is capable the use of autologous cells can provide more stimulation for additional antibody production.

Injection of antigen at a site removed from the tumor may stimulate an immune response through the local lymph nodes. When autologous cancer cells are used, the cell should be killed or inactivated to prevent growth at the site of inoculation. Allogeneic cells carry tumor-associated antigens, as well as strong HL-A antigens, on their surfaces. These antigens are recognized by the host, prompting vigorous immunologic rejection and increasing the immune response.

Crude tumor extracts are not effective because they contain only a small amount of antigen. In addition, some antigen is lost in preparation. Modified tumor cells are more effective than crude tumor extract. Whole, viable cells attenuated with radiation or chemical treatment (mitomycin C, neuraminidase) provide a higher antigen titer. Neuraminidase removes the sialic acid coating from the surface of the cells and makes them more immunogenic when reinoculated. The improved, enhanced immunogenicity may be related to a different form of processing by the immune system, as well as the uncovering of additional antigens on the surface of the cells.

Soluble cell-free antigen may be prepared from cancer cells. The antigen can be extracted as a soluble product, concentrated, and then stored for long periods. The advantage of growing cell cultures is that a large volume of cells can be obtained in an immune-free environment. The best source of immunizing material may ultimately be the surface membrane.

Modification of Antigenicity

Tumor antigens are weak and seldom are able to stimulate a strong immune response. Many attempts have been made to increase the antigenicity of the tumor cell. A variety of means, including coupling with foreign proteins, polysaccharides, or chemicals have been attempted. An effective antigen for immunotherapy may be purified cancer cell surface components coupled to a strong immunogenic substance. Work is in progress to increase antigenicity by using hybrid cells, which consist of normal cells of a different species (strongly antigenic) and cancer cells (presumed to be weakly antigenic). The purpose of this method is to produce a less malignant but more antigenic cancer cell. Preliminary work in animals has been promising but has not advanced beyond preliminary stages.

Passive Immunization

Antiserum directed against malignant disease also contains antibodies against normal cell surface antigens. This problem, combined with the possibility of serum sickness and the difficulty of obtaining a high titer antiserum, makes passive immunization an ineffective approach. It is also the problem of tumor enhancement. This humoral mechanism requires an antigen, antibody, and complement to destroy the cell. The body is unable to mobilize sufficient complement to carry this mechanism to its final goal of cell destruction. There is currently no method for producing complement. Therefore this method of cancer therapy has limited application.

If cancer is vertically transmitted (from parent to offspring), passive immunization is more effective than active immunization. The carcinogenic agent in vertical transmission resists the effect of active immunization because of immunologic tolerance.

In carefully controlled animal studies, injection of a specific antiserum inhibited the development of malignancy if given shortly after the inoculation with oncogenic virus. If given later, it delayed the appearance of the malignancy but did not result in cure.

If the principal reason for failure of the immune response proves to be immunologic tolerance, passive immunization may be one of the primary means chosen to control the malignancy. Unfortunately, the use of antibodies as a method of cancer control is unpredictable.

If the antibodies are cytotoxic and sufficient complement is present, control of the malignancy may be anticipated. However, if the antibodies are enhancing or blocking antibodies, the cancer cells may be tolerated and may even grow more rapidly.

Despite the potential for passive immunization, such a method cannot yet be tried in humans because highly specific antisera, comparable to those used in animals, are not yet available.

Adoptive Immunization

Cell Transfer (Allogeneic Lymphocyte Transfer)

Cell transfer involves the transfer of sensitized lymphoid cells from an actively immunized donor to a cancer patient. In humans this therapy must necessarily be allogeneic and is therefore subject to the homograft (allogeneic) rejection phenomenon. These transferred immunocompetent cells react against the patient's tumor cells.

Strictly defined, adoptive immunization refers to colonization of a recipient by live immunocompetent cells from an immune donor. This definition has now been extended to include transmission of the immune state through cell fractions derived from immune cells, such as immune RNA and transfer factors (TFs). The response is usually predictable and effective. Success is achieved by the development of an immune response directed against the recipient cells when intact live lymphocytes are used. Unless there is close tissue-matching, a graft-versus-host reaction may result.

It does not occur when TF and immune RNA are administered because the recipient is immunodeficient. The donor cells (live lymphocytes) may stimulate an antibody response to the antigens of the recipient, producing a graft-versus-host syndrome characterized by anorexia, diarrhea, wasting, loss of hair, skin rash, leukopenia, anemia, thrombocytopenia, and often death of the recipient. The graft-versus-host response may occur in young animals; and if they do not die, they suffer poor growth, susceptibility to infections, and diarrhea (runt disease).

Subcellular extracts (TF and immune RNA) have been demonstrated to transfer immunity to the recipient without initiating a graft-versus-host response.

When sensitized lymphocytes are cultured in the presence of antigens, at least four mediators of cellular immunity are produced, including TFs. Immune RNA, which has now been isolated, is a "hot" phenol extract of immune lymphoid cells that can transfer specific tumor immunity. Its action is similar to that of TF; their ultimate relation is unknown.

In another approach to adoptive immunotherapy, the patient's lymphocytes are activated in vitro with phytohemagglutinin for 24 to 48 hours. These cells are then reinfused with no ill effects. Studies have shown that pulmonary metastases regressed in most of these patients but that other lesions failed to respond to this therapy.

Adoptive immunotherapy describes the transfer of lymphocytes from a normal or immunized donor to a cancer patient to create activated killer (LAK) cells. In one variation, the lymphocytes removed from a patient are exposed to interleukin-2 in the laboratory and then transferred back into the same patient. The highly publicized interleukin-2 trial conducted by Steven Rosenberg of the National Cancer Institute is an example of this type of adoptive immunotherapy. Bone marrow transplantation also falls into this category because bone marrow contains a variety of mature immune cells and their forerunners.

Generally, the adoptive immunotherapy approach has not been promising and has no specific advantage over conventional therapy alone. However, most of the studies have been done with patients who had heavy tumor burdens that would obviate any form of immunotherapy.

Transfer Factors

Transfer factors comprise a group of low molecular weight antigen-specific factors that can transfer cutaneous delayed hypersensitivity. They are extracted from leukocytes.

Thymosin

Thymosin is under investigation for use in adoptive immunotherapy. It is an extract of calf thymus. The thymic hormone in this extract has been reported to confer immunocompetence on precursor T lymphocytes and to stimulate them to become T lymphocytes. When there is a thymosin deficiency in cancer patients, T-lymphocyte function is defective. In vitro studies have shown that the addition of thymosin to lymphocytes from these patients can restore normal T-lymphocyte-mediated immunity.

Bone Marrow Transplants

Many years ago it was found that if an animal had leukemia and received a transplant of bone marrow identical to its own (syngeneic marrow) the animal would, after irradiation fatal to the cancer, develop cancer again. However, when the marrow is foreign (allogeneic) to the host, the cancer may never recur. An immunologic mechanism is considered the explanation for this phenomenon.

In patients with primary immunodeficiency diseases it is possible to completely reconstitute the immune system by transplanting bone marrow cells from matched donors, a process called *cellular engineering*. Immunologic deficiencies have been quickly corrected in patients with absent or deficient thymus tissue by use of embryonal thymus transplant.

Mechanisms of Action

The approaches being undertaken in immunotherapy are directed toward increasing the resistance of the patient to her tumor, augmenting those components of the immune response that effectively combat the malignancy, and suppressing or eliminating those that interfere with immune resistance. The tumor has the ability to defend itself against host immunity by producing and shedding large amounts of antigen into the circulation. There are several methods for immunotherapy, as outlined above. At present, attention is being directed to the nonspecific methods for stimulating the immune mechanism. Among these methods, BCG has received the greatest amount of attention, and its mechanism of action is briefly reviewed.

The BCG induces a local, sustained, chronic granulomatous, inflammatory response. Lymphocytes, macrophages, and a variety of polymorphonuclear cells are attracted to the site of injection, and an immune response against the BCG organism is initiated. The lymphoid response releases a variety of lymphokines (transfer factor, lymphocyte transforming activity, migration inhibition factor, and lymphotoxin). Macrophages activated into a state of increased phagocytic and metabolic function seem able to kill tumor cells by as yet unknown mechanisms. The tumor cells may be killed as a result of the activated macrophages or by the local release of cytotoxic materials.

Optimum Requirements for Immunotherapy

1. The tumor must possess proved antigenicity. It must be sufficiently different from the corresponding normal cells of the host to be antigenic and capable of producing an immune response. Such tumors include melano-

ma, sarcoma, neuroblastoma, carcinoma of the breast, Burkitt's lymphoma, leukemia, colonic cancer, ovarian cancer, and others.

2. Identical antigens must be present when allogeneic tumors are used. It has been reported that melanomas, sarcomas, and common epithelial ovarian cancers share common tumor-specific antigens within their own group of tumors. If the tumors are processed, it is important to protect the tumor antigens so they are not altered.

3. Tumor cells must be free of blocking antibodies or antigen–antibody complexes that might inhibit production of an immune response.

4. Viable tumor cells should not be injected. Even though allogeneic cells with a different HL-A antigen may be rejected, the risk of dissemination is always present in the immunodepressed patient.

5. The patient must be immunologically capable of responding to the stimulus provided by immunotherapy. Tests employed include skin tests to common antigens, DNCB, or the responsiveness of lymphoid cells to mitogens. Surgery, irradiation, and chemotherapy may cause immunosuppression. Therefore if immunotherapy is to be employed it should be started before definitive therapy, as outlined above, and discontinued when the immunologic competence diminishes. It can be resumed when the competence increases. Reports indicate that the secondary immune response is more resistant to immunosuppression than is the primary response.

6. Immunotherapy is relatively ineffective in the presence of extensive tumor. It is therefore important to reduce the tumor mass to a minimum by conventional methods before instituting immunotherapy. A test that can indicate the critical volume of tumor before therapy is instituted is essential for selecting patients for this treatment.

7. The tumor itself acts as an immunosuppressant. It is obviously more likely to be effective when a large tumor is present. Therefore removal of tumor bulk by surgery, irradiation, or chemotherapy indirectly represents a method of immunotherapy.

8. A growing tumor puts the immune re-

sponse at a marked disadvantage. Therefore if immunotherapy is to be successful, it must be carried out early on a grand scale.

9. It is important to augment the cellular immunity while suppressing the production of antibodies. One of the theories advanced to explain the effect of chemotherapeutic agents is that they inhibit the action of the blocking antibodies and allow the killer lymphocytes to work. Work with killer (K) cells has caused this statement to be modified. The K cell is a variant of the B cell and is able to attack tumor target cells after they have been exposed to a specific antibody; it does not require the presence of complement.

Methods of Immunotherapy

The well-documented occurrences of spontaneous regressions of human neoplasms has led to widespread interest in host defenses against tumors, particularly the immune defense. The demonstration that cancers do arouse a specific immune response in the organism within which they appear has strengthened the evidence for an immune response to tumors. Tumor-associated antigens that stimulate an antibody response have been demonstrated in a variety of tumors. Attempts have been made to apply this knowledge to the control of tumors by employing immunotherapy. Immunotherapy is still in the embryonic and experimental stage. It is obvious from accumulated data that there are several ways in which it may be administered. Before discussing each type of immunotherapy it is important to point out the importance of the in vitro evaluation of immune responses. Immunotherapy should be monitored in the laboratory. In gynecologic cancer only BCG and *Corynebacterium parvum* have been subjected to extensive and intensive investigation. Therefore only these two agents are discussed as representative of the nonspecific and miscellaneous group.

Nonspecific and Miscellaneous

Coley, during the early part of this century, noted the regression of a malignancy in a patient whose course was complicated by erysipelas. He began to treat patients with various bacterial toxins (produced by streptococci and *Serratia marcescens*). Although there were a few promising results, there was no predictable cure rate among the patients treated with bacterial toxins. Other nonspecific methods of immunotherapy include *Corynebacterium parvum* and *Bordetella pertussis* vaccines, vaccinia, and poly-IC.

Bacille Calmette Guérin

Administration of BCG results in a nonspecific immunologic effect that has been shown to prevent neoplasia in animal tumor systems. It has been used increasingly for therapeutic trials in cancer patients. Nonspecific immunotherapy promotes cell-mediated immunity and antibody production, and it may be effective in partially reversing the immunosuppressive effects of the tumor and the conventional therapy.

The BCG may be administered orally, by scarification, or directly into the tumor (intralesionally). Its mechanism of action is unclear, although it induces a sustained, chronic granulomatous inflammatory response. Lymphocytes, macrophages, and polymorphonuclear leukocytes are attracted to the site of injection, and an immune response is thus initiated.

Cytotoxic factors, which damage not only cancer cells but normal cells as well, are produced. It appears that the sensitized lymphocytes release a nonspecific macrophage-activating factor (MAF) that creates a cytotoxic population of macrophages able to distinguish malignant from normal cells, killing only malignant ones. It increases the microbicidal and cytotoxic capacity of macrophages, which is now known to be partly due to interferon-gamma (IFN-γ).

Sensitized T lymphocytes also release a helper factor that enhances the response of immunocompetent B cells to antigens they otherwise would be unable to recognize. The establishment of a survival rate with the use of BCG must await the protocols to be established by the National Cancer Institute. Among them are draining abscesses, fever, malaise,

hypotension, bacteremia, granulomatous lesions of the liver, and even two fatalities thought to be due to hypersensitivity to the organism. The growth of the neoplasm is rarely accelerated after giving BCG. The complications of BCG immunotherapy can be classified as local or systemic.

Local complications
  Ulceration
  Induration
  Pruritus
  Serous drainage
  Regional lymphadenopathy

Systemic complications
  Fever, chills, malaise
  Nausea, myalgia
  Arthralgia
  Hepatitis
  Progressive mycobacterial infection
  Erythema nodosum
  Vitiligo
  Uveitis
  Thrombocytopenia
  Anaphylaxis
  Tuberculin shock
  Death

Terry reported that enthusiasm for the study of immunotherapy in patients with melanoma was enhanced by reports that intradermal injections of BCG prolonged survival in this disease. Unfortunately, subsequent randomized studies have not confirmed the observations of the original nonrandomized studies, a situation similar to that regarding treatment of ovarian cancer with BCG.

MER, a methanol extraction residue of BCG, is being tried as an immunopotentiator. It is part of an effort to develop nonliving derivatives of BCG that can be chemically defined and purified. The Maruyama vaccine is a water-soluble extract of human tuberculosis organism. Chemical trials are under way to evaluate its usefulness.

Cornybacterium parvum

Immunologic interest in the gram-positive anaerobe *Cornybacterium parvum* was stimulated after the demonstration of its remarkable stimulatory effect of the reticuloendothelial system when administered as a killed vaccine. There are several strains of *Cornybacterium* reported in the literature, but only two have been explored in current tumor work: *C. parvum* and *C. granulosum*. These strains have similar reticuloendothelial systems. The result is the emergence of a large number of highly activated macrophages. Macrophages activated by *C. parvum* show augmented phagocytic capability and increased lysosomal enzyme activity.

Corynebacterium parvum boosts the antibody response to a variety of antigens. Both IgM and IgG antibody levels are augmented, and relative binding affinities are enhanced. *C. parvum* can boost antibody levels to T cell-independent antigens as well as to T cell-dependent antigens. Evidence indicates that it is the activated macrophage that provides the added proliferative stimulus to the antigen-sensitive and ultimately antibody-producing B lymphocyte. In addition, the macrophages activated by *C. parvum* encourage chronic retention of lymphocytes within lymphoid organs. Because *C. parvum*-stimulated splenic macrophages may result in T-cell depression, the strategic local injection of *C. parvum* is important so the macrophages from the lymph nodes can carry out their antitumor effect. The macrophages from the stimulated spleen and lymph node cells have different responses. A pertinent finding relative to the delayed-type hypersensitivity following *C. parvum* therapy is that it must precede antigen sensitization to produce this effect. Because treatment of established tumors means that sensitization with tumor antigens must in large part precede *C. parvum*, the usual depression of cell-mediated immunity is circumvented.

Although it is not the intent of this section to be comprehensive, some other factors reported by *C. parvum* are listed: protection against viral infection and graft-versus-host disease, induction of autoimmunity evidenced by hemolytic anemia, fetal resorption, and an increased sensitivity to endotoxin and histamine.

Corynebacterium parvum has been reported to have its greatest effect when there is a reduced amount of tumor volume. It is more effective if the patient is immunocompetent and can respond to therapy. Intravenous *C. parvum* probably localizes in the lungs and liver and may prove to be highly effective against tumors or metastases in these organs, resulting in systemic immunity. It has been observed that there is at least a temporary drop in cell-mediated immunity following systemic (intravenous) injection of *C. parvum*.

Subcutaneous or intradermal injection of *C. parvum* is not toxic and may be highly effective if used strategically. It should be noted that too high a dose of *C. parvum* may overstimulate draining lymph nodes and impair their efficiency.

The most widely studied nonspecific stimulant in cancer therapy has been BCG. It is now apparent that BCG and *C. parvum* may be similar with respect to their modes of antitumor activity. Macrophages activated by either vaccine demonstrate nonspecific antitumor activity in vitro; in addition, the in vivo antitumor effects of each apparently result in part from the fallout from an immune response to the organisms themselves. It should be emphasized that augmentation of specific antitumor responses is common to the ways in which their antitumor activities are effected. *C. parvum* is fully effective when administered in the form of killed vaccine, whereas killed BCG is apparently ineffective. Hence BCG is difficult to control as far as the loss of viability during storage or transportation is concerned, whereas it is not a problem with *C. parvum*.

Considerable data are accumulating on the antitumor activities of various fractions of BCG (MER), which may be as effective as viable organisms. It is anticipated that material fractionated from *C. parvum* will become available, and time will determine if there is a relation between the nature and activity of *C. parvum* and BCG antitumor fractions. It has been shown that degrees of stimulation induced by both *C. parvum* and BCG are different in inbred strains of mice. It is also suggested that genetic constitution may be another intrinsic source of variability when using these agents.

Although immunotherapy offers an exciting approach to the control and treatment of cancer, it has not provided additional help to the conventional methods of treating cancer of the ovary. Currently, there is no method for monitoring the volume of cancer or the effect of treatment, which makes it difficult to know how much treatment should be given. In addition, the treatment is nonspecific, and the results are not predictable.

Müllerian Inhibiting Substance

A potentially specific biologic treatment for ovarian cancer is in progress. Donahue et al. carried out the initial experiments on müllerian inhibiting substance. They were based on the fact that epithelial ovarian cancers are related to tissues derived from the müllerian duct. Development of the genital duct system and external genitalia occurs under the influence of hormones circulating in the fetus during intrauterine life. The Sertoli cells in the fetal testis produce a nonsteroidal substance known as müllerian inhibiting substance, which causes regression of the müllerian duct system. Donahue et al. have demonstrated that the müllerian inhibiting substance is cytotoxic to a human serous cystadenocarcinoma cell line in vitro and inhibits the growth of the cell line in nude mice as well. Clinical trials of müllerian inhibiting substance await the development of new technology to prepare sufficient quantifies of this complex glycoprotein. Arlen Fuller at the Massachusetts General Hospital is carrying out this research.

Summary

Cancer-specific antigens were first identified in a little-quoted 1943 study by Gross. He described the failure of mice to accept transplants of a specific cancer after they had been immunized with material from the same cancer growing on pedigreed mice. Gross immunized mice by intradermal inoculation of tumor cells. These animals rejected a subcutaneous transplant of the same tumor, whereas nonimmunized animals did not. Unfortunately, Gross performed his experiments on a small number of animals. His report may have been ignored at that time because there was no scientific mind prepared to recognize its contribution and potential.

The rebirth of tumor immunology as an active field of research may be said to have occurred in 1957 when Prehn and Main observed that mice immunized against syngeneic methylcholanthrene-induced fibrosarcomas by inoculation of living sarcoma tissue followed by surgical removal of the growing tumor were resistant to subsequent grafts of the same tumor. In addition, immunization with normal tissue did not confer resistance to the tumor grafts. The mice that had become resistant to the tumor still accepted skin grafts from the primary host of these tumors. Different methylcholanthrene-induced sarcomas were found to have individually distinct antigens; mice that were immune to one tumor still accepted grafts of other tumors. Because the tumor-specific antigens were detected by transplantation techniques, they were referred to as tumor-specific transplantation antigens (TSTAs). The tumor antigens are now referred to as tumor-associated antigens (TAAs), as they are generally found in more than one tumor and occasionally even in normal tissue. Tumor-specific antigen is reserved for those situations in which the antigen has been identified with only one tumor.

The TSTAs have been demonstrated not only in chemically induced tumors but also in tumors induced by viruses. The latter were first demonstrated in mice that had been infected as adults with polyomavirus and so became resistant to transplants of tumors induced by that virus, presumably because the infection induced polyomavirus TSTAs in some of the infected cells. Immunization with polyomavirus tumor clones, which contained the polyomavirus tumor antigen but did not release infectious virus, also induced transplantation immunity. Although the polyomavirus TSTA was found to be shared by all tumors induced by the polyomavirus (in contrast to the TSTAs of chemically induced tumors, which are distinct for each individual tumor), it did not cross-react with the TSTAs of tumors induced by other viruses. As a rule, TSTAs of virus-induced tumors are the same for all tumors induced by the same virus but different in tumors induced by different viruses. This finding is true regardless of whether the oncogenic virus is of DNA or RNA type.

The well-documented occurrence of spontaneous regressions of human neoplasms has led to widespread interest in host defenses against tumors, particularly the immune defenses. The demonstration that cancers do arouse a specific immune response in the organism within which they appear has strengthened the evidence for an immune response to tumors. It has been demonstrated in a variety of tumors that they possess tumor-associated antigens that stimulate an antibody response. Attempts have been made to apply this knowledge to the control of tumors employing immunotherapy. Immunotherapy is still in an embryonic and experimental stage. It is obvious from accumulated data that there are different ways in which immunotherapy may be developed or given.

In general, immunization implies a method of protection, rather than an active form of treatment. Traditionally, an antigen has been given to stimulate an immune response to that antigen (*active immunity*). The administration of an antibody provides *passive immunity*. In work carried out in animals, immunization with an oncogenic virus provides complete protection against the later development of a tumor.

The long hoped for and ultimate goal of tumor immunology is effective immunization of cancer patients against their own tumor. The approaches being taken in immunotherapy are directed toward increasing the resistance of patients to their tumor, augmenting those components of the immune response that effectively combat the malignancy and suppressing or eliminating those that interfere with immune resistance. Attention is also being given to the possibility that the tumor may defend itself against host immunity by producing and shedding large amounts of antigen into the circulation.

It is important to evaluate the immunocompetence of the host when considering immunotherapy. In addition, one must select a form of immunotherapy based on clinical factors, including other modalities of therapy to be employed. Furthermore, immunotherapy has a practical role only when the amount of residual or remaining tumor cells is extremely small. In animal model systems, immunotherapy is most beneficial when fewer than 10^5 residual cells remain after surgery.

The following guidelines have been established for the clinical and practical application of immunotherapy based on human and animal studies.

1. A tumor should be entirely removed or debulked so the residual volume of cancer is small.
2. A method to judge the return of immunocompetence after surgery or irradiation will provide a timetable to help when administering the immunotherapy at the optimum time. The immunotherapy then provides even more resistance to disease.
3. The immunotherapy should be administered in areas where the lymphatic drainage is thought to be free of tumor. This method minimizes the chance of acquired tolerance and immunologic enhancement.
4. An attempt should be made to stimulate cell-mediated immunity without producing antibodies. T lymphocytes have the potential to act as killer lymphocytes, and the antibodies may be blocking or enhancing antibodies.
5. A method for monitoring the volume of cancer is necessary.
6. Methodology for monitoring both cell-mediated and humoral immunity, as well as blocking activity, should be available and utilized to ensure that the benefit outweighs any harm that may follow immunotherapy.

The application of immunotherapy is presently undergoing constant change. Advances are being made almost daily, although it is still considered experimental. With a few notable exceptions, a general comment can be made about all forms of immunotherapy for all types of cancer: No noteworthy benefit has been obtained, which does not mean that immunotherapy is an approach to cancer treatment whose time has passed. It merely reflects the fact that more work must be done to understand the cancer cell and antigens before immunotherapy can be employed as a predictable means of controlling the neoplastic cell. Additional progress could be made in this field if a test were devised that permitted evaluation of the tumor volume. It is evident that some progress has been made with immunopro-phylaxis, but use of immunotherapy in the presence of a large volume of tumor has not been successful.

Use of the cancer patient's immune system to control the growth of malignant cells is pre-dicated on the assumption that the surfaces of malignant cells contain antigens that are not present on normal cells. Although antigens have not been identified in pure form, when they are they must have certain properties to be effective for managing of the patient with cancer. These properties include the following: (1) They must be present when the cancer be-comes clinically apparent. (2) They must be recognizable by the immune system of the pa-tient with the cancer or by that of a representa-tive of some other species. (3) They must be capable of stimulating an effector, humoral, or cellular immune response. (4) They must be able to damage tumor cells. Currently, no such antigens with these characteristics have been identified on any cancer cell in humans.

Methods applied in the past, as well as those now under trial, may abe classified as active, adoptive, and nonspecific immunotherapy.

The body's inherent biochemical capacity for killing cancer cells may be combined with the new genetic technology. When they are put together, the result is biological response mod-ification (biomodulation). This subject has been covered in Chapter 27.

Bibliography

Alexander P: Immunotherapy of cancer: experi-ments with primary tumors and syngeneic tumor grafts. *Prog Exp Tumor Res* 10:23, 1968.

Anderson JM: *Immunotherapy of Cancer. Clinical Oncology.* Williams & Wilkins, Baltimore, 1972, p. 193.

Baldwin RW, Robins RA: Immune complexes in cancer. *Cancer Immunol Immunother* 4:1, 1978.

Barber HRK: Present status of tumor immunology in clinical gynecology. *Am J Reprod Immunol* 20:140, 1989.

Barber HRK, Dorsett BH: The immune system in gynecologic malignancies. *Mt Sinai J Med (NY)* 47:539, 1980.

Barber HRK, Ioachim HL, Dorsett BM: Common antigenic component in ovarian cancer. In deWat-teville HD (ed): *Diagnosis and Treatment of Ova-*

rian Neoplastic Alterations. Elsevier, Amsterdam, 1975, p. 107.

Bast RC Jr, Zbar B, Borson T, Rapp HL: BCG and cancer. *N Engl J Med* 290:1413, 1974.

Biggs PM, Churchill AE, Rootes DG, Chubb RC: The etiology of Marek's disease in oncogenic herpes-type virus. In Pollard M (ed): *Perspectives of Virology.* Academic Press, Orlando, Fl, 1968, p. 211.

Coley WB: The treatment of malignant tumors by repeated inoculations of erysipelas with a report of original cases. *Am J Med Sci* 105:487, 1893.

Coley WB: Late results of treatment of inoperable sarcoma with mixed toxins of erysipelas and bacil-lus prodigeons. *Trans Am Surg Ann* 19:27, 1901.

Cunningham TJ, Olson KB, Laffin R, et al: Treat-ment of advanced cancer with active immuniza-tion. *Cancer* 24:932, 1969.

Currie GA: Eight years of immunotherapy: a review of immunological methods used for the treatment of human cancer. *Br J Cancer* 26:141, 1972.

Currie GA, Bagshave KD: Active immunotherapy with *Cornybacterium parvum* and chemotherapy in murine fibrosarcoma. *Br Med J* 1:541, 1970.

Donahue PK, Swann DA, Hayashi A, Sullivan MD: Mullerian duct regression in the embryo corre-lated with cytotoxic activity against human ova-rian cancer. *Science* 205:913, 1979.

Ehrlich P: On immunity with special reference to cell life. *Proc R Soc Lond [Biol]* 66:424, 1906.

Foley EJ: Antigenic properties of methyl cholan-threne induced tumors in mice of the strain of ori-gin. *Cancer Res* 13:835, 1953.

Gross L: Intradermal immunization of C3H mice against a sarcoma that originated in an animal of the same line. *Cancer Res* 3:326, 1943.

Haddsen JW: Levamisole: a synthetic immuno-potentiator under evaluation. *Memorial Sloan-Kettering Cancer Center Clin Bull* 5:32, 1975.

Hellström KE, Hellström I: Immunological de-fenses against cancer. *Hosp Pract* 3:45, 1970.

Hollinshead A: *Active Specific Immunotherapy. Immunotherapy of Human Cancer.* Raven Press, New York, 1978.

Hollinshead A, Stewart T: Specific active im-munotherapy and specific active immunoprophy-laxis in lung cancer. Basis for cancer therapy 2. Reprinted from Moore M (ed): *Advances in Medical Oncology Research and Education.* Per-gamon Press, Oxford, 1979.

Hudson CN: Immunologic aspects of gynecological malignancy. *Br J Obstet Gynaecol* 86:154, 1979.

Hudson CN: Immunology and immunotherapy of ovarian cancer: ovarian cancer. *Adv Biosci* 26:1980.

Humphrey LJ, Jewell WR, Murray DR, et al: Immunotherapy for patients with cancer. *Ann Surg* 173:47, 1971.

Hunter-Craig I, Newton KA, Westburg G, et al: Use of vaccine virus in the treatment of metastatic malignant melanoma. *Br Med J* 2:512, 1970.

Isaacs A, Lindemann J: Virus interference: the interferon. *Proc R Soc Lond [Biol]* 147:258, 1957.

Israel L, Halpern B: Le *Cornybacterium parvum* dans les cancers avancés: première évaluation de pactirité therapeutique de cette immunostimuline. *Nouv Presse Med* 1:19, 1972.

Kersey JH, Spector BD, Good RA: Immunodeficiency and cancer. *Adv Cancer. Res* 18:211, 1973.

Klein E: Hypersensitivity reactions at tumor sites. *Cancer Res* 29:2351, 1969.

Knauf S, Auerbach GH: Purification of ovarian tumor associated antigen—in patients with advanced ovarian malignancy. *Am J Obstet Gynecol* 127:705, 1977.

Lawrence HS: Transfer factor. *Adv Immunol* 11:195, 1969.

Levi MM: Antigenicity of ovarian and cervical malignancy with a view towards possible immunodiagnosis. *Am J Obstet Gynecol* 109:687, 1971.

Levin L, McHardy JE, Kurling OM, et al: Tumor antigenicity in ovarian cancer. *Br J Cancer* 32:152, 1975.

Levis WR, Kraemer KH, Klinger WG, et al: Topical immunotherapy of basal cell carcinoma with dinitrochlorobenzene. *Cancer Res* 33:3036, 1973.

Male D: *Immunology—An Illustrated Outline.* Mosby, St. Louis, 1986.

Mandell GL, Fisher RI, Bostick F, Young RC: Ovarian cancer: a solid tumor with evidence of normal cellular immune function but abnormal "B" cell function. *Am J Med* 66:621, 1979.

Marligit G, Gutterman JN, Burgess MA, et al: Immunotherapy. Its possible application in the management of large bowel cancer. *Dig Dis* 19:1047, 1974.

Mathé G: Active immunotherapy for acute lymphoblastic leukemia. *Lancet* 1:697, 1969.

Mathé G, Weiner RS: *Investigation and Stimulation of Immunity in Cancer Patients.* Springer-Verlag, New York, 1974.

McKhann CF, Gunnarsson A: Approaches to immunotherapy. *Cancer* 34:1521, 1974.

Merigan TC, Regelson W: Interferon induction in man by a synthetic polyanion of defined composition. *N Engl J Med* 277:1283, 1967.

Miller JFAP, Basten A, Sprent J, Cheers C: Interaction between lymphocytes in immune response. *Cell Immunol* 2:469, 1971.

Mitchell MS, Kohorn EI: Cell mediated immunity and blocking factor in ovarian cancer. *Obstet Gynecol* 48:590, 1976.

Morton DL: BCG immunotherapy of malignant melanoma: summary of seven years experience. *Ann Surg* 180:635, 1974.

Nauts HC, Swift WZ, Coley BL: The treatment of tumor by bacterial toxins as developed by the late William B. Coley, M.D., reviewed in the light of modern research. *Cancer Res* 6:2303, 1946.

Oettgen HF, Old LJ, Farrow J, et al: Effects of transfer factor in cancer patients. *J Clin Invest* 50:71a, 1971.

Ohazaka W, Purchase HG, Burmaster BR: Protection against Marek's disease by vaccination with a herpes virus of turkeys. *Avian Dis* 14:413, 1970.

Order SE, Donahue V, Knapp R: Immunotherapy of ovarian carcinoma: an experimental model. *Cancer* 32:573, 1973.

Order SE, Kirkman R, Knapp R: Serologic immunotherapy: results and probable mechanism of action. *Cancer* 34:175, 1974.

Paluch E, Ioachim H: Lung carcinoma—reactive antibodies isolated from tumor tissues and pearl effusions of lung cancer patients. *J Natl Cancer Inst* 61:319, 1978.

Patillo RA, Storey MT, Rukert ACT: Expression of cell mediated immunity and blocking factor using a new line of ovarian cancer cells "in vitro." *Cancer Res.* 39:1185, 1979.

Pilch YH, Ramming KP: Transfer of tumor immunity with ribonucleic acid. *Cancer* 26:630, 1970.

Pilch YH, Ramming KP, Deckers PJ: Induction of anti-cancer immunity with RNA. *Ann NY Acad Sci* 207:409, 1973.

Plaque RE, Dray S: Monkey to human transfer for delayed hypersensitivity in vitro with RNA extracts. *Cell Immunol* 5:30, 1972.

Poulton T, Crowther ME, Hay FC: Immune complexes in ovarian cancer. *Lancet* 2:72, 1978.

Prehn RT, Main JM: Immunity to methycholanthrene-induced sarcomas. *J Natl Cancer Inst* 18:769, 1957.

Rigby PG: Prolongation of survival of tumor bearing animals by transfer of "immune" RNA with DEAE dextran. *Nature* 221:968, 1969.

Rosenberg B: Possible mechanisms for the antitumor activity of platinum coordination complexes. *Cancer Chemother Rep* 59:589, 1975.

Rosenberg B, Van Camp L, Trosko JE: Platinum compound: a new class of potent antitumor agents. *Nature* 22:385, 1969.

Ruckdeschel JC, Codish SD, Stranahan A, McKneally MF: Postoperative empyema improves survival in lung cancer: documentation and analysis of a natural experiment. *N Engl J Med* 287:1013, 1972.

Scott MT: *Corynebacterium parvum* as an immunotherapeutic anti-cancer agent. *Semin Oncol* 1:367, 1974.

Simmons RL: Immunospecific regression of methycholanthrene fibrosarcoma with the use of neuraminidase. *Surgery* 70:38, 1971.

Simmons RL, Rios A: Comparative and combined effect of BCG and neuraminidase in experimental immunotherapy. *Natl Cancer Inst Monogr* 39:57, 1973.

Simmons RL, Rios A, Ray PK, Lundgren G: Effect of neuraminidase on the growth of methylcholanthrene fibrosarcoma in normal and immunosuppressed syngeneic mice. *J Natl Cancer Inst* 47: 1087, 1971.

Sjögren HO, Hellstrom I, Bansal SC, Hellstrom KE: Suggestive evidence that "blocking antibodies" of tumor bearing individuals may be antigen-antibody complexes. *Proc Natl Acad Sci USA.* 68:1372, 1971.

Sokal JE, Aungst CW, Synderman, M.: Delay in

progression of malignant lymphoma after BCG vaccination. *N Engl J Med* 291:1226, 1974.

Sparks FC: Complications of BCG immunotherapy in patients with cancer. *N Engl J Med* 289:827, 1973.

Sparks FC, O'Connell TX, Lee Y-TN, et al: BCG therapy given as an adjuvant to surgery: prevention of death from metastases from mammary adenocarcinoma in rats. *J Natl Cancer Inst* 53:1825, 1971.

Stjeruswald J, Levin A: Delayed hypersensitivity: induced regression of human neoplasms. *Cancer* 28:628, 1971.

Terry WD: Immunotherapy of malignant melanoma. *N Engl J Med* 303:1174, 1980.

Thor DE, Dray S: Transfer of cell-mediated immunity by immune RNA assessed by migration inhibition. *Ann NY Acad Sci* 207:355, 1973.

Webb HE, Smith GCE: Viruses in the treatment of cancer. *Lancet* 1:1206, 1970.

Zbar B, Rapp HJ: Immunotherapy of guinea pig cancer with BCG. *Cancer* 34 (suppl):1532, 1974.

29

Directions in the Design of Clinical Trials, Present and Future

There are four chief avenues of advance toward the conquest of cancer: (1) cancer prevention—by eliminating from the external and internal environment chemical and other agents that cause or promote cancer; (2) earlier cancer detection—through improved methods, whose application allows earlier curative therapy; (3) more effective application of present treatment methods—by making more widely available the best present techniques of surgery, irradiation, and chemotherapy; and (4) development of new methods of cancer treatment and prevention—through research. It is becoming increasingly evident that major gains in the effort to eradicate cancer will come from developments achieved through research.

Clinical Investigation

Clinical investigation of cancer is essentially the culmination of the basic and preclinical studies in cancer research and the development from these studies of techniques useful for preventing, diagnosing, and treating cancer in humans. Clinical investigation can include such diverse investigations as the biochemical studies of purine metabolism in patients with leukemia; assays of enzyme differences between normal and neoplastic human cells; studies of cell kinetics in leukemia and solid tumors; the clinical pharmacology, absorption, excretion, and therapeutic effectiveness of new agents against cancer; clinical trials of radiation sensitizers; the use of im-

munologic methods for detecting or treating human cancer; and immunologic studies of organ transplants. Clinical investigations contributing directly to improvement in the main treatment modalities (surgery, radiation therapy, chemotherapy, and immunotherapy) must be restructured and pursued to achieve the goals of the directions and the designs of clinical trials, present and future.

The design of a clinical study is critical if reliable information is to be obtained. The homogeneity of the patient group in which the value of a certain treatment modality is to be assessed is of the utmost importance. In a heterogeneous group the possible advantage of a treatment form for a certain subgroup can be obscured owing to an insufficient or negative effect on the rest of the treated patients. Therefore it is important to have an accurate evaluation of all the factors that can affect the prognosis in ovarian cancer.

There are certain parameters that can readily be measured when evaluating the impact of therapy. Among the most important goals in ovarian cancer clinical trials is to answer the following: (1) What proportion of patients have been cured? (endpoint: cure). (2) What degree of palliation has been afforded those who died? (endpoints: duration and quality of life). (3) What work has been done to achieve any benefit? (endpoint: effective treatment, any complications).

By "cure" is meant that the life expectancy of the treated cancer patient is the same as "normal" life expectancy, specifically, the same as that of a matched cohort in the general population. It is more difficult to define palliation. Palliation includes both an objective and a subjective response. It usually means that the quality of life during and after treatment is infinitely better than it was prior to the treatment. The median survival time is usually included in this evaluation. In general, for ovarian cancer it usually means that there has been disease regression and improvement in the patient's physical and mental well-being; this state must remain usually for an arbitrary time, often designated to be 3 months.

Important developments have again stimulated interest in ovarian cancer, namely, new insights in the natural history of the disease, the discovery of more effective chemotherapeutic agents, and methods of individualizing radiation therapy with or without radiation sensitizers.

Evaluation of Patient Groups

It is important to keep the variables as even in each group as possible. The homogeneity of the patient group in which the value of a certain treatment modality is to be assessed is of utmost importance. Among these factors are the extent of disease and the histologic type of these tumors, the degree of differentiation, and the surgery that is carried out.

It is important to have an accurate clinical staging of the extent of the ovarian cancer. All too often these patients are understaged and therefore undertreated. The concept that peritoneal implantations progressively move from the pelvis to the upper abdomen and that a negative exploration of the peritoneal surfaces in the pelvis indicates a disease-free state in the entire peritoneal cavity are now known to be erroneous.

Meyers has shown that radioactive material injected into the pelvic cavity of humans ascends into the upper abdomen. The ascent of the fluid in the left pericolic gutter is blocked by the left phrenicolic ligament. Virtually all the flow is to the right subhepatic and subphrenic spaces, which may result in early tumor implantations in the upper abdomen and the di-

aphragmatic surfaces and involve the lymphatics of the diaphragm.

It is evident that invasion of the retroperitoneal nodes is not rare. The significance of ascitic fluid is constantly being reevaluated. The thinking has shifted from the concept that ascites results from irritation either by the mass of tissue itself or the peritoneal implants to a more sophisticated concept that lymphatics are blocked and therefore the capacity of reabsorption is decreased. This concept raises an interesting point about stage Ic: If ascites is due to the blockage of lymphatic capillaries in the diaphragm, the patient would rightfully belong in stage III. Time and additional work will determine if these patients should be treated as stage III patients.

The histologic types of tumor and the degree of differentiation have been covered in another chapter. It is accepted that the more differentiated the tumor, the better the prognosis. It is important to identify the low potential malignancy (borderline) tumors and to exclude them from studies on the treatment of ovarian cancer.

Although the common epithelial ovarian cancer does not lend itself well to surgical treatment, surgery remains the backbone of therapy. The most important factor in prognosis seems to be the bulk of disease left behind after surgery, particularly for patients with stage IIb and III lesions. It is important to know the extent and location of any residual carcinoma. Obviously, it is easier to treat localized disease in the pelvis or the paraaortic nodes than it is to treat peritoneal implants scattered throughout the upper abdomen.

Methods of Treatment

Surgery, radiation therapy, and chemotherapy are the modalities most often used. Immunotherapy is under active investigation, but at this time it contributes little to the management of patients with ovarian cancer.

Surgery

The goal of surgery is to excise all of the ovarian cancer; and if it is not possible, maximal debulking is attempted. Unless all or most of the disease is removed, there is little chance for cure or a prolonged tumor-free interval.

Radiation Therapy

It is accepted that external radiation therapy has limited application for the management of common epithelial ovarian cancer. Its application is limited by the volume and site of the residual tumor after surgery. There has been a revival of interest in radiation therapy for the treatment of common epithelial ovarian cancer. Clinicians from the Princess Margaret Hospital in Toronto have reported that they consider irradiation to be the postoperative treatment of choice for patients with poorly differentiated stage I and all those with stage II and III who have no gross residual disease or only a small amount of pelvic residual disease. When the disease is more extensive, they have obtained few cures with radiation therapy and prefer to use chemotherapy as the initial approach.

Chemotherapy

The questions to be asked regarding chemotherapy and possible trials are of a totally different nature from those for radiation therapy. In chemotherapy trials the target area is of less importance than it is for radiation therapy trials. However, the tumor mass is important for both modalities.

As cancer chemotherapy has developed, clinical trials of anticancer drugs have become more complex. Initial drug trials were relatively simple clinical experiments in which the endpoint was some evidence of anticancer activity with a reasonable level of toxicity. As more chemicals with anticancer activity were found, it became necessary to develop a clinical trial strategy for testing them; and a modification of the classic three phases of clinical trial utilized by the pharmaceutical industry for other areas of drug development became established.

For protocol design, a clinical trial can be defined as a carefully and ethically designed experiment with the aim of answering some precisely framed questions. Excellent guidelines for protocol writing had been presented by Gehan and Schneiderman. Clinical trials are divided into three phases: phase I, which is a therapeutic intent trial and tests acceptability of the drug; phase II, which is directed to screening for antitumor activity and has the imperfections of any screening system; and phase III, in which the drug is given to a large number of patients to determine if the activity seen in phase II can be confirmed, if unexpected events such as new types of activity or adverse effects occur, and if the drug has any value in relation to other potential treatments.

Cancer has been seen in humans since antiquity. It has been identified in fossil bones and recently in mummies. Tumors are currently identified according to their appearance, behavior, and location. A growing body of evidence indicates that although they look alike they may not act alike. Within any group of tumors and indeed any stage of a given cancer, there are different degrees of malignancy. These differences must be understood if advances are to be made in the field of anticancer drug therapy.

Tumors were finally identified and described according to their microscopic appearance. It became evident that cancer cells arise from normal cells, and that there are at least as many cancers as there are normal cells types. Currently, more than 100 human malignancies have been identified. Carcinogenesis is the change from a new cell to one endowed with new growth (neoplastic) properties. The neoplastic cell transmits to its descendants components of the neoplastic cell as well as those of the original cell. Their function is often at a more primitive level than that of the normal cell. The cancer cell grows in an uninhibited manner; and, unlike the normal cell, its growth is not controlled, resulting in a nodule of neoplastic cells and finally a tumor. The only control on the growth of a cancer is the death of its host. It does not respond to normal growth controls and is not influenced by contact inhibition; moreover, although its growth is inefficient, the cancer cell divides continuously. It possesses the characteristic properties of invasion and the ability to metastasize. Cartilage and dense fibrous tissues obstruct the easy spread of cancer, but bone is readily invaded. At the edge of most tumors there is a collection of lymphoid cells, representing an attempt at defense.

Cancer research has directed a great deal of energy, resources, and money toward finding specific and constant chemical, biologic, and immunologic differences between normal and cancer cells. It is important to identify the differences in the development and maintenance of the properties of cancer cells and, by understanding these differences, to control the cancer cell. It is hoped that the future reveals these differences and thus permits selective destruction of cancer cells by the use of chemicals.

The long-term future belongs to the immunologist and geneticist, and the intermediate future to the researchers; but the present and immediate future belongs to the surgeon and chemotherapist. To the extent that chemotherapy is developed first, surgery will be needed less; but in most fields in which early detection is developed first, it will be largely surgery that converts these gains and information into cured patients by extirpation of the cancer before it has spread. Currently, progress in making an early diagnosis of malignancy is limited because of the various epidemiologic factors and the question of whether ovarian cancer represents a metastatic disease or multiple primaries within the peritoneal cavity.

Surgery and irradiation are effective only for localized disease. Chemotherapy (drugs and hormones) can be used effectively for disseminated, as well as localized, cancer. Chemotherapy has become a reality only since the 1960s. It has been employed generally for palliation but has also proved its value as a primary therapeutic modality. Its prophylactic role after surgical removal or eradication of the cancer by radiation therapy has only recently been explored. A major goal of current chemotherapy is to achieve cures by prompt, vigorous treatment of cancer without producing inordinate morbidity and some mortality.

Combinations of chemotherapeutic agents have been used with considerable success, particularly when each of the drugs used acts on the cancer cells in a different way. Improved knowledge of cell kinetics or cell divisions, as well as of the life cycle of the cancer cell, has provided the basis for a more rational approach to the use of anticancer drugs. Major improvements in treating certain types of cancer have been achieved by using several anticancer drugs simultaneously and by using different drugs in sequence.

Cell Biology

Cell biology is complex and involves all of the metabolic, enzymatic, and hormone synthesis necessary for the cell to remain viable. The cells of the body have both internal and external functions. The individual functions in mature cells or parenchymatous tissues are concerned with the maintenance of metabolic cycles for energy and for the specialized synthesizing functions characteristic of differentiated tissues. These functions include the synthesis and maintenance of hemoglobin for gas transport; the synthesis of secretory products, such as insulin, mucin, casein, and steroids; and the synthesis of constructive products, such as cilia, keratin, and osteoid. The biochemical basis for these activities is the translation of genetic material contained in DNA to the specific RNA and proteins concerned in such specialized differentiated functions.

Certain tissues, such as the intestinal tract, skin, and bone marrow, require replacement of a large number of mature dying cells. There must be an internal function geared to rapid cell replication. It involves the cycle of DNA replication known as mitosis in mammalian cells. Because the neoplastic process involves replication of unwanted cells, much chemotherapy is directed toward inhibiting the mitotic cycle of such cells, especially the steps by which new DNA molecules are produced.

The external function of tissue growth relative to the cancer problem concerns the process by which cell, tissue, and organ growth is restricted after a critical volume is reached and stimulated to resume after death or removal of part of an organ. Knowledge of how to measure this parameter is vital to the judicious use of immunotherapy. Cell growth is limited and organ size controlled by a combination of local factors, such as contact inhibition (allogeneic inhibition) in which normal cells become inhibited in replication and migration by contact with other normal cells, and distant factors, such as humoral feedback mechanisms and controls. The latter is believed to result in the release of growth-inhibiting substances, "chalones," from normal tissue. The accidental death of tissue cells by injury results in changes in this homeostatic mechanism, with the result that certain clonogenic cells, which have retained the capacity to divide, begin to do so in order to regenerate the lost normal tissue.

Cancer is a disease of the cell. An understanding of the life cycle of a cell and, in this instance the cancer cell, is important when planning therapy for a given malignancy. Cellular reproduction occurs via a series of chemical steps known as the cell cycle (the cell cycle is measured from mitosis to mitosis). An understanding of the order of steps has allowed identification of the phase of cellular activity during which a specific anticancer drug acts. It is now evident that a drug for cancer must be defined not only by its chemical composition but also by its specific dosage, specific route, and schedule of administration, each of which significantly modifies its activity.

Cell Kinetics

A study of tumor cell kinetics confirms that only some of the tumor cells are in an active growth cycle at any one time, and the synthesis of critical cellular constituents is known to occur during specific phases of that cycle. It is important and necessary to explore and understand the selective toxicity of anticancer drugs during different phases of the cell cycle. This step is essential to a deeper understanding of a rational approach to chemotherapy. It is also important to elucidate the natural rate of the death of cells within a tumor and to exploit this knowledge of tumor cell death. For carrying out therapeutic options it is essential to know the fraction of cells in the tumor that have the ability to reproduce, as well as the selective killing of cancer cells, especially those that are not in the critical phases of synthesis. This

information is vital to understanding the cell kinetics of slow-growing tumors, particularly solid tumors such as ovarian carcinomas.

One important goal is to solve the problem of how to invade selectively the sanctuary of tumor cells. Malignant cells lodged at a distance from the closest capillaries or beyond the blood-brain barrier may enjoy a pharmacologic sanctuary where drug concentrations cannot reach them in concentrations that would have lethal effects. Experimental and clinical research must supply a method for eradicating the last cancer cell, no matter where it lodges or seeks sanctuary.

Anticancer Chemotherapy

Chemotherapy is no longer a modality reserved for palliation alone. It now constitutes a major and indispensable therapeutic approach capable of curing certain kinds of widespread cancer. The cancers that have been cured by drug therapy with a predictable rate are choriocarcinoma, metastatic hydatidiform mole, Burkitt's tumor, acute lymphatic leukemia of children, Hodgkin's disease, embryonal carcinoma of the testis and ovary, extraembryonal carcinoma of the ovary, adenocarcinoma of the uterine corpus, and cancers in the superficial layers of the skin.

Chemotherapy has been therapeutically beneficial in a significant number of cases but has not resulted in predictable cures (e.g., for the cancers listed above). Cancers that have been affected by chemotherapy are chronic myelocytic leukemia, chronic lymphatic leukemia, lymphosarcoma, reticulum cell sarcoma, multiple myeloma, polycythemia vera, mycosis fungoides, malignant melanoma, Wilms' tumor, and neuroblastoma.

There are other types of cancer that have been significantly affected by anticancer drug therapy. Clinical improvements occur, and sometimes the survival time is increased; but predictable long-term survival or long-term freedom from disease has not been observed. The cancers responding in this manner include cancer of the breast, large intestine, stomach, pancreas, prostate, head and neck, thyroid, ovary, and adrenal gland. Some cancers are notably not susceptible to the anticancer drugs used to date. Major clinical benefit has not usually followed treatment of cancer of the lung, cervix, kidney, or bladder.

Anticancer drugs occasionally produce cures in a broad spectrum of cancers. The cancers that can be cured by chemotherapy are not always those that grow most rapidly. Not all of the cancers are from the same primitive embryonic tissue; many organ classes and a variety of histologic types are represented. The chief blocks in the progress of anticancer chemotherapy are the lack of a predictable method for monitoring the volume of cancer and the inability to test in vitro the response of cancer cells to the actions of the anticancer drugs.

Furthermore, curative chemotherapy is not usually a product of a single drug (except for choriocarcinoma) or of a single technique of drug use. Rather, many drugs in a variety of combinations are used. Surgery and irradiation may be included in the therapy. It is obvious that no one drug, whether now in use or to be identified in the future, will serve as an overall cure. The number of combinations and regimens indicates that a drug that fails in the treatment of one kind of cancer may act against another.

There are many factors, not all of which are known, that play a role in the sensitivity of cancer cells to the action of anticancer drugs. It is logical to outline the path that an anticancer drug must take to effectively control a cancer cell (cancer cells divide continuously, though inefficiently). The anticancer drug must reach the surface of the cancer cell, enter the cell through its surface membrane, remain active or undergo activation by the necessary enzymes, reach a critical target site, and combine with it at a time when chemical processes on which the cell depends for its viability or reproduction are in progress. This complex process highlights the importance of a clear understanding of the life cycle of the cell or its kinetics.

Furthermore, competing and bypass pathways in the cell must not be able to compensate for the chemical injury the drug inflicts. It is important to measure the number of mutations in a given volume of tumor cells to predict the development of resistance so valuable time is not lost pursuing a drug regimen that has lost its ability to control the cancer cell. Failure of the whole chain of events can result from failure of any one step. Thus any drug given by the wrong regimen to a mass of cancer cells that are biologically not susceptible to its action at that time is a failure of chemotherapy. Better drug design and better understanding of the biologic characteristics of each cancer type, and indeed of each cancer, as well as a better understanding of the cell cycle will advance the effectiveness of chemotherapy.

The dramatic and persistent change that accompanies the development of cancer has supported the *somatic mutation theory* of carcinogenesis. This theory bolsters the concept that the cancer is caused by a change in the cellular genetic material itself. It is important to know whether cancer is the result of a change in the genetics of the cell or of a change in the nongenetic material (epigenetic). If it affects the genetic material, it is irreversible and can be controlled only by selective destruction, whereas if it affects the epigenetic material it may be reversible and controllable.

Since the 1960s more than 30 compounds have been developed that are useful in the control of cancer. It is obvious that many more drugs are available, and the best are yet to be found. So far, most of the drugs identified with anticancer properties have followed from empiric screening. Most of this work is carried out by drug companies, governmental agencies, and cooperative groups. The National Cancer Institute has a division that reviews and tests drugs from all kinds of sources throughout the world. The preparation and clinical use of these drugs are under the control of the Food and Drug Administration. (FDA). The question should be raised whether this authority, as it relates to cancer, would not better be transferred to the National Cancer Advisory Board.

The use of active drugs for cancer may bring success even before there is a clear understanding of the malignant process. Indeed their use may serve as a probe to explain the intricacies of neoplastic growth. In fact, other medications, often derived from plants, produced predictable therapeutic results against many disease processes before the mechanism of the disease was clearly understood.

After the development or isolation of a new drug, several steps must be carried out under controlled conditions before the drug can be used to treat cancer patients.

1. Antitumor activity must be demonstrated in the same screening system.
2. A broad-scale study in other known biologic screening systems is necessary.
3. After the activity of the drug has been confirmed, two general areas of study follow.
   a. It must be determined what the compound does and how it does it.
   b. The compound must be tested in animals.

Current research efforts that appear to have promise include the stem cell assay, the use of autologous bone marrow, and the testing of alternating non-cross-resistant drug combinations. More work is needed before statements can be made about the relative merits of combination drug therapy for the management of common epithelial ovarian cancer.

Preclinical Testing

Careful preclinical pharmacology and toxicology are necessary to arrive at the optimum dose and route of administration for a new agent. Various rapidly growing systems are used to determine drug activity (e.g., bacteria, viruses, mammalian cells in culture, and transplantable and spontaneous tumors of small rodents). Specific organ toxicity is also determined in larger animals, such as dogs and monkeys. General concepts of duration of action, blood levels achieved, tolerable routes of administration, usual routes of excretion, and possible modes of action are accumulated. At the end of each testing one should know, within 10%, the lethal dose in highly developed animals by single and repeated doses. This figure is often used as a basis for extrapolation to the first human trials; and hence every attempt should be

made to gather high-quality data on the animal species closest to man. Commonly, the first human dosage level is one-fifth to one-tenth the LD_0 in dogs.

Careful preclinical pharmacology and toxicity are necessary, but the time required for these observations should be modified when the observations indicate that a stated time is not necessary for completion of the study. For example, patients with advanced cancer have a finite life expectancy in the absence of effective treatment. One thousand cancer patients die in the United States every day. If a new compound shows appreciable activity against cancer, extensive pharmacologic studies can be made concomitantly with the clinical trials.

Clinical Trials

Study of a new compound in humans requires skill in clinical pharmacology.

Phase I

In general, the primary aim of a phase I trial is to determine clinically the tolerated regimens of a drug that will later be used in trials to determine antitumor action in humans. There should be no expectation that phase I patients will achieve remissions, although observations enabling a drug-induced remission to be recognized should be included as a matter of routine. Unfortunately, during most phase I trials the patients are normally those with far-advanced disease in whom chemotherapy has failed.

Phase I testing consists in toxicity trials of host responses rather than trials in which the antitumor effects of the drug are even roughly assessed. The information that is hopefully collected from phase I trials includes (1) an idea of useful routes of administration; (2) an idea of the doses tolerable during the period of time necessary to observe remission of the tumor types to be studied later, perhaps after 30 to 60 days; and (3) early identification of intolerably toxic drugs and unfeasible routes of administration. Such drugs should be discarded as soon as possible. No drug should complete phase I trial if it has not been tacitly committed to be carried through phase II.

The time required to deliver a drug from its conception of first recognition in a testing system to clinical usefulness depends on the biologic factors and ability to produce the drug. A minimum of 2 to 3 years may be required; and in some instances it takes a decade to ascertain the optimal method of using the drug.

The phase I study has the following endpoints: (1) establishment of a maximum tolerated dose on a given schedule and route of administration; (2) establishment of the toxicity patterns and determination of whether the toxicity is predictable, tolerable, and reversible; and (3) evidence of antitumor activity. It must be emphasized that a phase I trial is a therapeutic intent trial. Unfortunately, in many cases enthusiasm for pursuing further studies with a drug often wanes if the phase I trial gives no hint of activity.

One of the critical problems in a phase I study is how to reach the maximum tolerated dose (MTD) in the safest and most efficient fashion. The theoretic goal of a phase I study is to reach a single MTD for a particular schedule. In practice, the MTD reached is often a function of the degree of prior therapy to which patients have been exposed. For example, patients with extensive prior chemotherapy or radiation therapy tolerate less drug, particularly those who have marrow suppression, than patients without extensive prior treatment.

Phase II

Phase II is a trial period during which an attempt is made to use the dose or doses of the drug determined in the phase I trials in order to search for evidence of antitumor effect in man. A phase II trial requires about 20 patients with one type of tumor that can be evaluated for potential antitumor effect after treatment for a month or more at the maximum tolerated doses by the route administered. If several responses are observed among the 20 patients, further trials are in order; and if many responses are noted, a phase III trial may be designed. In addition, a spectrum of tumors must be screened. Remissions must be carefully defined for each experimental approach. Frequency, duration, and extent of remission should also be recorded.

Phase II trials are mainly concerned with establishing optimum dosage schedules and combinations for chemotherapeutic agents. This type of clinical trial has produced such outstanding achievements as increasing the cure rate of metastatic choriocarcinoma from 0% to more than 90%.

Phase II studies are investigations that determine if a new drug has antitumor activity worthy of further clinical evaluation. The phase II trial is not planned to give definitive answers on the ultimate value or role of a given drug, which is the purpose of the larger phase III studies. In a sense, the phase II trial is a screen for antitumor activity and has the imperfections of any screening system.

Phase III

The aim of phase III studies is to determine what should become standard therapy, usually by comparing a new agent showing promise at the completion of phase II trials with some standard form of therapy. In phase III trials, careful definitions of subjective and objective remissions and data on frequency, completeness, and duration of remission are mandatory.

It is a time for large-scale trials to compare the efficacy of different applications of the various therapeutic modalities. Each of these trials requires extensive evaluation in many patients, in different institutions, and with proper controls.

For a new drug, a phase III trial classically is a study in which the drug is given to a large number of patients to determine if: (1) the activity seen in phase II can be confirmed; (2) unexpected events, such as new types of activity of adverse effects occur; and (3) the drug has any value in relation to other potential treatments.

It is much more than an attempt to confirm the findings of phases I and II. It is an attempt to add total identification of the drug.

Immunochemotherapy

The property of specific recognition of the immune system is being evaluated in the field of antitumor chemotherapy. It is unnecessary to say that selective immunochemotherapy is of special therapeutic interest. However, it would represent a major advance in anticancer therapy if it could be achieved with a predictable chance to reach the cancer cell selectively. Most drugs effective in controlling the growth of cancer cells are also toxic to normal cells. It is the small margin of safety between inhibiting the growth of a cancer cell and damaging normal cells that greatly limits the use of antitumor chemotherapeutic drugs. However, by exploiting the known principles of immunology it is possible to attach antitumor drugs to antibodies prepared against specific or even tumor-associated antigens identified with that particular tumor. The antibodies directed against the antigen of the cancer cell would seek out the cancer cell or cells, attach to it or them, and thus deliver the drug selectively and in high concentrations where it is needed to carry out its lethal effect, while sparing completely the normal cells. It is now technologically possible to experiment with this method. The concept of this "magic bullet" as a therapeutic method for control of cancer has been resurrected.

New Drugs

It is important to pursue a planned, empiric search for new drugs that have anticancer effect. With our present knowledge of pharmacology and insights into cell kinetics, it is logical to pursue a program of chemical synthesis of compounds or polymers designed to interfere with critical steps in cancer cell biosynthesis and metabolism. A coordinated program involving chemists, biologists, and clinicians must be directed to the specific targets and techniques of selecting the compounds for trial. This cooperative endeavor will ensure immediate feedback and quick acceptance of drugs for clinical trial.

However, empiric screening of natural products (particularly plant extracts), soil, and antibiotics continues to provide compounds that have major usefulness in clinical oncology. Approximately a dozen compounds derived from plants and bacteria are now in clinical use and have demonstrated significant therapeutic benefit. This type of program should be encouraged and can run parallel to a program of chemical synthesis of compounds without being competitive. The cooperative programs obviously should be expanded. The results of such studies are urgently needed for the control and prevention of metastases.

Surgery and radiation therapy are already highly effective in controlling most primary cancers. Failure to prevent dissemination of the cancer or to provide effective treatment after the disease has become widespread accounts for the greatest number of deaths. Certain drugs are now under clinical investigation that in animals are more effective in preventing metastases than in inhibiting growth of the primary tumor. The routine prevention of metastases would be a significant advance, if not a landmark, in the control of cancer.

The search for botanic and antibiotic drugs against cancer should be extended in conjunction with relevant biologic screening. To expedite the production, testing and use of new drugs, it seems appropriate to charge the National Cancer Advisory Board with the responsibility and control of the use of new anticancer drugs and to keep the control of all other drugs under the jurisdiction of the FDA.

Ovarian Cancer Vaccine

In principle, the concept of an ovarian cancer vaccine has much merit. However, a great deal more basic and applied clinical research must be carried out before we can evaluate what an ovarian cancer vaccine would contribute to the overall management of patients with this disease.

The subject is reviewed in Chapter 28 but is outlined here for the sake of completeness. Tumor-associated antigens (TAAs), which are present on the cell in minute quantities, have been isolated from soluble products, including inhibitory antigens (IAs), obtained from separated membranes of common epithelial ovarian cancer. The inhibitors (IAs) prevent the induction of cell-mediated immune responses by TAAs. Current experiments suggest that IA are nucleoproteins that exist in plaques or patches at intervals along the ovarian cancer cell surface membranes. Hopefully, TAAs of the common epithelial ovarian cancer, which is about to be tested with a phase I study, will prove to have specific active immunotherapeutic potentialities. Lung studies, which have been under way for a long time, indicate that strong cell-mediated immune reactivity is present for at least 5 years following immunization and probably lasts much longer. Real benefit might result from public health programs or prophylactic immunization of women in high-risk groups for the development of common epithelial ovarian cancer. A program for evaluating immunization for the management of melanoma is currently under investigation.

Biologic Response Modification

The term biotechnology encompasses many activities that have in common the fact that they all possess the fundamental abilities of living organisms. One of the most impressive achievements of science has been the explosion of knowledge about the chemical composition of organisms and the way these chemicals interact to create the phenomena scientists recognize as life.

With genetic engineering there is a reweaving of the threads of life. The possibility of transferring genes from one organism to another is an alluring prospect, as genetic engineering can reduce the cost and increase the supply of an enormous range of materials now used in medicine, agriculture, and industry. Furthermore, there are many substances that occur naturally and only small quantities that might well prove invaluable if they were available in quantities sufficient for their potential to be examined.

The body's inherent biochemical capacity for carrying cancer cells combined with the new genetic technology provides a biologic response modification, or biomodulation. The new wave in cancer treatment is generating

a great deal of excitement among scientists, physicians, and patients. This technology has provided, in quantity, interleukins, thymic hormones, tumor necrosis factor, lymphotoxins, interferons, and a variety of other biologic response modifiers.

Monoclonal antibodies

Monoclonal antibodies are homogenous antibodies produced by a single clone. They are usually produced from hybridomas, which are prepared by fusing immunized mouse or rat spleen cells with a nonsecretory myeloma. When cloned, monoclonal antibodies represent a group of cells derived from a single original cell; hence they are genetically identical. Monoclonal antibody technology explodes a fundamental power of the body's immune system: the ability to recognize molecules of a specific shape and attack the cells that carry these molecular targets.

Monoclonal antibodies work by attaching to unique proteins on the surface of cancer cells. Once the cancer cell is coated with antibodies, cells of the immune system recognize that it should be destroyed, and the T cell or killer cell then attacks the cancer cell. Monoclonal antibodies can be used to carry drugs or toxins to a cancer cell while avoiding normal cells. The drug-laden antibody attaches to the cancer cell surface; and the drugs or toxins, though not necessarily the antibody, are engulfed by the cell. Once inside the cell, the drugs or toxins poison the cell. One toxin—Ricin, for example—destroys the ribosomes, the cell's protein factory. Radioactive particles can be attached to monoclonal antibodies. The antibodies carry the particles to cancer cells, where their radioactive material is then concentrated to kill the tumor.

These approaches have great promise for making a significant contribution not only to the diagnosis but to the therapy of cancer.

Müllerian Inhibiting Substance

The genital duct system and the external genitalia develop under the influence of hormone circulating in the fetus during intrauterine life.

Sertoli cells in the fetal testes produce a non-steroidal substance known as müllerian inhibiting substance (MIS), which causes regression of the paramesonephric duct (müllerian duct).

A potential specific biologic treatment for ovarian cancer is being developed from the experimental studies of Donahue. Epithelial ovarian cancers are related to tissues derived from the müllerian duct. MIS is a fetal testicular product that causes regression of the müllerian duct in male embryos. Using a partially purified fraction of MIS, it has been demonstrated that MIS is cytotoxic to the human serocystadenocarcinoma cell line in vitro and inhibits growth of the cell line in nude mice. Clinical trials of MIS are under way, and the development of new technology to prepare sufficient quantities of this complex glycoprotein is being explored. This work gives promise of adding another method for the treatment of common epithelial ovarian cancer.

Multiple-Drug Resistance in Cancer Patients

An ancient pump protein that flushes toxins from cells may be the problem when cancer chemotherapy fails. Its identification offers hope that multiple-drug-resistant cancers might be made vulnerable again. Data suggest that multiple-drug resistance is associated with elevated levels of P-glycoprotein, a cell membrane protein that may act as a pump to remove chemotherapeutic drugs from the cell. Many researchers believe that the higher the level of P-glycoprotein the greater is the drug resistance. Technology has produced P-glyco Chek-C219 tm, which is a fluorescein-labeled monoclonal antibody that directly measures P-glycoprotein through fluorescent flow cytometry and microscopy. Work has progressed to the point where it is possible to evaluate P-glyco Chek in patient populations as a possible means of determining levels of P-glycoprotein in order to optimize treatment protocols, predict therapeutic responsiveness, and identify candidates for alternative therapeutic approaches.

Oncogenes

Oncogenes traditionally have been defined as genes able to confer on cells the property of unregulated growth. All known oncogenes are derived from proto-oncogenes, their genetic counterparts, which are normally found in all mammalian cells and generally play a role in the normal process of cell growth and differentiation. In the past, oncogenes have been considered to be good genes that have gone bad, but this view has now been challenged. It is reported that oncogenes are not bad genes but good genes that have been altered, inappropriately expressed, or inappropriately inactivated.

Oncogenes fall into a few general categories: those involved in phosphorylation, those that regulate growth, those that play a role in protein transcription, and those involved in DNA replication. The protein product of each is found in that part of the cell best suited to its activity. The src protein, a protein kinase, spans the cell membrane; and the myc protein, which controls messenger RNA, operates in the nucleus.

When proto-oncogenes undergo certain genetic alterations (including point mutations, insertions, deletions, and translocations), the normal control of growth and differentiation may change to the promotion of neoplastic development. The presence of oncogenes was originally assessed on the basis of their ability to induce transformation to a malignant phenotype and tissue culture (elevated through morphologic changes) or tumorigenicity when cells expressing these genes were introduced into animals.

Although most studies have been directed to exploring the ability of oncogenes to cause uncontrolled growth of cells and development of tumors, it is now accepted that uncontrolled growth, taken alone, does not confer on a tumor the property of being benign or malignant. Other properties of malignant cells, including the ability to metastasize and their resistance to chemotherapy and radiation therapy, are more important than the simple growth properties in determining whether therapy of a patient with cancer will be successful.

The development of the changes in tumor cells that lead to a more malignant phenotype is known as tumor progression.

Investigators have studied the capacity of oncogenes to lead to two properties of malignant cells: (1) the ability to metastasize; and (2) the development of radiation resistance. Parallel to this research have been cytogenetic changes in the transformed cells that have been investigated in the sites of oncogene integration into the host genome, and there have been attempts to correlate such genetic events of the biologic properties of the transformed cells.

HER-2/neu oncoprotein (H2n) is an investigational assay for a protein product of the HER-2/neu oncogene. Amplification in this gene is significantly greater in patients with early relapse and poor survival. In patients with node-positive breast disease, this test may predict outcome better than either estrogen or progesterone receptors. The standard range for HER-2/neu is more than 5 femtomoles/milligram (fmol/mg) protein.

The HER-2/neu proto-oncogene is increased in 25 to 35% of human primary breast cancers, and this alteration is associated with disease behavior. In some studies several similarities were found in the biology of HER-2/neu in breast and ovarian cancer, including similar increase and direct correlation between increases and overexpression, evidence of tumors in which over expression occurs without an increase in HER-2/neu, and the association between gene alteration and clinical outcome.

Berchuck and colleagues have reported on the overexpression of HER-2/neu associated with poor survival in advanced epithelial ovarian cancer. They used the immunohistochemical technique involving a monoclonal antibody specifically reactive with the external domain of HER-2/neu to study expression of the HER-2/neu in frozen sections of normal ovary and advanced epithelial ovarian cancer. They found that survival with high HER-2/neu expression was significantly less than that of a control group; moreover, the patient was less likely to have a complete response to primary therapy. It is obvious from all of these findings that HER-2/neu deserves further evaluation as a prognostic marker in epithelial ovarian cancer.

GnRH Agonist

Work under way shows that the gonadotropin-releasing hormone (GnRH) agonist may play a role in the treatment of hormone-dependent cancers. To understand the great potential of GnRH, it is necessary to review the advances in reproductive neuroendocrinology. A vast amount of work done between 1937 and 1971 solved the mystery of a releasing factor secreted by the hypothalamus into the portal system at the pituitary level to regulate the release of tropic hormones. Evidence shows that a delicate balance is required to achieve the desired effect. Too much or too little GnRH destroys the intended clinical response. Under normal conditions, the pulsatile release of GnRH by the hypothalamus (one pulse every 1–2 hours) results in anterior pituitary production and release of follicle-stimulating hormone (FSH) and luteinizing hormone (LH). However, the continuous, excessive, absent, or more frequent release of GnRH inhibits FSH and LH production and release, which is called downloading. The decreased pulse level of GnRH lowers LH secretion but increases FSH secretion.

Application of this releasing factor to the treatment of carcinoma of the prostate has given encouraging results. In men, GnRH agonist causes a marked reduction in serum testosterone and mean sperm concentration. The testicular histologic examination reveals suppressed spermatogenesis in Leydig cell hyperplasia. Symptoms of androgen deficiency necessitate the administration of testosterone, which dampens the enthusiasm for using androgens as a male contraceptive. However, they are proving useful for the management of men with carcinoma of the prostate. Injections of leuprolide acetate produces a GnRH agonist effect for the palliative treatment of advanced prostatic cancer. This therapy provides an alternative when orchiectomy or estrogen administration is either contraindicated or unacceptable to the patient.

D-Trp-6-luteinizing hormone releasing hormone (D-Trp-6-LHRH) has proved useful for treating benign and malignant ovarian cancer. One report showed that, with advanced ovarian cancer, those treated monthly with a long-acting depot preparation of D-Trp-6-LHRH were improved. Much work is needed in this field, but at least an advance has been made.

Flow Cytometry

By providing multiple analyses on single cells, flow cytometry allows the description of cellular heterogenicity, establishing the biologic counterpart of clinical heterogeneity, to most tumors. Analysis of DNA content, a reflection of cell ploidy, is useful for establishing the prognosis of many solid tumors; and analysis of other markers has been crucial to increasing our knowledge of lymphoid differentiation, classifying hematologic malignancies, and detecting minimal residual disease. In studies that have been reported, there is significant evidence that the common epithelial ovarian cancer does not arise from a single clone but, rather, represents a multiple-clone cancer. This point may account for some of the complete eradication of ovarian cancer in some patients, whereas in others there is an initial good response with a plateau and then deterioration. It is obvious that widespread application of flow cytometry to ovarian cancer could make a significant contribution to identifying the constitution of these tumors.

Areas in Which Research is Needed

A great deal of research is needed to find the optimal use of the drugs that are available and to search for new drugs and the uses to which they can be put. Although little has been achieved in delineating metabolic or enzymatic differences between normal and malignant cells, renewed efforts should be directed to this end with the new and advanced technology available. A recognition of even a small difference between normal and cancer cells might lead to a new drug design. The advanced methods of testing drugs, particularly the many antibiotics identified, have revealed activity against many important biosynthetic enzymes. Drugs that may affect enzymes unique to oncogenic viruses hold particular promise for neoplasms found to be caused by viruses. Work with the reverse transcriptase enzyme may serve to unravel the mystery of the role of viruses in human cancer. Drugs that affect enzymes unique to oncogenic viruses could then be definitely applied to their control with a predictable response rate.

The pharmacology and metabolic disposition of known active compounds in human cancer patients must be explored in greater depth. Unfortunately, all anticancer drugs have an immunosuppressive effect. There is a small ratio between this effect and their cancer-controlling ability. This ratio must be explored or better drugs synthesized that have little or no immunosuppressive effect. The control of cancer would be advanced by (1) the synthesis and an understanding of the key structures of the compounds; (2) knowledge of how and where to inhibit key enzymes; and (3) discovery of species, tissues, or cell differences in regard to their affinities for the anticancer drugs.

Certain drugs now under clinical investigation in animals prevent metastases much more effectively than they inhibit growth of the primary tumor. It is the tendency to spread that often makes cancer incurable. In fact, metastases are the most important clinical feature of cancer because they usually determine whether the patient can be cured. An advance would be made by understanding the mechanism whereby certain drugs potentiate the destructive effects of heat on cancer cells. Research is needed to find new and effective drugs to produce radiosensitization of tumors that would kill cancer cells at a dose that would not destroy normal tissue.

Predictive testing of drugs before use in humans is mandatory, and better methods for such testing must be designed. The optimal dose, ideal route, schedule, and conditions of administration may be learned from experimental animals, as must the toxicities and side effects that may develop. Control of toxic effects is important. In addition, an in vitro test for the effectiveness of a drug on the patient's own cancer cells before its clinical use would help to select the proper drug for the cancer in that patient.

Current cooperative projects of clinical investigation of chemotherapy provide an essential link in cancer research, as the research is directed to the ultimate goal of prevention and control of cancer in humans. The input of these cooperative group studies permits a comparatively rapid evaluation of the results of treatment with greater precision and validity because of the variety and diversity of those investigators who have been screened for their material, program, and integrity by peer review. Accumulated data of this high quality with strict control provide a method of discarding the inferior plans of treatment and pursuing and expanding those that yield superior results.

Developing New Drugs for Ovarian Cancer: Future Directions

Today a specific magic bullet acting as an anticancer drug has not been found. Will one be found in the future? It is doubtful that a single drug will be found that cures all ovarian cancers. From past experience and fundamental considerations of cancer in a multiorgan creature such as humans, it seems improbable that such a specific drug could be found. However, it is possible that a drug will be found that acts on certain cell types, which is not dissimilar to antibiotic therapy where a panel of antibiotics are screened against a given bacterium.

Therapeutic and technologic advances have profoundly modified the parameters of new drug testing in ovarian cancer. The potential of compounds tested today for this disease therefore must be assessed according to this changing reality. Previous treatment with or without platinum is the criterion that had been applied in a review of single agent clinical data. Results obtained with older compounds have also been, when possible, reassessed in order to facilitate a comparative interpretation of recent trials.

Progress that hopefully may profoundly affect cancer chemotherapy comes from several areas:

Molecular biology
Immunology
Earlier detection
Amelioration of anticancer drug toxicity
Better supportive care
Antimetastatic drugs

That new and better anticancer drugs are required is accepted, but the nature of the best and most appropriate screening techniques that define such agents is not known. Little reliance can be placed on a specific experimental tumor, but neither is it certain that whole banks of screening tumors will lead to better results. In vitro tests against proliferating tumor cells, although of value for answering precise questions regarding mechanisms, have not been of great value for discovering new anticancer drugs. However, such systems may have a role as initial primary screens.

When studying the potential for developing new drugs for ovarian cancer, certain conclusions can be proposed. They are suggestive but not conclusive.

1. The rate of clinical response to single-agent first-line therapy is clearly reduced when comparing early historical data with more recent trials—a result of much more stringent criteria of evaluation as well as of technologic progress. The only exceptions—represented by high-dose intravenous cyclophosphamide, intravenous melphalan, and ifosfamide— probably suggest better drug bioavailability with these compounds.

2. The rate of clinical response after first line (alkylating drug-containing) therapy has failed and is generally followed by dismal results with additional treatment. The platinum compounds are the most active available agents in this situation. When studied in adequate numbers of patients and confirmed by a variety of investigators, antitumor activity of more than 20% per new agent can be considered of major interest. Carbo-platinum and ifosfamide are probably the compounds that deserve more attention; the accumulated data must be expanded.

When platinum compounds have failed, almost no other chemotherapeutic agent produces an additional response, at least for the management of ovarian cancer. Occasionally there is an objective response, and when it occurs it is considered a major achievement. Cis-platinum and carboplatinum given at increasingly higher doses have occasionally produced some response.

Taxol is a novel diterpene compound derived from the bark of the Western yew, Taxus brevifolia. A mitotic spindle poison, it is a potent inhibitor of cell replication in vitro. Projects are under way to evaluate its role in the treatment of ovarian cancer.

Hormonal therapy has produced unpredictable results. Because of different mechanisms of action in tumor heterogenicity, hormonal agents might have a role if combined with cytotoxic agents. More work is required in this field.

Preclinical screening models currently are crude and need to be improved. In particular, the cross-resistance of the dose-response issues still need to be reliably addressed in the laboratory in view of their clinical implications.

Although much progress has been made in the field of anticancer chemotherapy for ovarian cancer, much work remains. It appears obvious that these patients are living longer and more comfortably, but the 10-year survival has not significantly improved.

Summary

The finding that several disseminated human tumors can be cured by anticancer drugs alone demonstrates that selective toxicity does exist and that there is a potential cure. An effort must be made to understand the interaction of the drug, host, tumor, oncogenic agent, and host defense mechanisms. Research on which drugs to give for which tumors, in what combinations, and when in the course of the disease (e.g., before operation, after operation, with radio-therapy, after widespread metastases) are areas of great promise.

Only some of the tumor cells are in an active growth cycle at any one time, and the synthesis of critical cellular constituents is known to occur during specific phases of that cycle. The cell cycle is measured from mitosis to mitosis. It is important to accumulate knowledge on selective toxicity during different phases of the cell, to know the time of the natural death of cells within the tumor, and to know their regeneration time at the surface and the interior of the cancer in order to discover the means by which to maneuver cells into an active cycle or to kill them during the resting phase.

It has been shown that cells lodged at a distance from the closest capillary or beyond the blood-brain barrier enjoy a sanctuary from anticancer drugs. It is important to find means to deliver lethal doses of anticancer drugs to these areas.

A program to screen botanic and microbiologic substances for anticancer activity must be expanded. Chemical synthesis of compounds or polymers designed to interfere with critical steps in cancer cell biosynthesis and metabolism are important. The specific targets and techniques for selecting the compounds for trial must be coordinated by chemists and biologists. The program must be streamlined and coordinated so that rapid feedback occurs from an area of the project that demonstrates anticancer activity.

Much research is needed to (1) study the metabolic or enzymatic differences between normal and malignant cells in order to open programs for new drug designs; (2) design new and sophisticated methods that test drugs, particularly those that affect enzymes unique to oncogenic viruses (particularly important if viruses are ever identified as a causative agent in human cancers); (3) study and fractionate pharmacologic products known to be active in controlling human cancer; (4) study compounds that inhibit key enzymes with the aim of discovering species or tissue differences in affinities for drugs; (5) develop anticancer drugs that are not immunosuppressive; (6) explore new classes of drugs that would inhibit invasion or act specifically on metastases; (7) explore the mechanisms whereby certain drugs potentiate the lethal effects of heat on tumor cells; and (8) search for new drugs that effectively produce radiosensitization of tumors.

New and better ways for predictive testing of anticancer drugs are needed. A method by which a drug can be tested in the laboratory before its clinical use would be a great contribution. Cooperative group studies (e.g., the Gynecologic Oncology Group) bring earlier results of high precision and validity because of the positive intellectual input of several investigators in planning and reporting the research. It is hoped that clinical investigation in chemotherapy will provide an essential link in cancer research.

The decade of the 1990s undoubtedly will expand the work of Salmon et al. with chemo-sensitivity studies, as well as work done on the immune complexes and the use of plasmapheresis. Flow cytometry has shown that a certain number of common epithelial tumors are heterogeneous and contain more than one clone of cells. Expansion of work on the hybridomas offers the potential for a new approach to diagnosis and therapy for malignant disease. The success or failure of current ovarian cancer vaccines will be determined during the 1990s as well. All of these areas require structured trials to determine the role they will play in managing common epithelial ovarian cancer.

Progress that may profoundly affect cancer chemotherapy may come from several areas: molecular biology; genetic engineering and gene splicing; immunology; earlier detection; control of anticancer drug toxicity; better supportive care; and antimetastatic drugs. It is obvious that the doom and gloom of the 1970s and 1980s is being replaced with a spirit of optimism for the 1990s.

Bibliography

Bagley CM, Young RC, Schein PS, et al: *Ovarian carcinoma metastatic to the diaphragm—frequently undiagnosed laparotomy. Am J Obstet Gynecol* 116:397, 1973.

Barber HRK (ed): *Immunobiology for the Clinician.* John Wiley & Sons, New York, 1977, p. 9.

Bargmann CL, Hung MC, Weinberg RA: The new oncogene encodes an epidermal growth factor receptor-related protein. *Nature* 319:226, 1986.

Barnes DM, Lammil GA, Millis RR, et al: An immunohistochemical evaluation of c-erb B-2 expression in human carcinoma. *Br J Cancer* 58:448, 1988.

Bellman GB, Knapp RC, Order SE, Hellman S: The role of lymphatic obstruction in formation of ascites in a murine ovarian carcinoma. *Cancer Res.* 32:1663, 1972.

Berchuck A, Kamel A, Whitaker B, et al: Overexpression of HER-2 neu is associated with poor survival in advanced epithelial ovarian cancer. *Cancer Res* 50:4087, 1990.

Bloomfield RD: Current cancer chemotherapy in obstetrics and gynecology. *Am J Obstet Gynecol* 109:487, 1971.

Braylan RC: Flow cytometry. *Arch Pathol Lab Med* 107:1, 1983.

Bruce WR, Meeker BE, Valeriote FA: The comparison of the sensitivity of normal hematopoietic and transplanted lymphoma colony forming cells to chemotherapeutic agents administered in vivo. *J Natl Cancer Inst* 37:233, 1966.

Brule G, Eckhardt SJ, Hall TC, Winkler A: *Drug Therapy of Cancer.* World Health Organization, Geneva, 1973, p. 12.

Carter SK: Study design principles for the clinical evaluation of new drugs as developed by the chemotherapy program of the National Cancer Institute. In Staquet M (ed): *The Design and Clinical Trials in Cancer Therapy.* Editions Scientifiques Européenes, Brussels, 1972, p. 242.

Carter SK, Bakowski MT, Hellmann K: *Chemotherapy of Cancer.* John Wiley & Sons, New York, 1977.

Dembo AJ, Bush RS, Beale FA, et al: Ovarian carcinoma: improved survival following abdominopelvic irradiation in patients with a completed pelvic operation. *Am J Obstet Gynecol* 134(7): 793, 1979.

De Vita VT: Cell kinetics and chemotherapy of cancer. *Cancer Chemother Rep* 1:35, 1971.

Donahue PK, Swann DA, Hayashi A, Sullivan MD: Müllerian duct regression in the embryo correlated with cytotoxic activity against human ovarian cancer. *Science* 205:913, 1979.

Drebin JA, Link VC, Stern DF, et al: Down modulation of an oncogene protein product and reversion of the transformed phenotype by monoclonal antibodies. *Cell* 41:695, 1985.

Frei E III: Cytokinetics and clinical cancer. In *Chemotherapy Oncology.* Year Book Medical Publishers, Chicago, 1970, p. 131.

Gehan EA, Freireich EJ: Nonrandomized controls in cancer clinical trials. *N Engl J Med* 290:198, 1974.

Gehan EA, Schneiderman NA: Experimental design of clinical trials. In Holin JE, Frie III E (eds): *Cancer Medicine.* Lea & Febiger, Philadelphia, 1973.

Greenwald ES: Cancer Chemotherapy. *NY State J Med* 2:2641, 1972; 3:2757, 1972.

Greenwald ES: *Cancer Chemotherpay.* Medical Examination Publishing, Flushing, NY, 1973.

Hellmann K, Carter SK (eds): *Fundamentals of Cancer Chemotherapy.* McGraw-Hill, New York, 1987.

Hellmann K, Carter SK (eds): *Future Directions —Fundamentals of Cancer Chemotherapy.* McGraw-Hill, New York, 1989, p. 499.

Hoffman J, Post J: The effects of antitumor drugs on the cell cycle. In Zimmerman AM, Padilla GM, Cameron IL (eds): *Drugs and the Cell Cycle*. Academic Press, Orlando, FL, 1973, p. 219.

Knapp RC, Freedman EA: Aortic lymph node metastasis in early ovarian cancer. *Am J Obstet Gynecol* 119:1013, 1974.

Meyers MA: The spread and localization of acute intraperitoneal effusions. *Radiology* 95:547, 1970.

National Program for the Conquest of Cancer: *Report of the National Panel of Consultants on the Conquest of Cancer*. Report No. 91-1402. U.S. Government Printing Office, Washington, DC, 1970.

Parker RT, Parker CH, Wilbanks DD: Cancer of the ovary: survival studies based upon curative therapy, chemotherapy and radiotherapy. *Am J Obstet Gynecol* 108:878, 1970.

Raber MN: Clinical applications of flow cytometry. *Oncology* 2(3):35, 1988.

Salmon SE, Hamburger AW, Soehnlen B, et al: Quantitation of differential sensitivity of human-tumor stem cells to anticancer drugs. *N Engl J Med* 298:1321, 1978.

Schneiderman MA: How do you know if you have done any better? *Cancer* 35:64, 1975.

Skipper HE: Clowes memorial lecture. *Cancer Res* 31:1173, 1971.

Skipper HE, Schabel FM Jr: Quantitative and cytokinetic studies in experimental tumor models. In Holland JR, Frei III E (eds): *Cancer Medicine*. Lea & Febiger, Philadelphia, 1973, p. 629.

Smith JP, Rutledge FN, Declos L: Results of chemotherapy as an adjunct to surgery in patients with localized ovarian cancer. *Semin Oncol* 2:277, 1975.

VanderSchuerem E, Ang KK: Design and clinical trials for the treatment of ovarian cancer: ovarian cancer. *Adv Biosci* 26:79, 1980.

Webb MJ, Decker DG, Mussey E, Williams TJ: Factors influencing survival in stage I ovarian cancer. *Am J Obstet Gynecol* 116:222, 1973.

Zimmerman AM, Padilla GM, Cameron IL: *Drugs and the Cell Cycle*. Academic Press, Orlando, FL, 1973.

Addendum

It is difficult to devote a single chapter to new developments and the most important points related to the subject of ovarian cancer, even though these topics are important and should be presented to the clinician. To incorporate such topics into other chapters, it would be necessary to sacrifice the individual attention which each deserves. Therefore it was decided to group these subjects in a separate chapter.

Reverse Transcriptase

Reverse transcriptase is a newly isolated RNA-dependent DNA polymerase that can transcribe the base sequence of a viral RNA onto a DNA strand in vitro; hence it is now possible to synthesize relatively large quantities of such virus-specified DNA. If a virus is the cause of a particular cancer, its genetic material may be present in the cancer cells in the form of DNA, even though it may not reveal its presence. It is possible to extract cellular DNA from tumors, purify it, and separate its strands. This DNA can be mixed with synthetic single-stranded DNA, carrying the base sequence of the RNA virus. Should a complementary viral genome (i.e., DNA specified by the same virus) exist in the tumor extract, the two should bind together, reconstituting double-stranded molecules. Such molecules can be recognized. Thus the identification of these double-stranded "hybrid" molecules would, in itself, prove the existence of the same viral genome in the tumor and, on the basis of present evidence,

strongly indicate the tumor's viral etiology. Studies with retroviruses have opened up a new field of research and have supplied answers to questions which had previously puzzled scientists. A retrovirus is an RNA virus which encodes an enzyme that makes a DNA copy of its RNA and splices it into the host chromosome.

Cytogenetics of Ovarian Cancer

Definite patterns of numerical and structural chromosome changes in ovarian cancer have been described. These reports support the current concepts that such changes in gynecologic tumors are not random and that patterns for invasiveness appear to be tissue-specific or organ-specific. Information available at this time suggests that many of the chromosome abnormalities in cancer are most likely secondary or coincidental, but that primary, significant chromosome changes exist as well. Identifying such changes is difficult because of the variability of cytogenetic changes among cancers of the same histopathologic type, their obliteration by coexisting coincidental changes, and, particularly in the case of solid tumors, technical problems.

Cytogenetics is the study of the chromosome complement of cells. It is well known that the normal human chromosome number is 46. However, neoplasms have been shown to have a wide variation in chromosome number and structure (aneuploidy), often differing from cell to cell within the same tumor. *Karyotype* refers to the chromosome characteristics of an individual or of a cell line. The cells are arrested in metaphase for study. Banding of the chromosomes has enabled more accurate evaluation of the chromosomes being studied. Metaphase chromosomes, arrested by colchicine and recorded by microphotography of single-cell nuclei, are arranged in pairs in descending order of size and according to the position of the centromer. The Patau system, which is that most commonly used, arranges these pairs of chromosomes into seven groups, A to G.

Karyotypes of neoplastic cells are examined for variation from normal; that is, the overall number of chromosomes falling into each of seven Patau groups is determined, and changes in individual chromosome structures are evaluated. Such structurally abnormal chromosomes, referred to as *marker chromosomes*, result from gaps, breaks, deletions, or rearrangements. Those marker chromosomes that are recurrent are of particular interest because they most likely represent specific rather than coincidental chromosome changes—changes that may be involved in the causation or progression of cancer.

Ovarian cancers seem to differ from other gynecologic tumors in their ploidy distribution and their frequency of marker chromosomes. A variety of modes and consistent markers has been reported for primary ovarian cancers. In malignant ovarian tumors, the chromosome distribution varies with the degree of invasiveness.

Wakong-Vaartaja and Auersperg reported that 59% of the differentiated and undifferentiated cancers of the ovary were in the hypodiploid $(2n - x)$ group, and 41% were in the triploid $(3n \pm x)$ group, and 100% of the undifferentiated were in the triploid group. Ovarian cancers that were localized had a high diploid mode, whereas those that had metastasized had a high triploid mode. Evidence suggests that spread outside the ovary is associated with a change from the diploid to the triploid mode. The same authors reported a higher incidence of large marker chromosomes in ovarian cancer. Because benign, borderline, and invasive areas may be present in the same tumor, it is obvious that wide sampling must be carried out to determine accurately the chromosomal content of the cancer.

Certain projects have been aimed at identifying genes that contribute to the development of ovarian cancer. It has been shown that chromosomal analysis of tumor cells to document the consistent involvement of a specific chromosome or specific chromosomes in the structural rearrangement as likely sites of genes contributing to tumorigenesis is in progress. It has been demonstrated that there is a preferential involvement of chromosomes 1, 3, and 6 in the structural rearrangement in ovarian cancer. It has also been demonstrated that there is a loss of DNA sequences from chromosome 3 and especially from chromosome 6, confined to the tumor characterizing many ovarian cancers, which supports the conclusion that these chromosomes contain genes whose loss or inactivation contributes to ovarian tumorigenesis. It has been shown that abnormalities involving chromosomes 11 and 19 have been reported to occur commonly in the subset of ovarian cancers but at a frequency lower than that found for chromosomes 1, 3, and 6. The nonrandom involvement of chromosomes 1, 3, and 6 (and perhaps 11 and 19) in terms of structural rearrangement in ovarian cancer suggests that one or more of these segments contain genes whose loss of inactivation contributes to ovarian cancer tumorigenesis or progression (or both).

High-Risk Patients

The most logical definition of a high-risk patient would be any patient with an ovarian cancer or with an adnexal mass that becomes progressively larger or who has any of the pelvic findings listed in Chapter 7.

The first group of patients at high risk are those explored through an improper or inadequate incision. When dealing with ovarian cancer or a suspected malignancy of the ovary, it is important to operate through a vertical incision. The incision must not only be longer than the extent of the cancer but must allow easy access to the area between the liver and diaphragm. The initial operation often determines the success or failure of therapy. It is the height of professional integrity not to succumb to the wishes or demands of the patient but, rather, to advise the patient of the importance of the contemplated incision. Inability to communicate this vital information to the patient is not a license for poor and inadequate treatment, and the surgeon is morally bound to withdraw from the case if the patient insists on a surgically improper incision that may jeopardize her chance of survival.

The other groups at high risk for ovarian cancer are women with the following traits: nulliparity, involuntary infertility, group A blood type, positive family history, early menopause, severe dysmenorrhea, marked premenstrual swelling, spontaneous abortions, breast cancer, residence in highly industrialized countries, and incessant ovulators. These groups are discussed in Chapter 3.

Cadherin Cell Adhesion Receptors

Cadherins comprise a family of cell adhesion receptors that are crucial for the mutual association of vertebrate cells. Through their homophilic binding interaction, cadherins play a role in cell-sorting mechanisms, conferring adhesion specificities on cells. The regulated expression of cadherins also controls cell polarity and tissue morphology. Cadherins are thus considered to be the important regulators of morphogenesis. Moreover, pathologic examination suggests that the down-regulation of cadherin expression is associated with the invasiveness of tumor cells.

The first step of cancer metastasis is the detachment of cells from the primary tumor mass. In general, when cadherins are sufficiently active, cells, especially epithelial ones, are unable to disrupt their mutual connections; it is only when cadherins are inactivated that cells can be freed from their adhesive constraints and migrate out of their parent colonies. Therefore suppression of cadherin activity might trigger the release of tumor cells. It could occur either by suppression of cadherin gene expression or by loss of function of the expressed cadherin molecules.

Because it is accepted that metastasis of tumor cells is assumed to be initiated by the detachment of some cells from primary tumor sites, elucidating the mechanism of the tumor cell detachment should be important to understanding the initiation process of metastasis. The molecular basis of the detachment of tumor cells, however, remains to be solved. It has been shown that there is an unstable expression of E-cadherin adhesion molecules in metastatic and ovarian tumor cells. Immunofluorescence staining has revealed that cells of the highly metastatic line were heterogeneous; that is, their culture contained both E-cadherin positive and negative cells. In contrast, cells of the weakly metastatic lines homogeneously expressed E-cadherin. When the highly metastatic line was subcloned, all the subclones consisted of E-cadherin positive and negative cells. These results suggest that the expression of E-cadherin genes is not stably controlled in the highly metastatic line. Although additional work is necessary to confirm the causal relations between the altered cadherin activity and tumor invasiveness, the results presented indicate that consideration should be given to cadherins when elucidating the molecular basis of tumor invasion in metastases. This subject is receiving a great deal of attention.

Ovarian Cancer Masquerading as an Umbilical Hernia

Each year one to three patients who had been operated on for an umbilical hernia that proved to be an ovarian cancer are referred to me. The history of each is similar: The patient had a known history of umbilical hernia; there is an increase in the size of the abdomen that aggravates the hernia; and at the time of repair the surgeon was surprised to find an ovarian cancer. The message is obvious: Patients being operated on for an umbilical hernia with the above history should undergo thorough rectovaginal examination after an enema. Purists believe that all women undergoing abdominal surgery should have a preoperative pelvic and vaginal examination.

Ovarian Mesothelioma

J.D. Woodruff proposed the concept that the ovary and entire peritoneal cavity are mesothelial structures, and that whatever stimulates the ovary to produce a neoplastic change can also affect other parts of the peritoneal cavity. He believed that visceral and parietal peritoneal metastases of ovarian cancer are not actually metastases but represent multiple primary cancers. This concept is not universally accepted, but it is an exciting one that stimulates pathologists, gynecologists, and research scientists to rethink the traditional concepts of the pathogenesis of ovarian neoplasia. Woodruff stated that the advantages of the mesothelioma concept are the following: (1) to specify the epithelium of the ovary as mesothelium and identify it as a unique epithelial cell of the mesodermal origin; (2) to identify both epithelium and stroma as tissues of mesodermal origin and thus explain the origin of the mixed lesions of the uterus, tubes, ovaries, and peritoneal cavity; (3) to explain the common findings of multiple cell types in many ovarian tumors, that is, combinations of serous, mucinous, endometrioid, mesonephroid, and mesothelial cell types; (4) to note the similarity between lesions of the ovary and those arising in the endocervix, endometrium, and endosalpinx; (5) to explain the occurrence of multiple foci of neoplasia in the ovary and upper genital canal, both systems are of mesodermal origin; (6) to suggest a theory for genesis of ovarian mesothelioma.

Woodruff reviewed the literature of the last century and the early part of this century and found that in series reporting as many as 500 ovariotomies there were only seven malignancies, and in one review of 100 patients with ovarian cysts there were no malignancies. During this century there has been an increase in the malignancy rate of ovarian tumors, and Woodruff suggested that these statistics point to a carcinogen or carcinogens that have been introduced into industrialized urban communities. The increase in population and longevity probably plays some role in the increase of the common epithelial ovarian cancer. Because women who have incessant ovulation without the rest period provided by pregnancy have a higher incidence of ovarian malignancies than those who have had numerous children or who have been on long-term oral contraceptives, it seems that the process of ovulation with recurrent breaks in coelomic epithelium subjects the ovary to greater risk for the introduction of carcinogens into the ovary—in contrast to the undisturbed mesothelial surface of the ovary that is at rest and not ovulating.

There were 240 cases of ovarian malignancy at The Johns Hopkins Hospital over a 5-year period, but no malignant epithelial tumors of the testis were documented during this period of time. This difference calls for some interesting speculations. The testis has a capsule, or tunica albuginea, that is well developed at 8 to 10 weeks of embryonic life and separates the covering mesothelium from the underlying tissue; thus invasion into the matrix can occur only through trauma. In contrast, there is no capsule in the female gonad, and openings develop constantly during the process of ovulation. Because there are so few testicular neoplasms identified as malignant mesothelia (three or four) it must be concluded that the testis is protected from the intraabdominal environment and its associated irritants. An additional argument in favor of this concept is that female patients presenting with ascites and papillary abdominal carcinomatosis are generally assumed to have primary ovarian cancer even though the ovarian surfaces may be the last involved in the entire peritoneal cavity. It was Woodruff's opinion that these cases classically demonstrate the spectrum of cell types described for ovarian cancer and most dramatically defend the validity of this concept. Although neoplasms arising from the surface or lining cells of the ovary are classically referred to under such general terms as "cystadenocarcinoma," "papillary carcinoma," and "undifferentiated cancer," Woodruff presented evidence to support the thesis that such lesions are mesotheliomas; such a thesis can be defended embryologically, histologically, and clinically.

Areas of Future Promise in the Conquest of Ovarian Cancer

The number two killer in the United States is cancer. Cancer kills one man, woman, or child every 63 seconds in the United States. Among women, cancer far exceeds any other disease as a cause of "working years lost."

It was projected that in 1991 about 1.1 million people would be diagnosed as having cancer and about 514,000 would die of the disease: 1400 people a day, about 1 every 62 seconds. Of every five deaths from all causes in the United States, one is from cancer. However, when normal life expectancy is taken into consideration (factors such as dying of heart disease, accidents, and diseases of old age), a "relative" 5-year survival rate of 51% is seen for all cancers. Estimates of cancer incidence show that gynecologic malignancies are the third most common cancer type in women, after breast and gastrointestinal cancers, with approximately 175,000 and 115,400 deaths per year, respectively. Gynecologic cancers are also the third leading cause of cancer deaths in women; they cause an estimated 23,500 deaths per year. It was estimated that in 1992 there would be approximately 21,000 new cases of cancer of the ovary and about 13,000 ovarian cancer deaths, making it the fourth leading cause of death for women and yielding a crude death rate of 64%.

The Division of Cancer Treatment of the National Cancer Institute has been analyzing gynecologic cancers from the standpoint of requirements for developing an overall strategy for combining systemic therapy (e.g., chemotherapy, immunotherapy, or both) with the local modalities of surgery and radiation therapy in an attempt to increase the potential for long-term disease control. In an all-out attack on a specific cancer (by site), it is imperative to know the overall incidence of disease; the frequency of presentation at diagnosis of local, region, and metastatic stages; the patterns of failure; the prognostic variables; the therapy and survival by stage; and the potential for increased therapeutic efficacy with systematic therapy.

Ovarian cancer is difficult to diagnose early. It occurs in an organ that lies deep within the pelvis. In elderly, obese, tense women with an inelastic and conical vagina, it is difficult to palpate pathology until the disease is advanced. Methods for early diagnosis are therefore receiving high priority. Preliminary reports indicate that an antigen is present on the surface of the ovarian cancer cell and that it is capable of stimulating an antibody response. There is fairly solid additional data that an antigen-antibody complex is present on the surface of the ovarian cancer cell as well as in the positive ascitic fluid. The challenge is to translate this knowledge into a serologic diagnosis for early ovarian cancer by employing immunologic techniques—techniques that take advantage of the extraordinary power of discrimination of the immune defense mechanism itself. If the tumor sheds malignant cells before it releases antigens, such a test will have less value than if the tumor releases antigens before it releases intact cancer cells. There is evidence that the antigen is released before intact cancer cells. Another question concerns the volume of tumor necessary before the release of tumor antigens. If the volume of cancer must reach a size of 1 cm^3 or more before shedding its antigen, the tumor at that time would contain a billion cells capable of originating a new focus of disease and would no longer be an early stage of cancer.

A serologic test may prove to be an all-or-nothing test: The patient either would have cancer or would not. Inability to detect precursors of cancer would reduce the significance of the serologic test as a method of early diagnosis, if it is assumed that ovarian cancer is a continuum of diseases progressing from atypia to dysplasia, to cancer in situ, to invasive cancer. The serologic test would still serve to detect ovarian cancer in stages I or II instead of stages III and IV, where 70% of the cases of ovarian cancer are now diagnosed. This test may not provide the hoped-for early diagnosis, but at least it would be an *earlier* diagnosis. In any event, it would provide a method for monitoring the cancer patient and could serve as the keystone of therapy.

Ovarian Cancer as an Autoimmune Disorder

Ovarian cancer not only acts like an immunosuppressive agent, it produces a secondary type of autoimmune disorder or disease in a large number of patients with cancer. Nonspecific hemagglutinating antibodies have been identified in these patients, and their presence makes it difficult to cross-match the patients. They often respond within a relatively short time to cortisone therapy and are then cleared of these antibodies after successful treatment with surgery, irradiation, or chemotherapy.

The polyglandular imbalances seen with certain endocrine syndromes may have a counterpart in the cancer patient, that is, the multi-immunologic syndrome that accounts for the variety of problems that arise in the cancer patient. Stage III and IV ovarian cancer have characteristics similar to those found in autoimmune disorders and indeed in autoimmune disease. Whether there is a clear-cut relation between ovarian cancer and immunodeficiency diseases remains to be seen.

Augmenting the Immunity of Patients with Ovarian Cancer

Ovarian cancer is associated with an immunosuppressive state, and methods to reverse this state would make a significant contribution to its control. As a corollary, selective immunosuppression and strengthening of the immune responses would be an ideal modality of treatment. A method that would selectively suppress the enhancing and blocking antibodies while stimulating the production of a strong cell-mediated response would be an advance in the control of this cancer.

A possible mechanism of action is the arming of nonsensitized cells. Certain sera taken from either animals or human patients during the period of tumor remission have been found to increase the cytotoxic effect of immune lymphocytes. This process has been referred to as *potentiation*. One may speculate that potentiation is related to the unblocking phenomenon and operates by removing (or neutralizing the action of) blocking serum factors present in the lymphocyte suspensions tested, but other mechanisms, including the arming of nonsensitized cells, are equally possible.

The origin, nature, function, chemical composition, and role of complement must be explored. Although the cell-mediated response is the primary path to tissue rejection and tumor control, additional work remains to be done with cytotoxic antibodies and complement. Even a sufficient supply of cytotoxic antibodies is not able to kill tumor cells unless an ample supply of complement is present. Perhaps an understanding of the nature and function of complement could expand its role in tumor control.

Theoretically, immunotherapy is potentially the perfect therapeutic modality for the treatment of cancer. An important distinction must be made between *immunotherapy*, (the treatment of established tumors and their metastases) and *immunoprophylaxis* (the induction of transplantation resistance by immunization prior to tumor cell grafting). The development of more precise techniques for measuring the presence of small numbers of cancer cells would be useful for detecting cancer and for quantitating the response to various types of therapy. It has been shown that immunotherapy can eradicate a small volume of tumor, but even a strong and maximally magnified tumor rejection mechanism cannot eradicate large, established tumors.

Because the immune mechanism is depressed in the very young and the very old and parallels the level of hormone production, the relation between these two mechanisms should be explored. Most of the antigenic determinants are on the cell surface membrane, and the hormone receptors are found in the same place. The role and interaction of immunology and endocrinology remain to be explored.

New Antiovarian Cancer Drugs

New anticancer drugs must be found, and those available must be explored in greater detail. Attack on the DNA of a tumor cell stands at the forefront of tumor therapeutic models: The use of antimetabolites introduces the wrong building blocks or prevents synthesis of the correct ones, and alkylating agents simply hammer away at the completed DNA. Perhaps methods may be evolved to starve the cancer cell in the same way that asparaginase starves the leukemia cell. The role of combination therapy should be expanded with prospective protocols. The basic principle of multistep therapy is to set off cytolytic mechanisms that are strictly localized in cancer tissue. This approach should be explored. *Cis*-platinum is currently one of the most promising drugs for the management of common epithelial ovarian cancer. It is discussed in detail in Chapter 22.

Knowledge that may be contributed by applying the reverse transcriptase enzyme to the identification of viruses in human cancer is accumulating. If a virus is identified, antiviral remedies may work preventively but probably have no effect on gross tumor.

Cellular engineering has been employed by Robert Good for the treatment of leukemias. In patients with primary immunodeficiency diseases, Good was able to completely reconstitute the immune system by transplanting bone marrow cells from matched donors. It is conceivable that this approach, coupled with aggressive chemotherapy, can provide powerful new approaches to the management of solid tissue cancers.

Woodruff reported that the ovary and the peritoneum of the abdominal cavity are mesothelial tissues. The question of whether the millet seed implants represent metastatic disease or multiple primaries has not yet been answered. Because the latter theory suggests a common stimulus to produce the multiple primaries, it is important to explore this suggestion. The common stimulus may enter the peritoneal cavity by way of the cervix, endometrial cavity, and tubes; or perhaps there is another common etiologic explanation.

Epidemiologic evidence suggests that environmental factors are major etiologic factors in ovarian cancer. Because the highest rates for ovarian cancer are recorded in highly industrialized countries, it has been suggested that physical or chemical products of industry are major causes of these neoplasms. A major exception is highly industrialized Japan, which has one of the lowest rates of ovarian cancer in the world. A possible explanation is that the causative factors are present in higher concentrations in the environment in the United States than in Japan. This possibility is supported by the higher rates of cancer of the ovary in Japanese migrants and their offspring in the United States. The search for causative carcinogens is being focused on the immediate environment: Food, personal customs, and the chemical carcinogens used in industry are being investigated. Of the main industrial products known or suspected to have human carcinogenic activity, only asbestos and talc have been seriously considered. There are no hard data at this time, however, to implicate them in ovarian cancer.

Palpation of an Ovarian Cancer

It is commonly reported that an ovarian cancer is hard, knobby, fixed, and bilateral. I have found that there is indeed characteristic findings when palpating a growing ovarian cancer. Ovarian cancers usually grow rapidly and often grow away from their blood supply, which explains why they are prone to rupture and at the time of surgery have often reached the point where they have necrotic areas that rupture at the time of removal. I have found that on careful palpation of an ovarian tumor there are areas that are hard, cystic, soft, and rubbery, as well as knobby and occasionally smooth. Such palpatory characteristics have proved to be invaluable for diagnosing ovarian cancer.

Major Prognostic Factors for Ovarian Carcinoma

There are prognostic variables predictive of survival in ovarian carcinoma. Univariate analysis showed that clinical stage (FIGO), the presence of ascites, age of the patient, histologic type and grade, cellular DNA content, morphometric grade, mitotic activity index, and volume-corrected mitotic index (M/b index) were prognostic. However, there are other prognostic factors that are important.

DNA index (DI): Aneuploid cells with a DI of more than 1.0 indicate an unfavorable prognosis.

Cell cycle distribution (CCD): A high percentage of S phase (more than 10%) indicates an unfavorable prognosis.

Synthesis index (SI): High numbers of S-A cycling cells (more than 6.0%) indicate an unfavorable prognosis.

Estrogen receptor assay: An estrogen receptor-negative assay of less than 10 femtomoles (fmol)/mg cytosol protein indicates an unfavorable prognosis.

Progesterone receptor assay: A progesterone receptor-negative assay of less than 10 fmol/mg cytosol protein indicates a favorable prognosis.

Epidermal growth factor receptor (EGFR) assay: An EGFR-negative assay of less than 5 fmol/mg protein indicates a favorable prognosis.

HER-2/neu oncoprotein (H2n) assay: An assay of more than 5 fmol/mg protein indicates an unfavorable prognosis.

A histogram of these seven tests can give a good indication of the prognosis.

Peritoneovenous Shunting

LeVeen has devised a peritoneovenous shunting approach. The technique, in summary, is carried out by making a transverse incision 2 to 3 inches long over the anterior axillary line about 3 inches below the costal margin on the right side. A transverse incision is made 1 inch above the medial third of the clavicle. The internal jugular vein is exposed between the two heads of the sternocleidomastoid muscles.

A long, slender bronchial alligator or rectal biopsy forceps is passed subcutaneously from below and brought out through the neck incision. A long line of heavy sutures are attached to the forceps and pulled from the neck to the abdomen just underneath the skin. The sutures are tied to the silicone tubing, which is pulled upward by gentle traction until it is delivered into the cervical wound. The silicone rubber tubing is measured so the tip corresponds with the subsequent location in the superior vena cava, 1 inch below the manubriosternal junction.

In the abdomen the external and internal oblique muscles are separated in the direction of their fibers. Two purse-string sutures of 00 Dacron are inserted through the transversalis muscle, transversalis fascia, and peritoneum. A stab wound is made in the center of the purse-string and the perforated abdominal collecting tube is inserted. The purse-string is tightened around the valve stem, the venous tubing is pulled through a stab wound in the muscles, and the musculature is closed over the surface of the valve.

Although the concept is a good one and the technical aspects are easy, the nature of ovarian cancer is such that fragments of the tumor often block the tubing and prevent escape of the ascitic fluid from the abdomen into the venous system. The wide perforated tubing that is inserted into the peritoneal cavity has a valve in it.

Neumann attempted to treat ascites by everting a loop of small intestine (ileoentectropy) to augment absorption of ascitic fluid. This procedure works much better in patients with ascites secondary to cirrhosis than it does in those with ascites due to ovarian cancer.

Familial Ovarian Cancer

Women with two first degree blood relatives (mother, sister, or daughter) are at high risk to develop ovarian cancer. There is a familial Ovarian Cancer Registry at the Roswell Park Memorial Institute, New York State Department of Health [Elm and Carlton Streets, Buffalo, NY 14263; (716) 845-3110]. Dr. M. Steven Piver is the Director of this registry. In the *Newsletter* of April 1989, Piver stated, "Moreover, the history of the Registry has demonstrated very clearly that familial ovarian cancer should no longer be looked on as a rare occurrence. In addition to the 413 cases in the

Registry, we are made aware almost weekly of cases which require consultative counselling for proposed prophylactic oophorectomy in the family of two or more first-degree relatives who have had ovarian cancer."

Genetic counseling for a prophylactic oophorectomy should be done at the time a woman has completed her family but no later than age 35. It is crucial to all women with a family history of ovarian cancer because the disease occurs most commonly in sister/sister and mother/daughter pedigrees. Sisters and daughters in families with a history of ovarian cancer have a 50% chance of developing the disease. This figure compares to the 1.4% chance of women without this family history, or only one of every 70 newborn females in the United States.

Because of this 50% risk that first-degree relatives could develop ovarian cancer; genetic counseling should begin during the early twenties and physical surveillance during the early thirties. Physical surveillance consists in pelvic and abdominal examinations, a CA 125 assay every 6 months, and pelvic ultrasonography every year.

The quality of α-L-fucosidase activity in the serum of humans is determined by heredity. An individual may inherit low, intermediate, or high activity of α-L-fucosidase in serum. About 8% of the general population has low enzyme activity in serum. Low serum α-L-fucosidase activity was three times more prevalent among ovarian cancer patients than among healthy females, suggesting that low serum α-L-fucosidase activity in females may be a hereditary condition associated with increased risk for developing ovarian cancer.

Cancer Nursing

The oncology nurse has become a vital member of the cancer care team. Nurse-oncologists place emphasis not only on how to manage problems but, equally important, on the human values of cancer nursing. They are assuming an increasingly important role in the management of patients with gynecologic cancer. The oncology nurse usually carries out all of the treatments, relates well to the patient, and helps the patient adjust to the diagnosis of cancer. They assume an active role in the rehabilitation of these patients and on many services are charged with the responsibility of follow-up and maintaining the statistics relating to the oncology service. Clinical cancer nurse specialists provide expertise in cancer nursing to patients, families, and other nurses regarding the initiation, planning, implementation, and evaluatation of nursing care for cancer patients; they collaborate with physicians and other health care workers. The oncology nurses have been able to share and support one another and be sensitive to their own physical and emotional needs; the latter need is particularly in evidence during periods of heavy stress, such as that resulting from the death of a favorite long-term patient, a high patient census, or heavy activity.

Hospice Concept

The hospice concept, taking its name from the medieval way stations for weary pilgrims, seeks to discover and provide humane ways of caring for the contemporary cancer patient who has reached a terminal phase of the disease. The hospice concept of care for the terminally ill, long practiced in Europe, has recently been gaining acceptance in the United States. St. Christopher's Hospice in England is one of the most famous in the world.

Those working in a hospice talk of death as the last frontier, where physical, mental, and spiritual needs come together. Changing attitudes toward health care in general and toward the care of the dying in particular have created an environment favorable to the development of programs based on the hospice model. The hospice concept is dedicated to making possible something that all patients seek, that is, a dignified and honorable death. Because approximately 70% of the ovarian cancer patients are in stages III and IV when they present for treatment and the survival rate is low despite all the modern advances, the hospice provides an opportunity for the care of these patients.

Bibliography

Barber HRK (ed): *Immunobiology for the Clinician*. John Wiley & Sons, New York, 1977.

Barber HRK: New frontiers in ovarian cancer diagnosis and management. *Yale J Biol Med* 64:127, 1991.

Blumenfeld D, Braly PC, Ben-Ezra J, Klevecz RR: Tumor DNA content as a prognostic feature in advanced epithelial ovarian carcinoma. *Gynecol Oncol* 27:389, 1987.

DeBoer CH: Transport of particulate matter through the human female genital tract. *J Reprod Fertil* 28:295, 1972.

De Vita VT, Todd H, Wasserman HR, et al: Prospectives on research in gynecologic oncology. *Cancer* 38(suppl):509, 1976.

DiCioccio RA, Barlow JJ, Matta KL: Properties of alpha-L-fucosidase from sera of a healthy female and ovarian cancer patients with low enzyme activity. *Obstet Gynecol* 11:355, 1988.

DiCioccio RA, Brown KS: Biosynthesis, processing and extracellular release of alpha-L-fucosidase in lymphoid cell lines of genetic origins. *Biochem Genet* 26:401, 1988.

Edelman GM: Morphoregulatory molecules. *Biochemistry* 27:3533, 1988.

Fraccaro M, Mannini A, Tiepolo L: Karyotypic clonal evolution in a cystic adenoma of the ovary. *Lancet* 1:613, 1968.

Gelender AB, Cohen JA: A review of cytogenetic studies of gynecologic neoplasms. *Chicago Med School Q* 32:59, 1973.

Good RA, Prehn RT, Lawrence HS: Evaluation of evidence for immune surveillance. In Smith RT, Landy M (eds): *Immune Surveillance*. Academic Press, Orlando, FL, 1970, p. 438.

Good RA: Relations between immunity and malignancy. *Proc Natl Acad Sci USA* 69:1026, 1972.

Greene WH, Marsh JC: Infection in malignant disease: Diagnosis and treatment; forum on infection. *Clin Views Res Pract* 3:3, 1977.

Haapasalo H, Collan Y, Atkins NB: Major prognostic factors in ovarian carcinomas. *Int J Gynecol Cancer* 1:155, 1991.

Hashimoto M, Niwa O, Nitta Y, et al: Unstable expression of E-cadherin adhesion molecules metastatic ovarian tumor cells. *Jpn J Cancer Res* 80:459, 1989.

Julian CG, Goss J, Blanchard K: Biologic behavior of primary ovarian malignancy. *Obstet Gynecol* 44:873, 1974.

Kayayama KP, Toews HA: Chromosomes of metastatic ovarian carcinoma treated with a progestogen and alkylating agents. *Am J Obstet Gynecol* 104:997, 1969.

Knobil E: The neuroendocrine control of the menstrual cycle. *Recent Prog Horm Res* 36:53, 1980.

Kübler-Ross E: *On Death and Dying*. Macmillan, New York, 1973.

LeVeen HH, Christoudias G: IPM peritoneovenous shunting for ascites. *Ann Surg* 180:580, 1974.

Lynch HT, Albano WA, Black L, et al: Familial excess of cancer of the ovary and other anatomic sites. *JAMA* 245:261, 1981.

Lynch HT, Albano WA, Lynch JE, et al: Surveillance and management of patients at high genetic risk for ovarian carcinoma. *Obstet Gynecol* 59:589, 1982.

Lynch HT, Harris RE, Guirgis H, et al: Familial association of breast/ovarian carcinoma. *Cancer* 41:1543, 1978.

National Health Education Committee: *The Killers and Cripplers—Facts on Major Diseases in the United States Today*. David McKay, New York, 1976, p. 51.

Neumann CG, Adie GC, Hinton JW: The absorption of ascitic fluid by means of ileoentectropy in patients with advanced cirrhosis. *Ann Surg* 146:700, 1957.

Newhouse ML, Berry G, Wagner JC: A study of the mortality of female asbestos workers. *Br J Ind Med* 29:134, 1972.

Newhouse ML, Pearson RM, Fullerton JM, Bolsen EA, Shannon, HS: A case control study of carcinoma of the ovary. *Br J Prev Soc Med* 31:148, 1977.

Palmerly TH, Woodruff JD: The ovarian mesothelioma. *Am J Obstet Gynecol* 120:234, 1974.

Patau K: Identification of individual chromosomes, especially in man. *Am J Genet* 12:250, 1960.

Piver SM: *Newsletter—Familial Ovarian Cancer Registry*, April 1989.

Piver SM, Mettlin CG, Tsukada Y, et al: Familial ovarian cancer registry. *Obstet Gynecol* 64:195, 1984.

Proceedings of the National Conference on Cancer Nursing sponsored by the American Cancer Society, September 1973, Chicago. American Cancer Society, New York.

Rapp F: Herpes viruses and cancer. *Adv Cancer Res* 19:265, 1974.

Rashad MN, Fathalla MF, Kerr MG: Sex chromatin and chromosome analysis in ovarian teratomas. *Am J Obstet Gynecol* 96:461, 1966.

Rodenburg CJ, Cornelisso CJ, Heintz PAM, et al: Tumor ploidy as a major prognostic factor in advanced ovarian cancer. *Cancer* 59:317, 1987.

Rossman P (ed): *Hospice*. Fawcett Columbine, New York, 1977.

Silverberg SG: Prognostic significance of pathologic features of ovarian carcinoma. In Nogales F (ed): *Ovarian Pathology*. Springer-Verlag, Berlin, 1989, pp. 85–109.

Slot E: Karyologic study of the cancer of the ovary and the cancer cells in the ascitic effusion. *Neoplasma* 14:3, 1967.

Slotman BJ, Rao BR: Ovarian cancer (review). *Anticancer Res* 8:417, 1988.

Spiegelman S, Axel R, Baxt W, et al: Human cancer and animal viral oncology. *Cancer* 34:1406, 1974.

Süss R, Kinzel V, Scribner JD: *Cancer Experiments and Concepts*. Springer-Verlag, New York, 1973.

Takeichi M: The cadherins: cell-cell adhesion molecules controlling animal morphogenesis. *Development* 102:639, 1988.

Takeichi M: Cadherin cell adhesion receptors as a morphogenetic regulator. *Science* 251:1451, 1991.

Tobacman JK, Tucker MA, Kase R, et al: Intraabdominal carcinomatosis after prophylactic oophorectomy in ovarian cancer-prone families. *Lancet*, 2:795, 1982.

Wakonig-Vaartaja T, Auersperg N: Cytogenetics of gynecologic neoplasms. *Clin Obstet Gynecol* 13:813, 1970.

Wakonig-Vaartaja R, Hughes DT: Chromosome studies in 36 gynecological tumors of the cervix, corpus uteri, ovary, vagina and vulva. *Eur J Cancer* 3:263, 1967.

Weiss RR, Richart RM, Okagaki T: DNA content of mucinous tumors of the ovary. *Am J Obstet Gynecol* 103:409, 1969.

Woodruff JD: History of ovarian neoplasia: facts and fancy. *Obstet Gynecol Annu* 5:331, 1976.

Woodruff JD: The pathogenesis of ovarian neoplasia. *Johns Hopkins Med J* 144:117, 1979.

Glossary

Accessible antigens. Antigens of self that are in contact with antibody-forming tissues and with the host, which is normally tolerant.

Active immunization. Direct immunization of the intact individual or immunocompetent cells derived from the individual and returned to him.

Active immunotherapy. May be divided into two groups: specific immunogens and nonspecific adjuvants. Active specific immunotherapy is attempted by immunization of a tumor-bearing patient with autologous tumor cells that have been altered chemically or by irradiation. Nonspecific immunotherapy attempts to augment antitumor immunologic activity with nonspecific stimulants such as BCG or phytohemagglutinin.

Adaptation. Process whereby protection accorded to a foreign graft from the immune reaction of the recipient renders the graft less vulnerable to immunologic attack by the host.

Adjuvant. Substance that, when mixed with an antigen, enhances its antigenicity.

Adoptive immunization. Transfer of immunity from one individual to another by means of specifically immune lymphoid cells or materials derived from such cells capable of transferring specific immunologic information to the recipients' lymphocytes.

Agglutinin. Antibody that produces aggregation or agglutination of a particulate or insoluble antigen.

Allergy. Specifically altered state of reactivity of a host following exposure to an allergen. The term applies to either hypersensitivity or immunity.

Allogeneic. Pertaining to genetically dissimilar individuals of the same species or referring to tissues originating in different individuals of the same species or in members of a different inbred strain.

Allogeneic inhibition. In vitro damage to cells caused by contact with genetically dissimilar cells. When two antigenetically different lymphocytes

are cultured in the presence of phytohemagglutinin (a substance that activates lymphocytes), there is a mutually damaging effect—the opposite of syngeneic preference.

Allotype. Genetically determined, polymorphic, antigenic variations in a given plasma protein that occurs within a species.

α-Fetoprotein (AFP). Serum protein synthesized in the fetus by perivascular hepatic parenchymal cells and found in a high percentage of patients with hepatomas and malignant teratomas, especially of the endodermal sinus type. It is present in concentrations up to 400 mg/dl during early fetal life, falling to less than 3 μg/dl ml in adults. Increased levels may be detected in the serum of adults with hepatoma (80% positive) or teratoma (40% positive) and may be used to follow the progress of the disease.

Alpha ray. Stream of alpha particles, which are helium nuclei.

Anamnestic response. Recall mechanism; the accelerated response of antibody production to an antigen in an animal that previously responded to the antigen; synonymous with secondary immune response.

Anergy. Deficiency in the response to agents that normally induce an immune response, especially delayed hypersensitivity.

Aneuploid. Having a chromosome number that is not an exact multiple of the haploid number; associated with invasive cancer.

Antibody. Specific globulin (immunoglobulin) produced in response to stimulation by an antigen and capable of reacting specifically with that antigen. A paratope is the site or area on an antibody molecule complementary to the epitope on the antigen molecule. The number of paratopes per molecule is the valence of the antibody.

Antigen. Substance capable of inducing the production of specific immunity. The antigens may be extrinsic (not a constituent of the cell), intrinsic (constituent of the cell), or occult (self-antigen that does not reach antibody-forming tissues).

Antigen determinant (epitope). Small three-dimensional configuration of the everted surface of the antigen molecule that combines with a specific antibody. The total number of antigen determinants per antigen molecule is the valence of that antigen.

Antiserum. Serum containing antibodies and obtained from animals exposed to antigen(s) of a certain nature.

Atopy. Hereditary predisposition to develop immediate-type hypersensitivity on contact with certain antigens (atopens or reagins).

Autoantigen. Substance in a person's tissue to which he or she is immunologically sensitive.

Autochthonous. Tissues of any sort originating in the same host or tumor borne by the host of origin.

Autologous. Derived from the subject itself.

Axiom. Established principle (e.g., that a neoplasm is named from its most differentiated portion and graded from its least differentiated parts).

Bacteriophage. Virus that uses bacteria as host cells.

B cell, B lymphocyte. Bone marrow cell. These cells mediate humoral immunity and are thymus-independent. In the avian species, B cells are derived from the bursa of Fabricius. In man, no discrete bursa has been identified.

Bergonie and Tribondeau 1906. Radiosensitivity of cells and tissues in proportion to their reproductive capacity and in inverse proportion to their degree of differentiation.

Beta particle. Comes from a neutron in the nucleus. A neutron may split into a proton and an electron. The electron is then ejected from the nucleus as a beta particle.

Binding site. Antibody-combining sites and other sites of specific attachment of macromolecules to one another.

Biologic response modifiers (BRM). Compounds that modify an immune response, usually enhancing it. They include immunopotentiating bacterial products, chemicals such as polynucleotides, physiologically active molecules such as thymic hormones and interferon, and the two adjuvants administered with the antigen. A number of these substances have been used in an attempt to potentiate immune reactions in cancer patients and those with immunodeficiency. The body's inherent biochemical capacity for killing cancer cells is combined with the new genetic technology to produce biologic response modification, or biomodulation.

Blast transformation. Transformation of small lymphocytes with minimal cytoplasm, condensed nuclei, and few cytoplasmic organelles into a lymphoblast characterized by abundant cytoplasm, numerous organelles, and a large nucleus with multiple nucleoli. Blast transformation may be induced by a number of mitogens.

Blocking antibody. Antibody of the IgG class that combines with allergen and prevents it from reacting with cell-fixed IgE.

Blocking factor (enhancement antibody). Humoral antibody or antigen–antibody complex that acts as a noncytotoxic antibody. Instead of damaging the cell, it coats it with a protective covering so neither complement nor killer lymphocytes can attack the cell.

Brachytherapy. (Greek *brachy*: short; and *therapy*: treatment) Term used to distinguish the therapeutic use of encapsulated radionuclides close to the tumor from their use at a distance from the tumor. For the latter, the term *teletherapy* (Greek *tele*: far) has been used.

Cadherins. Family of glycoproteins involved in the calcium-dependent cell–cell adhesion mechanism that is detected in most tissues. Cadherins play a crucial role in construction of tissues and the whole animal body. Almost no other biochemical event bridges so many levels of biologic organization as cell adhesion. Cadherins are thus considered to be important regulators of morphogenesis. Moreover, pathologic examinations suggest that down-regulation of cadherin expression is associated with the invasiveness of tumor cells.

CA 15-3 (breast antigens 115D8/DF3). Used in an immunoradiomimetic assay with monoclonal antibodies to breast carcinoma cell lines MCF-7 and defatted milk fat globules. Preliminary clinical data indicate a sensitivity of 57% in primary lesions preoperatively and 79% in metastatic breast cancer.

Cathepsin D. Estrogen-induced lysosomal enzyme. Overexpression of cathepsin D is an independent predictor for tumor recurrence and death among node-negative breast cancer patients.

Cancer. (Latin *cancri*: crab). An inclusive term used to describe a variety of malignant neoplasms.

Cancer antigen 125 (CA 125). The 125th monoclonal antibody screened was designated OC 125 and its antigenic determinant was called CA 125. The presence of the CA 125 antigenic determinant in serum can be identified only by the OC 125 antibody. CA 125 is used in an immunoradiomimetic assay with a monoclonal antibody (OC 125); it has 88% sensitivity for detecting nonmucinous epithelial ovarian carcinoma and 60% sensitivity for detecting uterine cancer.

Cancerous growth. Cancerous growth measuring 1 cc (approximately $\frac{1}{16}$ cubic inch) and weighing about 1 g (approximately $\frac{1}{30}$ ounce) is about the smallest that can be detected by palpation or roentgenography, yet it contains about one billion cancer cells, each perhaps capable of originating a new focus of disease.

Carbohydrate antigen 19-9 (CA 19-9). Used in an immunoradiomimetic assay with a monoclonal antibody against sialylated Lewis[a] antigen (blood group substance); useful in pancreatic, gastric, hepatic, and recurrent colorectal carcinoma. This antigen is also termed gastrointestinal cancer-associated antigen (GICA). Patients who are Le[a-b-] test negative with this assay.

Carboplatin. White to off-white crystalline powder with the molecular formula of $C_6H_{12}M_2O_4Pt$ and a molecular weight of 371.25 daltons. It is soluble in water at a rate of approximately 14 mg/ml, and the pH of a 1% solution is 5 to 7. It is virtually insoluble in ethanol, acetone, and dimethylacetamide. Carboplatin, like cisplatin, produces predominantly interstrand DNA cross-links rather than DNA–protein cross-links. This effect is apparently cell-cycle-nonspecific. The aquation of carboplatin, which is thought to produce the active species, occurs at a slower rate than in the case of *cis*-platinum. Despite this difference, it appears that both carboplatin and *cis*-platinum induce equal numbers of drug–DNA cross-links, causing equivalent lesions and biologic effect. The difference in potencies for carboplatinum and *cis*-platinum appear to be directly related to the difference in aquation rates.

Carcinoembryonic antigen (CEA). Antigen found originally in fetal tissues of endodermal origin as well as in malignant tumors of adult tissues of endodermal origin. It probably results when a gene is derepressed by some stimulus. Because other tissues have been found to contain CEA, it is possible that the CEA molecule has more than one antigenic surface determinant.

Carcinoma. In modern medicine: all malignant tumors.

Cell cycle distribution (CCD). Cell cycle distribution analysis of a specimen measures the proportion of cells in the proliferative phase of the cell cycle (S, G2, and M phases). Survival is significantly better from tumors with a low proliferative activity. A high S-phase fraction indicates a poorly differen-

tiated, aneuploid tumor likely to be estrogen receptor-negative and progesterone receptor-negative. Prognosis is poor if the high cell cycle distribution for S phase is greater than 10.

Cell-mediated immunity (CMI). Specific immunity mediated by small lymphocytes. They are thymus-dependent cells and are referred to as T cells, in contrast to the thymus-independent cells, which are called B cells. The T cells are probably the most important cells of cancer immunity and organ rejection.

Central venous pressure. The following data have been helpful for interpreting central venous pressure (measured in centimeters of water), assuming there is no significant abnormality of cardiac output:

0–5 cm H_2O pressure = hypovolemia
6–12 cm H_2O pressure = normovolemia
>12 cm H_2O pressure = hypervolemia

Chalones. Group of naturally occurring substances that are sensitized by cells and appear to be importantly involved in the regulation of cell division as well as in the differentiation of such normal cell types as epidermal cells, liver and kidney cells, granulocytes, and certain other cell types. Because the antimitotic effect of these substances is tissue-specific and they are essentially nontoxic, they appear to represent an almost ideal group of substances for use in the suppression of growth of those tumors that have lost the ability to synthesize their own chalones but remain sensitive to their inhibitory effects.

Chimerism. State in which two or more genetically different populations of cells coexist.

Chromosome. Carriers of genetic information composed of DNA on a framework of protein. They are in the cell nucleus and are visible in a dividing cell as deeply staining rod-shaped or J-shaped structures.

Cis-platinum   (*cis*-diamminedichloro-platinum). Heavy metal complex containing a central atom of platinum surrounded by two chloride atoms and two ammonia molecules in a *cis* position. It is a white, lyophilized powder with the molecular formula $PtCl_2H_6N_2$ and molecular weight 300.1 daltons. It is soluble in water or saline at 1 mg/ml and in dimethylformamide at 24 mg/ml. It has a melting point of 207°C.

Citrate intoxication. Intoxication characterized by hypotension, narrow pulse pressure, and elevated left ventricular end-diastolic and central venous pressures.

Clonal selection theory of acquired immunity of Burnet. Theory suggesting that immunity and antibody production are functions of clones of mesenchymal cells. Each clone is able to react immuno-logically with a small number of antigens, and each cell is immunologically competent because it carries on its surface a receptor that is able to react with a given antigen.

Clone. Group of cells derived from single original cells by asexual division; they are therefore genetically identical.

Cobalt 60. Radioactive isotope with a half-life of 5.3 years that emits beta and gamma radiations (1.17 and 1.33 MeV); used as teletherapy.

Common epithelial ovarian cancers. Cancers composed of one or more of several types of epithelium and stroma in a variety of combinations. They are generally considered to be derived from the surface epithelium (mesothelium) covering the ovary and from the underlying ovarian stroma. The word *common* has been applied because most ovarian tumors belong in this general category.

Serous tumors. Composed of epithelium resembling that of the fallopian tube or the surface epithelium of the ovary. Ciliated epithelium is found on the benign tumors but rarely in the presence of cancer. Psammoma bodies may be present, and any mucus produced is extracellular.

Mucinous tumors. Composed of tumors whose epithelial element includes a prominent component of mucin-filled cells. The epithelium may resemble endocervical or enteric epithelium, occasionally containing argentaffin cells and rarely Paneth cells. From time to time the question is raised whether these tumors should be included among the germ cell tumors as teratomas. The differential diagnosis should include metastatic adenocarcinoma from the large bowel.

Endometrioid tumors. Have microscopic features of one or more of the typical forms of endometrial neoplasia. A small number of endometrioid tumors can be shown to arise in endometriosis, but the demonstration of such an origin is not required for the diagnosis. Endometrioid carcinomas may have a markedly papillary pattern, which is unusual in carcinomas of the endometrium.

Clear-cell (mesonephroid) tumors. Composed of cells that contain glycogen and resemble cells of renal cell carcinoma or the hobnail or peg-shaped cells lining small cysts and tubules. Hobnail cells are characterized by scant cytoplasm and large nuclei that project into the lumen. The clear-cell tumor must be distinguished from the endodermal sinus tumor, dysgerminoma, and lipid cell tumor.

Common language. Until the International Federation of Gynecology and Obstetrics (FIGO) established a histologic classification and clinical staging for ovarian cancer in 1971, there was no common language.

Complement. System of serologically nonspecific proteins present in fresh normal serum that are necessary for the lysis or death of cellular antigens in the presence of antibody.

Concomitant tumor immunity. Ability to reject a second tumor graft while the first tumor graft continues to grow. A piece of a tumor removed and implanted close to the original tumor usually continues to grow, whereas the same piece of tumor transplanted at a distance from the original tumor may be rejected.

Coombs test. Use of antiglobulin antiserum produced in a heterologous species to detect non-agglutinating antibodies on the surface of red blood cells.

Cosmid. Genetically engineered plasmid that can be packaged in a bacteriophage code and introduced into host bacterial cells by a process of phage infection.

Curie. Quantity of any radioisotope that disintegrates at the rate of 3.7×10^{10} disintegrations per second. Subunits of the curie (Ci) unit are the millicurie (mCi) = 1/1000 of a curie; microcurie (μCi) = 1/1000 of a millicurie; millimicrocurie (mμCi) = 1/1000 of a microcurie.

Cycling index (CI). Measures the rate of cellular proliferation in most tumor activity. The CI distinguishes G0 (resting) cells from S, G2, M, and G1 phases of the cell cycle. Recurrence is significantly more frequent, with more active tumors having high proliferative rates regardless of stage.

Cytophilic antibody. Globulin component of immune serum that becomes attached in vitro to certain normal cells in such a way that these cells are subsequently capable of specifically absorbing antigens.

Deblocking antibody. Antibody capable of overcoming the inhibitory effect of blocking factor, thereby permitting immunologic destruction of malignant cells.

Delayed hypersensitivity. See *Cell-mediated immunity.*

Dinitrochlorobenzene (DNCB). Drug used to test for cell-mediated immunity. When applied to the skin it acts as a hapten, attaching to a protein in the skin and producing an antigen that has the potential to sensitize lymphocytes. Within 2 weeks the challenge produces a marked local response in patients with good cell-mediated immunity.

Disseminated intravascular coagulation (DIC). Characterized by a triad of thrombocytopenia, hypofibrinogenemia, and lysis of a blood clot within 2 hours.

DM/70K (dianon marker NB/70K). Marker used in a radioimmunoassay for detecting human ovarian tumor-associated antigen NB/70K using the monoclonal antibody NB12123. Sensitivity of 70% is found for ovarian carcinoma. Elevated levels have also been associated with other gynecologic malignancies, as well as carcinoma of the lung and breast.

DNA index (DI). The DNA index of a tumor cell indicates the degree of aneuploidy (aneuploid cells have an abnormal number of chromosomes). Highly aneuploid tumors have the worst prognosis and diploid tumors the best.

DNA ligase. Enzyme that covalently joins two pieces of double-stranded DNA.

DNA probes. Direct approach to medical diagnosis by going right to the patient's or the infecting microorganism's genes. Methods for cutting, reproducing, and selecting links of DNA are allowing biologists to do just that. The method is based on the strong bonding between strands of DNA molecules with complementary sequences. Of the four types of DNA subunits that form each strand, adenosine on one strand tends to line up with a thymidine on the other strand, and guanine pairs with cytosine. This binding of strands is called *hybridization*. It depends on the same forces that hold together the two strands of the DNA helix. Although the match of complementary bases does not need to be perfect for hybridization to occur, the better the match the tighter the binding.

Electrophilic atom. Electron-deficient atom, e.g., a carcinogen. See *Nucleophilic atom*.

Enhancement antibody. See *Blocking factor*.

Epidemiology. Cancer epidemiology seeks to correlate differences in the incidence of different types of cancer with already established differences in the external or internal environment of the persons developing these cancers, e.g., the relation identified between cigarette smoking and lung cancer.

Epidermal growth factor receptor (EGFR). Used in an investigational assay. EGFR-negative tumors carry a prognosis similar to that for estrogen receptor (ER)-positive disease, even in ER-negative tumors; 90% of EGFR-positive tumors are ER-negative. EGFR-negative status may best define a subgroup of ER-negative patients with better survival.

Epigenetic change. Change due to an alteration of a nongenetic biochemical process that sometimes affects the hereditary material. It is theoretically a reversible process.

Epithelial ovarian cancers. See *Common epithelial ovarian cancers*.

Epitope. Part of an antigen that directs specificity. Antibodies produced in response to antigen react specifically with each individual determinant group of epitope.

Established tumor. In tests of substances for antigrowth activity against transplantable tumors in animals, the test substance is sometimes given before there is any visible growth of the tumor. If, on the other hand, the tumor implant is allowed to grow before the test substance is administered, it is referred to as "established."

Etiology. Cancer etiology is the study of the causes of cancer. Its ultimate goal is cancer prevention. Three agent have now been shown to cause cancers: chemicals, radiation, and viruses. Of these agents, two (chemicals and radiation) clearly cause cancer in humans, and the third (virus) is highly suspect on the basis of present knowledge.

Ewing's histologic grading. Ewing influenced many pathologists when he presented material using only three grades. Using Ewing-inspired grades, Broders' grades III and IV are combined and called grade III. The histologic classification is based on the uniformity or lack of uniformity of the cells, whether the nucleus is regular, the nucleus/cytoplasm ratio, the number and size of the nucleoli, and the number of mitoses per high-power field.

Familial ovarian cancer. Patients at high risk for familial ovarian cancer include those with two first-degree blood relatives who have ovarian cancer or if the patient's mother had ovarian cancer before the menopause. A first-degree blood relative is identified as a mother, sister, or daughter. Aunts and grandmothers are considered second-degree blood relatives.

Favored or privileged site. Anatomic region where foreign tissues tend to survive because of the diminished ability of an immunologic reaction to be incited there.

Ferritin. Used for a radioimmunoassay measuring a dimeric iron-storage protein containing sialic acid. With head and neck cancers, decreasing ferritin levels are prognostic of successful therapy. With neuroblastoma, ferritin levels are used to monitor the course of the disease.

Forbidden clone. Hypothetical clone of immunologically competent cells with specificity for self-antigens that, according to the clonal selection theory, has been suppressed during fetal life but may regain activity during adult life and cause autoimmune disease.

Freund's adjuvant. *Complete*: Freund's water-in-oil emulsion of mineral oil, plant waxes, and killed tubercle bacilli used to incorporate with antigen to stimulate antibody production. *Incomplete*: Freund's mixture without tubercle bacilli.

Gene. Elementary germinal unit, situated in chromosomes, that carries a hereditary transmissible character. It is composed of distinctly arranged deoxyribonucleic acid chains. Histocompatibility genes are special entities, the nature of which determines the fate of grafts.

Genome. Complete set of hereditary factors of an organism, as contained in the haploid assortment of chromosomes.

Genotype. Sum of the genes of an organism.

Germ cell tumors. Undifferentiated tumors; in some, extraembryonic structures predominate; in others, the predominant structures are immature or mature structures that may be derived from any or all of the three embryonic layers (ectoderm, mesoderm, endoderm).

Dysgerminoma. Composed of germ cells that have not differentiated to form embryonic or extraembryonic structures. The tumor has a uniform appearance and is composed of large, rounded, clear cells that resemble primordial germ cells morphologically and histochemically. Its stroma is almost always infiltrated with lymphocytes and often contains granulomas similar to those of sarcoid.

Teratomas

Extraembryonal forms. Endodermal sinus tumor is composed of embryonal cells lining a network of spaces. The most specific feature is the presence within some of the spaces of isolated papillary projections containing single blood vessels and having a peripheral lining of neoplastic cells. The tumor resembles the endodermal sinuses of the rat placenta. It contains intracellular and extracellular hyaline bodies resembling Russell bodies. When, on rare occasions, these vesicles form a major portion of the neoplasm, it is called a polyvesicular vitelline tumor.

Choriocarcinoma. Rare tumor composed of both cytotrophoblast and syncytiotrophoblast. It may be associated with precocious puberty.

Adult teratoma. Composed exclusively of mature (adult) structures. It may be solid or cystic. The cystic is commonly called a dermoid. It is made up mainly of ectodermal elements but

may contain endodermal and mesodermal tissue.

Embryonal teratoma. Contains immature (embryonal) structures. Mature tissue may be present as well. The tumor is highly malignant and usually radioresistant. *Polyembryonic embryoma* is an unusual and poorly differentiated form of embryonal teratoma. Myriad early embryos make up a large portion of the tumor.

Struma ovarii. Thyroid tissue is exclusively present or constitutes a grossly recognizable component of a more complex teratoma.

Carcinoids. Arise most often from respiratory or gastrointestinal epithelium in a dermoid cyst but may develop within a solid teratoma or a mucinous cystic tumor.

Gonadal stromal tumors

Female type. Granulosa cell tumor is the most common. It may contain not only granulosa cells but also varying numbers of spindle-shaped, collagen-producing cells, elements resembling theca cells, and lutein cells. A variety of microscopic patterns may be encountered: microfollicular, macrofollicular, trabecular, cyclindromatous, insular, gyriform, solid-tubular, and sarcomatoid or diffuse.

Male type. Sertoli-Leydig cell tumor contains Sertoli and Leydig cells of varying degrees of maturity; indifferent gonadal cells of embryonal appearance are present in certain cases. The designation *arrhenoblastoma* has been abandoned because not all of these tumors produce masculinization.

Gynandroblastoma. Rare tumor in which collections of granulosa cells with typical Call-Exner bodies coexist with hollow tubules lined by Sertoli cells.

Gonadoblastoma. Rare ovarian cancer composed of germ cells (dysgerminoma) and gonadal stromal cells (granulosa-Sertoli). Sex chromatin studies usually show a negative nuclear pattern (46,XY) or sex chromosome mosaicism (XO/XY). Most patients are intersexual with phenotype female habitus, amenorrheic, and possibly virilized. The malignancy rate is very low.

Gold, radioactive (^{198}Au). Radioactive isotope with a half-life of 2.7 days that emits beta (960 KeV) and gamma (412 KeV) radiation; used in small sources in a colloidal form to suppress malignant serous effusions and to control free-floating cancer cells in the peritoneal cavity.

Graft-versus-host reaction. In the presence of an immunodeficient host, the graft may produce lymphocytes that react to the host antigen, producing hepatosplenomegaly, lymphopenia, diarrhea, and skin rash. In the very young *runt disease* (allogeneic disease), which develops after injection of allogeneic lymphocytes into immunologically immature experimental animals, produces a picture similar to the one outlined above plus failure to thrive and often death.

Granulosa cell tumor of juvenile type. Characterized by macrofollicular or diffuse pattern of growth often with extensive luteinization and hyperchromatic nuclei, features giving it a somewhat malignant appearance that is not supported by its generally benign pattern of clinical behavior.

Half value layer (HVL). The thickness of a specific material that reduces the flux of radiation by one-half; a function of voltage, filtration, and target material, it is used as a rough gauge of radiation quality.

Haploid. Having a single set of unpaired chromosomes in each nucleus, a characteristic of gametes.

Hapten. Partial antigen that contains at least one of the determinant groups of an antigen. It can react specifically with antibodies but does not itself induce the formation of antibodies unless it is complexed with a carrier molecule such as a protein.

Helper factor. Sensitized T-lymphocyte subpopulations release a helper factor that enables immunocompetent B cells to respond to antigens that they otherwise would be unable to recognize. The stimulated B lymphocytes differentiate into plasma cells, which are the main producers of antibody. Helper factor also stimulates the B lymphocyte to produce a variant of the B cell, the *killer (K) cell*, which is able to attack tumor cells only after the tumor cells have been exposed to specific antibody. Complement is not required for this action. See *Killer cell.*

Hepatitis-associated antigen (Australian antigen). This antigen (Au antigen), first detected in the serum of an Australian aborigine, has been detected in the sera of patients during the incubation period and early clinical course of serum or transfusion hepatitis, but not in the sera of patients with a short incubation form of infectious hepatitis. The serum of patients carrying the antigen has been shown, by electron microscopy, to contain aggregates of pleomorphic particles and tubules. The aggregates have been interpreted to be antigen–antibody complexes, and the particles are thought to be antigen derived from the virus that caused the infection.

HER-2/neu oncoprotein (H2n). Used in an investigational assay for the protein product of the HER-2/neu oncogene. Amplification of this gene is significantly greater in patients with early relapse and poor survival. With node-positive disease this test may predict outcome better than either estrogen receptors or progesterone receptors.

Heterophil. Pertaining to antigenic specificity shared among species.

Heterozygosity. Occupancy of dissimilar genes in the same chromosome.

Histocompatibility. Ability to accept transplants of tissue from another animal of the same species. Such ability depends on the identical genetic constitution of donor and recipient.

Histologic grading. Broders classification consisted of four numerical grades (I, II, III, IV) for both epidermoid and adenocarcinoma of the cervix. The basis for this classification is the well-known observation that the degree of malignancy keeps pace with the degree of cell differentiation, grade I being the most highly differentiated and grade IV the most immature. The original Broders grading method is cumbersome to apply because as many as 13 cytologic characteristics must be observed and evaluated. The following factors are recorded for each grade: epithelial pearls, individual keratinized cells, intercellular bridges, tumor giant cells, and mitoses per high-power field. Most pathologists now use a simplified version. See *Ewing's histologic grading.*

Histologic type and grading. Parameters used to classify the microscopic characteristics of the tumor.

HL-A antigen (human leukocyte antigen). Genetic locus containing two closely linked groups of several alleles, i.e., subloci. It is present on the cell membranes of all nucleated cells and plays a major role in determining graft rejection.

Horizontal transmission of viruses. Transmission among individual hosts of the same generation. See *Vertical transmission of viruses.*

Host. Organism whose body serves to sustain a graft; loosely interchangeable with *recipient.*

Human chorionic gonadotropin, β-subunit (β-hCG). Ordinarily made by the placenta and used as an indicator of pregnancy. Measured in an enzyme immunoassay. β-hCG is also produced by tumors of germ cell origin, such as testicular and ovarian cancers, as well as some lung cancers.

Humoral immunity. Any immune reaction that can be transferred with immune serum is termed humoral immunity (in contrast to cell-mediated immuniy). In general, this term refers to resistance that results from the presence of specific antibody. It is initiated by the thymus-independent B cells. These B lymphocytes proliferate and differentiate into plasma cells that secrete immunoglobulins (IgG, IgM, IgA, IgD, IgE).

Hybrid. Animal whose parents belong to different species. Ordinarily, procreation depends on a fixed sexual role of one or the other species' partners. When it occurs, regardless of the sexual identity of the mated species, the offspring is a reciprocal hybrid (mutual hybrid).

Hybridomas. Cells produced by the physical fusion of two different cells. Although normal cells are mortal, tumor cells may be immortal. Therefore selected mouse myeloma cells are fused with lymphocytes from the spleen of mice immunized with a particular antigen, with the result being a hybrid myeloma, or "hybridoma." Hybridomas express the lymphocytes' property of specific antibody production and the immortal character of the myeloma cells. Individual hybrid cells can be cloned, and each clone produces large amounts of identical antibody to a single antigenic determinant. The individual clones can be maintained indefinitely.

Idiotype. Unique antigenic determinant on the antigen-binding region of an immunoglobulin molecule.

Immunogen. Antigen that induces a specific immunologic response.

Immunologic surveillance. Described by Sir F. Mac-Farlane Burnet, effective immunologic surveillance depends on the presence of tumor-specific antigenic determinants on the surfaces of neoplastic cells, which enable these altered cells to be recognized as nonself and to be destroyed by immunologic reactions.

Immunoreaction. Reaction between antigen and its antibody.

Interferon. Protein released by cells in response to virus infection. It represents nonspecific immunity.

Interleukins. Group of antigen nonspecific factors involved in lymphocyte activation and differentiation. Interleukin 1 (IL-1)/lymphocyte activating factor (LAF) is produced by macrophages and other antigen-producing cells. It acts on T cells to induce interleukin 2 (IL-2) receptors. IL-2/T cell growth factor (TCGF) is produced by activated T cells. It is necessary for the long-term proliferation of T cells and can also act on previously stimulated B cells. Interleukin 3 (IL-3) is one of the colony-stimulating factors (CSF) produced by cell lines of several lineages that induces proliferation of lymphocytes.

Killer cell (K cell). Sensitized T lymphocytes produce a helper factor that acts on the immunocompetent cell to produce a population of cells, possibly variants of the B cell, termed killer cells, which are able to attack tumor cells that have been exposed to a specific antibody. Unlike the usual humoral antibody (immunoglobulin) response, complement is not needed to destroy the cell.

Krükenberg tumor. Metastatic lesion of distinctive appearance characterized by the presence of mucus-filled signet-ring cells accompanied by sarcoma-like proliferation of the ovarian stroma. This tumor is usually secondary to gastric cancer but may originate in any organ in which mucinous carcinomas arise, including the breast and intestine. On rare occasions a tumor with the pattern of a Krükenberg tumor appears to be primary in the ovary.

Line. Group of cells grown under defined conditions from initially heterogeneous populations. Only occasionally is such a line monoclonal.

Linear energy transfer (LET). Measure of the average rate of energy loss along the track of an ionizing particle, expressed as energy units per unit track length. It is the energy released (usually in kiloelectron volts) per micrometer of medium (tissue) along the track of any ionizing particle.

Lipid-associated sialic acid in plasma (LASA-P). Biomarker useful in a wide range of malignancies; it reflects alteration in the surface membrane of malignant cells. The LASA-P test measures total gangliosides and glycoproteins by the biochemical extraction and partition method of Katopodis et al. Sensitivities range between 77 and 97%, depending on the cell origin of the neoplasm. Studies have shown improved predictive value when the LASA-P test is combined with other biomarkers and biomarker profiles.

Locus. Precise location of a gene on a chromosome. Different forms of the gene (alleles) are always found at the same position on the chromosome. A complex locus is a locus within which mutation and recombination can occur at more than one site.

Lymphokine. Substances released by sensitized lymphocytes when they come in contact with the antigen to which they are sensitized. There are at least four mediators of cellular immunity, including transfer factor, lymphocyte-transforming activity, migration inhibition factor, and lymphotoxins.

Lymphotoxins. Family of glycoproteins. The various lymphocyte populations release different forms of lymphotoxin, generally under stimulation by an antigen lectin. The molecules have cytostatic or cytotoxic capabilities and may be involved in various T-cell cytotoxic reactions.

Lysogeny. Virus joins up with the DNA of the cell and is carried along through many generations. It is inactive unless some noxious agent stimulates it to become active. *Lysogeny:* The virus is part of the DNA of the cell. *Transduction:* Some of the DNA is carried along as part of the virus.

Macrophage. Large mononuclear phagocyte. In tissues this cell may be designated a histiocyte and in blood a monocyte. Macrophages in the spleen, lymph nodes, and thymus are known as sinus-lining macrophages (sometimes called reticulum cells). An antigen must contact or pass through a macrophage before it can become a processed antigen with the ability to encounter and then sensitize a small lymphocyte.

Macrophage-activating factor (MAF). Increases microbicidal and cytotoxic capacity of macrophages; it is now known to be partly due to interferon-gamma (IFN-γ). Activated macrophages have the capacity to kill tumor cells nonspecifically but selectively. They recognize transform (malignant) cells as foreign and are selectively cytotoxic to them but not to nonmalignant cells.

Major histocompatibility complex (MHC). Also known as the human leukocyte antigen (HLA) system, the MHC comprises a group of genes located on the short arm of chromosome 6. These genes coat for surface antigens on many kinds of cell. They are critical to the recognition of self versus nonself, as the MHC defines what is self. Thus HLA antigens are important to tissue cross-matching procedures and are partially responsible for tissue transplant rejection, which occurs when a donor MHC and recipient MHC do not match.

Meson. Particle 200 times heavier than the electron that was found among cosmic rays. According to the two meson theories, the heavier mesons would be found at high altitudes in the earth's atmosphere, where cosmic rays had knocked them out of the nuclei. The decay products, the lighter mesons, would be found at lower altitudes.

Migration inhibition factor (MIF). Lymphokine produced when a sensitized lymphocyte is cultured in the presence of an antigen to which it is sensitized. It inhibits the migration of these lymphocytes.

Mitogen. Substance that induces lymphocytes to undergo blast transformation, mitosis, and cell division (causing mitosis or cell division).

Mixed lymphocyte (leukocyte) culture (MLC). Results from transformation of small lymphocytes to blast cells, with synthesis of DNA, in mixed cultures of blood leukocytes from normal allogeneic individuals. The magnitude of the reaction reflects the degree of disparity between histocompatibility antigens of the two donors. In identical twins neither set stimulates the other, whereas in unrelated pairs there is almost always stimulation of each cell by the other. The degree of stimulation is analyzed either morphologically by blast transformation or biochemically by measuring tritiated thymidine incorporation into newly synthesized DNA.

Monoclonal antibodies. Homogenous antibodies produced by a single clone. They are usually from hybridomas, which are prepared by fusing immunized mouse or rat spleen cells with a nonsecretor myeloma using polyethylene glycol or Sendai virus. The fusion mixture is plated out in HAT medium (hypoxanthine/aminopterin/thymidine). Aminopterin blocks a metabolic pathway that can be bypassed if hypoxanthine and thymidine are present, but the myeloma cells lack this bypass and consequently die in HAT medium. Spleen cells also die naturally in culture after 1 to 2 weeks; a few cells survive, as they have the immortality of the myeloma and the metabolic bypass of the spleen cells. Some of the fused cells secrete antibody, and the supernatants are tested in a specific assay. The desired antibody is then fused and can be maintained indefinitely.

Monoclonal, oligoclonal, polyclonal. Derived according to whether it is due to one, a few, or many clones.

Mosaic. Individual composed of two or more cell lines from the same species. It can come about either through somatic mutation or by grafting cells between individuals of a close genetic constitution, such as dizygotic twins.

Müllerian inhibiting substance (MIS). Fetal testicular product that produces regression of the müllerian ducts in male embryos. It is manufactured by Sertoli cells in the fetal testes, producing a nonsteroidal substance know as MIS.

NB/70K (Dianon marker NB/70K-DN/70K). Human ovarian tumor-associated antigen. It is measured in a radioimmunoassay using the monoclonal antibody NB12 123. Sensitivity of 70% for ovarian cancer.

Nuclear grade. Nuclei of the tumor cells are graded from 1 to 3 according to the classification of Black and Speer. Grade 1: markedly enlarged, irregular in outline, chromatin clumping, and prominent nucleoli. Grade 2: intermediate degree of differentiation. Grade 3: in terms of size and appearance, similar to each other and to normal ovarian tissue when present. Grade 1 is the most anaplastic and grade 3 the least anaplastic.

Nucleophilic atom. Atom with excess electrons. The information-containing macromolecules of the cell (DNA, RNA, protein) are relatively rich in nucleophilic sites; and in cases that have been adequately studied, derivates of chemical carcinogens have been found to be firmly bound to the DNA, RNA, and protein of target tissues. Furthermore, in some cases susceptibility to cancer formation by chemical carcinogens has been correlated with the kinds and amounts of these macromolecule-bound carcinogens. See *Electrophilic atom*.

Nude mice (nu nu mice). Mice born with a congenital absence of the thymus. The blood and thymus-dependent areas of the lymph nodes and spleen are depleted of lymphocytes. These mice are homozygous for the gene "nude"—abbreviated *Nu*, hence *nu nu*—and they have no hair. They should be distinguished from mice carrying other genes that cause a lack of hair (e.g., shaven, *sha*; hairless, *hr*; bare, *br*; hair loss, *hl*). All of the latter strains have a normal thymus.

Ovary. Female gonad.

Supernumerary ovary. Independent of and equal in size to the normal ovary. It is rare.

Accessory ovaries. Usually attached to the normal gland by peritoneal bands in the mesovarium or adjacent part of the broad ligament, near the hilum of the ovary. They have clinical significance if they undergo pathologic changes or when bilateral oophorectomy is carried out; their presence may result in continued ovarian activity. Accessory ovaries *occur in about 3% of women*.

Ectopic ovaries. May be congenital or acquired; acquired type is much more common. Congenital displacement may be due to nondescent, a phenomenon by which the ovary remains above the pelvic brim, or it may be due to the ovary having been pulled into the inguinal canal or large labia by the gubernaculum. The acquired type is common and may follow pregnancy with prolapse of the ovary into the cul-de-sac.

Overgrowth stimulating factor (OSF). Can cause normal cells in culture to adopt the appearance and growth habit of the transformed cell. Stimulated cells revert to normal when the overgrowth stimulating factor is removed.

Oxygen enhancement ratio (OER). Radiation dose under anoxic conditions/dose under fully oxygenated conditions required to produce an equivalent effect. OER for most mammalian cells is about 3.

P-170 glycoprotein. Resistant cells express a distinct transmembrane protein called P-glycoprotein (molecular weight 170,000 daltons). It can be measured with the monoclonal antibody C219. P-glycoprotein acts as a toxin pump, clearing chemotherapeutic agents from the cell before they can kill it. It is of interest as an early warning of developing resistance, allowing the oncologist to quickly redirect therapy.

Paratrope. See *Antibody*.

Passive transfer of immunity. The transfer of specific antibody from one individual to another.

Penumbra. Radiation just outside and adjacent to the full beam arising from the finite size of the source; its usage usually includes components from scatter in tissue or from incomplete beam collimation.

Phosphorus 32 (^{32}P). Beta emitter with a maximum energy of 1.7 MeV and a half-life of 14.2 days. It may be given orally, intravenously, or intraperitoneally. It is maximally incorporated into cells with short turnover times and is used to suppress malignant serous effusions and to control free-floating cancer cells in the peritoneal cavity.

Phytohemagglutinins. Lectins extracted from the red kidney bean *Phaseolus vulgaris* or *Phaseolus communis*. They can be purified to yield a glycoprotein mitogen, which stimulates lymphocyte transformation and causes agglutination of certain red blood cells. Phytohemagglutinins provide a method for estimating the pool of thymus-dependent lymphocytes (T cells).

Pi mesons (pions). Heavy mesons, they can be positive, negative, or neutral. They are 270 times heavier than the electron.

Plasmid. Small, circular, extrachromosomal, self-replicating piece of DNA found in some bacteria.

PMPO syndrome (postmenopausal ovary syndrome). Palpation of what is interpreted as a normal-sized ovary in the premenopausal woman represents an ovarian tumor in the postmenopausal woman.

Pneumocystis *carinii*. Example of a parasite of low-grade virulence that presents a clinical problem only in the *immunologically compromised* host. The organism induces a pneumonitis with characteristic clinical and pathologic findings. Three groups of susceptible hosts have been defined: (1) premature or debilitated infants; (2) individuals with primary immunodeficiency disorders; and (3) individuals with a malignancy or who are receiving immunosuppressive therapy and who demonstrate an immunologic deficit. There is increasing dyspnea, progressive cyanosis, and a dry, nonproductive cough. Most remarkable is the lack of systemic reaction to this infection, and many patients are usually dyspneic and cyanotic, even in the absence of fever, malaise, or anorexia. The laboratory findings include demonstration of a ventilation perfusion deficit, with a relatively normal pH and PCO_2 and a low PCO_2. Serologic techniques for the diagnosis of the diseases are hindered in humans because most affected individuals have immunodeficiency states and are therefore incapable of an antibody response.

Pokeweed mitogen (PWM). Mitogen extracted from the pokeweed plant that can be purified to yield a glycoprotein. The pokeweed mitogen stimulates blast formation of both B and T cells.

Prophylactic immunization. Immunization of an individual against a causative agent (e.g., a virus) or tumor-specific antigen before any natural encounter with the agent or tumor.

Proto-oncogene. Normal gene that is modified and becomes an oncogene.

Rad. Unit of absorbed dose of ionizing radiation equivalent to the absorption of 100 ergs per gram of irradiated material.

Radioactivity, artificial. Emission of radiant energy arising from the breakdown of nuclei that have been energetically unstable, e.g., ^{60}Co and ^{137}Cs.

Radioactivity, natural. Emission of radiant energy arising from the breakdown of nuclei that are unstable in their natural states, e.g., radium.

Receptors. Specific molecules on the surface or within the cytoplasm of a cell that recognizes and binds with other specific molecules.

Estrogen receptors (ERs). ER test measures receptor expression and reports a tumor as ER-positive or ER-negative. ER-negative tumors are aggressive and rarely respond to endocrine therapy. ER status is a strong, independent predictor of recurrence and survival. ER-negative means that there is less than 10 femtomoles (fmol) ER/mg cytosol protein.

Progesterone receptors (PRs). PR expression is reported as positive or negative. PRs have greater predictive value than ERs and are better correlated with the outcome of endocrine therapy. PR-positive may indicate false-negative ER results. PR-negative means that there is less than 10 fmol PR/mg cytosol protein.

Epidermal growth factor receptors (EGFRs). EGFR-negative tumors carry a prognosis similar to that of ER-positive disease, even in ER-negative tumors. Ninety percent of EGFR-positive tumors are ER-negative. EGFR-negative status may thus define a subgroup of ER-negative patients with better survival. EGFR-negative means that there is less than 5 fmol/mg protein.

Restriction endonuclease. Enzyme that cleaves double-stranded DNA at or near recognition sites of specific base sequences.

Retrovirus. RNA virus encoding an enzyme that makes a DNA copy of its RNA and splices it into the host chromosome.

Reverse transcriptase (RNA-dependent DNA polymerase). This recently isolated factor can transcribe the base sequence of a viral RNA onto a DNA strand in vitro. It is now possible to test human cancers for association with any one of a number of RNA viruses.

Second look operation. Reoperation of a patient at a stated time who has no evidence of clinical disease.

Selective IgG deficiency. Associated with a variety of disorders but most frequently with diseases of an autoimmune nature. It affects 1 in 700 individuals. The immunoelectrophoretic pattern shows an absence of IgA. Cellular immunity is intact, and all other immunoglobulins are present, e.g., IgG, IgM, IgD, and IgE.

Sequestered antigen. Any antigen or antigenic determinant that is hidden from contact with immunologically competent cells or antibody and thus cannot stimulate an immune response. They may be intracellular antigens or hidden determinants on cell surfaces or on soluble molecules.

Serology. Study of antigen–antibody reactions in vitro.

Serum sickness reaction. Systemic allergy to the administration of a large amount of serum or purified foreign protein. Its appearance coincides with, and is caused by, the interaction of newly formed antibody with excess antigen circulating in the blood and tissue fluids.

Sex cord tumor with annular tubules (SCTATs). Characterized by simple and complex ring-shaped tubules, with a pattern intermediate between that of a granulosa cell tumor and a Sertoli cell tumor. It resembles a gonadoblastoma except for the absence of a germ cell component.

Shock lung. Long confused with such pathologic diagnoses as bronchopneumonia, patchy atelectasis, and agonal changes and now known as Adult Respiratory Distress Syndrome (ARDS). Pulmonary edema can be the result of sepsis, fat embolism, cardiac failure, lung contusion, or oxygen toxicity. The resulting pulmonary insufficiency is a major cause of death in injured patients and those receiving intensive care. A single cause for shock lung has not been described, and any or all of the above may be implicated.

Specific stimulation. Utilization of tumor cells or their antigenic products for immunization directed specifically toward that tumor or other tumors sharing the same antigens.

Staging of ovarian cancer. Clinically determined estimate of the extent of the disease and the size of the tumor. (Histologic type and grading classify the cancer's microscopic character.)

Stem (primitive) cell. Cell capable of proliferation, sometimes giving rise to differentiated cells.

Stromal reactions. Chabon, Takenchi, and Sommers employed a stromal evaluation in a breast study. The stroma of each epithelial ovarian cancer was graded according to the number of lymphocytes, plasma cells, and polymorphonuclear leukocytes (PMNs) present. Lymphocyte, plasma cell, and PMN infiltration in the stroma and around small veins was graded 0 to 3: 0 = none, 1 = minimal, 2 = moderate, 3 = marked.

Supervoltage radiation. High-energy radiation with ill-defined limits usually extending beyond energies that no longer are preferentially absorbed in bone (i.e., 500 KeV) to peak energies of several millielectron volts.

Suppressor T cells. Important set of feedback controls, centered around sensitized T lymphocytes, through which inhibitory populations of these cells suppress the production of sensitized lymphocytes and antibody-forming cells.

Swan-Ganz catheter. Pulmonary arterial pressure and pulmonary wedge pressure may be monitored by the Swan-Ganz catheter to give an index of left ventricular competence. Central venous pressure monitoring measures only the function of the right side of the heart.

Syngeneic. Pertaining to genetically identical or nearly identical animals, such as identical twins or highly inbred animals.

Syngeneic preference. Unlike allogeneic inhibition, syngeneic preference represents improved growth in syngeneic recipients.

Synthesis Index (SI). Or Cycling Index (CI). Measures the rate of cellular proliferation and thus tumor activity. CI distinguishes G_0 (resting) cells from S, G_2, M, and G_1 phases of the cell cycle. Recurrence is significantly more frequent with more active tumors having high proliferative rates, regardless of stage.

Teletherapy. Treatment with the radiation source at a distance from the body. See *Brachytherapy*.

Template theory. Instructive theory of antibody production in which it was supposed that an antigen was taken into a cell and acted directly as a template that determined the shape of the combining site of the antibody produced by that cell. The theory was originally proposed by Haurowitz, Mudd, and Alexander.

Tests for evaluating a clotting disorder. Several tests may be helpful.

Bleeding time. May be unreliable because of variations in puncture technique. It may also be abnormal because of platelets deficient in number or function or because of von Willebrand's disease. Normal = <4 minutes.

Clotting time (glass). Insensitive test. It does, however, test for all intrinsic coagulation factors except factors VII and XIII and platelets. Normal = <15 minutes (usually <10 minutes).

Prothrombin time (one-stage). Reliable and sensitive test for the extrinsic system coagulation factors (V, VII, X), as well as for fibrinogen (factor I) and prothrombin (factor II). Normal = <20 seconds (check control value).

Prothrombin consumption test. Reliable test of platelet function (unlike the bleeding time) that has acceptable sensitivity for the intrinsic system coagulation factors (unlike the clotting time). It checks factors V, VIII, IX, X, XI, and XII. Normal = <20% (alternatively expressed as >80%).

Partial thromboplastin time, activated (PTT). Sensitive screening test for detecting alterations in the coagulation mechanism, such as previously undiagnosed hemophilia, various coagulation deficiencies, and circulating anticoagulants. Normal = 20 to 45 seconds.

Thrombin time. When prolonged, indicates overheparinization, defibrination, or fibrinolysis.

Platelet count. Quantity of platelets can be rapidly estimated from a smear. Platelet counts considerably below 100,000/mm^3 may implicate massive banked blood transfusions as a cause of bleeding. Normal = >100,000/mm^3.

Tetraploid. Having four times the haploid number of chromosomes.

Therapeutic immunization. Any therapy initiated after the patient shows clinical manifestations of malignancy.

T lymphocyte (T cell). Lymphocytes that have matured and differentiated under thymic influence are termed thymic-dependent lymphocytes. These cells are primarily involved in the mediation of cellular immunity, as well as in tissue and organ rejection.

Tissue polypeptide antigen (TPA). Molecules derived from the cytoskeleton of epithelial cells. TPA, measured in an immunoradiomimetic assay, is useful for the management of many carcinomas. In prostate cancer, for example, TPA has been shown to be a reliable marker for estimating prognosis: Patients with normal TPA values at the time of diagnosis have a longer survival than those with elevated values.

Tolerance. Failure of the antibody response to a potential antigen after exposure to the antigen. Tolerance commonly results from prior exposure to antigens.

Transcription stage. Transcribing of genetic information from nucleus to cytoplasm, i.e., from DNA to RNA by messenger RNA.

Transduction. Form of recombination that depends on bacteriophage for its completion. A phage particle can carry some DNA from the lysed cell in which it was formed to the new cell it infects. There, instead of multiplying, it remains inactive; and the transferred bacterial DNA may become incorporated into the DNA of the new host. Apparently only a small portion of the genetic material undergoes transduction at any one time. In *Salmonella*, a genus of bacteria to which many pathogenic intestinal bacteria belong, the ability to resist certain drugs can be transferred by transduction. See *Lysogeny*.

Transfer factor. Heat-labile, dialyzable extract of human lymphocytes that is capable of conferring specific antigen reactivity to the donor. See *Lymphokine*.

Transformation. Process that occurs when one bacterium absorbs the DNA of another, dead bacterium and incorporates some of it into its own genetic constitution. The incorporated DNA is then transmitted to later generations. Usually only a small part of the genetic material is involved in transformation, and usually the process occurs only between members of the same species; however streptomycin resistance has been transferred in this way from pneumococci to streptococci.

Translation stage. Translation of the base sequence code in RNA into an amino acid sequence in proteins.

Tumor angiogenesis factor (TAF). Represents induction of the growth of blood vessels by a stimulant released by tumor cells. The growth of the tumor parallels the development of new blood vessels.

Tumor necrosis factor (TNF). Produced by macrophages, TNF is cytotoxic for some tumor cells and some parasites.

Vector molecule. Plasmid, cosmid, or virus that carries formed DNA into a host organism.

Vertical transmission of viruses. Transmission from one generation to the next, i.e., from mother to offspring. See *Horizontal transmission of viruses*.

Xenogeneic (heterologous). Pertaining to individuals of different species.

Index